CLINICAL OBESITY

EDITED BY

PETER G.KOPELMAN
Medical Unit
St. Bartholomew's and Royal London School of Medicine and Dentistry
Queen Mary and Westfield College
Turner Street
London E1 2AD

AND

MICHAEL J.STOCK
Department of Physiology,
St George's Hospital Medical School
Cranmer Terrace
London SW17 0RE

b

Blackwell
Science

© 1998 by
Blackwell Science Ltd
Editorial Offices:
Osney Mead, Oxford OX2 0EL
25 John Street, London WC1N 2BL
23 Ainslie Place, Edinburgh EH3 6AJ
350 Main Street, Malden
  MA 02148 5018, USA
54 University Street, Carlton
  Victoria 3053, Australia
10, rue Casimir Delavigne
  75006 Paris, France

Other Editorial Offices:
Blackwell Wissenschafts-Verlag GmbH
Kurfürstendamm 57
10707 Berlin, Germany

Blackwell Science KK
MG Kodenmacho Building
7–10 Kodenmacho Nihombashi
Chuo-ku, Tokyo 104, Japan

First published 1998

Set by Setrite Typesetters, Hong Kong
Printed and bound in Great Britain at
the University Press, Cambridge

The Blackwell Science logo is a
trade mark of Blackwell Science Ltd,
registered at the United Kingdom
Trade Marks Registry

For further information on Blackwell Science,
visit our website:
www.blackwell-science.com

DISTRIBUTORS

Marston Book Services Ltd
PO Box 269
Abingdon, Oxon OX14 4YN
(*Orders*: Tel: 01235 465500
          Fax: 01235 465555)
USA
Blackwell Science, Inc.
Commerce Place
350 Main Street
Malden, MA 02148 5018
(*Orders*: Tel: 800 759 6102
                781 388 8250
          Fax: 781 388 8255)
Canada
Login Brothers Book Company
324 Saulteaux Crescent
Winnipeg, Manitoba R3J 3T2
(*Orders*: Tel: 204 224–4068)

Australia
Blackwell Science Pty Ltd
54 University Street
Carlton, Victoria 3053
(*Orders*: Tel: 3 9347 0300
          Fax: 3 9347 5001)

A catalogue record for this title
is available from the British Library

ISBN 0-632-04198-6

Library of Congress
Cataloging-in-publication Data

Clinical obesity/edited by Peter G. Kopelman
and Michael Stock.
        p.   cm.
    Includes bibliographical references.
    ISBN 0-632-04198-6
    1. Obesity.   I. Kopelman, Peter G.
    II. Stock, Michael. J.
    [DNLM: 1. Obesity.   WD 210 C6415 1998]
RC628.C56   1998
616.3'98 — dc21
DNLM/DLC
for Library of Congress   97-46120
                                              CIP

Contents

List of Contributors

GEORGE A. BRAY, MD, *Pennigton Biomedical Research Center, Baton Rouge, Louisiana 70808–4124, USA*

PETER S.W. DAVIES, MPhil, PhD, *School of Human Movement Studies, Faculty of Health, Queensland University of Technology, Brisbane, Australia*

JEAN-PIERRE DESPRÉS, PhD, *Lipid Research Center, Laval University Medical Research Center, 2705 Laurier Boulevard (TR-93), Ste-Foy (Québec), Canada, G1V 4G2*

NICK FINER, FRCP, *Centre of Obesity Research, Luton and Dunstable Hospital, Lewsey Road, Luton LU4 0DZ*

STEVEN FRANKS, MD, FRCP, *Unit of Metabolic Medicine and Department of Obstetrics and Gynaecology, St Mary's Hospital Medical School, Norfolk Place, London W2 1NY*

KEITH N. FRAYN, ScD, PhD, FRCPath, *Oxford Lipid Metabolism Group, Nuffield Department of Clinical Medicine, University of Oxford, Radcliffe Infirmary, Oxford OX2 6HE*

RONALD R. GRUNSTEIN, MD, PhD, FRACP, *Centre for Respiratory Failure and Sleep Disorders, Royal Prince Alfred Hospital, Camperdown 2050, Sydney, Australia*

CATHERINE R. HANKEY, MSc, SRD, *University Department of Human Nutrition, Queen Elizabeth Building, Glasgow Royal Infirmary Glasgow G31 2ER*

ANDREW J. HILL, PhD, *Division of Psychiatry & Behavioural Sciences, School of Medicine, University of Leeds, 15 Hyde Terrace, Leeds LS2 9LT*

GRAHAM A. HITMAN, MD, FRCP, *Medical Unit, St Bartholomew's and The Royal London School of Medicine and Dentistry, The Royal London Hospital, Whitechapel, London E1 1BB*

SUSAN A. JEBB, PhD, SRD, *MRC Dunn Clinical Nutrition Centre, Addenbrooke's Hospital, Hills Road, Cambridge CB2 2DH*

ROLAND T. JUNG, MA, MD, FRCP, *Tayside NHS Consortium, Diabetes Centre, Ninewells Hospital, Dundee DD1 9SY*

PETER G. KOPELMAN, MD, FRCP, *Medical Unit, St. Bartholomew's and Royal London School of Medicine and Dentistry, Queen Mary and Westfield College, Turner Street, London E1 2AD*

JOHN G. KRAL, MD, PhD, *SUNY Health Science Center at Brooklyn, Department of Surgery, 450 Clarkson Avenue, Box 40, Brooklyn, New York 11203–2098, USA*

MICHAEL E.J. LEAN, MA, MD, FRCP, *University Department of Human Nutrition, Queen Elizabeth Building, Glasgow Royal Infirmary, Glasgow G31 2ER*

IAN A. MacDONALD, PhD, *School of Biomedical Sciences, University of Nottingham Medical School, Queen's Medical Centre, Nottingham NG7 2UH*

ILSE L. MERTENS, RD, MSc, *Department of Endocrinology, Metabolism and Clinical Nutrition, University Hospital Antwerp, Wilrijkstraat 10, B-2650 Edegem, Antwerp, Belgium*

LORNA RAPOPORT, SRD, *Health Behaviour Unit, Department of Epidemiology and Public Health, University College London Medical School, 2–16 Torrington Place, London WC1E 6BT*

AILA RISSANEN, MD, *Obesity Research Unit, Helsinki University Central Hospital, Paasikivenkatu 4, FIN-00250 Helsinki, Finland*

STEPHEN ROBINSON, MB BChir, MA, MRCP, *Unit of Metabolic Medicine and Department of Obstetrics and Gynaecology, St Mary's Hospital Medical School, Norfolk Place, London W2 1NY*

PETER J. ROGERS, PhD, *Consumer Sciences Department, Institute of Food Research, Earlygate, Whiteknights Road, Reading RG6 6BZ*

WIM H.M. SARIS, MD, PhD, *Department of Human Biology, Universiteit Maastricht, P.O. Box 616, 6200 MD Maastricht, The Netherlands*

JACOB C. SEIDELL, PhD, *Department of Chronic Disease and Environmental Epidemiology, National Institute of Public Health and the Environment, P.O. Box 1, 3720 BA Bilthoven, The Netherlands*

MICHAEL J. STOCK, PhD, *Department of Physiology, St George's Hospital Medical School, Cranmer Terrace, London SW17 0RE*

CAROLYN D. SUMMERBELL, SRD, PhD, *Systematic Reviews Training Unit, Department of Primary Care and Population Sciences, Royal Free Hospital School of Medicine, Rowland Hill Street, London NW3 2PF*

LUCINDA K.M. SUMMERS, MB BS, MRCP, *Oxford Lipid Metabolism Group, Nuffield Department of Clinical Medicine, University of Oxford, Radcliffe Infirmary, Oxford OX2 6HE*

ANDRÉ TCHERNOF, PhD, *Lipid Research Center, Laval University Medical Research Center, 2705 Laurier Boulevard (TR-93), Ste-Foy (Québec), Canada, G1V 4G2*

MARLEEN A. van BAAK, PhD, *Department of Human Biology, Universiteit Maastricht, P.O. Box 616, 6200 MD Maastricht, The Netherlands*

LUC F. van GAAL, MD, PhD, *Department of Endocrinology, Metabolism and Clinical Nutrition, Universal Hospital Antwerp, Wilrijkstraat 10, B-2650 Edegem, Antwerp, Belgium*

JANE WARDLE, PhD, FBPS, C PSYCHOL, *Health Behaviour Unit, Department of Epidemiology and Public Health, University College London Medical School, 2–16 Torrington Place, London WC1E 6BT*

JOHN WILDING, DM, MRCP, *Diabetes and Endocrinology Clinical Research Unit, University Clinical Departments at Aintree, Fazakerley Hospital, Longmoor Lane, Liverpool L9 7AL*

GARETH WILLIAMS, MD, FRCP, *Diabetes and Endocrinology Clinical Research Unit, University Clinical Departments at Aintree, Fazakerley Hospital, Longmoor Lane, Liverpool L9 7AL*

Introduction

Clinical Obesity originates from the editors' perception of a need for a textbook on obesity emphasizing obesity as a disease entity by reviewing the more clinical and practical aspects of the condition and addressing its scientific basis. The recent advances in our knowledge about obesity and its related conditions have reinforced this need. We believe that the original objectives for the book have been achieved and that *Clinical Obesity* will prove very relevant to clinicians, and postgraduate and undergraduate medical students, as well as being valuable to newcomers to the research area. Readers should find the information in each chapter up-to-date and easily accessible: the choice of chapter headings is intended to facilitate cross-reference between sections.

We are witnessing an epidemic of overweight and obesity across the world. Jaap Seidell's introductory chapter on Epidemiology details the global increase in the prevalence of obesity and draws particular attention to the rapid rise in prevalence in Europe during the past two decades. This increase is having a major influence on the health of populations. Both overweight and obesity are associated with increasing mortality and morbidity and may account for as much as 30% of coronary heart disease and 75% of new cases of type 2 diabetes. In addition, other associated and equally disabling conditions should not be ignored — osteoarthritis, respiratory complications with impaired quality of life are just a few examples. Jaap Seidell makes the telling point that small changes in energy balance, undetectable by epidemiological measures, may nevertheless have profound effects for the longer term on the prevalence of overweight and obesity.

When assessing populations, body-weight alone, or after adjustment (e.g., body mass index, BMI), is the most common yardstick used for assessing the degree of obesity and the effectiveness of treatment. However, as Susan Jebb points out in her chapter on Measuring Body Composition, knowing the size of the fat reserves and the fat-free mass tells us considerably more about what is going on, both in terms of the understanding the pathophysiology of obesity and monitoring treatment. Not so long ago these measurements were rarely seen outside the research laboratory, but many of the techniques are now becoming increasingly common in clinical practice. Jebb reviews all the methods, from the simplest to the most sophisticated, and helps the potential user make the difficult choice between what they can afford and what they need in terms of accuracy and detail. Towards the end of the chapter, she compares the various methods for measuring regional fat distribution—the importance of which become obvious in several subsequent chapters.

Many textbooks on obesity include several chapters examining animal models which focus on information largely derived from laboratory-bred, genetically manipulated rodents. In *Clinical Obesity* there is a single chapter, Energy Balance and Animal Models of Obesity, in which Michael Stock questions the validity of animal models to the human situation. He suggests that many erroneous suppositions have been made in humans as a consequence of extrapolation from animals but concludes that there is still a large amount which can be learnt from animals. He reviews the mechanisms in the animals involved in regulating energy balance and discusses areas which have lost favour with researchers during recent years such as set-point theories, diet-induced thermogenesis and the regulation of energy balance by hypothalamic centres. Stock emphasizes that much may be gained from animal studies providing the influence on energy intake and expenditure of physiological mechanisms is clearly distinguished from those related to behaviour.

The role of genes and genetic inheritance on obesity has puzzled generations of scientists. Recent findings have begun to put genetic influences into perspective and, indeed, have provided a new 'respectability' for obesity research. Nevertheless, the identification of genes involved in the predisposition to the condition and the associated complications will continue to perplex and challenge researchers given the heterogeneous nature of obesity. Graham Hitman suggests in Molecular Genetics of Obesity that the complexity of obesity means that there are several genes predisposing an individual to excessive corpulence which, importantly, require prolonged exposure to critical environmental factors for the condition to manifest. Hitman reviews the approaches molecular scientists are applying to identify the genes involved; these include studies of monogenic human syndromes and candidate genes. The chapter concludes with a review of strategies likely to succeed for the future in identifying major genes involved in obesity.

Although genes are undeniably important, the escalating population levels of obesity cannot be attributed to recent changes in genetic characteristics of a population. This emphasizes the great importance which should be placed on understanding the processes that govern food intake and eating behaviour. Hill and Rogers suggest in their chapter on Food Intake and Eating Behaviour in Humans that the limitations of much of the research into eating behaviour is because it has concentrated on the physiology of appetite in animals with extrapolation to humans. If such mechanisms are to be relevant to humans, they need to be integrated into a wider context which considers learned and cognitive influences on eating and the constraints and opportunities provided by the social setting. Such an approach offers a much broader framework and acknowledges the interplay of events 'beneath and outside the skin'. The chapter includes both an overview of the control of human food intake from this perspective and a review of current methods for assessment.

Following on from considerations of food intake, Ian MacDonald's chapter on Energy Expenditure in Humans considers the fate of the energy consumed. Obviously, any food energy not retained in the body has to be expended, and MacDonald explains the principles behind the measurements of energy expenditure before describing the various components making up daily heat production. By far the largest component is the resting metabolic rate, which comprises the fasting rate plus the smaller component resulting from the thermic effect of feeding (diet-induced thermogenesis). The energy cost of activity is considered next, but because this is covered in greater detail in a later chapter, he moves on to discuss the interesting, albeit controversial, issue of the origins of thermogenesis in humans and the role of the sympathetic nervous system. In the final section, it is pointed out that weight-stable obese subjects have, if anything, a higher energy expenditure than normal due to their higher fat-free mass. However, given the very small daily positive energy balance required to produce the slow, yearly gain typical of the dynamic phase, it is unsurprising that a low energy expenditure, particularly when activity is low, is associated with high weight gains: a point which reiterates the concerns about the accuracy of epidemiological measures for population energy intake and expenditure.

Given the large mass of skeletal muscle, 40% of normal body-weight, it is not surprising to learn from Keith Frayn and Lucinda Summers that it is a major route for the disposal of carbohydrate and lipid. This has important effects on the size of the energy reserves in adipose tissue, which in turn helps regulate plasma triglyceride and fatty acid levels. When reviewing Substrate Fluxes in Skeletal Muscle and White Adipose Tissue, Frayn and Summers emphasize the dramatic shifts in the flux of carbohydrate and lipid handled by muscle (mainly) and adipose tissue between the fed and fasting state, and between rest and exercise. However, even though these fluxes account for much of the body's energy turnover, a careful review of the evidence fails to identify any specific defect in muscle or adipose tissue metabolism as the cause of obesity. Nevertheless, the authors explain how derangement in both tissues as a consequence of obesity have detrimental effects, most notably on insulin sensitivity.

Apart from the very recent advances in our understanding of the molecular biology of obesity, one of the most important advances in the past decade has been the realization that body fat distribution may be almost as important (i.e., dangerous to health) as the overall degree of obesity. The differences between visceral/intra-abdominal and subcutaneous adipose tissue depots and their impact on various metabolic and endocrine functions feature in several chapters, but forms the central theme in Peter Kopelman's chapter on Effects of Obesity on Fat Topography. Apart from the obvious gender differences in fat distribution, various metabolic and endocrine influences affect the distribution of body fat as well being affected themselves by fat distribution. This makes the unravelling of cause from effect very difficult, but this chapter should help to resolve much of the confusion in this area. André Tchernof and Jean-Pierre Després review in the following chapter, Obesity and Lipoprotein Metabolism, the compelling evidence which confirms that upper body obesity, or more particularly intra-abdominal visceral adipose tissue, is closely linked to the medically important syndrome of insulin resistance and dyslipidaemia. This syndrome is an important cause of coronary heart disease although, once again, the precise cause and effect relationship continues to be unravelled. Unquestionably, individuals with upper body obesity need early treatment and Tchernof and Després provide information not only about the identification of those at particular risk but also the therapeutic alternatives. The latter is further considered in later chapters.

Luc van Gaal and Ilse Mertens in their chapter on the Effects of Obesity on Cardiovascular System and Blood Pressure Control, Digestive Disease and Cancer highlight the seriousness of excessive body fatness in relation to many important diseases. Such conditions commonly lead to the obese patient seeking medical advice: the chapter includes a description of the possible pathophysiological mechanisms linking obesity with diseases providing a rationale for treatment and evidence of benefit.

Fertility and the general health of women are compromised by obesity. Stephen Robinson and Steven Franks in Obesity, Infertility, Contraception and Pregnancy describe the association between obesity, the polycystic ovary syndrome and the detrimental effect of increasing body-weight on reproductive function. All too often body-weight is overlooked by those managing clinical aspects of reproductive function: this chapter underlines its importance of overweight and obesity. Maternal obesity carries implications both for the mother and the developing fetus and has profound effects on metabolic processes including glucose turnover. This may result in the development of gestational diabetes as an additional complicating factor. Weight loss and appropriate contraception are important management considerations in the circumstances which are considered by Robinson and Franks.

Proper recognition of the strong links between obesity and disordered pulmonary function including obstructive sleep apnoea has occurred only recently. Ronald Grunstein in Pulmonary Function, Sleep Apnoea and Obesity provides a comprehensive outline of the pathophysiological mechanisms of the changes resulting in alterations of breathing, which are of considerable clinical significance in the obese. The key features in disordered sleep breathing, snoring and daytime somnolence, are often overlooked by clinicians despite the increasing availability of non-invasive investigations and effective treatment with nasal continuous positive airway pressure. Grunstein reviews pulmonary function, gas exchange and respiratory mechanics in the awake and sleeping obese subject and indicates the clinical sequelae. He emphasizes the frequency of the problem based on epidemiological surveys and suggests several alternative treatment regimens.

When reviewing Obesity in Childhood, Peter Davies confirms that not only is the prevalence increasing, but also there appears to be a large increase in the degree of obesity, i.e., we are now seeing more 'super-obese' children with skinfolds > 95th centile. Because children grow, assessing obesity using BMI has to be based on age-related data, but skinfold measures are also useful. As with adults, it is difficult to ascribe the cause of obesity simply to an increase in energy intake since (i) it is difficult to assess, and (ii) it appears that, on average, intakes have been decreasing over the years. This suggests that decreased physical activity is responsible for the rising incidence of childhood obesity: once again this is difficult to accurately assess. Treatment also has to acknowledge that a child is growing, but Davies points out that this can be used to allow children to 'grow into their weight', i.e., maintaining weight while they increase in stature will result in a decreased BMI.

In Diabetes and Obesity, John Wilding and Gareth Williams point out that one does not have to be obese to be diabetic, or vice versa, but the risk of non-insulin-dependents diabetes mellitus (NIDDM) at BMI > 35 is 80-times that of someone with a BMI < 23 — hence the importance of this chapter in a book on obesity. After discussing in detail the evidence and various theories linking the two conditions, the authors draw on their clinical experience to describe the various management strategies available, with emphasis being given to the benefits of weight loss, provided, of course, that this can be maintained. Although the chapter is devoted to NIDDM, the authors take time to point out the problems caused by obesity in IDDM — particularly in young women.

Nick Finer in Clinical Assessment, Investigation and Principles of Management highlights an essential need for a structured approach to obesity management. The nature of the condition requires this to be step-wise and to include several health care professionals, each having particular experience and skills. The setting for care will originate within the community and primary care but will, on occasions, involve hospital-based units for more specialized management programmes. The fundamental principles of management should incorporate a comprehensive clinical assessment with an estimate of risk and a realistic weight goal negotiated with the patient. Goal setting should not just apply to weight but to other desirable behaviours such as increasing exercise and assertiveness, and can also relate to direct health benefits, for example blood pressure reduction or improved control of diabetes.

Carolyn Summerbell tackles the difficult subject of the Dietary Treatment of Obesity, highlighting that the elusiveness of success is because too much attention is given to the diet, and not enough attention given to understanding and helping the patient deal with the problems of changing eating habits. Thus, even though the bulk of her chapter provides useful information on basic principles and relative merits of different dietary regimens, one of the most stimulating sections is that dealing with the need to improve the way in which dietary treatments are delivered. This chapter should encourage more physicians to take dietary treatment more seriously, and make more use of the nutritional and dietetic expertise of other health professionals.

The lack of success of simple psychological treatments for obesity is explained by the implausibility that population levels of psychopathology have risen by such a degree to explain the increased prevalence of obesity. By contrast, behavioural methods for managing obesity have met with success when they are applied to alter eating habits regardless of the origin of such habits. Jane Wardle and Lorna Rapoport discuss in Cognitive–Behavioural Treatment its principal components for the management of obesity. They suggest, once again, that animal models do have relevance when designing human treatment programmes and illustrate how the use of self-administered rewards in humans can improve compliance. Nevertheless, these programmes require careful regulation of the exposure to food or stimuli leading to eating in order to prevent the subjects inadvertently eating excessively. The successful application of such techniques do result in modest weight loss which, importantly, is maintained for the longer term. As with all therapies, patients must undergo a comprehensive assessment prior to starting treatment. Wardle and Rapoport describe this assessment and detail the essential elements of cognitive behaviour therapy.

When it comes to Exercise and Obesity, Marleen van Baak and Wim Saris describe how high levels of physical activity protect against obesity as well as other co-morbidities. Although exercise increases daily energy expenditure, more often than not this is compensated, particularly in the lean, by increases in food intake. Thus, it would seem that the protective effects of exercise may be due simply to fine tuning between intake and expenditure to give better control of energy balance. This does not help the obese to lose weight, but better control of energy balance helps weight maintenance and is particularly useful in helping to prevent regain after weight loss. Combining exercise with dietary restriction results in only small additional losses in weight, but it does help maintain fat-free mass, improve psychological functions and introduces exercise as part of a lifestyle change to give better control over body-weight.

In the Drug Treatment of Obesity, Roland Jung considers that most doctors are resistant to the idea of using drugs to treat obesity, but are quite happy to prescribe drugs for the long-term treatment of associated diseases (e.g., hypertension, NIDDM, hypertriglyceridaemia, etc). Jung argues that one way to help overcome this resistance is to conduct drug trials with better designs and higher standards, and to provide better evidence and information to the prescribing physician. He then goes on to briefly review three categories of drugs, those that decrease absorption, suppress appetite or increase metabolic rate (thermogenesis), but focuses on the appetite suppressants since this is where clinical experience is greatest. Even here, the number of suitable drugs that can be recommended is currently limited to no more than one or two compounds, and this lack of choice is probably another reason why physicians are reluctant to resort to drugs when attempting to treat their obese patients. However, the scope for developing new drugs is increasing rapidly as more basic information about how energy balance and body composition becomes available. As George Bray points out when reviewing Strategies for Discovering Drugs to Treat Obesity, much of this new information is based on animal studies. Unfortunately, in addition to the problems of bridging the species gap, many of the newer, potential treatments will also require a good deal of pharmaceutical ingenuity to produce clinically acceptable, orally active compounds. Nevertheless, a lot of effort and investment is going into developing new agents and no doubt the next decade will see several of those described by Bray appearing in the clinic.

Obesity is a chronic condition which requires life-long management. John Kral argues in Surgical Treatment of Obesity that operative intervention is the only proven way to achieve this. Surgery, he maintains, is the most powerful method to alter behaviour: 'traditional' forms of dietary, behavioural and drug treatment fail because they are unable to change eating behaviour for the long term. Indeed, no non-surgical method has been conclusively shown to achieve a medically significant degree of weight loss sustained for a meaningful period of time (>5 years). The National Institute for Health Consensus Development Conference recognized the potential importance of surgery in 1991 by concluding that gastric restrictive or bypass procedures were justified as effective treatments for obesity. Since this statement, techniques have further advanced, safety has improved and substantial additional long-term data has become available to confirm the durable effectiveness of surgical intervention for patients appropriately selected. Moreover, the indications for surgery have widened with the introduction of laparoscopic techniques. Kral pointedly emphasizes that surgical failures result largely from poor patient selection rather than technical faults and concedes that there are still no absolute predictors of outcome for the individual obese patient nor valid methods for patient selection. He concludes that a prerequisite for any surgical programme is pre-operative education and meticulous follow-up—for the long term.

When considering the Benefits and Risks of Weight Loss, Michael Lean and Catherine Hankey point out that although the usual clinical experience is that only modest amounts of weight are lost, this is accompanied by significant improvements in a whole range of associated risk factors. Apart from the direct improvements in health that follow, an added benefit is reduced reliance on drugs to treat these co-morbidities, which in turn decreases costs and side-effects. The hazards of weight loss, in otherwise healthy subjects, are considered to be infrequent and/or relatively minor, although the chances of developing gallstones increases significantly with larger losses in weight. Nevertheless, Lean and Hankey consider the hazards of weight loss are far outweighed by the benefits. Due to a paucity of good, reliable data, these authors' conclusions about the hazards of weight cycling are more circumspect. On balance, however, they tend to ascribe any adverse health effects of weight cycling to pre-existing disease, either as a cause of unintentional weight loss or as a reason for intentional weight loss.

Obesity is now a major economic burden to most developed countries, accounting for between 4 and 8% of the total health care expenditure. These figures do not include indirect costs arising from loss of productivity. Aila Rissanen puts these costs into perspective in Public Health Strategies and the Economic Costs of Obesity and draws on her considerable experience in Finland to paint a grim prospect for the future. She suggests that public health strategies for the prevention of weight gain and overweight must be directed both at the community level and into primary care and should be combined with community campaigns and media publicity about the importance of physical activity and diet. The concern shared by many about the inevitable health outcome of overweight and obesity means that any programme of prevention must also include an approach to identify who are at high risk.

Obesity research and the management of overweight and obesity have reached a watershed. The recognition of the importance of excessive weight as a public health issue, and the identification of potential genetic mechanisms, have stimulated considerable concern about the problem in future generations and interest in developing more effective methods for prevention and therapeutic intervention. *Clinical Obesity* provides a timely review of current knowledge and, using scientific and clinical evidence, makes predictions about future directions— essential information for all with an interest in obesity.

Peter G. Kopelman
Michael J. Stock

CHAPTER 1

Epidemiology: Definition and Classification of Obesity*

JACOB C. SEIDELL

How to measure obesity

When we speak about the prevalence of obesity in populations we actually mean the fraction of people who have an excess storage of body fat. In adult men with an average weight the percentage body fat is in the order of 15–20%. In women this percentage is higher (about 25–30%). Because differences in weight between individuals are only partly due to variations in body fat, many people object to the use of weight or indices based on height and weight (such as the body mass index, BMI) to discriminate between overweight and normal-weight people. There are always examples which illustrate the inappropriate use of BMI certain individuals such as an identical BMI in a young male body builder and a middle-aged obese women. The facts are, however, that despite these obvious extremes there is a very good correlation between BMI (weight/height^2) and the percentage of body fat in large populations. Deurenberg *et al.* (1991) established that one can quite accurately estimate the body fat percentage in adults with the following equation:

Body fat percentage = 1.2 (BMI) + 0.23 (age) – 10.8 (gender) – 5.4

About 80% of the variation in body fat between (Dutch) individuals could be explained by this formula. The standard error of estimate was about 4%. In this equation the value for gender is 1 for men and 0 for women. It follows from this equation that for a given height and weight the body fat percentage is about 10% higher in women compared to men. In addition, people get fatter when they get older even when their body-weights are stable. The correlation between BMI and fat percentage implies that in populations BMI can be used to classify people in terms of excess body fat. In practice, people or populations are usually not classified on the basis of the body fat percentage but on the basis

*Parts of this chapter have been previously published as: Seidell, J.C. & Flegal, K.M. (1997) Assessing obesity: classification and epidemiology. *British Medical Bulletin* 53, 238–252.

of their BMI. Usually, the same cut-off points are applied for men and women and for different age-groups. This is done because the relationships between BMI and mortality are similar (i.e., the relative mortality associated with obesity is similar in men and women, in most age-groups the absolute mortality is much lower). The same relative risk and lower absolute risk associated with overweight and obesity among women compared to men implies that women can probably tolerate body fat better than men. The reason in women could be that their excess body fat is usually distributed as subcutaneous fat and mainly peripherally (thighs, buttocks and breasts) and in men there is a relative excess of body fat stored in the abdominal cavity and as abdominal subcutaneous fat. It has been suggested that optimal BMI (i.e., the BMI associated with lowest relative risk) increases with age (Andres, 1985). The reasons why older people seem to tolerate an excess body fat better than younger people are manifold and range from selective survival to decreased lipolysis of adipose tissue in older people.

The cut-off points in Table 1.1 have been proposed by a WHO Expert Committee for the classification of overweight (WHO, 1995): These apply to both men and women and to all adult age-groups. There are limitations in the interpretation of BMI in very old subjects as well as in certain ethnic groups with deviating body proportions (e.g. in populations where stunted growth is common or in those with relatively short leg length compared to sitting height).

How to measure fat distribution

Since the pioneering work of Jean Vague in the 1940s it has slowly become accepted that different body morphology or types of fat distribution are in-dependently related to the health risks associated with obesity (Vague, 1956). Starting with Jean Vague's brachio-femoral adipo-muscular ratio as an index of fat distribution (which was based on ratios of skinfolds and circumferences of the arms and thighs) more recent indices have been designed specifically to be good predictors of intra-abdominal fat. The most popular among all measures is the waist/hip circumference ratio. The simplest of these measures is the waist

Table 1.1 WHO classification of overweight.

BMI	WHO classification	Popular description
$<18.5\text{kg/m}^2$	Underweight	Thin
$18.5-24.9\text{kg/m}^2$	—	'Healthy', 'normal' or 'acceptable' weight
$25.0-29.9\text{kg/m}^2$	Grade 1 overweight	Overweight
$30.0-39.9\text{kg/m}^2$	Grade 2 overweight	Obesity
$\geq40.0\text{kg/m}^2$	Grade 3 overweight	Morbid obesity

circumference (Table 1.2), which has been suggested to predict intra-abdominal fat at least as accurately as the waist/hip ratio (Pouliot *et al.*, 1994) and to predict levels of cardiovascular risk factors and disease as well as BMI and waist/hip ratio (Han *et al.*, 1995). It has also been suggested that waist circumference could possibly be used to replace classifications based on BMI and the waist/hip circumference ratio (Lean *et al.*, 1995). More complex measures, such as the sagittal abdominal diameter, the ratio of waist/thigh circumference, the ratio of waist/height or the conicity index, have also been proposed to perform even better than waist circumference for one or more of these purposes. However, the differences among these measures are small and the use of ratios may complicate the interpretation of associations with disease and their consequences for public health measures. For instance, the waist/height ratio may be a better predictor of morbidity because the waist is positively associated with disease and because height, for reasons unrelated to body composition or fat distribution, is inversely associated with disease.

Replacing BMI and waist/hip ratio by simple cut-off points which are optimal for each sex, age-group, population and relationship with specific diseases may, however, be too simple. Still, as suggested by Lean *et al.* (1995), some cut-off points may be of guidance in interpreting values of waist circumference for adults. Other cut-off points, based on classification of subjects on a 'critical level' of intra-abdominal fat, have been proposed by investigators from Québec (Lemieux *et al.*, 1996).

Who is obese?

Very little is known about the factors that may explain the large differences between populations in the distributions of BMI (see next section). Obviously, overweight in individuals in any population is the result of a long-term positive energy balance. Just to say that overweight is characterized by physical inactivity or ingestion of large quantities of food is an oversimplification. Several epidemiological studies have shown that the following factors are associated with overweight in the population.

Table 1.2 Sex-specific cut-off points for waist circumference. Level 1 was initially based on replacing the classification of overweight (BMI $\geq 25\,kg/m^2$) in combination with high waist/hip ratio (WHR ≥ 0.95 in men and ≥ 0.80 in women). Level 2 was based on classification of obesity (BMI $\geq 30\,kg/m^2$) in combination with high waist/hip ratio (10,12).

	Level 1 ('alerting zone')	Level 2 ('action level')
Men	$\geq 94\,cm$ (~37 inches)	$\geq 102\,cm$ (~40 inches)
Women	$\geq 80\,cm$ (~32 inches)	$\geq 88\,cm$ (~35 inches)

Demographic factors

- Age: increasing with age at least up till age 50–60 years in men and women. Figures 1.1(a) and (b) show the relationship between age and prevalence of obesity in the U.K., the Netherlands and the U.S.A. (NHANES III, 1988–1994) (Department of Health, 1993; Seidell, 1997, Flegal *et al.*, 1997).
- Gender: women have generally higher prevalences of obesity compared to men especially when older than 50 years of age.
- Ethnicity: large usually unexplained variations between ethnic groups. Figure

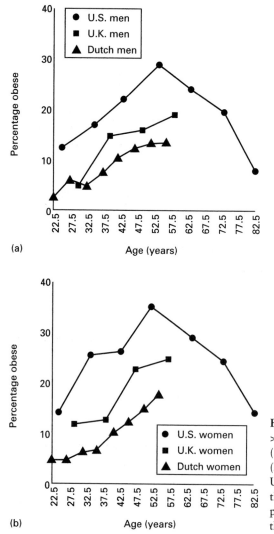

(a)

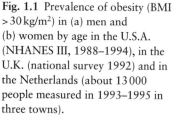

(b)

Fig. 1.1 Prevalence of obesity (BMI > 30 kg/m²) in (a) men and (b) women by age in the U.S.A. (NHANES III, 1988–1994), in the U.K. (national survey 1992) and in the Netherlands (about 13 000 people measured in 1993–1995 in three towns).

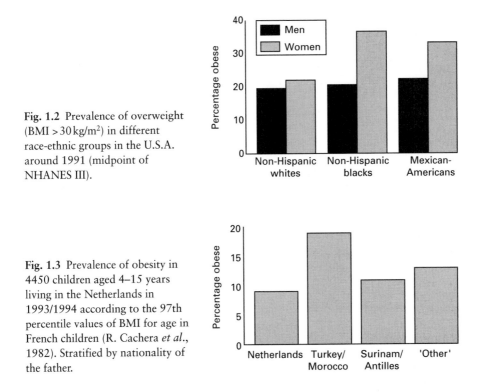

Fig. 1.2 Prevalence of overweight (BMI > 30 kg/m²) in different race-ethnic groups in the U.S.A. around 1991 (midpoint of NHANES III).

Fig. 1.3 Prevalence of obesity in 4450 children aged 4–15 years living in the Netherlands in 1993/1994 according to the 97th percentile values of BMI for age in French children (R. Cachera *et al.*, 1982). Stratified by nationality of the father.

1.2 shows that in the U.S.A. there is little variation for men by race-ethnic group but much larger differences for women by race-ethnic group.

Figure 1.3 shows the prevalence of overweight among Dutch children by ethnic group and illustrates the higher prevalence among children of immigrants compared to 'native' Dutch children (Brugman *et al.*, 1995).

Socio-cultural factors

• Educational level and income: in industrialized countries, higher prevalence in those with lower education and/or income.
• Marital status: usually increasing after marriage.

Biological factors

• Parity: it has been claimed that BMI increases with increasing number of children but recent evidence suggests that this contribution is, on average, likely to be small, less than 1 kg per pregnancy. Many study designs confound the changes in weight with ageing and changes in weight with parity (Williamson *et al.*, 1994).

Behavioural factors

• Dietary intake: although it is clear that nutrition is of critical importance in establishing a positive energy balance, research on this topic has not been easy to interpret because of confounding and of increased under-reporting with increasing degrees of obesity. Another reason may be that only small deviations in energy balance are necessary to yield large differences in body-weight in the long term. The methodological errors in determining energy intake may be too large to allow detection of the nutritional determinants of obesity. In particular it has been suggested that the fat percentage of the diet is associated with higher prevalence of obesity although the epidemiological evidence may be flawed or biased (Seidell, 1997b).

• Smoking: smoking lowers body-weight and cessation of smoking increases body-weight. The associations between smoking and obesity may, however, vary considerably among populations (Molarius et al., 1997).

• Alcohol consumption: unclear in most populations, moderate alcohol consumption sometimes associated with higher BMI (Prentice, 1995).

• Physical activity: those who remain or become inactive are usually heavier than those who are physically active. Similar limitations apply as for the interpretation of the evidence of nutritional determinants of obesity: methodological problems such as confounding and biased reporting as well as measurement error make it difficult to interpret the literature.

Prevalence of obesity in Europe and the U.S.A.

Obesity, defined as a BMI $\geq 30 \, kg/m^2$ is a common condition in Europe and the U.S.A. (Seidell, 1995). In order to make a comparison possible between countries it is necessary to compare population-based data on measured height and weight in which identical protocols for measurement were applied and which were collected in the same period. The most comprehensive data on the prevalence of obesity in Europe are from the WHO MONICA study (WHO MONICA, 1989). The majority of these data were collected between 1983 and 1986. The populations are not necessarily representative of the countries in which they are located.

Tables 1.3 and 1.4 show the age-standardized prevalence of overweight and obesity in 39 European centres participating in this study (WHO MONICA, 1989). Only in three centres the prevalence of obesity was slightly lower than 10% (Gothenburg in Sweden (men and women); Toulouse in France (men); Catalonia in Spain (men)) and, on average, the prevalence of obesity was about 15% in men and 22% in women. Overweight, on the other hand is much more common among men than women. More than half of the people aged 35–65

Table 1.3 Prevalence of overweight (BMI 25–30 kg/m^2) and obesity (BMI $\geq$ 30 kg/m^2) in European men aged 35–64 years. Data from the WHO MONICA (first round 1983–1986) populations (8).

| Country | Centre | Prevalence | | |
		Overweight	Obese	Overweight + obese
Iceland	Iceland	44	11	55
Sweden	Northern Sweden	45	12	57
Sweden	Gothenburg	44	7	51
Finland	Kuopio Province	50	18	68
Finland	North Karelia	51	17	68
Finland	Turku-Loima	49	19	68
Denmark	Glostrup	44	11	55
U.K.	Glasgow	46	11	57
U.K.	Belfast	45	11	56
Germany	Bremen	53	14	67
Germany	Rhein-Neckar	52	14	66
Germany	Augsburg (urban)	56	18	74
Germany	Augsburg (rural)	56	20	76
Germany*	Halle County	51	18	69
Germany*	Karl-Marx-Stadt	50	15	65
Germany*	Cottbus County	51	17	68
Germany*	'Rest of DDR MONICA'	54	19	73
Belgium	Ghent	50	11	61
Belgium	Charleroi	48	20	68
Belgium	Luxembourg Province	45	14	59
France	Lille	44	14	58
France	Bas Rhin/Strasbourg	52	22	74
France	Haute Garonne/Toulouse	51	9	60
Switzerland	Vaud-Fribourg	49	12	61
Switzerland	Ticino	51	19	70
Russia	Novosibirsk (2 samples)	46	14	60
Russia	Moscow (2 samples)	45	13	58
Lithuania	Kaunas	54	22	76
Poland	Warsaw	48	17	65
Poland	Tarnobrzeg Voivodship	39	13	52
Czech Rep.	'Czechoslovakia'	51	21	72
Hungary	Pecs	42	19	61
Hungary	Budapest	46	15	61
Serbia	Novi Sad	50	18	68
Spain	Catalonia	57	9	66
Italy	Area Brianza	44	11	55
Italy	Friuli	49	17	66
Italy	Area Latina	52	18	70
Malta	Malta	46	25	71
95% CI of mean		46.2–51.4	14.2–16.8	62.1–66.3
Mean $\pm$ SD		48.8 $\pm$ 4.1	15.5 $\pm$ 4.2	64.2 $\pm$ 6.8

* Formerly German Democratic Republic.

Table 1.4 Prevalence of overweight (BMI 25–30 kg/m²) and obesity (BMI ≥ 30 kg/m²) in European women aged 35–64 years. Data from the WHO MONICA (first round 1983–1986) populations (8).

Country	Centre	Prevalence		
		Overweight	Obese	Overweight + obese
Iceland	Iceland	30	11	41
Sweden	Northern Sweden	33	14	47
Sweden	Gothenburg	25	9	34
Finland	Kuopio Province	39	20	59
Finland	North Karelia	37	23	60
Finland	Turku-Loima	37	17	54
Denmark	Glostrup	25	10	35
U.K.	Glasgow	38	16	54
U.K.	Belfast	34	14	48
Germany	Bremen	37	18	55
Germany	Rhein-Neckar	31	12	43
Germany	Augsburg (urban)	36	15	51
Germany	Augsburg (rural)	36	22	58
Germany*	Halle County	36	25	61
Germany*	Karl-Marx-Stadt	31	19	50
Germany*	Cottbus County	36	23	59
Germany*	'Rest of DDR MONICA'	35	27	62
Belgium	Ghent	37	15	52
Belgium	Charleroi	35	26	61
Belgium	Luxembourg Province	33	18	51
France	Lille	30	18	48
France	Bas Rhin/Strassbourg	34	23	57
France	Haute Garonne/Toulouse	25	11	36
Switzerland	Vaud-Fribourg	30	12	42
Switzerland	Ticino	29	14	43
Russia	Novosibirsk (2 samples)	38	44	82
Russia	Moscow (2 samples)	39	34	73
Lithuania	Kaunas	38	45	83
Poland	Warsaw	39	26	65
Poland	Tarnobrzeg Voivodship	36	32	68
Czech Rep.	'Czechoslovakia'	37	31	68
Hungary	Pecs	34	26	60
Hungary	Budapest	36	18	54
Serbia	Novi Sad	40	30	70
Spain	Catalonia	44	24	68
Italy	Area Brianza	28	15	43
Italy	Friuli	37	19	56
Italy	Area Latina	43	30	73
Malta	Malta	32	41	73
95% CI of mean		33.2–36.0	18.8–24.6	52.5–60.1
Mean ± SD		34.6 ± 4.5	21.7 ± 9.1	56.3 ± 12.2

* Formerly German Democratic Republic.

years in Europe seem to be either overweight or obese. Given the large within- and between-country estimates of the prevalence of obesity, it is difficult to derive an overall prevalence figure for Europe as a whole from these data. It is fairly safe to assume that such an overall prevalence figure would be in the range of 10–20% in men and 15–25% in women.

The study of explanations for the large diversity in prevalence data, on the other hand, could give important clues to the understanding of the origins of common obesity. Striking, for example, are the very high BMIs in the women from Eastern European countries. There is only a moderate association ($r = 0.39$, $P = 0.02$) of the prevalence between men and women (Seidell & Rissanen, 1997). The distributions of the BMI values in men seem to be rather homogeneous over Europe despite large socio-economic and cultural differences between the countries. In addition, it is clear that there are major differences in the mortality rates of cardiovascular disease which, at least in men, cannot be explained by differences in BMI (Seidell & Rissanen, 1997).

Trends in obesity prevalence in Europe and the U.S.A.

Table 1.5 shows some of the available recent trend data on obesity in Europe and the U.S.A. The prevalence has increased by about 10–40% in most countries in the past decade, for instance the prevalence in the U.K. has doubled during this period. It seems that in most countries an increasing prevalence was observed although preliminary data from Denmark (Mikkelsen *et al.*, 1995) suggests that the prevalence increased in men but decreased in women in the period 1960–80.

Subgroup analyses by sex, age and educational level with regard to time-trends yielded different results in different countries. In some studies the increase in the prevalence of obesity was most pronounced in young adults whereas in others it was more pronounced in older subjects. Usually, there was a stronger increase in the prevalence of obesity in those with relatively low educational levels compared to those with higher education. Figure 1.4 illustrates with data from the Netherlands (Seidell, 1997a) that changes in BMI may be different between levels of education.

National Surveys in the U.S.A. have shown a marked increase in the prevalence of obesity over time. From 1960 to 1978 there was only a slight increase in overweight. However, between 1978 and 1991 a striking increase in the prevalence of overweight occurred. This increase was seen for all age groups, for both men and women, and for non-Hispanic whites, non-Hispanic blacks and Mexican-Americans. The magnitude of the increase was similar for all these groups. The U.S.A. experience shows that a population-wide increase in the prevalence of overweight may occur relatively quickly after a

Table 1.5 Recent trends in obesity prevalence in some European countries and the U.S.A.

Country	Obesity definition (BMI cut-off point)	Year	Ages	Men (%)	Women (%)
England	30 kg/m²	1980	16–64	6	8
		1986–87		7	12
		1991		13	15
		1993		13	16
Sweden	Men: 30 kg/m²	1980–81	16–84	4.9	8.7
	Women: 28.6 kg/m²	1988–89		5.3	9.1
Finland	30 kg/m²	1978–79	20–75	10	10
		1985–87		12	10
		1991–91		14	11
Germany	30 kg/m²	1985	25–69	15.1	16.5
		1988		14.7	17.2
		1990		17.2	19.3
East Germany	30 kg/m²	1985	25–65	13.7	22.2
		1989		13.4	20.6
		1992		20.5	26.8
Netherlands	30 kg/m²	1987	20–59	6.0	8.5
		1988		6.3	7.6
		1989		6.2	7.4
		1990		7.4	9.0
		1991		7.5	8.8
		1992		7.5	9.3
		1993		7.1	9.1
		1994		8.8	9.4
		1995		8.4	8.3
U.S.A.	30 kg/m²	1960	20–74	10.0	15.0
		1973		11.6	16.1
		1978		12.0	14.8
		1991		19.7	24.7

long period during which the prevalence of overweight is fairly stable (Flegal *et al.*, 1997).

Causes of time trends in obesity

Diminished physical activity, high-fat diets and inadequate adjustments of energy intakes to the diminished energy requirements are likely to be major determinants of the observed changes. Prentice and Jebb (1995) have proposed that, on a population level, limited physical activity may be more important than energy

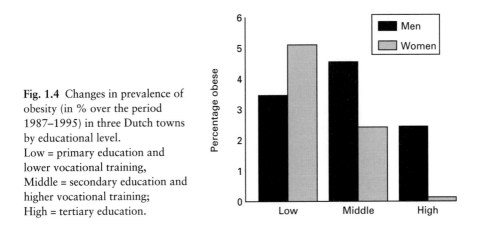

Fig. 1.4 Changes in prevalence of obesity (in % over the period 1987–1995) in three Dutch towns by educational level.
Low = primary education and lower vocational training,
Middle = secondary education and higher vocational training;
High = tertiary education.

or fat consumption in explaining the time trends of obesity in the U.K. Their analyses were based on aspects of physical activity (such as number of hours spent watching television) and household consumption survey data. Although such data may be indicative such analyses may also be biased. Particularly, energy and fat consumption are under-reported with increasing degrees of overweight (Seidell, 1997b). Changes in smoking behaviour may also contribute to changes in body-weight on a population level. Data from the U.S.A. showed that although smoking cessation could explain some of the increase in the prevalence of overweight, smoking cessation alone could not account for the major portion of the increase (Flegal *et al.*, 1995). In other studies it was also shown that the increase in the obesity prevalence may be independent of smoking status (Boyle *et al.*, 1994; Wolk & Rössner, 1995).

Epidemiological methods that can be used to assess energy intake and energy expenditure may be subject to bias but, in addition, they also have considerable ratio of within- to between-subject variation. It should be noted that only small changes in energy balance are needed to increase average BMI by one unit. Depending on the distribution of BMI in the population this may greatly increase the prevalence of obesity. These small changes in energy balance may not be detectable by epidemiological measures of energy expenditure and intake.

It was previously shown (Seidell, 1997c) that dramatic increases in the prevalence of obesity in the Netherlands (about 37% in men and 18% in women over a period of 10 years) can be the consequence of relatively minor changes in average body-weight. If height had remained constant an average weight increase of slightly less than 1 kg over 10 years could be pushing the prevalence of obesity upward as much as was observed. This could reflect only minute changes in energy balance on a daily basis. Experimentally, over-feeding with about 7000 kcal will result in a weight gain of, on average, about 1 kg. If we neglect all metabolic adaptations to over-feeding and increases in body-weight we can calculate that a constant positive energy balance of about 2 kcal/day may be sufficient to increase the average body-weights of individuals by about 1 kg in 10 years resulting in a substantial increase in the prevalence of obesity. It is clear that such small persistent changes in energy balance are not detectable by existing methods for measuring energy expenditure and energy intake in populations.

In the Netherlands, data from two identical nutrition surveys performed in 1987–88 and 1993 suggested that energy intake decreased from 2329 kcal/day (9746 kJ) in 1987–88 to 2216 kcal/day (9278 kJ) in 1993 (Voorlichtingsbureau voor de Voeding, 1993). This reduction of about 113 kcal/day was attributable to a decrease in fat consumption (protein intake increased and carbohydrate and alcohol consumption remained constant). Smoking behaviour had changed, particularly in men, since the 1970s but in the 1980s no further decrease was observed. This may imply that daily energy expenditure has decreased during the same period with the same order of magnitude. It is not uncommon in societies which are in a phase of 'post-modernization' to see simultaneous improvement in dietary intakes (reduction in fat and energy) and increases in the prevalence of obesity (Seidell, 1997b).

Impact of obesity and associated diseases on morbidity and mortality

BMI is probably linearly related to increased mortality in men and women. In many studies a U- or J-shaped association between BMI and mortality was observed (Troiano *et al.*, 1996) but some recent large studies have suggested that much of the increased mortality at low BMI is due to smoking and smoking-related disease as well as other clinical disorders causing weight loss (Lee *et al.*, 1993; Manson *et al.*, 1995; Jousilahto *et al.*, 1996; Seidell *et al.*, 1996). Figure 1.5 shows the effect of weight instability, smoking and early mortality on the shape of the association between BMI and total mortality in U.S. women (Manson *et al.*, 1995). It is clear that the U-shaped curve has disappeared after exclusion of women who were ill, had unstable weights or died early. The figure only shows the relative mortality risks. The absolute mortality rates in the women who were non-smokers and had stable weights were much lower than the mortality rates in the total group.

Obesity is related to diabetes mellitus and coronary heart disease (CHD) in men and women. In addition, increasing degrees of overweight are associated with an increased incidence of arthritis of hands and knees, gallbladder disease, sleep apnoea and certain types of cancer (breast cancer and endometrial cancer in women, colon cancer in men). In Tables 1.6 and 1.7 the relative impact of overweight (BMI ≥ 25 kg/m^2) and obesity (BMI ≥ 30 kg/m^2) were calculated for

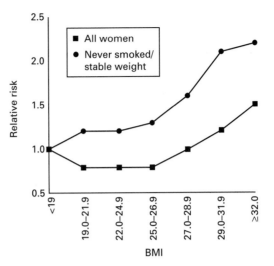

Fig. 1.5 Relationship between BMI (adjusted for smoking, menopause, hormone use and parental history of myocardial infarction) and relative risk of all-cause mortality in U.S. women (Manson *et al.*, 1995).

Table 1.6 Relative impact of overweight and obesity on coronary heart disease mortality in some recent large prospective studies in men and women.

	Jousilahti *et al.* (1996)		Willett *et al.* (1995)	Seidell *et al.* (1996)	
	Men	Women	Women	Men	Women
n	7740	8373	115 818	23 306	25 540
Follow-up (years)	15	15	14	12	12
Age at baseline (years)	30–59	30–59	30–55	30–54	30–54
% subjects with BMI ≥25 kg/m²	58	58	28	40	30
Relative risk BMI ≥25 vs BMI <25 kg/m²	1.3	1.5	2.2	1.7	2.3
PAR (BMI ≥25 kg/m²)	15%	22%	25%	20%	28%
% subjects with BMI ≥30 kg/m²	11	20	11	4	6
Relative risk BMI ≥30 vs BMI <30 kg/m²	1.4	1.3	2.6	2.5	2.3
PAR (BMI ≥30 kg/m²)	4%	6%	15%	6%	8%

* PAR (Population Attributable Risk). Fatal and non-fatal coronary heart disease combined.

CHD (Willett *et al.*, 1995; Jousilahti *et al.*, 1996; Seidell *et al.*, 1996) and diabetes mellitus (Chan *et al.*, 1994; Colditz *et al.*, 1995). From these studies performed in Finland, the U.S.A. and the Netherlands it can be shown that BMI in the range

Table 1.7 Relative impact of overweight and obesity on diabetes mellitus in some recent large prospective studies in men and women.

	Colditz et al. (1994)	Chan et al. (1995)
	Women	Men
n	114281	51529
Follow-up (years)	14	5
Age at baseline (years)	30–55	40–75
% subjects with BMI $\geq 25\,kg/m^2$	35	50
Relative risk BMI ≥ 25 vs BMI $< 25\,kg/m^2$	10.3	4.6
PAR* (BMI $\geq 25\,kg/m^2$)	77%	64%
% subjects with BMI $\geq 30\,kg/m^2$	8	7
Relative risk BMI ≥ 30 vs BMI $< 30\,kg/m^2$	10.6	8.3
PAR* (BMI $\geq 30\,kg/m^2$)	44	33

* See footnote to Table 1.6.

of $25–30\,kg/m^2$ is responsible for the major part of the impact of overweight on CHD mortality. If in these populations no one increased their weight to levels of BMI over $25\,kg/m^2$ about 15–30% of all deaths of CHD could theoretically have been prevented. It will be difficult to see the impact of the increased prevalence of obesity on CHD mortality because CHD mortality rates have been steadily decreasing in most affluent countries since the 1970s due to better hypertension control, cholesterol lowering, smoking cessation, improved diagnosis and treatment of patients with CHD, etc. The impact of obesity on diabetes mellitus is much larger than for CHD. If these figures are correct then about 64% of male and 77% of female cases of non-insulin-dependent diabetes mellitus (NIDDM) could theoretically have been prevented if no one had had a BMI over $25\,kg/m^2$. In contrast to CHD, interventions have had a much lower impact on the incidence of diabetes mellitus. In countries such as the Netherlands an increase in the prevalence of NIDDM of about 12% has been observed during the last decade or so (Ruwaard et al., 1996) which may have well been caused by the increased prevalence of obesity in the same period.

The impact of the increase on other diseases such as breast cancer and cerebrovascular disease may not be noticeable for the next few decades because the increased prevalence of obesity in young adults may not be reflected in an increase in these diseases until they reach their seventies. There are no sensitive monitoring systems for other health consequences such as arthritis and it will be difficult to directly observe the consequences of an increased proportion of obese subjects in society. Particularly because intervention studies aimed at changing body-weights in the general population have been quite unsuccessful (Williamson, 1996) more attention should be given to the prevention of obesity. Action should be directed not only to food habits of the general population but also to sedentary activity. Specific subgroups such as people who stop smoking, women who are pregnant and those with a family history of obesity and NIDDM should be targeted separately. Issues of safety, town planning and education are all of great importance and should not be limited to ministries of public health. For these and other reasons, the WHO launched a Task Force of Obesity (James, 1996; Woodman, 1996).

Conclusions

Overweight and obesity are common in Europe and the U.S.A. and the prevalence seems to be increasing in most countries where reliable data are available. Obesity is associated with a increased mortality and incidence of CHD and diabetes mellitus. The relative risks for moderate overweight and morbidity and mortality risks are usually only slightly elevated but because of its very high prevalence moderate overweight is a major contributor to the total burden of disease associated with increased body-weights.

Targets to reduce the prevalence of obesity to acceptable levels will not be reached in most countries (Russel et al., 1995; Smith, 1996). International guidelines for the treatment and, in particular, the prevention of obesity are urgently needed (Woodman, 1996). They should be aimed at high-risk groups for weight gain. These include those who have a genetic predisposition for weight gain and obesity but also those who change their lifestyle (e.g., those who stop smoking or those who reduce their physical activity) and, perhaps, women who become pregnant. Special targets should be developed to reach specific socio-economic and ethnic groups which have a high prevalence of obesity. Efforts to prevent excessive weight gain in children and adolescents should be balanced against the possibility of inducing unnecessary dieting behaviour and eating disorders in girls.

Promoting physical activity is a priority in this context and attention should not just be focused on more participation in sports clubs but should also stimulate normal outdoor activities such as walking and cycling and discouragement of 'sedentary behaviour'. International guidelines such as those prepared by the International Task Force on Obesity (Woodman, 1996) can only be implemented when sufficient input and commitment from governments and health professionals is obtained.

References

Andres, R. (1985) Mortality and obesity: the rationale for age-group specific weight–height tables. In: Andres, R., Bierman, E.L. & Hazzard, W.R. (eds) *Principles of Geriatric Medicine*, pp. 311–318. New York: McGraw Hill.

Boyle, C.A., Dobson, A.J., Egger, G. & Magnus, P. (1994) Can the increasing weight of Australians be explained by the decreasing prevalence of cigarette smoking? *International Journal of Obesity* **18**, 55–60.

Brugman, E., Meulmeester, J.F., Spee-van der Wekkes, J., Beuker, R.J. & Radder, J.J. (1995) *Peilingen in de jeugdgezondheidszorg: PGO-peiling 1993/1994*. TNO Preventie en Gezondheid, report nr. 95.061.

Chain, J.M., Rimm, E.B., Colditz, G.A., Stampfer, M.J. & Willett, W.C. (1994) Obesity, fat distribution, and weight gain as risk factors for clinical diabetes in men. *Diabetes Care* **17**, 961–969.

Colditz, G.A., Willett, W.C., Rotnitzky, A. & Manson, J.E. (1995) Weight gain as a risk factor for clinical diabetes mellitus in women. *Annals of Internal Medicine* **122**, 481–486.

Department of Health (1993) *The Health of the Nation: one year on … a report on the progress of the Health of the Nation*. London: HSMO.

Deurenberg, P., Weststrate, J.A. & Seidell, J.C. (1991) Body mass index as a measure of body fatness: age- and sex-specific prediction formulas. *British Journal of Nutrition* **65**, 105–114.

Flegal, K.M., Troiano, R.P., Pamuk, E.R., Kuczmarski, R.J. & Campbell, S.M. (1995) The influence of smoking cessation on the prevalence of overweight in the United States. *New England Journal of Medicine* **333**, 1165–1170.

Flegal, K.M., Carrol, M.D., Kuczmarski, R.J. & Johnson, C.L. (1998) Overweight and obesity in the United States: prevalence and trends 1960–1994. *International Journal Of Obesity* **22**, 39–47.

Han, T.S., van Leer, E.M., Seidell, J.C. & Lean, M.E.J. (1995) Waist circumference action levels in the identification of cardiovascular risk factors: prevalence study in a random sample. *British Medical Journal* **311**, 1401–1405.

James, W.P.T. (1996) The International Obesity Task Force: obesity at the World Health Organization. *Nutr Metab Cardiovasc Dis* suppl. **6**, 12–13.

Jousilahti, P., Tuomilehto, J., Vartiainen, E., Pekkanen, J. & Puska, P. (1996) Body weight, cardiovascular risk factors, and coronary mortality: 15 year follow-up of middle-aged men and women in eastern Finland. *Circulation* **93**, 1372–1379.

Lean, M.E.J., Han, T.S. & Morrison, C.E. (1995) Waist circumference indicates the need for weight measurement. *British Medical Journal* **311**, 158–161.

Lee, I-M., Manson, J.E., Hennekens, C.H. & Paffenbarger, R.S. (1993) Body weight and mortality: a 27 year follow-up of middle aged men. *Journal of the American Medical Association* **270**, 2823–2828.

Lemieux, S., Prud'homme, D., Bouchard, C., Tremblay, A. & Despres, J-P. (1996) A single threshold value of waist girth identifies normal-weight and overweight subjects with excess visceral adipose tissue. *American Journal of Clinical Nutrition* **64**, 685–693.

Manson, J.E., Willett, W.C., Tanpfer, M.J. *et al.* (1995) Body weight and mortality among women. *New England Journal of Medicine* **333**, 677–685.

Mikkelsen, K.L., Heitmann, B.L. & Sörensen, T.I.A. (1995) Secular changes in mean body mass index and its prevalence of obesity—three Danish population studies of 31,000 subjects. *International Journal of Obesity* **19** (suppl. 2), 30 (abstract).

Molarius, A., Seidell, J.C., Kuulasmaa, K., Dobson, A. & Sans, S. (1997) Smoking and body weight: WHO MONICA Project. *Journal of Epidemiology and Community Health* **51**, 252–260.

Pouliot, M.C., Despres, J.P., Lemieux, S.L. *et al.* (1994) Waist circumference and abdominal sagittal diameter: best simple anthropometric indexes of abdominal visceral adipose tissue accumulation and related cardiovascular risk in men and women. *American Journal of Cardiology* 73, 460–468.

Prentice, A.M. (1995). Alcohol and obesity. *International Journal of Obesity* 19 (suppl. 5), S44–S50.

Prentice, A.M. & Jebb, S.A. (1995) Obesity in Britain: gluttony or sloth? *British Medical Journal* 311, 437–439.

Russel, C.M., Williamson, D.F. & Byers, T. (1995) Can the year 2000 objective for reducing overweight in the United States be reached? A simulation study of the required changes in body weight. *International Journal of Obesity* 19, 149–153.

Ruwaard, D., Gijsen, R., Bartelds, A.I.M., Hirasing, R.A., Verkley, H. & Kromhout, D. (1996) Is the incidence of diabetes increasing in all age-groups in the Netherlands? *Diabetes Care* 19, 214–218.

Seidell, J.C. (1995) Obesity in Europe — scaling an epidemic. *International Journal of Obesity* 19 (suppl. 3), S1–S4.

Seidell, J.C. (1997a) Lichaamsgewicht. In: Maas, I., Gysen, R., Loberoo, I.E. *et al.* (eds) *Determinanten van Gezondheid.*, pp. 654–662. VTV.

Seidell, J.C. (1997b) Dietary fat and obesity: an epidemiological perspective. *American Journal of Clinical Nutrition* (in press).

Seidell, J.C. (1997c) Time trends in obesity: an epidemiological perspective. *Hormone and Metabolic Research* 29, 155–158.

Seidell, J.C. & Rissanen, A. (1997) Global prevalence of obesity and time trends. In: Bray, G.A., Bouchard, C. & James, W.P.T. (eds) *Handbook of Obesity*, pp. 79–91. New York: Dekker.

Seidell, J.C., Verschuren, W.M.M., van Leer, E.M. & Kromhout, D. (1996) Overweight, underweight, and mortality: a prospective study of 48,287 men and women. *Archives of Internal Medicine* 156, 958–963.

Smith, S.J. (1996) Britain is failing to meet targets on reducing obesity. *British Medical Journal* 312, 1440.

Troiano, R.P., Frongillo, E.A., Sobal, J. & Levitsky, D.A. (1996) The relationship between body weight and mortality: a quantitative analysis of combined information from existing studies. *International Journal of Obesity* 20, 63–75.

Vague, J. (1956) The degree of masculine differentiation of obesity — a factor determining predisposition to diabetes, atherosclerosis, gout and uric calculus. *American Journal of Clinical Nutrition* 4, 20–34.

Voorlichtingsbureau voor de Voeding (1993) *Zo eet Nederland 1992: Resultaten van de Voedselconsumptiepeiling 1992*, Den Haag.

Willamson, D.F. (1996) The effectiveness of community-based health education trials for the control of obesity. In: Angel, A., Auderson, H., Bouchard, C. *et al.* (eds) *Progress in Obesity Research 7*, pp. 331–335. London: John Libbey.

Williamson, D.F., Madans, J., Pamuk, E., Flegal, K.M., Kendrick, J.S. & Serdula, M.K. (1994) A prospective study of childbearing and 10-year weight gain in US white women 25 to 40 years of age. *International Journal of Obesity* 18, 561–569.

Willett, W.C., Manson, J.E., Stampfer, M.J. *et al.* (1995) Weight, weight change, and coronary heart disease in women. Risk within the 'normal' range. *Journal of the American Medical Association* 273, 461–465.

WHO MONICA (1989) Project: Risk Factors. *International Journal of Epidemiology* 18 (suppl. 1), S46–S55.

WHO Expert Committee. (1995) *Physical Status: the Use and Interpretation of Anthropometry.* WHO Technical Report Series no. 854. Geneva: WHO.

Wolk, A. & Rössner, S. (1995) Effects of smoking and physical activity on body weight: developments in Sweden between 1980 and 1989. *Journal of Internal Medicine* 237, 287–291.

Woodman, R. (1996) WHO launches initiative against obesity. *Lancet* 347, 751.

CHAPTER 2

....

Measuring Body Composition:
from the Laboratory to the Clinic

SUSAN A. JEBB

....

Background

Weight is a crude measure of the body's energy reserves, yet it is without doubt the most common method by which obesity is documented. It is also used as a proxy for the successful reduction of fat stores during obesity treatment programmes. More specific measurements of body fat have been common-place in specialized research laboratories since the 1950s, but the greatest change we see today is their emergence from the laboratory into the clinic. This is due in part to a growing awareness of the imprecision of body-weight as an index of adiposity and in parallel the development of other techniques, which are suitable for use in clinical practice. There has also been a rise in interest in fat distribution, with the focus on abdominal fat as a site of particular metabolic importance.

Measurements of body composition have yielded new insights into the pathophysiology of obesity. Although it has been apparent for many years that obesity is characterized by an excess of body fat we now recognize that obese individuals also have increases in other tissues. Fat-free mass (FFM) is enlarged, including both skeletal muscle and visceral organs, and bone mineral mass is increased. Together they explain the increased energy requirements of obese individuals relative to their lean counterparts (Prentice et al., 1996). Accurate measurements of body composition are necessary to make comparisons of energy expenditure data between lean and obese individuals. For example Fig. 2.1 shows that when expressed on an absolute basis the energy expenditure of obese individuals is significantly greater than that of lean subjects, but when corrected for differences in FFM there is no significant difference (Prentice et al., 1986).

In an epidemiological context the increased health risks associated with excess body-weight are largely attributable to excess fat. However, the site of fat deposition also plays an important role in determining co-morbidity and mortality. Thus, measurements of fat mass and its distribution can be a useful predictor of health risks. Likewise, monitoring changes in total body fat or in fat distribution as a consequence of anti-obesity interventions can provide a

18

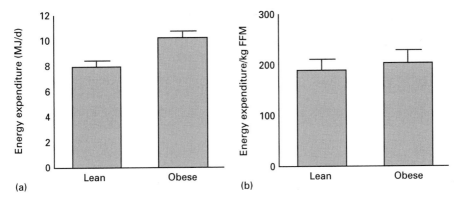

Fig. 2.1 Energy expenditure in lean and obese subjects, expressed in (a) absolute terms ($P < 0.001$) and (b) per kg FFM (NS). Data from Prentice *et al.* (1986).

useful marker of success before longer-term outcomes are apparent in terms of morbidity and mortality. Methods to measure the body composition of large groups of individuals, often in the field, or in mobile research stations requires a simple, practical method, capable of ranking individuals in the correct order of fatness.

In clinical practice the need to measure individual patients places the emphasis on measurement precision, to document small changes in fat mass or distribution in response to a variety of interventions. The time and facilities available for this purpose will depend on the nature of the investigation. If it forms part of routine clinical care, it is important that the method must not add to the overall consultation time, in a multi-centre clinical trial inter-centre reproducibility is vital, whilst for a specific research investigation, e.g., examining the effect of two different dietary regimens on the proportion of weight lost as fat, the accuracy and precision of the method must be of the highest quality to ensure reliable information on which to base public health recommendations or develop new physiological concepts.

This chapter will discuss each of the methods available to measure body composition, outlining their individual strengths and weaknesses and illustrating some of the insights they have given into human obesity and its treatment.

Measurement of gross body composition

Classical reference methods

The classical methods to measure body composition are based on a two-compartment model, in which the body is assumed to be composed of fat and FFM alone, where FFM is the difference between body-weight and fat mass.

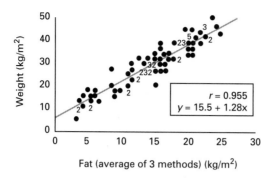

Fig. 2.2 Relationship of fat mass (mean of measurements by density, total body water and total body potassium methods) to body-weight. Measurements are divided by height² to correct for differences in stature. Reproduced from Webster *et al.* (1984).

This is therefore a very heterogeneous compartment comprising bone mineral, water, protein, glycogen and other minor constituents. However, data from direct cadaver analysis suggest that the composition of FFM is relatively constant with respect to its density, proportion of water and potassium concentration (Widdowson & Dickerson, 1964). This yields the three classical reference methods to measure body composition: total body water, total body potassium and body density.

Studies of the composition of excess weight change in 104 obese subjects using the mean of measurements by body density, total body water and total body potassium techniques suggest that the composition of weight loss is 74.1 ± 0.02% fat (Webster *et al.*, 1984) (Fig. 2.2). This has been popularly interpreted as 75% fat and has become a widely used standard in obesity treatment. The use of the mean of the three techniques represented an attempt to overcome the specific assumptions of each individual method, but as will become apparent this approach has now been superseded by more sophisticated multicompartment analysis of the body.

Body density

Assuming that the density of fat and FFM are known, the proportion of each constituent may be calculated from measurements of body density. Typically fat is assumed to have a density of 0.9 kg/L and FFM 1.1 kg/L (Siri, 1956), thus:

$$\% \text{ fat} = \frac{4.95}{d} - 4.50 \cdot 100$$

Density is calculated as body mass/volume. Traditionally the measurement of body volume requires complete submergence under water. Volume is measured either directly by water displacement or calculated as the difference between the weight of the subject under water and in air. In either case a correction must

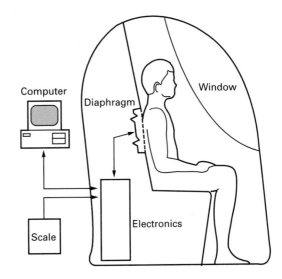

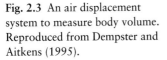

Fig. 2.3 An air displacement system to measure body volume. Reproduced from Dempster and Aitkens (1995).

be made for the volume of air in the lungs and in the gut. Many obese patients find this procedure difficult and frightening and some underwater weighing systems are unable to accommodate obese subjects. These problems can be minimized by careful attention to the design of the tank, but the method will still be unacceptable to a significant number of subjects. A method has been described to calculate body composition without the need for head submergence but this has not been widely used (Evans *et al.*, 1989). Recently a novel device to measure body volume has been produced which uses an air displacement technique (Fig. 2.3) (Dempster & Aitkens, 1995). The diaphragm oscillates between the two chambers to create sinusoidal volume perturbations in the two chambers which leads to complementary pressure fluctuations. The pressure and volume changes produced in the outer chamber by the presence of the subject allow the volume of the subject to be calculated. This commercial system, BOD POD, shows excellent agreement with classical underwater weighing with improved reproducibility and enhanced patient acceptability (McCrory *et al.*, 1995). This may overcome the significant practical limitations of underwater weighing and increase the usefulness of this technique, although direct experience of the method is still limited.

Body density can be measured with a high degree of precision and accuracy, but the principal scientific limitation of this method is the error incurred by the assumption of a known density of FFM. Deviations in body density can occur because of changes in hydration or the proportion of bone mineral. As yet there is little evidence of systematic differences in obese subjects but the variability is likely to be at least as great if not more than in individuals within the healthy weight range.

Total body water

Assuming that fat is anhydrous and that FFM contains a known proportion of water it is possible to estimate FFM from measurements of total body water, and fat can be calculated by difference from body-weight. Today the tracer of choice must be stable, non-radioactive and mix freely with all body water compartments. In practice deuterium or 18-oxygen are most commonly used with the former favoured since it is several-fold cheaper. The isotope can be administered orally or intravenously and a sample of body water, usually saliva, urine or plasma, collected before dosing and after equilibration of the isotope. This simple procedure makes the method suitable for almost all subjects in almost all circumstances.

The measurement of the isotope in body water is more complex, although some commercial laboratories offer an analytical service. Both deuterium and 18-oxygen can be measured by mass spectrometry, but a technique to measure deuterium using infra-red spectrophotometry has also been described (Jennings *et al.*, 1995). The precision is analogous to that obtained by mass spectrometry, although a much larger dose is recommended, approximately 0.5 g deuterium/kg body-weight. Nonetheless, this procedure is within the capability of most basic laboratories whereas mass spectrometry is generally confined to specialist centres.

The precision of measurements of total body water is 1–2% (Coward *et al.*, 1988). However, the error in determinations of body fat will be much greater if the assumed hydration fraction of FFM is incorrect. A recent study in healthy non-obese individuals showed a mean of 73.8% with a range of 69.4–78.4% (Fuller *et al.*, 1992). For a 90-kg subject with 50 litres of body water this will give rise to a range in body fat of 18–26 kg. In obese subjects it has been suggested that there may be a systematic increase in the hydration of fat-free tissue (Deurenberg *et al.*, 1989b) and in addition many obese people suffer from oedema, so it is difficult to accurately estimate the true hydration fraction of FFM in any given circumstance. There may also be particular problems in estimating changes in composition by this technique during periods of weight reduction since the loss of water, in association with glycogen during the early phase of weight loss, will be interpreted as a loss of 1.37 kg lean tissue for each kilogram of water which is lost.

Total body potassium

Potassium is an intracellular cation found exclusively in FFM. Measuring the concentration of potassium in the body allows the estimation of FFM. Whole-body counters are used to estimate the amount of 40-potassium, a naturally occurring radioactive isotope of potassium. Assuming this represents a known proportion of total body potassium, typically 0.012%, total body potassium can be calculated. Measurements of the potassium concentration of FFM in animal and human cadavers yields typical values of 2.46–2.66 mEq/kg for men and 2.28–2.5 mEq/kg in women (Lukaski, 1987).

Unfortunately, the potassium content of FFM is variable with more found in muscle than other lean tissues (Snyder et al., 1975), it changes with age (Dickerson & Widdowson, 1960) and can be distorted by disease and some drugs treatment, notably diuretics (Morgan et al., 1978). This makes total body potassium measurements an unreliable measurement of FFM in many situations. The technique is also limited by practical difficulties. Whole-body counters are only available in specialist centres and the measurement can take up to 1.5 hours since the body must be repeatedly scanned in order to detect the very low levels of 40-potassium. Subjects are confined to an enclosed whole-body counter, shielded from background radiation sources and this can be intimidating, particularly to those who have a history of claustrophobia.

In the obese there are two important limitations to this method. The potassium concentration of lean tissue varies with adiposity such that the concentration of potassium is lower in obese subjects than their lean counterparts (Colt et al., 1981; Morgan & Burkinshaw, 1983). Furthermore, adipose tissue exerts a shielding effect on the underlying lean tissue compartment, such that a lower potassium content will be recorded in an obese subject relative to their lean counterpart with a similar FFM. Adjustments can be made for the effect of body composition based on the attenuation of counts from the injection of a known amount of radioactive 42-potassium. However, the derivation of these calibration factors is often limited because of the technical and ethical difficulties of administering 42-potassium. One of the most sophisticated whole-body counters at the Brookhaven National Laboratory in New York uses a 137-caesium source, which is briefly placed under the scanning table and the gamma emissions recorded (Cohn et al., 1969). This allows an individual attenuation factor to be calculated to take into account the body geometry of the subject and the shielding effect of adipose tissue. In these circumstances the precision of the measurement of body fat is approximately 3%. In practice the performance of whole-body counters varies considerably as a consequence of both differences in hardware and attenuation calibrations. These have implications for both the precision and absolute accuracy of the method in addition to the errors attributable to the variable potassium content of FFM.

There is some debate about the validity of measurements of whole-body potassium during periods of weight change. Some studies suggest that the depletion of potassium during severe energy deficits exceeds the loss of nitrogen, thus exacerbating the apparent loss of lean tissue and minimizing fat loss (Archibald *et al.*, 1983).

Multicompartment models

In recent years it has become increasingly apparent that the inaccuracies of the classical reference methods relate to the limitations of the two-compartment model rather than errors in the measurement of the physical properties of the body. This has led to the development of more sophisticated models of the body in which some of the components of FFM are measured independently.

In 1961, Siri proposed the simultaneous measurement of body water and body density to yield a three-compartment model (fat, water and dry FFM) (Siri, 1961). However, this takes no account of bone mineral. Murgatroyd and Coward proposed that for the measurement of short-term changes in body composition bone mineral could reasonably be assumed to remain constant and derived a model to measure changes in fat and protein also based on total body water and density measurements (Murgatroyd & Coward, 1989). A comparison of these indirect techniques to measure changes in fat mass compared to fat balance studies demonstrated the improved precision of this approach (Jebb *et al.*, 1993). Figure 2.4 shows the change in body composition measured in this way during three periods of weight cycling. The loss of fat represents 82% of the weight loss during the initial 2-week period of very-low-calorie dieting and 88% over the full 18-week period (Jebb *et al.*, 1991).

In recent years the development of dual energy X-ray absorptiometry systems (DXA) to measure whole-body bone mineral has facilitated the measurement of bone as an additional compartment. Four-compartment models now combine measurements of bone mineral by DXA, water by deuterium

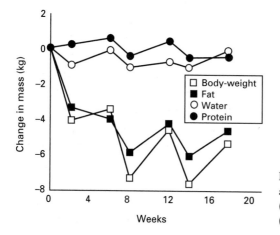

Fig. 2.4 Changes in body fat, water and protein during 'yo-yo' dieting (*n* = 6). Data from Jebb *et al.* (1991).

dilution and hence allow the calculation of the true density of the FFM. In this way the remaining compartment can be divided into fat and protein on the basis of body density. Glycogen is included as part of the protein compartment since it has a very similar density to protein. This is theoretically one of the most accurate methods to assess body composition *in vivo* (Fuller *et al.*, 1992). The propagated measurement error is 0.75 kg fat in 'reference man' (Snyder *et al.*, 1975). This approach has not yet been widely applied, which perhaps reflects the practical limitations of a method which involves a multitude of techniques, some of which may be particularly difficult in obese subjects.

Using this method it is possible to calculate the true hydration and density of FFM (Jebb & Elia, 1995). A study which has used this approach in a group of obese women (BMI > 30 kg/m²) has shown the mean hydration of FFM to be $71.2 \pm 1.6\%$ (range 68.2–75.1%) and the density of FFM 1.104 ± 0.006 kg/L (range 1.093–1.117 kg/L) (Fuller *et al.*, 1994). As more data accumulate on obese subjects it will be possible to redefine the assumptions about the composition of FFM which are used in traditional two-compartment models and hence improve their accuracy.

Novel techniques

In vivo *neutron activation analysis*

The multicompartment models described above represent a new approach to the calculation of body composition rather than truly novel measurement techniques. *In vivo* neutron activation analysis (IVNAA), however, is a new method pioneered by medical physicists which is able to analyse the body at molecular level. Most IVNAA systems involve prompt gamma neutron activation (Beddoe & Hill, 1985). The patient is first injected with tritium to measure hydrogen and then exposed to gamma radiation emitted by radionuclides specific for various elements. The complex spectrum of radiation from the patient is measured and analysed to determine nitrogen (for the measurement of body protein), hydrogen (for the measurement of body water), carbon (for the measurement of fat) and calcium (for the measurement of bone mineral). Other elements such as chlorine, phosphorus, magnesium and sodium can also be measured to estimate other specific compartments of the body. The quoted precision of measurements of both total body nitrogen and carbon is approximately 3% (Heymsfield *et al.*, 1993). Comparative studies between IVNAA and chemical dissection in two cadavers have shown good agreement (Knight *et al.*, 1986).

The drawback to this method is that the total radiation dose is approximately 50 mSv per patient for a full elemental analysis, approximately 6 times that of a cardioangiogram and its applications have therefore been limited. IVNAA measurements in obese subjects have generally been confined to measurements of total body nitrogen for which the radiation exposure is 0.26–0.50 mSv per measurement (Beddoe & Hill, 1985). The future of IVNAA depends on the development of methods which minimize the radiation exposure but maintain the precision.

Dual energy X-ray absorptiometry

DXA is widely used for the measurement of bone mineral and forms an integral part of the four-compartment model described previously. In recent years the software has been developed to divide the soft tissue into fat and FFM (Jebb, 1997). In its own right DXA therefore provides an example of a three-compartment model (bone, fat and fat-free soft tissue) and, with the additional measurement of total body water, an alternative four-compartment model can be derived (bone, water, fat and dry fat-free soft tissue).

Soft tissue composition is measured in a whole-body scan, which takes between 5 and 20 minutes depending on the particular machine (Fig. 2.5). The

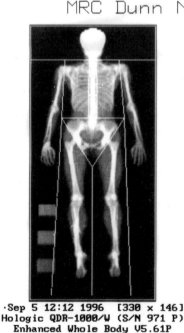

MRC Dunn Nutrition Unit.

```
A08259303      Wed Aug 25 09:04 1993
Name:
Comment:                         Comparison
I.D.:                       Sex:      F
S.S.#:            -  -     Ethnic:
ZIPCode:              Height: 163.00 cm
Scan Code:            Weight:  48.00 kg
BirthDate: 08/29/64          Age:   28
Physician:
Image not for diagnostic use
   TBAR227
   F.S.  68.00%  0(10.00)%
   Head assumes 17.0% brain fat
   LBM 73.2% water

   Region     Fat      Lean+BMC   % Fat
            (grams)    (grams)     (%)
   -------  --------  ---------  -------
   L Arm      543.8     1639.1    24.9
   R Arm      712.1     1696.9    29.6
   Trunk     2235.4    19618.9    10.2
   L Leg     2168.4     6457.0    25.1
   R Leg     2341.5     6747.3    25.8
   SubTot    8001.2    36159.2    18.1
   Head       650.1     3536.8    15.5
   TOTAL     8651.3    39695.9    17.9
```

·Sep 5 12:12 1996   [330 x 146]
Hologic QDR-1000/W (S/N 971 P)
Enhanced Whole Body V5.61P

HOLOGIC

Fig. 2.5 Soft tissue composition measured by DXA.

body is scanned in a rectilinear manner using two low-dose X-rays at different energies, typically 70 and 140 kev. The effective dose equivalent is similar to a day's background radiation and this low dose makes the procedure suitable for most groups of subjects including babies and children, although it remains prudent not to scan pregnant women. It is also acceptable to make longitudinal measurements in individual subjects. DXA is one of the very few techniques to bridge the gap between body composition analysis in the laboratory and the clinic. Although the capital costs are high (approximately £50 000) DXA machines are now available in many medium-to-large hospitals and the running costs are very modest. A wider group of researchers than ever before now have access to relatively sophisticated body composition analysis and this is likely to increase the applications of this methodology in clinical studies.

Unfortunately there are a number of difficulties in the measurement of obese subjects. Firstly the scanning area is relatively small (approximately 190×60 cm) and inadequate for most obese subjects. A method has been described for half body scans in obese subjects (Tataranni & Ravussin, 1995) but this is not ideal since patients inevitably feel embarrassed by the cumbersome procedure. Additionally there are concerns that there may be a confounding effect of tissue thickness on the measured fat mass. This has been clearly demonstrated in *in vitro* systems, although the physiological significance is unclear (Tothill *et al.*, 1994a; Jebb *et al.*, 1995).

One of the greatest advantages of DXA is the excellent precision of the measurement. The coefficient of variation for body fat mass is approximately 2%, which in theory makes it particularly suitable for the measurement of relatively small changes in composition (Tothill *et al.*, 1994b). Koyama *et al.* have compared changes in lean tissue mass measured by DXA with nitrogen balance studies in three obese women studies over two periods of treatment with a very low-energy diet (1.8 MJ/day) (Koyama *et al.*, 1990). Although there was a correlation between the changes in lean tissue measured by the two methods ($r = 0.40$, $P < 0.05$), there was considerable individual variability which the investigators attribute to the effect of changes in hydration on the DXA-measured loss of lean tissue.

Imaging

Imaging techniques have taken an anatomical approach to body composition analysis. Computed tomography (CT) and more recently magnetic resonance imaging (MRI) allow the examination of the composition of the body by tissue, organ or region (Van der Kooy & Seidell, 1993). CT is an X-ray based technique, whilst for MRI the subject is placed in a strong magnetic field and irradiated with radiofrequency pulses. The signal intensity is determined by the concentration and relaxation properties of water and fat in the tissues being studied. Adipose tissue has a much shorter relaxation time than other tissues and can be accurately identified. In both cases it is possible to measure total body composition by interpolating between sequential slices, however, this is rarely the most appropriate method to measure whole-body composition because of the limited availability of machines, cost, analysis time and in the case of CT a significant radiation exposure, of up to 5 mSv (Kvist *et al.*, 1986). In obese patients these measurements present practical problems since many patients may exceed the capacity of the machines.

Prediction techniques

Weight for height indices

In routine clinical practice there is a need for simple, practical methods which require the minimum time, experience and expenditure. Simple measures of weight and height are often deemed to be sufficient and the body mass index (BMI, weight/height^2) is the most widely used of these indices. It is extremely precise and there is minimal measurement error (Fuller *et al.*, 1991). However, self-reported measures may be biased towards under-estimation of BMI since there is a tendency to over-estimate height and under-estimate weight.

The BMI gives a measure of relative weight, adjusted for height which allows direct comparisons between individuals of different stature. In practice the BMI is widely used as an index of the degree of overweight, and serves as a useful classification procedure. However, a cautious practitioner will always interpret the BMI in the light of a clinical impression which may reveal alternative explanations for apparently high BMIs. For example, decreases in adult stature such as those due to kyphosis and increases in body-weight due to oedema or enhanced muscularity will all tend to increase BMI and will be interpreted as implying an elevated body fat mass. Although the BMI may generally rank groups of individuals in order of fatness, considerable absolute errors are possible in individual patients.

Correlation of BMI with other specific measures of fat mass has led to a number of prediction equations to transform BMI into an estimate of fat mass (e.g. Webster *et al.*, 1984). However, this procedure offers little or no further advantage and the absolute estimate of fat mass varies with the prediction equation employed (Elia, 1992). The estimate of fat mass based on BMI should not be used to estimate changes in fat mass. Since height may be assumed to remain constant in adults the changes in body composition will always be a function of the change in weight and will only vary with the prediction equation employed. Changes in BMI in adults are simply a more complicated version of changes in weight.

Skinfold thicknesses

The measurement of skinfold thicknesses at a number of sites has been used for many years to estimate body fat stores. Subcutaneous fat is measured using calipers which exert a standard pressure and it is assumed that the thickness of subcutaneous fat at the selected sites is representative and that there is a known relationship between subcutaneous fat and total fat mass, after allowing for gender differences and changes with age. The most commonly used method involves measurements at four sites: triceps, biceps, subscapula and suprailiac. Following log transformation of the data there is a linear relationship between the sum of the skinfold thickness at these sites and body density, which is age and gender specific (Durnin & Womersley, 1974). Thus, skinfold thickness measurements can be used to predict body density and hence body fat is calculated according to Siri's equation. Different prediction equations are needed for children and for specific racial groups.

It will be apparent that this technique combines the error associated with the prediction of body density with the uncertainties regarding the density of FFM, inherent to the density method. Nonetheless, we have repeatedly demonstrated that with a single observer the measurements can give good agreement with reference methods and may be more accurate than other prediction techniques (Fuller et al., 1992). Measurements of changes in body fat by skinfold thicknesses may be less reliable than the absolute estimates of fat mass. Ballor and Katch have demonstrated that seven out of 10 anthropometric prediction equations were significantly different from measurements of fat change by densitometry (Ballor & Katch, 1989). This is partly because of the measurement error on the pre- and post-weight-loss assessments and also because changes in subcutaneous fat may not fully represent the changes in total body composition.

One of the greatest drawbacks to this method is the poor reproducibility of the technique, particularly between different observers. The coefficient of variation for measurements made in six non-obese individuals by six experienced observers was 11, 16, 13 and 18 for triceps, biceps, subscapula and suprailiac respectively, although when summed and translated into an estimate of body fat the coefficient of variation was only 4.6% (Fuller et al., 1991). In the obese there may be specific problems; some patients may be too large for the jaws of the calipers and it is more difficult to locate the correct anatomical site than in lean individuals. Large subcutaneous fat deposits tend to be very compressible and so the measured thickness will vary with the time taken to make the measurement, which may impair the precision even further. Oedema can lead to an over-estimation of body fat, partly because the thickness of the skinfold may be increased, but also because of the increased body-weight. Finally this measurement can be very distressing to some obese patients since it makes such a direct measure of their overt fat stores.

Bioelectrical impedance

This method rests on the principle that fat is a poor conductor of an applied current whereas FFM, with its water and electrolyte content, is a good conductor. A small current is passed between tetrapolar electrodes on the hand and foot to measure the body impedance, which is proportional to the conducting volume, i.e. body water (Hoffer *et al.*, 1969). At high frequencies, typically 50 kHz, the current is able to overcome the capacitance of cell membranes and to fully penetrate the cells giving a measure of total body water, whereas at low frequencies, e.g. 1 kHz, it cannot enter the cells and hence measures only extracellular water. Although machines operating at a single high frequency are the most common, an increasing number are able to operate at a variety of different frequencies to assess extracellular water too (Tagliabue *et al.*, 1996). Recently a swept frequency has been used which makes multiple measurements across a spectrum of frequencies up to 1 MHz and this may provide a more accurate assessment of the two water compartments by allowing a mathematical integration of the measurements to zero frequency and infinity (Cornish *et al.*, 1993).

Prediction equations to convert the measured impedance into an estimate of body composition have been developed by comparison with isotope dilution studies. Although there is a good relationship between the measured impedance and total body water (with correction for height, as a proxy for conductor length) the standard error of the estimate is typically about 2 litres. This reflects the complex geometry of the body which cannot be adequately described using the model of a simple cylinder. Furthermore it is then necessary to assume the hydration fraction of FFM (as for the isotope dilution measurements of body water) to extrapolate to soft tissue composition. Thus, the prediction errors are again combined with those of the technique from which it was derived.

In practical terms the tetrapolar method is relatively straightforward. The patient must be supine with the limbs slightly abducted. Electrodes are carefully positioned at specific sites (Fig. 2.6), a small current applied and the voltage drop across the body measured. The impedance is calculated as voltage/current. Impedance represents the sum of the resistive and reactive components of the body; some machines measure only resistance, but since the reactive component in the human body is extremely small the difference between impedance and resistance is usually insignificant. Since this is essentially a measure of body

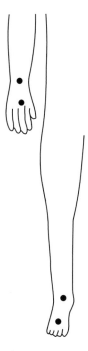

Fig. 2.6 Position of electrodes for the measurement of 'whole-body' impedance.

water patients should be normally hydrated. In patients with oedema the increased body water volume will be interpreted as an expansion of lean tissue mass and hence body fat will be under-estimated. In these patients a multifrequency technique will be more useful since it allows the calculation of intracellular water from the difference between total and extracellular volumes and hence a more accurate measure of the true soft tissue composition can be made (Cornish *et al.*, 1995).

There are a host of commercial impedance machines available and some centres have built their own devices. The cost is generally related to the associated software, which may also make predictions of basal metabolic rate, total energy expenditure, etc., based on data on weight, height, gender, physical activity, etc., which are inserted into the programme. Cautious investigators should always record the raw impedance measurement and select the most appropriate prediction equation for their group of subjects from the literature to convert the impedance measurement into an estimate of fat or FFM. There are relatively few multifrequency machines available at the present time and they tend to be significantly more expensive, reflecting their electronic complexity.

This year a new device based on the impedance principles has been introduced into the U.K. from Japan. This resembles a set of bathroom scales on which the patient stands bare-footed on two metal sole plates. The machine measures body-weight and records the impedance from foot to foot. An alternative model includes a hand-held module to mimic the conventional tetrapolar system. The reproducibility of the method is extremely good and studies are underway to compare the absolute accuracy with data obtained from reference methods (S.A. Jebb, unpublished). Although it is likely to suffer from similar limitations to traditional impedance systems this may be a practical method for patients to make some estimate of changes in body fat at home.

The absolute accuracy of impedance depends on the prediction equation employed (Elia, 1992). In obesity studies there is a particular problem since few prediction equations have included a significant number of obese subjects in their derivation. Studies have shown better agreement between impedance and reference methods in obese subjects following a period of weight loss (Van der Kooy et al., 1992; Webber et al., 1994), suggesting that some feature of the obese body composition may be directly contributing to the observed error such as the expansion of the extracellular water space (Deurenberg et al., 1989a). A recent analysis of a variety of prediction equations to estimate body fat in obese women, as measured by a multicompartment model, showed that the bias of percentage body fat relative to a three-compartment model (density plus total body water) ranged from –6.7% to +7.8% with 95% limits of agreement of up to 25% depending on the prediction equation employed (Fuller et al., 1994). The smallest errors (0.1 ± 6.5%) were seen for the equation of Segal (Segal et al., 1988).

Changes in composition may also be measured differentially by different equations, particularly between those which use Ht^2/R only and those which include additional anthropometric measures such as weight (Kushner et al., 1990). In weight loss studies a further problem arises in relation to the sites of fat loss. In the human body the arms and legs make a disproportionately large contribution to the measured impedance on account of their length and cross-sectional area, whereas the shorter, broader trunk makes a much smaller contribution (Fig. 2.7). Despite accounting for around 45% of body-weight the trunk contributes less than 10% to the measured impedance (Fuller & Elia, 1989). Thus, the measured decrease in total body fat in an individual subject will depend on the site of fat loss. This may be overcome in the future by the development of specific prediction equations for different segments of the body; however, their development is hindered by the lack of access to imaging techniques which provide the only appropriate reference method for segmental body composition measures.

Changes in the hydration fraction of FFM will also have an important impact on measured changes in composition by impedance such that short-term changes in body composition cannot be accurately measured. This has been documented in a study in which volunteers consumed a very-low-energy diet for 2 days and

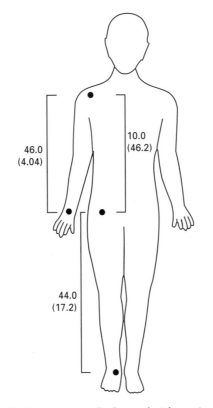

Fig. 2.7 Contribution of body segments to body-weight (shown in parentheses) and 'whole-body' impedance. Reproduced from Jebb and Elia (1994).

lost 1.3 ± 0.5 kg (Deurenberg *et al.*, 1989c). This weight loss is likely to be almost entirely composed of water and glycogen (FFM) with only minimal losses of body fat. Whole-body density measurements showed a decrease in FFM of 1.2 ± 0.8 kg, but losses measured by impedance were only 0.5 ± 0.8 kg, implying that 0.8 kg fat had also been lost. However, over a longer period of time the changes in glycogen become small in relation to the loss of body fat and the validity of this method may improve. Impedance-based methods may prove a useful technique for routine measurements in clinical practice since it minimizes the effects of observer error which can be a particular problem in a clinic setting if skinfold thickness measurements are used.

Near infra-red interactance

This technique uses a beam of near infra-red radiation to irradiate the underlying tissues. The measured optical density depends on the specific absorption characteristics of the underlying tissue. A commercial instrument emits two wavelengths of near infra-red radiation at 940 and 950 nm. A prediction equation interprets the optical density measured over the biceps muscle to give an estimate of whole-body fat mass (Conway et al., 1984).

There is a general concern that the composition of tissue overlying the biceps is unlikely to be representative of total body fat in all individuals. To some extent this is overcome since the prediction equation also includes measurement of weight, height, gender, age and physical activity which all contribute to the estimated fat mass. Indeed, measurements of the optical density at different sites of the body make only a small difference to the measured fat mass implying that most of the inter-individual variance is accounted for by the other factors in the equation (S.A. Jebb, unpublished). A specific difficulty in using this method in obese subjects is the poor penetration of the near infra-red beam into soft tissue. Since this is limited to about 1 cm it is probable that erroneous estimates will be made in obese subjects and comparisons of measurements by near infra-red with reference methods have demonstrated the extent of this under-estimation (Elia et al., 1990; Fuller et al., 1994).

There is some observer error associated with the method which is probably midway between skinfold thickness and impedance methods (Fuller et al., 1991). Otherwise it has similar advantages to other prediction techniques in terms of simplicity of measurement and relatively low cost. However, it offers few if any advantages over the other prediction methods and most studies have concluded that its absolute accuracy is poor (Fuller et al., 1992).

Accuracy and precision

One of the difficulties in evaluating the *in vivo* body composition techniques is that there is no true 'gold standard'. Although cadaver analysis is often cited as the ultimate reference method, in practice this is impossible and is not devoid of its own errors, not least the problems associated with accurately handling such large quantities of material, without loss of solids or water. In recent years it has been recognized that complex multicompartment models can act as accurate reference methods for absolute measures of body composition since they do not carry the errors of traditional two-compartment models with respect to the assumed composition of FFM. A number of studies have used the four-compartment model to determine the accuracy of other simpler techniques (Friedl et al., 1992; Fuller et al., 1992; Guo et al., 1992; Bergsma-Kadijk et al., 1996; Forslund et al., 1996).

Body composition techniques are frequently compared using correlation analysis. This is inadequate since methods may often show a good relationship with each other, but may not always agree (Jebb & Elia, 1994). Table 2.1 shows the correlation between individual methods and a four-compartment model for the measurement of absolute fat mass in studies at the MRC Dunn Nutrition

Table 2.1 Correlation, mean bias and 95% confidence limits of agreement for methods to measure percentage body fat relative to a four-compartment model ($n = 145$).

	Correlation coefficient	Bias	95% confidence limits
Density	0.926	1.51	5.39
Total body water	0.923	1.30	5.71
DXA	0.895	3.75	7.61
Skinfolds	0.870	1.72	7.33

Centre. It also includes the mean bias of the methods and 95% limits of agreement for individual subjects. This demonstrates clearly that good correlation coefficients can conceal considerable inter-individual variability. For example in a group of 145 subjects the correlation coefficient for DXA versus a four-compartment model is 0.9, the bias across the group as a whole is small yet the limits of agreement ($\pm 2\,SD$) are 7.61% (S.A. Jebb, unpublished).

Some of the deviations in the composition of FFM from the assumed value may be an individual characteristic and hence methods may be able to measure changes in composition more accurately than absolute values. Differences between regression equations in the case of the prediction methods may also become less significant. Nevertheless, results from one method may still not agree with another, because of the differences in their fundamental assumptions. For example the measurement of changes in fat mass in six subjects who lost $15.04 \pm 1.5\,kg$ weight estimated the proportion of weight lost as fat by DXA, skinfolds and impedance to be 92, 70 and 66%, respectively (Webber et al., 1994). To minimize potential errors repeated measurements must be made using the same method, by the same observer and under standardized conditions, but even this cannot prevent errors introduced by changes in the composition of FFM. This may be a particular problem in patients losing weight.

Short-term changes in fat mass can only be accurately measured by careful substrate balance studies. Measurements in our whole-body calorimeters can detect changes in fat balance with a precision of only $\pm 9\,g$ fat/day. In a study in which a group of six men were either over- or under-fed we compared a variety of methods to estimate the change in fat mass. The limits of agreement for individual subjects were smaller for the multicompartment models ($0.01 \pm 0.77\,kg$) than traditional two-compartment techniques (density $-0.28 \pm 0.99\,kg$, total body-weight (TBW) $0.33 \pm 1.48\,kg$). Skinfold thicknesses (measured by a single observer) showed good agreement ($-0.58 \pm 0.62\,kg$), whilst bioelectrical impedance was poorer (0.68 ± 3.03) (Jebb et al., 1993).

Table 2.2 Observer error in the measurement of body composition. Data from Fuller *et al.* (1991).

	Residual CV (%)	
	Raw measurement	Body fat mass
Weight (kg)	0.01	
Height (cm)	0.4	0.8
Skinfold thicknesses (mm):		
Triceps	11	
Biceps	16	
Subscapula	13	
Suprailiac	18	
Sum of 4 sites	9	4.6
Bioelectrical resistance (Ω)	1.2	2.6
Near infra-red interactance		
od 1	5.6	
od 2	6.2	4.2

CV, co-effecient of variation

It is also possible to use multicompartment models to assess the error in two-compartment techniques as a consequence of changes in the composition of FFM, e.g., changes in the proportion of water or mineral (Jebb & Elia, 1995). In this way it will ultimately be possible to redefine more accurate assumptions for methods such as body density and TBW techniques. For example, a better understanding of the loss of bone mineral associated with ageing will allow a more accurate estimate of FFM which is perhaps age and sex specific.

The importance of measurement precision cannot be over-estimated, both for absolute measurements and changes in composition. This includes both inter- and intra-observer reproducibility. The extent of inter-observer variability associated with each of the methods has been previously discussed and is summarized in Table 2.2 (Fuller *et al.*, 1991). Intra-observer variability varies but it is important that it is documented by each observer in their own study sample to ensure that measured changes in composition are outside the limits of precision of the measurement instrument. For example, a change of only 1% in fat mass cannot be accurately measured by skinfold thicknesses with a precision of approximately 5%.

Clinical applications

Techniques to measure gross body composition may be used to identify obese patients or to monitor the effect of anti-obesity interventions. In practice, patients requiring treatment are almost always identified on the basis of BMI, possibly with additional measurements of fat distribution (see below). Other specific measurements of body composition may also be made at an initial consultation if they form part of a baseline measure for the subsequent evaluation of progress. For routine clinical purposes this is likely to be one of the prediction techniques. However, if patients are participating in a specific research project to document the effect of a particular intervention or to compare two regimens it is possible that a 'reference' method will be employed. As reference methods become more practical, e.g., DXA and BOD POD, this will become increasingly common. More detailed research investigations are likely to use the most accurate tools available including multicompartment models, imaging and IVNAA. In some circumstances nitrogen balance studies may also be performed to measure small changes in lean tissue, although these measurements have their own inherent error associated with the complete collection of urine samples. For the most detailed studies full substrate balances must be performed within the confines of a whole-body calorimeter. Here changes in fat mass can be measured with considerable accuracy and precision (Jebb et al., 1993).

Measurements of changes in body composition during weight loss have provided the basis for much of our understanding of the physiology of weight loss under different circumstances. Forbes has undertaken a comprehensive analysis of body composition at a range of body-weights using a variety of two-compartment methods (Forbes, 1987). This demonstrates that there is a curvilinear relationship between body fat and lean tissue which becomes linear on log transformation (Fig. 2.8). This implies that as weight is gained there is an increase in the relative proportion of fat to lean tissue. As weight is lost the reverse must be true if the post-obese subject is to achieve a body composition similar to that of the never-obese individual of similar weight. Thus, the

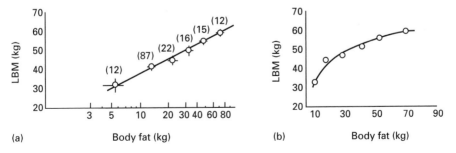

Fig. 2.8 Relationship between body fat and lean tissue mass in women of different body-weight. (a) Lean body mass (LBM) vs $\log_{10}$ body fat (kg), data shown are mean $\pm$ 2SEM and (b) LBM vs body fat. Reproduced from Forbes (1987).

appropriate composition of tissue lost will depend in part upon the initial fat mass of the subject. Nonetheless, the general estimate of 25:75% lean/fat tissue lost will be appropriate for severely obese patients.

There is considerable interest in the factors which may affect the composition of weight loss, particularly the extent of the energy deficit and the effect of exercise. A combined analyses from a number of studies, using a variety of two-compartment methods to measure changes in body composition, suggests that the greater the energy deficit the greater the losses of lean tissue (Prentice et al., 1991). This is consistent with classical nitrogen balance studies and a clinical trial which demonstrated greater losses of nitrogen on a very-low-energy diet than a 3.3 MJ/day diet (Garrow et al., 1989). However, there is not universal agreement; a complex analysis using IVNAA shows that the loss of lean tissue on a very-low-energy diet to be only $78 \pm 8.0\%$ (range 68.1–89.6%) (Ryde et al., 1993).

The macronutrient composition of the diet may also influence the relative proportion of fat and FFM which is lost. Most of the studies which have considered the effect of high-protein diets have been based on nitrogen balance. The classic work of Calloway and Spector suggest that if energy intake is kept constant nitrogen balance can be improved by increasing the nitrogen intake, although there is little improvement at intakes in excess of 6–7 g/day (Calloway & Spector, 1954). Hoffer et al. showed a significant improvement in nitrogen balance when dietary nitrogen was increased from 7 to 13.6 g/day with energy intakes of 2–2.3 MJ/day (Hoffer et al., 1984), but a number of other studies in subjects receiving very-low-energy diets (< 3.3 MJ/day) have shown no further improvement in nitrogen balance with intakes in excess of 6–10 gN/day (de Haven et al., 1980; Yang et al., 1981; Hendler & Bonde, 1988). Less data is available from studies using in vivo techniques, although measurements of total body nitrogen by IVNAA in obese adolescents on a high-protein (2.5 g/kg ideal body-weight (IBW)), low-energy (3.7 MJ/day) reducing diet showed weight losses of 15% of initial body-weight ($P < 0.001$) and only a 4.8% decrease in total body nitrogen (NS) (Archibald et al., 1983).

There are also comparisons of low-carbohydrate vs low-fat diets on the basis that ketogenic low carbohydrate diets may be 'protein sparing'. However, a recent study conducted with rigorous dietary supervision showed no difference in weight or fat loss between the two isoenergetic diets, providing 15 vs 45% carbohydrate (Golay et al., 1996). The only caveat to this conclusion is that measurements were made with skinfold thickness measurements and bioelectrical impedance analysis, which may not be sufficiently sensitive to detect small differences between groups. A study using IVNAA to measure total body nitrogen on an 800 kcal/day diet showed a smaller decrease in lean tissue in the group where 3.5% of energy was provided as carbohydrate, compared to 35%, although there was no significant difference when the data was expressed as the percentage change from the baseline values (Vaswani et al., 1983).

There is increasing evidence that the addition of exercise to an energy-restricted diet may minimize the loss of lean tissue (Prentice et al., 1991). A meta-analysis including measurements made by a variety of two-compartment methods showed that although total weight loss was not significantly different in diet only and diet plus exercise groups the loss of FFM was approximately halved in both men and women by the addition of exercise (Ballor & Poehlman, 1994). A study in which changes were measured using MRI has confirmed these findings. Twenty-four women participated in a randomized study of diet only (DO) versus diet plus exercise (DE) regimens. Mean weight loss was similar in both groups (DO = −10.0 ± 4.0 kg; DE = −11.7 ± 3.0kg), but the DE group lost more fat than the DO group (−11.3 ± 3.8 vs −8.3 ± 3.6; $P < 0.05$). Lean tissue and skeletal muscle mass were preserved in the DE group but reduced in the DO group ($P < 0.01$) (Ross et al., 1995).

The cumulative evidence from studies of the changes in body composition during assorted weight loss programmes has provided the basis for conventional treatment practices for the management of obese patients which have evolved to encourage moderate energy restriction, with a minimum of about 40 g protein per day and increased levels of physical activity to minimize the loss of lean tissue. Future analysis using more sophisticated multicompartment analyses of body composition will undoubtedly continue to refine these concepts and underpin the development of treatment programmes.

Fat distribution

Imaging

Imaging techniques can provide a direct measure of fat mass at specific sites of the body. CT and MRI have both been used to measure fat distribution, typically in the abdominal or intra-abdominal region. A particular advantage of these techniques is that it is also possible to discriminate between omental, mesenteric and retroperitoneal fat depots, which may be associated with independent metabolic effects. The absolute accuracy of the methods have been tested by comparison with sections from cadavers with correlation coefficients for adipose tissue volumes of greater than 0.9 (Van der Kooy & Seidell, 1993). The two methods do give different absolute values for abdominal fat mass although the ranking of subjects is similar by each method (Seidell et al., 1990).

Ideally visceral fat volume is calculated from multiple scans across the abdomen. This gives maximum precision, but increased measurement time and in the case of CT, increased exposure to ionizing radiation (approximately

25–50 mSv per slice (Kvist *et al.*, 1986)). There is, however, a good correlation between the fat area measured in a single CT slice at the level of L4 to L5 with total visceral fat volume ($r > 0.95$) (Kvist *et al.*, 1986) and the precision is estimated to be 1.9% for subcutaneous fat area and 3.9% for visceral fat (Thaete *et al.*, 1995). Measurements of intra-abdominal visceral fat and subcutaneous abdominal fat by CT show a significant increases in obese subjects relative to lean controls ($P < 0.001$) although the ratio was not significantly different (Wajchenberg *et al.*, 1995).

A limited number of studies have measured changes in regional body composition during weight loss (Fig. 2.9). The study of Hendler *et al.* demonstrated that in subjects who lost a mean of 24.5 kg to reach IBW, there was a decrease of 66% in intra-abdominal fat, 56% in subcutaneous fat at the waist and 51% in subcutaneous fat at the hip, such that the intra-abdominal fat area and hip subcutaneous fat area were reduced to that seen in never-obese individuals at IBW, although the waist subcutaneous fat area remained significantly elevated (Hendler *et al.*, 1995). It is not yet clear whether these differences in composition in the reduced-obese have any impact on subsequent health risks. Measurements made over a period of weight loss -12.9 ± 3.3 kg) followed by regain have shown no difference in the sites of deposition following a weight cycle compared to baseline values (Van der Kooy *et al.*, 1993).

Although imaging techniques are the reference method for visceral fat mass their use is generally confined to small-scale studies because of the practical limitations of these methods in terms of cost and machine availability.

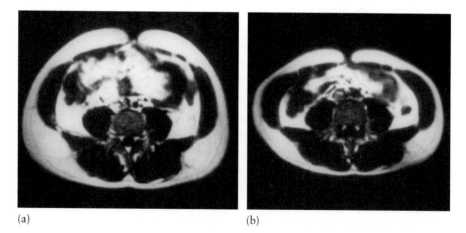

(a)   (b)

Fig. 2.9 Abdominal MRI scan before (a) and after (b) 10% weight loss. Courtesy of Dr J. Seidell.

Dual energy X-ray absorptiometry

In addition to the measurement of gross body composition by DXA it is possible to analyse specific regions of the body, e.g., arms, legs and trunk, with a coefficient of variation of approximately 5% (Jebb, 1997). This can give a very crude guide to fat distribution. However, in obese subjects the cramped nature of the scanning position makes regional divisions difficult or even impossible. Absolute measurements of regional body composition in obese and normal-weight subjects by DXA shows significant increases in fat in the whole body, arms, legs and trunk in obese subjects relative to lean controls, although as a percentage of body-weight the regional distribution of fat was not significantly different (Wajchenberg et al., 1995).

It is also possible to define a specific abdominal site, usually between L2 and L4 to measure the total fat mass in this region, including both the intra-abdominal and subcutaneous fat deposits, with a coefficient of variation of approximately 3% (Schlemmer et al., 1990; Svendsen et al., 1993b). If subcutaneous fat around the abdomen is estimated from simple anthropometric measures of the sagittal diameter and abdominal skinfold thickness it is possible to estimate intra-abdominal fat (Svendsen et al., 1993b; Jensen et al., 1995; Treuth et al., 1995). Although the correlation of abdominal fat measured by CT vs DXA is good ($r = 0.9$) the SEE is 7% and this increases to 15% for the estimation of intra-abdominal fat in a construct which includes DXA, waist/hip ratio and trunk skinfold thicknesses (Svendsen et al., 1993a).

DXA measurements have not yet been widely used to measure fat distribution. This is partly because it is a novel technique, but also because it does not have either the accuracy of imaging techniques or the convenience of anthropometric measurements. Its clinical potential for measurements of visceral fat has yet to be defined.

Anthropometry

Measurements of body dimensions can be used to give a rough estimate of body shape and it is generally concluded that increasing size reflects increasing fat mass. Skinfold thicknesses, circumferences and more recently abdominal diameters have all been used to define increasing abdominal fatness. None of these anthropometric measurements alone can distinguish between visceral and subcutaneous abdominal fat, but they do correlate with risk factors for diabetes and cardiovascular disease and they are advocated as suitable proxy measures for public health initiatives.

The interpretation of these proxies in terms of absolute measurements varies: a waist/hip ratio of 0.95 in men and 0.80 in women is usually deemed to be indicative of central obesity (National Academy of Sciences, 1991), whilst a waist circumference in excess of 89 cm in women and 102 cm in men has been suggested to identify individuals requiring anti-obesity interventions (Lean *et al.*, 1995). In general the validity of these proxy measures has been evaluated on the basis of correlation coefficients in relation to visceral fat measurements by imaging techniques. One of the most comprehensive studies in 213 men and 190 women showed that a waist girth of 95 cm in both sexes, a waist/hip ratio of 0.94 cm in men and 0.88 cm in women, and sagittal diameters of 22.8 cm in men and 25.2 cm in women corresponded to a visceral adipose tissue area of 130 cm^2 (Lemieux *et al.*, 1996).

The measurement of sagittal diameter as an index of abdominal fat is based on the premise that the accumulation of visceral fat will lead to increases in the sagittal diameter in a supine subject, whilst increases in subcutaneous adipose tissue will reduce sagittal diameter due to the effects of gravity (Sjöström, 1991). Correlations between the visceral fat area measured by CT or MRI and sagittal diameters range from 0.46 to 0.96 (Van der Kooy & Seidell, 1993). The relationship can be improved by adjusting for the thickness of the abdominal subcutaneous fat layer; however, the poorest correlations are seen in obese subjects where subcutaneous fat skinfold thicknesses may be particularly difficult to obtain.

The waist/hip ratio has been widely used as a proxy measure of visceral fat based on studies which have compared the ratio with CT-measured visceral fat (Ashwell *et al.*, 1985). However, the waist/hip ratio predicts less than half the variance in visceral adipose tissue in men and even less in women (Seidell *et al.*, 1987) and after adjustments for total body fat and age there is not always a significant independent association with visceral fat (Seidell *et al.*, 1988). In a study of obese women who succeeding in slimming to IBW, intra-abdominal fat (measured by MRI) was not significantly different from never-obese controls at IBW, but the waist/hip ratio remained elevated, implying that this ratio is a poor marker of intra-abdominal fat stores (Hendler *et al.*, 1995). This is in part due to using a ratio to measure small changes. More recently it has been suggested that waist alone, waist/thigh, or waist/height ratios may be more suitable. In a group of 20 male and 38 female subjects who lost 12.2 ± 3.5 kg and 10.2 ± 3.5 kg, respectively (11.5% body-weight for each group), MRI measurements of visceral fat decreased by 40.5 ± 17.1% and 31.7 ± 16.4% in men and women whilst waist circumference decreased by 11 and 8%, respectively. There was a significant correlation between changes measured by the two methods ($r = 0.66$, $P < 0.001$) such that a 1-cm reduction in waist circumference corresponded with a 5-cm^2 (3.5%) reduction in visceral adipose tissue. However, the standard deviation of 4% limits the usefulness of this method in individual subjects. One of the strengths of this type of measurement is that the coefficient of variation for body circumferences is <2% (Bray *et al.*, 1990) and the validity of self-reported measures is good (Kushi *et al.*, 1988).

The measurement of skinfold thicknesses represents an attempt to make a direct measure of fat mass at a particular site (Mueller & Stallones, 1981). A variety of skinfold thickness ratios have been proposed to reflect central versus peripheral fat distribution such as the trunk/extremity skinfold ratio ({supra-iliac + subscapula + abdominal}/{medial calf + triceps + biceps}) (Rice *et al.*, 1995). These measurements are limited by the same practical drawbacks associated with the prediction of total fat by this method, including inter- and intra-observer variability and the difficulties in actually measuring the thicknesses in obese individuals. However, this approach has been widely used in population-based studies of the genetic component of obesity and fat distribution, e.g., Bouchard *et al.* (1988) Comuzzie *et al.* (1994) and Rice *et al.* (1995).

Comparisons of these proxy measures with direct measurements of intra-abdominal fat are limited, but in general highlight the limitations. Anthropometric analyses provide a convenient method of patient assessment but as yet their clinical value is unclear, particularly for the measurement of changes in composition.

Conclusions

Body composition measurements form an integral part of obesity research both in the laboratory and in the clinic. Methods which have been developed and tested in the laboratory are increasingly making their way into the clinic. This progression is partly a consequence of a simplification of the methodology but it also reflects the recognition of their importance in the clinical management of patients.

Obesity is not a condition of excess weight but of excess body fat, which in turn contributes to the co-morbidity of the disease. The site of fat deposition may be particularly important in this respect, but more data is needed in which direct measures of fat distribution are combined with accurate measurements of total body fat to fully understand the complex interaction, including the effect of other confounding factors such as smoking, alcohol consumption and inactivity. Understanding this relationship will ultimately allow a more accurate assessment of the patients at greatest risk and hence help to target limited treatment resources most effectively.

However, we already know that a successful obesity treatment programme must reduce total and abdominal fat. In the clinic, measurements of changes in composition in individual patients provide a valuable method to monitor the efficacy of treatment interventions and to design treatment programmes which maximize the loss of fat tissue. To date there is no evidence that any particular anti-obesity treatment will produce proportionally greater losses at any particular site. Changes in total body fat will give a good guide to changes in fat at the abdominal site. The key issue is therefore to select a method with the necessary accuracy and precision yet which is suited to the practical difficulties encountered in routine clinical practice.

Unfortunately, as yet there are few studies in obesity research which have fully exploited the available methodology. Many studies have examined only small groups of subjects, often with inadequately sensitive methods. In many cases there is too little evidence to achieve a consensus and important physiological questions remain to be answered. This is partly because of limitations in the body composition methodology but also reflects the heterogeneity of the obese condition and individual responses to treatment. The situation will only be resolved by large, carefully controlled studies using accurate and precise techniques. This needs a firm link between laboratory research, both methodological and conceptual, and the practical needs of clinicians and their patients.

References

Archibald, E., Harrison, J. & Pencharz, P. (1983) Effect of a weight reducing high protein diet on the body composition of obese adolescents. *American Journal of Diseases in Childhood* **137**, 658–662.

Ashwell, M., Cole, T. & Dixon, A. (1985) Obesity: new insights into the anthropometric classification of fat distribution shown by computed tomography. *British Medical Journal* **290**, 1692–1694.

Ballor, D. & Katch, V. (1989) Validity of anthropometric regression equations for predicting changes in body fat of obese females. *American Journal of Human Biology* **1**, 97–101.

Ballor, D. & Poehlman, E. (1994) Exercise-training enhances fat-free mass preservation during diet-induced weight loss: a meta-analytical finding. *International Journal of Obesity* **18**, 35–40.

Beddoe, A. & Hill, G. (1985) Clinical measurement of body composition using *in vivo* neutron activation analysis. *Journal of Parenteral and Enteral Nutrition* **9**, 504–520.

Bergsma-Kadijk, J., Baumeister, B. & Deurenberg, P. (1996) Measurement of body fat in young and elderly women: comparison between a four-compartment model and widely used reference methods. *British Journal of Nutrition* **75**, 649–657.

Bouchard, C., Perusse, L., Leblanc, C., Tremblay, A. & Theriault, G. (1988) Inheritance of the amount and distribution of human body fat. *International Journal of Obesity* **12**, 205–215.

Bray, G., Greenway, F. & Molitch, M. (1990) Use of anthropometric measures to assess weight loss. *American Journal of Clinical Nutrition* **31**, 769–773.

Calloway, D. & Spector, H. (1954) Nitrogen balance as related to calorie and protein intake in active young men. *American Journal of Clinical Nutrition* **2**, 405–412.

Cohn, S., Dombrowski, C., Pate, H. & Robertson, J. (1969) A whole-body counter with an invariant response to radionuclide distribution and body size. *Physics in Medicine and Biology* **14**, 645–658.

Colt, E., Wang, J., Stallone, F., Itallie, T.B. & Pierson, R.N. (1981) A possible low intracellular potassium concentration in obesity. *American Journal of Clinical Nutrition* **34**, 367–372.

Comuzzie, A., Blangero, J., Mahaney, M., Mitchell, B., Stern, M. & MacCluer, J. (1994) Genetic and environmental correlations among skinfold measures. *International Journal of Obesity* **18**, 413–418.

Conway, J., Norris, K. & Bodwell, C. (1984) A new approach for the estimation of body composition: infra-red interactance. *American Journal of Clinical Nutrition* **40**, 1123–1130.

Cornish, B., Thomas, B. & Ward, L. (1993) Improved prediction of extra-cellular fluid balance measured by multiple frequency bio-electrical impedance analysis. *Physics in Medicine and Biology* **38**, 337–346.

Cornish, B., Ward, L., Thomas, B., Jebb, S.A. & Elia, M. (1995) Evaluation of multiple frequency impedance and Cole–Cole analysis for the assessment of body water volumes in healthy humans. *European Journal of Clinical Nutrition* **50**, 159–164.

Coward, W.A., Parkinson, S.A. & Murgatroyd, P. (1988) Body composition measurements for nutrition research. *Nutrition Research Reviews* **1**, 115–124.

de Haven, J., Sherwin, R., Hendler, R. & Felig, P. (1980) Nitrogen and sodium balance and sympathetic venous-system activity in obese subjects treated with a low calorie protein or mixed diet. *New England Journal of Medicine* **302**, 477–482.

Dempster, P. & Aitkens, S. (1995) A new air displacement method for the determination of human body composition. *Medicine and Science in Sports and Exercise* **27**, 1692–1697.

Deurenberg, P., Van der Kooy, K., Leenen, R. *et al.* (1989a) Body impedance is largely dependent on the intra- and extra-cellular water distribution. *European Journal of Clinical Nutrition* **43**, 845–853.

Deurenberg, P., Leenen, R., Van der Kooy, K. & Hautvast, J. (1989b) In obese subjects the body fat percentage calculated with Siri's formula is an overestimation. *European Journal of Clinical Nutrition* **43**, 569–575.

Deurenberg, P., Westrate, J. & Van der Kooy, K. (1989c) Body composition changes assessed by bioelectrical impedance measurements. *American Journal of Clinical Nutrition* **49**, 401–403.

Dickerson, J. & Widdowson, E. (1960) Chemical changes in skeletal muscle with development. *Biochemical Journal* **74**, 142–144.

Durnin, J. & Womersley, J. (1974) Body fat assessed from total body density and its estimation from skinfold thickness measurement in 481 men and women aged 16 to 72 years. *British Journal of Nutrition* **32**, 77–97.

Elia, M. (1992) Body composition analysis: an evaluation of 2 component models, multicomponent models and bedside techniques. *Clinical Nutrition* **11**, 114–127.

Elia, M., Parkinson, S.A. & Diaz, E. (1990) Evaluation of near infra-red interactance as a method for predicting body composition. *European Journal of Clinical Nutrition* **44**, 113–121.

Evans, P., Israel, R., Flickinger, E., O'Brien, K. & Donnelly, J. (1989) Hydrostatic weighing without head submersion in morbidly obese females. *American Journal of Clinical Nutrition* **50**, 400–403.

Forbes, G. (1987) Lean body mass–fat interrelationships in humans. *Nutrition Reviews* **45**, 225–231.

Forslund, A., Johansson, A., Sjodin, A., Bryding, G., Ljunghall, S. & Hambraeus, L. (1996) Evaluation of modified multicompartment models to calculate body composition in healthy males. *American Journal of Clinical Nutrition* **63**, 856–862.

Friedl, K., de Luca, J., Marchitelli, L. & Vogel, J. (1992) Reliability of body fat estimations from a four-compartment model by using density, body water and bone mineral measurements. *American Journal of Clinical Nutrition* **55**, 964–770.

Fuller, N. & Elia, M. (1989) Potential use of the bio-electrical impedance of the 'whole-body' and of body segments for the assessment of body composition: comparison with densitometry and anthropometry. *European Journal of Clinical Nutrition* **43**, 779–791.

Fuller, N., Jebb, S.A., Goldberg, G. *et al.* (1991) Inter-observer variability in the measurement of body composition. *European Journal of Clinical Nutrition* **45**, 43–49.

Fuller, N., Jebb, S.A., Laskey, M., Coward, W. & Elia, M. (1992) Four component model for the assessment of body composition in humans: comparison with alternative methods and evaluation of the density and hydration of fat free mass. *Clinical Science* **82**, 687–693.

Fuller, N., Sawyer, M. & Elia, M. (1994) Comparative evaluation of body composition methods and predictions, and calculation of density and hydration fraction of fat-free mass, in obese women. *International Journal of Obesity* **18**, 503–512.

Garrow, J., Webster, J., Pearson, M., Pacy, P. & Harpin, G. (1989) Inpatient–outpatient randomised comparison of Cambridge diet versus milk in 17 obese women over 24 weeks. *International Journal of Obesity* 13, 521–529.

Golay, A., Allaz, A.F., Morel, Y., de Tonnac, N., Tankova, S. & Reaven, G. (1996) Similar weight loss with low- or high-carbohydrate diets. *American Journal of Clinical Nutrition* 63, 174–178.

Guo, S., Chumlea, W., Wu, X., Wellens, R., Siervogel, R. & Roche, A. (1992) A comparison of body composition models. In: Ellis, K. & Eastmann, J. (eds) *Human Body Composition: In vivo Methods, Models and Assessment*, pp. 27–30. New York: Plenum Press.

Hendler, R. & Bonde, A. (1988) Very-low-calorie diets with high and low protein content: impact on triiodothyronine, energy expenditure and nitrogen balance. *American Journal of Clinical Nutrition* 48, 1239–1247.

Hendler, R., Welle, S., Scott, M., Barnard, R. & Amatruda, J. (1995) The effects of weight reduction to ideal body weight on body fat distribution. *Metabolism* 44, 1413–1416.

Heymsfield, S., Wang, Z., Baumgartner, R., Dilmanian, F., Ma, R. & Yasumura, S. (1993) Body composition and ageing: A study by *in vivo* neutron activation analysis. *Journal of Nutrition* 123, 432–437.

Hoffer, E., Meador, C. & Simpson, D. (1969) Correlation of whole-body impedance with total body water volume. *Journal of Applied Physiology* 27, 531–3534.

Hoffer, L., Bistrian, B., Young, V., Blackburn, G. & Matthews, D. (1984) Metabolic effects of very low calorie weight reducing diets. *Journal of Clinical Investigation* 73, 750–758.

Jebb, S.A. (1997) Measurement of soft tissue composition by dual energy X-ray absorptiometry. *British Journal of Nutrition* 77, 151–163.

Jebb, S.A. & Elia, M. (1994) Measurement of body composition in clinical practice. In: Heatley, R., Green, J. & Losowsky, M. (eds) *Consensus in Clinical Nutrition*, pp. 1–21. Cambridge: Cambridge University Press.

Jebb, S.A. & Elia, M. (1995) Multicompartment models in health and disease. In: Davies, P. & Cole, T. (eds) *Body Composition Techniques in Health and Disease*, pp. 240–254. Cambridge: Cambridge University Press.

Jebb, S.A., Goldberg, G.R., Coward, W., Murgatroyd, P. & Prentice, A.M. (1991) Effects of weight cycling caused by intermittent dieting on metabolic rate and body composition in obese women. *International Journal of Obesity* 15, 367–374.

Jebb, S.A., Murgatroyd, P., Goldberg, G.R., Prentice, A.M. & Coward, W.A. (1993) *In vivo* measurement of changes in body composition: description of methods and their validation against 12-d continuous whole-body calorimetry. *American Journal of Clinical Nutrition* 58, 455–462.

Jebb, S.A., Goldberg, G.R., Jennings, G. & Elia, M. (1995) Dual energy X-ray absorptiometry measurements of body composition: effects of depth and tissue thickness, including comparisons with direct analysis. *Clinical Science* 88, 319–324.

Jennings, G., Bluck, L., Chowings, C., Podesta, D. & Elia, M. (1995) Evaluation of an infra-red method for the determination of total body water in a clinical context. *Clinical Nutrition* 14 (suppl. 2), 53.

Jensen, M., Kanaley, J., Reed, J. & Sheedy, P. (1995) Measurement of abdominal and visceral fat with computed tomography and dual energy X-ray absorptiometry. *American Journal of Clinical Nutrition* 61, 274–278.

Knight, G., Beddoe, A., Streat, S. & Hill, G. (1986) Body composition of two human cadavers by neutron activation and chemical analysis. *American Journal of Physiology* 250, E179–E185.

Koyama, H., Nishizawa, Y., Yamashita, N. *et al.* (1990) Measurement of composition changes using dual photon absorptiometry in obese patients undergoing semi-starvation. *Metabolism* 39, 302–306.

Kushi, L.H., Kaye, S.A., Folsom, A.R., Soler, J.T. & Prineas, R.J. (1988) Accuracy and reliability of self-measurement of body girths. *American Journal of Epidemiology* 128, 740–748.

Kushner, R., Kunigk, A., Alspaugh, M., Andronis, P., Leitch, C. & Schoeller, D. (1990) Validation of bioelectrical impedance analysis as a measurement of change in body composition in obesity. *American Journal of Clinical Nutrition* 52, 219–223.

Kvist, H., Sjostrom, L. & Tylen, U. (1986) Adipose tissue volume determinations in women by computed tomography. *International Journal of Obesity* 10, 53–67.

Lean, M., Han, T. & Morrison, C. (1995) Waist circumference as a measure for indicating need for weight management. *British Medical Journal* 311, 158–161.

Lemieux, S., Prud'homme, D., Bouchard, C., Tremblay, A. & Depres, J.P. (1996) A single threshold value of waist girth identifies normal weight and overweight subjects with excess visceral adipose tissue. *American Journal of Clinical Nutrition* 64, 685–693.

Lukaski, H. (1987) Methods for the assessment of human body composition: traditional and new. *American Journal of Clinical Nutrition* 46, 537–556.

McCrory, M., Gomez, T., Bernauer, E. & Mole, P. (1995) Evaluation of a new air displacement plethysmograph for measuring human body composition. *Medicine and Science in Sports and Exercise* 27, 1686–1691.

Morgan, D. & Burkinshaw, L. (1983) Estimation of non-fat body tissues from measurements of skinfold thickness, total body potassium and total body nitrogen. *Clinical Science* 65, 407–414.

Morgan, D., Burkinshaw, L. & Davidson, C. (1978) Potassium depletion in heart failure and its relation to long term treatment with diuretics: a review of the literature. *Postgraduate Medical Journal* 54, 72–79.

Mueller, W. & Stallones, L. (1981) Anatomical distribution of subcutaneous fat: skinfold site choice and construction of indices. *Human Biology* 53, 321–335.

Murgatroyd, P. & Coward, W.A. (1989) An improved method for estimating changes in whole-body fat and protein mass in man. *British Journal of Nutrition* 62, 311–314.

National Academy of Sciences (1991) *Diet and Health*. Washington DC: National Academy of Sciences Press.

Prentice, A.M., Black, A., Coward, W. *et al.* (1986) High levels of energy expenditure in obese women. *British Medical Journal* 292, 983–987.

Prentice, A.M., Goldberg, G., Jebb, S.A., Black, A., Murgatroyd, P. & Diaz, E. (1991) Physiological response to slimming. *Proceedings of the Nutrition Society* 50, 441–458.

Prentice, A.M., Black, A., Coward, W.A. & Cole, T. (1996) Energy expenditure in affluent societies: an analysis of 319 doubly-labelled water measurements. *European Journal of Clinical Nutrition* 50, 93–97.

Rice, T., Bouchard, C., Perusse, L. & Rao, D. (1995) Familial clustering of multiple measures of adiposity and fat distribution in the Québec Family Study: A trivariate analysis of percent body fat, body mass index and trunk-to-extremity skinfold ratio. *International Journal of Obesity* 19, 902–908.

Ross, R., Pedwell, H. & Rissanen, J. (1995) Effects of energy restriction on skeletal muscle and adiopose tissue in women as measured by magnetic resonance imaging. *American Journal of Clinical Nutrition* 61, 1179–1185.

Ryde, S., Saunders, N., Birks, J. *et al.* (1993) The effects of VLCD on body composition. In: Kreitzman, S. & Howard, A. (eds) *The Swansea Trial*, pp. 31–54. London: Smith-Gordon.

Schlemmer, A., Hassager, C., Haaarbo, J. & Christiansen, C. (1990) Direct measurement of abdominal fat by dual photon absorptiometry. *International Journal of Obesity* 14, 603–611.

Segal, K., Loan, M. van., Fitzgerald, P., Hodgdon, J. & van Itallie, T.B. (1988) Lean body mass estimation by bioelectrical impedance analysis: a four-site cross validation study. *American Journal of Clinical Nutrition* 47, 7–14.

Seidell, J., Oosterlee, A., Thijssen, M. *et al.* (1987) Assessment of intra-abdominal and subcutaneous abdominal fat: relation between anthropometry and computed tomography. *American Journal of Clinical Nutrition* 45, 7–13.

Seidell, J., Oosterlee, A. & Deurenberg, P. (1988) Abdominal fat depots measured with computed tomography: effects of degree of obesity, sex and age. *European Journal of Clinical Nutrition* 42, 805–815.

Seidell, J., Bakker, C. & Van der Kooy, K. (1990) Imaging techniques for measuring adipose tissue distribution—a comparison between computed tomography and 1.5-T magnetic resonance. *American Journal of Clinical Nutrition* 51, 953–957.

Siri, W. (1956) *The Gross Composition of the Body.* New York: Academic Press.

Siri, W. (1961) *Body Composition from Fluid Spaces and Density: A Combined Analysis of Methods.* Washington, DC: National Academy of Sciences–National Research Council.

Sjöström, L. (1991) A computer-tomography based multi-compartment body composition technique and anthropometric predictions of lean body mass, total and subcutaneous adipose tissue. *International Journal of Obesity* 15, 19–30.

Snyder, W., Cook, M., Nasset, E., Karhausen, L., Parry-Howells, G. & Tipton, I. (1975) *Report of the Task Force on Reference Man.* Oxford: Pergamon Press.

Svendsen, O., Haarbo, J., Hassager, C. & Christiansen, C. (1993a) Accuracy of measurements of body composition by dual energy X-ray absorptiometry *in vivo*. *American Journal of Clinical Nutrition* 57, 605–608.

Svendsen, O., Hassager, C., Bergmann, I. & Christiansen, C. (1993b) Measurement of abdominal and intra-abdominal fat in post-menopausal women by dual energy X-ray absorptiometry and anthropometry: comparison with computerised tomography. *International Journal of Obesity* 17, 45–51.

Tagliabue, A., Cena, H. & Deurenberg, P. (1996) Comparative study of the relationship between multi-frequency impedance and body water compartments in two European populations. *British Journal of Nutrition* 75, 11–19.

Tataranni, P. & Ravussin, E. (1995) Use of dual energy X-ray absorptiometry in obese individuals. *American Journal of Clinical Nutrition* 62, 730–734.

Thaete, F., Colberg, S., Burke, T. & Kelley, D. (1995) Reproducibility of computed tomography measurement of visceral adipose tissue area. *International Journal of Obesity* 19, 464–467.

Tothill, P., Avenell, A., Love, J. & Reid, D. (1994a) Comparisons between Hologic, Lunar and Norland dual energy X-ray absorptiometers and other techniques used for whole-body soft tissue measurements. *European Journal of Clinical Nutrition* 48, 781–794.

Tothill, P., Avenell, A. & Reid, D. (1994b) Precision and accuracy of measurements of whole-body bone mineral: comparisons between Hologic, Lunar and Norland dual energy X-ray absorptiometers. *The British Journal of Radiology* 67, 1210–1217.

Treuth, M., Hunter, G. & Kebes-Szabo, T. (1995) Estimating intrabdominal adipose tissue in women by dual energy X-ray absorptiometry. *American Journal of Clinical Nutrition* 62, 527–532.

Van der Kooy, K., & Seidell, J. (1993) Techniques for the measurement of visceral fat: a practical guide. *International Journal of Obesity* 17, 187–196.

Van der Kooy, K., Leenen, R., Deurenberg, P., Seidell, J., Westerterp, K. & Hautvast, J. (1992) Changes in fat-free mass in obese subjects after weight loss: a comparison of body composition measures. *International Journal of Obesity* 16, 675–683.

Van der Kooy, K., Leenen, R., Seidell, J., Deurenberg, P. & Hautvast, J. (1993) Effect of a weight cycle on visceral fat accumulation. *American Journal of Clinical Nutrition* 58, 853–857.

Vaswani, A., Vartsky, D., Ellis, K., Yasumura, S. & Cohn, S. (1983) Effects of caloric restriction on body composition and total body nitrogen as measured by neutron activation. *Metabolism* 32, 185–188.

Wajchenberg, B., Bosco, A., Marone, M. *et al.* (1995) Estimation of body fat and lean tissue distribution by dual energy X-ray absorptiometry and abdominal body fat evaluation by computed tomography in Cushing's disease. *Journal of Endocrinology and Metabolism* 80, 2791–2794.

Webber, J., Donaldson, M., Allison, S. & Macdonald, I. (1994) A comparison of skinfold thickness, body mass index, bioelectrical impedance analysis and dual energy X-ray absorptiometry in assessing body composition in obese subjects before and after weight loss. *Clinical Nutrition* 13, 177–182.

Webster, J., Hesp, R. & Garrow, J. (1984) The composition of excess weight in obese women estimated by body density, total body water and total body potassium. *Human Nutrition: Clinical Nutrition* **38C**, 299–306.

Widdowson, E. & Dickerson, J. (1964) Chemical composition of the body. In: Comar, C. & Bronner, F. (eds) *Mineral Metabolism. An Advanced Treatise*, pp. 2–210. New York: Academic Press.

Yang, M., Barbosa-Saldivar, J., Pi-Sunyer, X. & Itallie, T.V. (1981) Metabolic effect of substituting carbohydrate for protein in a low-calorie diet: a prolonged study in obese individuals. *International Journal of Obesity* **5**, 231–236.

CHAPTER 3

Energy Balance and Animal Models of Obesity

MICHAEL J. STOCK

Why study animals?

It may seem a trifle odd to find a chapter on animal models of obesity in a book on clinical obesity, and it would not be surprising to find many readers skipping this section in order to get to those dealing with human aspects of the problem. However, for those who have stopped to find out what this chapter is all about, it is hoped that they will see how dependent we are on animal studies for our basic understanding of the biology of human energy metabolism and body composition. Moreover, the animal models of obesity are constantly providing a fresh source of ideas about the possible origins of obesity in humans, and how novel, innovative strategies might be devised to help prevent or cure this problem. In some ways, therefore, this chapter is a little like the preclinical component of the typical medical student's degree, the relevance of which is often not appreciated until the student is exposed to real-life clinical situations. So, perhaps the same applies here, with readers of later chapters coming back to see what lessons can be learned from animal studies. Those that do can be instantly rewarded by learning that the first description of a human single-gene obesity (Montague *et al.*, 1997) was entirely dependent on knowledge gained from studying a genetically obese mouse.

Given the target audience this book is designed for, no attempt will be made in this chapter to list all the available experimental models of obesity, or to compare their advantages and disadvantages. For those contemplating using animal models for research on obesity, detailed reviews covering these models have been published recently (Caterson *et al.*, 1996; Hansen, 1996; Stock, 1996; York & Bray, 1996). Instead, the animal literature will be reviewed in order to deal with several key, fundamental questions about energy balance and obesity. These questions are:

- Is energy balance regulated?
- Is energy balance regulated by the control of intake?
- Is energy balance regulated by the control of energy expenditure?

- How might the controls of intake and expenditure be integrated to achieve energy balance?
- To what extent do the physiological mechanisms observed in animals help explain human energy balance and obesity?

Is energy balance regulated?

When physiologists talk about regulation, there is a certain inevitability that they will frame their description around the concept of homeostasis. Energy balance, or body energy content, is no exception, and the example most often used to support this is the observation that many adult humans can control their body-weight to within a few kilograms over 40 or more years in spite of having eaten in excess of 20 000 kg (20 tonnes) of food. However, these individuals appear to be a minority, and the rest gain weight with advancing years and, if not obese, are certainly heavier and fatter in middle age than they were in their early 20s. This progressive increase in body energy content together with quite large variations in body fat between individuals would suggest that energy balance is not regulated in the same precise way as other, much more important physiological functions (e.g., blood pressure, blood glucose, body temperature, etc.) that have an immediate impact upon function. However, the fact that fatness can vary considerably between and within individuals does not mean necessarily that it is not regulated, any more than the increase in blood pressure which commonly accompanies advancing age.

The same changes with age in body fat are seen in the common laboratory animals (rats and mice) used for experimental studies on energy balance, and in these we certainly do have evidence that their body energy is still being regulated. The evidence comes from a variety of studies, but the essential feature is that the animals are shown to 'defend' a certain body-weight or energy content when energy balance has been deliberately perturbed or disrupted. This defence of body-weight has sometimes been cited as evidence for a set-point for body-weight regulation (i.e., a 'ponderostat', or a 'lipostat'), and the trend for body-weight to increase with advancing years as being due to a programmed change in the set-point, i.e., there is a 'sliding' set-point.

There are two obvious experimental paradigms for testing the regulation of energy balance to see if animals will defend a certain body-weight. These are to produce either a depletion or an excessive over-filling of body energy stores, and then to observe any compensatory responses that help return body stores and body-weight to normal. For example, short-term restriction of food intake in laboratory rodents results in a depression of body-weight or body-weight gain that is followed by a rapid compensation such that body-weight will return to normal (Hirsch & Han, 1969). As an alternative to food restriction, Baile *et al.* (1970) caused weight loss in rats by exercise or injection of lipolytic agents, and this was followed by a rapid regain in body-weight when treatment was withdrawn. However, longer periods of deprivation, particularly at an age before the animals have finished growing, can result in a permanent depression of body-weight, even though there may have been a period of rapid 'catch-up' growth. This catch-up phase is, in itself, evidence of regulation of body-weight, although it is more concerned with musculoskeletal growth than with energy balance in terms of fat reserves. This illustrates one of the problems of using changes in body-weight as an index of change in body fatness, particularly as most experimental studies are carried out on animals that are still capable of growth.

Food restriction is a simple and reversible way to deplete body energy reserves, but a permanent reduction can be produced by placing bilateral lesions in the lateral hypothalamus (LH). The LH, together with the ventromedial hypothalamus (VMH), forms the basis of the original 'dual-centre' theory of appetite control, with the VMH being a satiety centre and the LH being thought of as the hunger centre. The reason for considering LH as a hunger centre was that stimulation caused a satiated animal to eat or over-eat (hyperphagia), whereas lesioning resulted in complete cessation of feeding (aphagia). Usually, the LH-lesioned animal escapes from the aphagia and, after a catch-up period, settles at a steady body-weight, but always lower than that of control animals. In other words, it appeared as if the animals were now defending a new set-point (Corbett & Keesey, 1982). Further evidence for a reset set-point comes from experiments where rats were food-restricted to reduce body-weight before having LH lesions placed. In this situation, where body-weight had already been depressed to the new set-point, there was no aphagia due to the LH lesions, and the rats simply continued to defend their new body-weight (Keesey & Powley, 1986).

Another way to observe compensatory responses to reduced energy reserves is to surgically remove large amounts of the fat by performing a lipectomy. The responses to lipectomy reported in the literature are variable, with an almost equal division between those reporting compensatory responses and those reporting a failure of the lipectomized animals to restore their body fat reserves. This is perhaps not surprising given the sometimes quite major surgery involved, and the fact that different animals (e.g., normal, dietary-obese or genetically-obese) and different diets (e.g., normal or high-fat diets) have been used by different workers. It would certainly seem that compensatory responses are more readily seen in animals starting off with large fat depots and/or being allowed access to high-fat diets (e.g., Liebelt *et al.*, 1965; Taylor *et al.*, 1973; Chlouverakis & Hojniki, 1974). However, even in some of the papers where the authors claim that animals failed to compensate for the loss of fat (e.g., Faust *et al.*, 1976; Kral, 1976), careful analysis of their results shows that some compensation did occur. Given the recent excitement about the possible role of leptin as a lipostatic signal secreted by adipose tissue (see later), these older studies, now buried in the literature, begin to take on a new significance.

Unlike food restriction, persuading rats and mice to overeat was always thought to be difficult, if not impossible, simply because for many years it was believed that these animals exerted precise control over their energy intake such as to match exactly intake to their energy expenditure. As a result, most of the early literature on over-feeding involves fairly drastic techniques, such as force-feeding, induction of hypoglycaemia with insulin or placing bilateral lesions in the VMH (Table 3.1). Few of these studies investigated as to whether body-weight was defended in any way. However, electrical stimulation of the LH to induce hyperphagia results in an increase in body fat which returns to its previous level when stimulation is discontinued (Steinbaum & Miller, 1965). Likewise, feeding supplements by stomach tube will result in increased body-weight gain, and this is reversed when tube-feeding is discontinued (Fig. 3.1). The cafeteria feeding system is a more physiological, and much less stressful way to induce excessive weight gain that relies on producing voluntary hyperphagia in rodents by offering them a variety of highly palatable human food items. When the cafeteria diet was withdrawn, the accumulated excess body fat was lost and the rats returned to the same weight as control rats (Fig. 3.1). Reversible weight gains are also seen after infusion of neuropeptide Y (NPY) into the paraventricular nucleus (PVN) of the hypothalamus to induce hyperphagia (Stanley *et al.* 1986).

Table 3.1 Rodent models of hyperphagia.

Dietary	Force-feeding (gastric intubation) High-fat diets Sucrose solutions Cafeteria diets
Hypothalamic	Surgical lesions (VMH, PVN) Chemical lesions (goldthioglucose, monosodium glutamate, bipideryl mustard, ibotenic acid) Electrical stimulation (lateral hypothalamus) NPY (intracerebroventricular or PVN injection)
Metabolic	2-deoxyglucose 2-mercaptoacetate Insulin hypoglycaemia

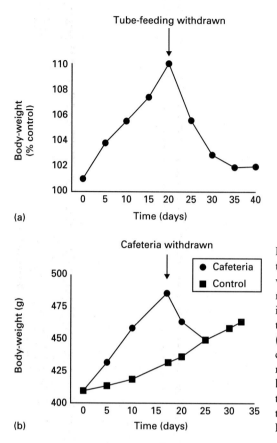

Fig. 3.1 Reversible weight gains in two models of obesity. (a) Excess weight gained as a result of feeding rats 47% of total energy by gastric intubation; total energy intake was the same as in free-feeding controls. (b) Weight gain of rats offered a cafeteria diet compared to that in rats eating the normal stock diet. In both examples, withdrawal of treatment results in a rapid loss of the excess weight. Adapted from Rothwell and Stock (1979a).

Evidence for humoral factors that control energy balance comes from parabiotic experiments, where genetically lean and obese animals (e.g., *ob/ob* and *db/db* mice, and *fa/fa* rats) are surgically joined together such that they share the same circulation (e.g., Coleman, 1973). The suppression of body-weight of the *ob/ob* mouse by its lean partner, and the suppression of the body-weight of its lean partner by the *db/db* mouse and *fa/fa* (Zucker) rat can now be explained in terms of circulating leptin levels (no leptin in *ob/ob*; high leptin in *db/db* and *fa/fa*), but still remains one of the most important pieces of evidence to show that energy balance is regulated.

By moving out of the laboratory and into the natural world one can find several examples, such as hibernation and the premigratory hyperphagia of birds, where regulatory mechanisms come into play to increase body energy reserves in anticipation of increased requirement. More importantly, there is evidence to show that if hibernation or migration is prevented, these increases in energy reserves are subsequently reversed and the animal returns to its normal posthibernation or postmigration body-weight even though it has not hibernated or migrated (Mrosovsky & Powley, 1977).

Table 3.2 Rodent obesity genes.

Gene	Protein	Function
ob	Leptin	Fat-cell hormone
db	Leptin receptor	Hormone receptor
fa	Leptin receptor	Hormone receptor
fat	Carboxypeptidase E	Peptide hormone processing
tub	Tubby	Apoptosis?
agouti	Agouti	Antagonist of MSH (MC-4) hypothalamic receptor

MSH, melanocyte-stimulating hormone; MC-4, melanocortin-4.

Finally, the most powerful evidence for energy balance and body fat being regulated by a homeostatic-like system comes from the examples of genetic obesity seen in rodents. Apart from the *ob/ob*, *db/db* and *fa/fa* mutants, there are several other single-gene obese mutants (Table 3.2) available for study, and there have been some very exciting and rapid advances made in our understanding of energy balance regulation following identification of these genes and their gene products. These will be mentioned again in this and other chapters, but the important point to note here is that if a mutation in a single gene can have such a profound effect upon energy balance, such that a mouse bearing the mutation (e.g., *ob/ob*) can be four times heavier than its normal, wild-type sibling, it is very obvious that there are some very powerful mechanisms controlling energy balance that depend on that gene. Even though we now know the genes responsible for most of these rodent obesities, we are only just beginning to unravel the physiological mechanisms they control. Moreover, we have to bear in mind that, with probably only a few exceptions, human obesity does not present with the same phenotypic expression as these simple single-gene defects. Thus, even though many individuals may have a genetic predisposition to excessive weight gain, obesity is not inevitable and, conversely, those without a genetic predisposition can still become obese. Likewise the normal, wild-type rat and mouse is quite capable of becoming obese, and in the sections discussing mechanisms that follow it is important to bear in mind that it is just as important to understand how obesity is *acquired*, as it is to understand how it is *inherited* as a result of a single-gene mutation. In this respect, emphasis will be given to mechanisms that operate to maintain leanness and resist obesity, since it is here that the pathophysiological defects that give rise to obesity are most likely to arise.

Is energy balance regulated by the control of intake?

It would seem almost heretical, if not simply naive, to suggest that energy balance regulation could be achieved without controlling food intake. However, there are a disturbing number of studies which suggest that intake control can be dissociated from energy balance regulation. In spite of this, many researchers have, and continue to assume that intake is being controlled simply because body-weight remains constant following some kind of experimental intervention. In other words, the dogma that body-weight regulation depends entirely upon control of intake is so ingrained that some workers simply rely on tracking body-weight as a proxy measure of energy intake.

Along with the need to drink, reproduce and avoid pain, the drive to eat is one of the most powerful influences on behaviour, and so it is quite surprising to find that researchers have resorted to quite drastic experimental procedures, such as most of those listed in Table 3.1, to produce hyperphagia and obesity. As noted in the previous section, the need to use such extreme techniques has been used as evidence for the robust, accurate control of food intake, but two points have to be emphasized about such studies in laboratory rodents. Firstly, most of these animals are used when they are still growing, and the dominant physiological drive is to attain a sufficient intake of nutrients to ensure adequate growth. Secondly, standard laboratory diets for rodents are consistently dull and unpalatable, which means that having met their nutritional requirements, the animals are unlikely to overeat. Even then, the very low fat content of these diets imposes a physical limit on the amount (bulk) of food that can be ingested. This explains why it is actually very easy to induce large increases in voluntary food intake simply by offering the animals a cafeteria diet consisting of a varied choice of highly palatable food items, many of them with a high fat content. This voluntary hyperphagia also shows that intake is not so robust as first thought, and in this respect the laboratory rodents are no different from humans where the physiological controls on energy intake often fail to compete with the psychosocial influences that drive people to eat more than they require. Smaller increases in voluntary energy intake can be achieved by feeding rodents high-fat or high-sucrose diets, but whether these, or cafeteria diets, result in obesity depends very much upon the age and strain of the animal used. The capacity for dissipating the excess energy via diet-induced thermogenesis (DIT — see next section) is highly variable, and this means that when the capacity for DIT is high, it is possible to find animals that maintain weight and resist obesity, even though they are hyperphagic (Rothwell & Stock, 1979b).

Apart from experimentally induced hyperphagia, there are several other situations where control of intake seems to fail, or becomes uncoupled from the control of energy balance. One such situation is pregnancy, where it is possible for an animal to meet the entire cost of pregnancy without any increase in energy intake (Quek & Trayhurn, 1990). Another example is in rats that reduce voluntary food intake so as to compensate for varying and quite large amounts of the same diet that was fed to them by gastric intubation. The compensation is remarkably precise and results in the same total energy intake as free-feeding controls. Unfortunately, this apparently powerful demonstration of precision in energy intake control cannot be reconciled with the observation that the tube-fed animals became obese (see Fig. 3.1 for an example), with the degree of obesity being related to the amount that was fed by stomach tube (Rothwell & Stock, 1978; Rothwell & Stock, 1979a). Thus, to conclude this section, it is possible to have hyperphagia without increased adiposity (e.g., cafeteria diets), but it is also possible to have increased adiposity without hyperphagia (e.g., pregnancy and tube-feeding). This implies that energy balance can be regulated by some means other than by controlling energy intake and, given the First Law of Thermodynamics, this can only be achieved by controls operating on energy expenditure.

Is energy balance regulated by the control of energy expenditure?

The idea that energy expenditure decreases when food intake is restricted is well accepted, and seen as part of the body's defence against starvation that helps protect its energy reserves and prevent emaciation. However, the idea that expenditure could increase to dissipate or 'waste' energy consumed in excess of requirements has had a turbulent history ever since it was first mooted at the turn of the century. Originally called *luxoskonsumption*, the idea that heat production could be stimulated by hyperphagia (now known as diet-induced thermogenesis; DIT) did not really gain hold until the advent of the cafeteria feeding system in the late 1970s. By performing precise, quantitative measurements of energy balance in cafeteria-fed rats it was possible to show that the large increases in voluntary energy intake could result in equally large increases in heat production, such that the animals failed to gain any more body energy than the controls (Table 3.3). These cafeteria feeding experiments

Table 3.3 Energy balance and DIT in cafeteria-fed rats. Data from Rothwell and Stock (1982).

	Control diet	Cafeteria diet
Intake (kJ)	4990	8640***
Gain (kJ)	790	1180
Expenditure (kJ)	4200	7460***
Net efficiency (%)	34	20***
% Excess intake expended		89

*** P<0.001 vs control.

are better known for first implicating brown adipose tissue (BAT) thermogenesis in body-weight regulation and obesity (Rothwell & Stock, 1979b), but they deserve at least as much recognition for establishing DIT as a major component in the regulation of energy balance.

Following this, and many subsequent studies with the cafeteria diet, it became obvious that most of the anomalous and paradoxical findings in the literature dealing with the control of intake could be resolved if account was taken of DIT. For example, it is possible for VMH-lesioned rats to get fatter with no increase in food intake (Bernardis & Goldman, 1976), and if VMH-lesioned rats are pair-fed to controls they still become obese (Han & Liu, 1966). In other words, it would seem that these animals become obese not because they are eating more, but because they are expending less energy, i.e., VMH lesions decrease or abolish DIT. The opposite appears to happen in rats with LH lesions, since even though these animals exhibit aphagia they still lose weight at a faster rate than food-deprived controls. The reason for this is that the LH-lesioned animals have much higher rates of heat production than non-lesioned animals (Keesey *et al.*, 1984). Another example where changes in DIT explain alterations in energy balance independently of energy intake is the tube-fed rat, where simply tube-feeding exactly the same amount of food in a reduced number of meals compared to the normal *ad-libitum* feeding pattern results in reductions in DIT and, consequently, increased metabolic efficiency (Rothwell & Stock, 1984). However, apart from the resistance to obesity seen in the cafeteria-fed young rat, the most powerful evidence for a role of thermogenesis in the control of energy balance comes from the study of the genetically obese rodent models.

There had been several indirect hints that metabolic heat production was impaired in some of the genetically obese models, particularly in the *ob/ob* mouse which was known to exhibit hypothermia due to impaired metabolic responses to the cold (Trayhurn *et al.*, 1977). However, it was not until this same group (Trayhurn *et al.*, 1982) undertook a full energy balance study using the cafeteria diet that the full extent of this thermogenic defect could be quantified in terms of its impact on energy balance. The key features in this very important paper are as follows, but the energy balance data have also been summarized in Table 3.4.

• Genetically lean mice on the cafeteria diet exhibit large increases in energy intake and heat production (DIT), and do not gain any more body energy or fat than lean mice on the control diet, i.e., hyperphagic cafeteria-fed mice increase DIT and exhibit a marked decrease in energetic efficiency.

• The energy intake of the genetically obese (*ob/ob*) mice on the standard diet is about the same as that of the lean mice on the cafeteria diet, but they deposit much more fat, i.e., they are metabolically more efficient. This means that a far

Table 3.4 Cafeteria feeding in genetically lean and obese (ob/ob) mice. Adapted from Trayhurn et al. (1982).

	Lean		Obese	
	Control	Cafeteria	Control	Cafeteria
Intake (kJ/day)	65	109***	104	154*
Gain (kJ/day)	9	11	31	58***
Expenditure (kJ/day)	56	98***	73	96**
Net efficiency (%)	24	13***	44	50*

* $P<0.05$, ** $P<0.01$, *** $P<0.001$ vs control.

greater proportion of ingested energy is deposited as fat, and much less dissipated as heat.

• When these ob/ob mice are put on a cafeteria diet, they increase their intake even further and, not surprisingly, deposit even more fat. The high rate of fat deposition is exacerbated by a further increase in metabolic efficiency.

Thus, the difference in the response to hyperphagia in the two genotypes is that the lean mouse decreases energetic efficiency, whereas the obese mouse increases its metabolic efficiency: the difference is due to a failure to increase DIT in the obese mutant. This study remains one of the best illustrations of the impact of a thermogenic defect on energy balance regulation. It was a forerunner of many similar studies in other genetically obese mutants showing similarly high energetic efficiencies. Moreover, it now seems that defective or depressed DIT is the primary cause of most animal models of obesity, be they dietary, surgical, chemical or genetic. Thermogenic defects often appear before hyperphagia develops, and the increased metabolic efficiency can still result in obesity even when food intake is restricted to the same level as control animals.

It is regrettable that the number of well-controlled, full energy balance studies to measure DIT in some of the newer models of obesity (e.g., tub and fat) are somewhat limited, but probably this is because (i) they are very difficult and somewhat tedious to undertake, and (ii) most researcher's attention and interest is easily diverted towards understanding the mechanisms responsible for DIT and the defects that lead to obesity. The suggestion that the sympathetic nervous system (SNS) could be involved in DIT actually pre-dates the studies on DIT in cafeteria-fed and with genetically obese rodents (see Stirling & Stock, 1968), but it was not until these later studies were undertaken, over a decade later, that it was realized that the SNS was activating BAT thermogenesis (Rothwell & Stock, 1979b). Since then, there have been innumerable studies demonstrating the role of sympathetic activation of BAT in mediating DIT, and the reduced sympathetic activation of BAT that is seen in most models of obesity. As a result, there is now a very large literature on this aspect of energy metabolism (e.g., see review by Himms-Hagen, 1990), but the important features to note are the following.

• Sympathetic stimulation of BAT thermogenesis involves the activation by noradrenalin of an atypical or β_3-adrenoceptor (β_3AR), which was first pharmacologically identified in BAT (Arch et al., 1984).

• β_3AR activation in BAT results in increased lipolysis and fatty acid oxidation by the mitochondria, which are uncoupled.

• The uncoupling of oxidative phosphorylation in BAT mitochondria is due to an uncoupling protein (UCP) unique to BAT.

• The rich sympathetic innervation, high blood flow and dense population of uncoupled mitochondria explains the phenomenally high capacity of BAT to produce heat.

In spite of the numerous studies that followed the suggestion that BAT was involved in the regulation of energy balance, resistance to the idea persisted for some time. However, any remaining doubts were dispelled by a study involving the production of a transgenic mouse with a genetic ablation of BAT (Lowell et al., 1993). The genetic ablation of BAT was achieved by linking the gene for diphtheria toxin to the promoter for the gene for UCP, which meant that any cell expressing UCP would also express diphtheria toxin and effectively self-destruct. Since UCP is unique to BAT, this was the only tissue to be disrupted in the transgenic mouse bearing the toxigene. These transgenic mice became obese, and did so without becoming hyperphagic, although hyperphagia did develop at a later stage. Moreover, these 'BAT-less' mice showed all the other features associated with obesity—hyperglycaemia, hyperinsulinaemia and elevated plasma lipids and cholesterol. Thus, this transgenic mutant provides a very powerful demonstration of the importance of BAT in the regulation of metabolism, at least in the mouse. Table 3.5 summarizes the relationship between BAT, the SNS and DIT in lean and genetically obese rodents.

Before concluding this section, it has to be pointed out that the genes for the β_3AR and UCP exist on the human genome and, as this chapter was being prepared, two more genes coding for uncoupling proteins have been identified. Unlike UCP in BAT (now known as UCP1), UCP2 (Fleury et al., 1997) appears to have a ubiquitous tissue distribution, whereas UCP3 (Boss et al., 1997) seems to be confined to skeletal muscle and BAT. Quite how they fit in with DIT, energy balance and obesity remains to be seen, but it is clear that evolution has ensured that more than one biochemical pathway exists for thermogenesis, and suggests that 'wasteful' heat production has an important biological survival value.

Table 3.5 DIT, BAT and the SNS.

---

1 Young over-fed rodents increase metabolic rate and dissipate excess energy intake via DIT; energetic efficiency decreases

2 Genetically obese rats (*fa/fa*) and mice (*ob/ob*) are energetically more efficient than the lean
Obese rodents fail to increase DIT when over-fed; energetic efficiency increases

3 Increased DIT in over-fed animals results from SNS activation of BAT thermogenesis
Feeding fails to increase SNS activation of BAT in obese rats and mice

4 Chemical sympathectomy increases body-weight and fat
Genetical ablation of BAT increases body-weight and fat

How might the controls of energy intake and expenditure be integrated to achieve energy balance?

It is tempting to conclude from the preceding section that most experimental and genetic rodent obesities are due to thermogenic defects in the regulation of energy balance rather than to hyperphagia. However, if the mechanisms for controlling energy intake in these animals are intact, then one would expect to see reductions in food intake to compensate for the positive energy balance and greater fat deposition in these animals. Clearly, this does not happen since food intake is more often than not increased above normal and exacerbates, rather than ameliorates, the development of obesity. Thus, although defects in appetite control may not be the primary or most obvious cause of the obesity in these animal models, the fact that these control mechanisms fail to counteract the effects of defective thermogenesis on energy balance suggests that both sides of the energy balance equation (intake and expenditure) are compromised and contribute to the obesity.

Given that energy intake can influence energy expenditure (e.g., DIT in hyperphagic cafeteria-fed rodents), and that expenditure can affect intake (e.g., stimulation of appetite by exercise or cold exposure), it seems obvious that the two must be tightly coordinated and that, as described above, defects in one are inevitably associated with defects in the other. This implies a common, central control centre, and the most obvious site for such regulation is the hypothalamus. All the early experimental work on hypothalamic mechanisms concentrated on how areas such the VMH, LH and PVN influence food intake, but it was soon realized that these same areas influence thermogenesis. For example, Perkins *et al.* (1981) showed that electrical stimulation of the VMH resulted in increased sympathetic activation of BAT thermogenesis, and likewise Seydoux *et al.* (1981)

showed that the obese VMH-lesioned rat failed to activate BAT thermogenesis. This explains how VMH-lesioned animals can become obese without necessarily becoming hyperphagic. As with food intake, the effects of LH lesions on energy expenditure are opposite to those of VMH lesions, i.e., the weight loss of LH-lesioned animals is due to increased energy expenditure as well as to reduced energy intake (Keesey *et al.*, 1984).

The PVN may be an exception to this tight linkage between intake and expenditure, since the obesity that results from PVN lesions seems to be almost entirely due to hyperphagia (Bray *et al.*, 1989). However, one cannot rule out an influence of the PVN on thermogenesis, since the PVN is probably the predominant site of action of some very important neurotransmitters and neuropeptides that affect the regulation of energy balance via effects on both energy intake and expenditure. For example, corticotrophin-releasing factor (CRF) reduces food intake while increasing thermogenesis (LeFeuvre *et al.*, 1987; Arase *et al.*, 1988), and the increased CRF levels resulting from bilateral adrenalectomy are sufficient to completely eradicate the development of obesity in the *ob/ob* mouse and the *fa/fa* rat (Marchington *et al.*, 1983; Feldkircher *et al.*, 1996). Likewise, NPY is an exceptionally potent stimulus to feeding, but at the same time depresses thermogenesis (Billington *et al.*, 1991). One can see similar reciprocal effects (i.e., decreased intake, increased expenditure) with other neurotransmitter systems, such as serotonin (Rothwell & Stock, 1987), and a synergistic interaction between serotonin and noradrenalin using a neuronal reuptake inhibitor for both monoamines (Stock, 1997).

Thus, it is obvious that both the anatomical structures and the neural and neuroendocrine mechanisms for controlling energy balance via intake and expenditure are essentially the same. Of course, this does not rule out functionally distinct influences on other important aspects of eating behaviour (e.g., nutrient selection, taste preferences, etc.) or energy expenditure (e.g., locomotor activity, thermoregulation, etc.). Moreover, it has to be emphasized that the hypothalamic control mechanisms involved in energy balance have evolved from very basic, primitive systems dedicated to ensuring adequate nutrition for growth and reproduction, and the extent to which they are involved in the fine control of energy balance may be limited. For example, although NPY is one of the most potent stimulators of feeding known, the food intake and body-weight of the NPY-knockout transgenic mouse is perfectly normal (Erikson *et al.*, 1996). This suggests that NPY may not be involved in normal, meal-to-meal or day-to-day control of food intake, but acts as an urgent signal to direct behaviour towards feeding when body energy reserves become severely depleted. In this respect, both angiotensin-II (thirst) and NPY (hunger) could be considered emergency hormones responsible for protecting the body against severe hypovolaemia and emaciation, respectively.

The idea of the hypothalamus integrating and controlling energy intake and expenditure via behavioural, autonomic and neuroendocrine mechanisms fits neatly with other homeostatic controls originating from the hypothalamus and lower brainstem. However, what has not been so obvious is the nature of the sensory input to this system. Unlike other control systems where there are known sensors (e.g., thermoreceptors, baroreceptors, chemoreceptors, etc.), it has never been quite clear what aspect of energy balance is being 'sensed' and how that sensory information is relayed to the hypothalamus. There have been many 'sensors' suggested, but one of the earliest and most enduring theories is the glucostatic theory of Jean Mayer (1953) which proposes that food intake is controlled by the availability of glucose. This in turn will depend upon circulating levels of glucose and insulin, as well as the liver glycogen reserve. There have been innumerable studies investigating and, on the whole, confirming a glucostatic component to feeding behaviour. At various times the theory has been modified to move away from consideration of absolute circulating levels of plasma glucose to take into account rates of cellular glucose utilization and availability, as well as subtle effects in the rate of change in circulating levels (for a recent review, see Campfield & Smith, 1990). There is evidence that peripheral glucoreceptors in the liver (and possibly in the intestine) monitor the influx of glucose following a meal and relay this information via the vagus to the hypothalamus. However, there is also very good evidence for central glucoreceptors, particularly in the VMH. One of the essential requirements of a glucoreceptor that is monitoring the body's utilization of glucose energy is that it should be insulin sensitive. This is implicit in Mayer's original hypothesis, and unlike the rest of the brain, it turns out that the VMH and a few other discrete areas exhibit a weak blood–brain barrier to insulin, and neuronal glucose uptake is insulin dependent—as it is in the peripheral tissues.

The role of insulin in controlling energy intake has taken on a greater significance with the realization that levels in the cerebrospinal fluid (CSF) may play an important role, particularly as CSF levels of insulin tend to provide a more integrated indication of peripheral glucose status than the rapid, transient fluctuations plasma levels seen after every meal (Woods et al., 1996). Given the link between the VMH and the sympathetic activation of BAT thermogenesis, any influences of glucose and insulin on energy intake will obviously have effects on DIT. This would explain why, for example, carbohydrate feeding has greater effects on DIT in experimental animals (Stock & Rothwell, 1982) and why central injections of insulin alone will increase BAT thermogenesis (Müller et al., 1997).

The problem with the glucostatic control of food intake and/or thermogenesis is that because of the limited glycogen stores it can operate only over a relatively short time scale, i.e., responding to meal-to-meal fluctuations in glucose/glycogen availability. Likewise, the afferent vagal and gut-related hormonal signals (e.g., cholecystokinin, enterogastrin, glucagon, glucagon-like peptide (GLP-1), etc.) are transient influences that are difficult to fit into any theory of long-term energy balance regulation. The distinction between short- and long-term regulation explains why Kennedy first proposed the lipostatic theory (Kennedy, 1953) to relate the control of energy balance to the fat reserves, rather than to the glycogen reserves. Unfortunately, in spite of many intriguing suggestions over the intervening 40 years, the nature of the lipostatic signal remained elusive, at least until recently.

The best candidate so far for the lipostatic signal emerged in 1994 when the *Ob* gene was identified (Zhang *et al.*, 1994). This gene was shown to be almost exclusively expressed in adipose tissue, and it has been shown subsequently that circulating levels of the gene product (leptin) reflect the size of the fat stores—in other words it is a circulating hormone that signals to the brain the size of the body's major energy reserve. As pointed out earlier, the importance of this hormone in the regulation of energy balance becomes all to obvious in the *ob/ob* mouse which, because of a mutation resulting in a premature stop codon, fails to produce leptin and becomes massively obese. Injecting these *ob/ob* mice with recombinant leptin, however, restores the signal and they rapidly lose weight (Campfield *et al.*, 1995; Halaas *et al.*, 1995; Pelleymounter *et al.*, 1995). The weight loss is due to a marked decrease in food intake, but there are also increases in body temperature and oxygen consumption and, as one might expect, leptin has now been shown to increase the sympathetic activation of BAT (Collins *et al.*, 1996). Another, very important effect of leptin is to restore fertility in the female *ob/ob* mouse (Chehab *et al.*, 1996), and is consistent with the idea that the ability of females to reproduce (i.e., exhibit oestrus/menstrual cycling) requires adequate energy reserves to support pregnancy (Frisch & McArthur, 1974). In other words, the lack of leptin in the *ob/ob* female mouse is interpreted by the hypothalamus as indicating a complete absence of fat stores. This, and other features of the *ob* gene and leptin are summarized in Table 3.6, and a simplified view of its main actions shown diagrammatically in Fig. 3.2.

The leptin-receptor gene (*Ob-R*) has now been identified (Tartaglia *et al.*, 1995), but there appears to be six spliced-variants (Lee *et al.*, 1996) labelled *Ra* to *Rf* (see Table 3.7), only one of which (*Rb*) appears to be a full-length receptor, complete with an intracellular signalling sequence. The structure has all the characteristics of a cytokine receptor, and is expressed in a variety of tissues, but most importantly in the hypothalamus, particularly in the arcuate nucleus (Mercer *et al.*, 1996). Activation of these receptors results in increased neural activity in areas (e.g., PVN, VMH) known to be involved with the control of food intake and thermogenesis (Woods & Stock, 1996; Elmquist *et al.*, 1997). Mutations in the *Rb* receptor are responsible for the obesity (and infertility) of

Table 3.6 The mouse obese gene (*ob*) and gene product (leptin).

18-kDa (167-amino-acid) gene product; 84% homology with human *ob*

ob/ob mutation = premature stop codon

Expressed in adipose tissue

Expression rapidly decreased/increased by fasting/refeeding

16-kDa secreted protein (leptin) in plasma; absent in *ob/ob*; elevated in *db/db*

Leptin injection in *ob/ob*:
   Decreases weight, fat, intake, blood glucose and insulin
   Increases metabolic rate, body temperature and activity
   Restores fertility in females

Leptin sensitivity: *ob/ob* > > lean; no effect in *db/db* or *fa/fa*

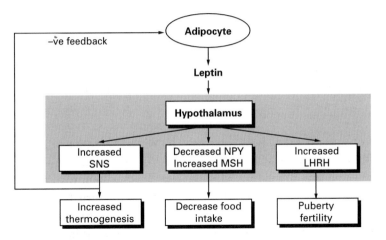

Fig. 3.2 A simplified model of how the leptin system may work. Preliminary evidence suggests that increased SNS activity may act as the negative-feedback signal (via the adipocyte β$_3$AR) to inhibit leptin release. Failure to produce leptin (e.g., *ob/ob* mice) causes hyperphagia, reduced thermogenesis and infertility. Failure of the hypothalamus to detect leptin due to leptin-receptor mutations (e.g., *db/db* mice, *fa/fa* rats) has the same effects, and the lack of the SNS negative feedback on adipocytes results in very high leptin levels.

both the *db/db* mouse and the *fa/fa* rat (Chua *et al.*, 1996; Lee *et al.*, 1996), and explains why they have high circulating levels of leptin, and why they fail to respond to injection of recombinant leptin (Campfield *et al.*, 1995; Halaas *et al.*, 1995; Chua *et al.*, 1996).

    Given a mutated, non-functional leptin receptor, the leptin resistance of the *db/db* mouse and *fa/fa* rat is understandable, but this cannot explain why

Table 3.7 Splice variants of the leptin receptor.

Variant	Function	Tissues
Ob-Ra	Transporter?	Ubiquitous
Ob-Rb (long form)	Intracellular signalling	Hypothalamus, cortex, thalamus, kidneys, adrenals
Ob-Rc	?	Testis, adipose tissue
Ob-Rd	?	Testis, adipose tissue
Ob-Re	Binding protein?	Blood?
Ob-Rf	?	Liver, spleen

non-genetic models of obesity have high circulating levels of leptin (Frederich *et al.*, 1997). Like most obese humans, who also have high plasma leptin levels, this has been explained as being due to leptin resistance. However, there is also a marked degree of leptin resistance in normal animals in which very high doses of leptin are required to produce responses, and this has prompted the idea that leptin functions mainly to protect the body fat reserves against depletion rather than preventing excessive accumulation of fat (Ahima *et al.*, 1996; Friedman, 1997). This would be consistent with the inhibitory effects of leptin on hypothalamic NPY (Stephens *et al.*, 1995), since low leptin levels following starvation and fat depletion would result in release of NPY and, consequently, inhibition of thermogenesis and increased food intake. As fat stores are refilled, leptin levels will rise, inhibit NPY release, and food intake and DIT return to normal. The delayed ovulation in fasted female mice, and its restoration with an injection of leptin (Ahima *et al.*, 1996) further supports a role for leptin as a hormone that signals when energy reserves are adequate. Thus, unlike most other hormonal controls, it would appear that its physiological role is most obvious when levels are low (e.g., fasting) or absent (e.g., *ob/ob* mouse). In other words, it is a hormone that signals when the fat stores are full, and its main function is to switch off mechanisms that compensate for a negative energy balance when fat stores are replete, rather than switching on responses to the overfilling of fat stores. It seems that leptin levels have to increase a lot to influence energy balance in well-fed animals (and humans), and even then it is possible that it is exerting some hitherto unidentified regulatory response or protective influence.

The above description of how leptin may fit in to the physiological control of energy balance has to be treated with a great deal of caution, particularly as the literature on leptin and its receptors is expanding exponentially, and by the time this book is published it is likely that the picture could have changed dramatically. Already, for example, there is evidence to suggest that melanocyte-stimulating hormone (MSH), acting via the hypothalamic melanocortin-4 (MC-4) receptor (see Table 3.2), might be almost as important as leptin in controlling energy balance (Fan et al., 1997; Huszar et al., 1997). However, it is worth emphasizing that leptin probably represents one of the most important advances in the past 50 years in our understanding of the control of energy metabolism, and that it, together with the short-term controls exerted by glucose, insulin and other gut-related signals, provides a firm foundation on which we can refine our understanding of the basic, physiological controls operating on energy intake and expenditure.

To what extent do physiological mechanisms observed in animals help explain human energy balance and obesity?

The question posed in this final section takes us back to the introduction to this chapter where it was claimed that our understanding of the basic, biological controls involved in the regulation of energy balance in humans depends on knowledge gained from animal studies. Any attempt to defend this claim has to recognize the distinction between the strictly physiological influences on energy intake and expenditure and the behavioural influences. There is no doubt that there is a mutual dependence and interaction between the two in both animals and humans, but it is quite obvious that psychosocial influences on feeding patterns and activity levels are far greater in humans, to the extent that they can completely over-ride the physiological controls. However, the opposite could also apply when survival is threatened as, for example, during starvation when powerful physiological mechanisms take over and dominate behaviour.

If the response to starvation in animals is due to low leptin levels disinhibiting the effects of NPY on intake and thermogenesis (see previous section), perhaps this also explains the hunger and the lowering of metabolic rate seen in starving or food-restricted humans. It would certainly explain the marked hyperphagia seen in the two massively obese children recently identified as having undetectable levels of leptin due to a mutation in the ob gene (Montague et al., 1997). Like the ob/ob mouse, it would seem that the lack of leptin in these children is interpreted as an absence of fat stores (i.e., the hypothalamus assumes they are starving) and, also like the ob/ob mouse, it is presumed that injections of recombinant leptin will inhibit food intake, stimulate thermogenesis and restore body-weight to normal. If only for these two children, the knowledge gained from animal studies is of obvious benefit, since not only the diagnosis (ob gene mutation), but also the cure (recombinant leptin) of their condition would not have been possible without research on animals.

Based mainly on the dramatic anti-obesity effects of leptin in ob/ob mice, there has been considerable research and financial interest into manipulating the leptin system to help treat human obesity. However, there are lessons from other animal studies that suggest this effort might bring few returns. For example, if leptin only functions to protect against starvation (see previous section) and has little physiological impact when plasma leptin levels are at, or above normal, then raising levels further with exogenous leptin is unlikely to have any effect. Whether this apparent 'leptin resistance' reflects the physiological limits of leptin's actions or is a pathophysiological manifestation is a moot point, but it does suggest that leptin treatment would be most effective in those that have lost excess fat and whose plasma leptin levels were below normal. In other words, leptin treatment should be quite effective at preventing regain, but ineffective at producing weight loss.

The preceding discussion is probably a good example of how knowledge gained from animal research never quite meets the expectations of the clinical researchers, i.e., most human obesity is not due to a deficiency of leptin, and leptin treatment to induce weight loss does not look very promising. However, the *ob/ob* mouse is not the only, or the most appropriate, model of human obesity, and those that are (e.g., high-fat or cafeteria dietary obese models) have high circulating levels of leptin, just like most obese humans. What is important is that the normal rat or mouse is quite capable of becoming obese, just like most humans, but also like humans, there is a very large genetic influence on the susceptibility to obesity. Furthermore, even in those hyperphagic animals that resist obesity by increasing DIT, prolonged exposure to high-fat or cafeteria diets results in obesity in later life (Connoley *et al.*, 1989), just as it does in very many adult humans eating similar diets. In other words, 'middle-age spread' in animals and humans is as much an age-related failure in physiology as it is a weakening in behavioural control.

The important lesson to be learned from all this is that clinical research has to identify and concentrate on those subtle genetic and/or acquired differences that cause some individuals to get obese easier, or earlier than others. With the non-genetic animal models, it required a lot of effort and ingenuity to identify the mechanisms underlying these differences, and given the difficulties in undertaking similar investigations in humans, it is perhaps not surprising that little progress has been made. Thus, negative findings should not be construed as evidence that mechanisms operating in animals do not exist or are not important in humans. For example, nobody should yet discount the importance of physiological factors influencing food intake (e.g., blood glucose and amino acids, body temperature, insulin, NPY, cholecystokinin, enterogastrin, MSH, opioids, serotonin, etc.), and those determining energetic efficiency (e.g., the role of DIT, BAT, UCP, β_3AR, etc.). The fact that these influences can be over-ridden and swamped by psychosocial influences on feeding behaviour and activity does not negate their influence on susceptibility to weight gain.

This is borne out to some extent by recent findings showing weak associations between human gene polymorphisms for the β_3AR (Clément *et al.*, 1995; Walston *et al.*, 1995; Widén *et al.*, 1995) and UCP genes (Oppert *et al.*, 1994; Fumeron *et al.*, 1996) and susceptibility to early and/or morbid obesity, with far greater risks if patients possess mutations in both genes (Clément *et al.*, 1996). These associations are very weak, but given the relative small contribution that BAT thermogenesis is likely to make to human expenditure, the fact that any association between BAT genes and obesity can emerge from an epidemiological survey is remarkable. This means that clinical researchers must take more notice of what has been discovered in animals, but they should not to expect it to be at all easy to detect the influence of mechanisms that can have very subtle, but very important cumulative effects on energy balance and the propensity to obesity.

References

Ahima, R., Prabakaran, D., Mantzoros, C. *et al.* (1996) Role of leptin in the neuroendocrine response to fasting. *Nature* 382, 250–252.

Arase, K., York., D.A., Shimizu, H., Shargill, N. & Bray, G.A. (1988) Effects of corticotropin releasing factor on food intake and brown adipose tissue thermogenesis in rats. *American Journal of Physiology* 255, E255–E259.

Arch, J.R.S., Ainsworth, A.T., Cawthorne, M.A. *et al.* (1984) Atypical β-adrenoceptor on brown adipocytes as a target for anti-obesity drugs. *Nature* 309, 163–165.

Baile, C.A., Zin, W.M. & Mayer, J. (1970) Effects of lactate and other metabolites on food intake. *American Journal of Physiology* 219, 1026–1034.

Bernardis, L.L. & Goldman, J.K. (1976) Origin of endocrine-metabolic changes in the weanling rat ventromedial syndrome. *Journal of Neuroscience Research* 2, 91–116.

Billington, C.J., Briggs, J.E., Grace, M. & Levine, A.S. (1991) Effects of intracerebroventricular injection of neuropeptide Y on energy metabolism. *American Journal of Physiology* 260, R321–R327.

Boss, O., Samec, S., Paolini-Giacobino, A. *et al.* (1997) Uncoupling protein-3: a new member of the mitochondrial carrier family with tissue-specific expression. *Federation of European Biochemical Societies Letters* 408, 39–42.

Bray, G.A., York, D.A. & Fisler, J. (1989) Experimental obesity: a homeostatic failure due to defective nutrient stimulation of the sympathetic nervous system. *Vitamins and Hormones* 45, 1–125.

Campfield, L.A. & Smith, F.J. (1990) Systemic factors in the control of food intake: evidence for patterns as signals. In: Stricker, E.M. (ed.) *Handbook of Behavioural Biology*, Vol. 10, pp. 183–206. New York: Plenum.

Campfield, L.A., Smith, F.J., Guisez, Y., Devos, R. & Burn, P. (1995) Recombinant mouse *Ob* protein: evidence for a peripheral signal thinking adiposity and central neural networks. *Science* 269, 546–549.

Caterson, I.D., Atkinson, R.L., Bray, G.A. *et al.* (1996) Group Report: What are the animal and human models for the regulation of body weight and what are their respective strengths and limitations. In: Bouchard, C. & Bray, G.A. (eds) *Regulation of Body Weight: Biological and Behavioral Mechanisms*, pp. 85–110. Chichester: Wiley.

Chehab, F.F., Lim, M.E. & Lu, R. (1996) Correction of the sterility defect in homozygous obese female mice by treatment with the human recombinant leptin. *Nature Genetics* 12, 318–320.

Chlouverakis, C. & Hojniki, D. (1974) Lipectomy in obese hyperglycaemic mice (*ob/ob*). *Metabolism* **23**, 133–137.

Chua, S.C., Chung, W.K., Wu-Peng, X.S. *et al.* (1996) Phenotypes of mouse 'diabetes' and rat 'fatty' due to mutations in the OB leptin receptor. *Science* **271**, 994–996.

Clément, K., Vaisse, C., Manning, B.StJ. *et al.* (1995) Genetic variation in the β_3-adrenergic receptor and an increased capacity to gain weight in patients with morbid obesity. *New England Journal of Medicine* **333**, 352–354.

Clément, K., Ruiz, J., Cassard-Doucier, A.-M. *et al.* (1996) Additive effect of A→G(−3826) variant of the uncoupling protein gene and the Trp64Arg mutation of the β_3-adrenergic receptor gene on weight gain in morbid obesity. *International Journal of Obesity* **20**, 1062–1066.

Coleman, D.L. (1973) Effects of parabiosis of obese with diabetes and normal mice. *Diabetologia* **9**, 294–298.

Collins, S., Kuhn, C.M., Petro, A.E., Swick, A.G., Chrunyk, B.A. & Surwit, R.S. (1996) Role of leptin in fat regulation. *Nature* **380**, 677.

Connoley, I.P., Rothwell, N.J., Sheen, C.L. & Stock, M.J. (1989) Effects of cafeteria feeding from weaning on body composition, lipofuscin accumulation and longevity in male and female rats. In: Bjorntorp, P. & Rossner, S. (eds) *Obesity in Europe 88*, pp. 127–131. London: Libby.

Corbett, S.W. & Keesey, R.E. (1982) Energy balance of rats with lateral hypothalamic lesions. *American Journal of Physiology* **242**, E273–E279.

Elmquist, J.K., Rexford, S.A., Maratos-Flier, E., Flier, J.S. & Saper, C.B. (1997) Leptin activates neurons in ventrobasal hypothalamus and brainstem. *Endocrinology* **138**, 839–842.

Erickson, J.C., Clegg, K.E. & Palmiter, R.D. (1996) Sensitivity to leptin and susceptibility to seizures of mice lacking neuropeptide-Y. *Nature* **381**, 415–418.

Fan, W., Boston, B.A., Kesterson, R.A. & Cone, R.D. (1997) Role of melanocorticogenic neurons in feeding and the agouti obesity syndrome. *Nature* **385**, 165–168.

Faust, I.M., Johnson, P.R. & Hirsch, J. (1976) Non-compensation of adipose tissue mass in partially lipectomized mice and rats. *American Journal of Physiology* **231**, 538–544.

Feldkircher, K.M., Mistry, A.M. & Romsos, D.R. (1996) Adrenalectomy reverses pre-existing obesity in adult genetically-obese (*ob/ob*) mice. *International Journal of Obesity* **20**, 232–235.

Fleury, C., Neverova, M., Collins, S. *et al.* (1997) Uncoupling protein-2: a novel gene linked to obesity and hyperinsulinemia. *Nature Genetics* **15**, 269–272.

Frederich, R.C., Hamann, A., Anderson, S., Lollman, B., Lowell, B.B. & Flier, J.S. (1997) Leptin levels reflect body lipid content in mice: evidence for diet-induced resistance to leptin action. *Nature Medicine* **12**, 1311–1314.

Friedman, J.M. (1997) The alphabet of weight control. *Nature* **385**, 119–120.

Frisch, R. & McArthur, J.W. (1974) Menstrual cycles: fatness as a determinant of minimum weight for height necessary for their maintenance or onset. *Science* **185**, 949–951.

Fumeron, F., Durack-Brown, I., Betoulle, D. *et al.* (1996) Polymorphisms of uncoupling protein (UCP) and β_3-adrenoceptor genes in obese people submitted to a low-calorie diet. *International Journal of Obesity* **20**, 1051–1054.

Halaas, J.L., Gajiwala, K.S., Maffei, M. *et al.* (1995) Weight-reducing effects of the plasma protein encoded by the obese gene. *Science* **269**, 543–545.

Han, P.W. & Liu, A.C. (1966) Obesity and impaired growth of rats force-fed 4 days after hypothalamic lesions. *American Journal of Physiology* **211**, 229–231.

Hansen, B.C. (1996) Animal models of the aging-associated metabolic syndrome of obesity. In: Bouchard, C. & Bray, G.A. (eds) *Regulation of Body Weight: Biological and Behavioural Mechanisms*, pp. 48–60. Chichester: Wiley.

Himms-Hagen, J. (1990) Brown adipose tissue thermogenesis: role in thermoregulation, energy regulation and obesity. In: Schönbaum, E. & Lomax, P. (eds) *Thermoregulation: Physiology and Biochemistry*, pp. 327–414. New York: Pergamon.

Hirsch, J. & Han, P.W. (1969) Cellularity of rat adipose tissue, effects of growth, starvation and obesity. *Journal of Lipid Research* **10**, 77–82.

Huszar, D., Lynch, C.A., Fairchild Huntress, V. *et al.* (1997) Targeted disruption of the melanocortin-4 receptor results in obesity in mice. *Cell* **88**, 131–141.

Keesey, R.E. & Powley, T.L. (1986) The regulation of body weight. *Annual Reviews of Psychology* 37, 109–133.

Keesey, R.E., Corbett, S.W., Hirvonen, M.D. & Kaufman, L.N. (1984) Heat production and body weight changes following lateral hypothalamic lesions. *Physiology and Behavior* 32, 309–317.

Kennedy, G.C. (1953) The role of depot fat in the hypothalamic control of food intake in the rat. *Proceedings of the Royal Society*, B 140, 578–592.

Kral, J.G. (1976) Surgical removal of adipose tissue in the male Sprague-Dawley rat. *American Journal of Physiology* 231, 1090–1096.

Lee, G.H., Proenca, R., Montez, J.M. *et al.* (1996) Abnormal splicing of the leptin receptor in diabetic mice. *Nature* 379, 632–638.

LeFeuvre, R.A., Rothwell, N.J. & Stock, M.J. (1987) Activation of brown fat thermogenesis in response to central injection of CRF in the rat. *Neuropharmacology* 26, 1217–1221.

Liebelt, R.A., Ichinoe, S. & Nicholson, N. (1965) Regulatory influences of adipose tissue on food intake and body weight. *Annals of the New York Academy of Science* 131, 559–582.

Lowell, B.B., Susulic, V.S., Hamann, A. *et al.* (1993) Development of obesity in transgenic mice after genetic ablation of brown adipose tissue. *Nature* 366, 740–721.

Marchington, D., Rothwell, N.J., Stock, M.J. & York, D.A. (1983) Energy balance, diet-induced thermogenesis and brown adipose tissue in lean and obese (fa/fa) Zucker rats after adrenalectomy. *Journal of Nutrition* 113, 1395–1402.

Mayer, J. (1953) Glucostatic mechanism of regulation of food intake. *New England Journal of Medicine* 249, 13–16.

Mercer, J.G., Hoggard, N., Williams, L.M., Lawrence, C.B., Hannah, L.T. & Trayhurn, P. (1996) Localization of leptin receptor nRNA and the long form splice variant (Ob-Rb) in mouse hypothalamus and adjacent brain regions by *in-situ* hybridization. *Federation of European Biochemical Societies Letters* 387, 113–116.

Montague, C.T., Farooqi, I.S., Whitehead, J.P. *et al.* (1997) Congenital leptin deficiency is associated with severe early-onset obesity in humans. *Nature* 387, 903–908.

Mrosovsky, N. & Powley, T.L. (1977) Set-points for body weight and fat. *Behavioural Biology* 20, 205–223.

Müller, C., Voirol, M.J., Stefanoni, N. *et al.* (1997) Effect of chronic intracerebroventricular infusion of insulin on brown adipose tissue activity in fed and fasted rats. *International Journal of Obesity* 21, 562–566.

Oppert, J.-M., Vohl, M.-C., Chagnon, M. *et al.* (1994) DNA polymorphism in the uncoupling protein (UCP) gene and human body fat. *International Journal of Obesity* 18, 526–531.

Pellymounter, M.A., Cullen, M.J., Baker, M.B. *et al.* (1995) Effects of the obese gene product on body weight regulation in *ob/ob* mice. *Science* 269, 540–542.

Perkins, M.N., Rothwell, N.J., Stock, M.J. & Stone, T.W. (1981) Activation of brown adipose tissue thermogenesis by the ventromedial hypothalamus. *Nature* 289, 401–402.

Quek, V.S. & Trayhurn, P. (1990) Calorimetric studies on the energetics of pregnancy in golden hamsters. *American Journal of Physiology* 259, R807–R812.

Rothwell, N.J. & Stock, M.J. (1978) A paradox in the control of energy intake in the rat. *Nature* 273, 146–147.

Rothwell, N.J. & Stock, M.J. (1979a) Regulation of energy balance in two models of reversible obesity in the rat. *Journal of Comparative Physiology and Psychology* 93, 1024–1034.

Rothwell, N.J. & Stock, M.J. (1979b) A role for brown adipose tissue in diet-induced thermogenesis. *Nature* 281, 31–35.

Rothwell, N.J. & Stock, M.J. (1982) Effects of feeding a palatable 'cafeteria' diet on energy balance in young and adult lean (+/?) Zucker rats. *British Journal of Nutrition* 47, 461–471.

Rothwell, N.J. & Stock, M.J. (1984) Energy balance, thermogenesis and brown adipose tissue activity in tube-fed rats. *Journal of Nutrition* 114, 1965–1970.

Rothwell, N.J. & Stock, M.J. (1987) Effect of diet and fenfluramine on thermogenesis in the rat: possible involvement of serotonergic mechanisms. *International Journal of Obesity* 11, 319–324.

Seydoux, J., Rohner-Jeanrenaud, F., Assimacopoulos-Jeannet, F., Jeanrenaud, B. & Girardier, L. (1981) Functional disconnection of brown adipose tissue in hypothalamic obesity in rats. *Pflügers Archive* **390**, 1–4.

Stanley, B.G., Kyrkouli, S.E., Lampert, S. & Liebowitz, S.F. (1986) Neuropeptide-Y chronically injected into the hypothalamus: a powerful neurochemical inducer of hyperphagia and obesity. *Peptides* **7**, 1189–1192.

Steinbaum, E.A. & Miller, N.E. (1965) Obesity from eating elicited by daily stimulation of the hypothalamus. *American Journal of Physiology* **208**, 1–5.

Stephens, T.W., Basinski, M., Bristow, P.K. *et al.* (1995) The role of neuropeptide-Y in the anti-obesity action of the obese gene product. *Nature* **377**, 530–532.

Stirling, J.J. & Stock, M.J. (1968) Metabolic origins of thermogenesis induced by diet. *Nature* **220**, 801–802.

Stock, M.J. (1996) Models of nutrient partitioning. In: Bouchard, C. & Bray, G.A. (eds) *Regulation of Body Weight: Biological and Behavioural Mechanisms*, pp. 33–43. Chichester: Wiley.

Stock, M.J. (1997) Sibutramine: a review of the pharmacology of a novel anti-obesity agent. *International Journal of Obesity* **21** (suppl. 1), S25–S29.

Stock, M.J. & Rothwell, N.J. (1982) Obesity thermogenesis and carbohydrate metabolism. In: Birch, G.G. & Parker, K.J. (eds) *Nutritive Sweeteners*, pp. 23–246, London: Applied Science Publishers.

Tartaglia, L.A., Dembski, M., Weng, X. *et al.* (1995) Identification and expression cloning of a leptin receptor OB-R. *Cell* **83**, 1263–1271.

Taylor, A.W., Garrod, J., McNally, M.E. & Seard, D.C. (1973) Regeneration of epididymal fat pad cell size after exercise training and three different feeding patterns. *Growth* **37**, 345–354.

Trayhurn, P., Thurlby, P.L. & James, W.P. (1977) Thermogenic defect in pre-obese *ob/ob* mice. *Nature* **266**, 60–62.

Trayhurn, P., Jones, P.M., McGuckin, M.M. & Goodbody, A.E. (1982) Effect of overfeeding on energy balance and brown fat thermogenesis in obese (*ob/ob*) mice. *Nature* **295**, 323–325.

Walston, J., Silver, K., Bogardus, C. *et al.* (1995) Time of onset of non-insulin diabetes mellitus and genetic variation in the β_3-adrenoceptor gene. *New England Journal of Medicine* **333**, 343–347.

Widén, E., Lehto, M., Kanninen, T., Walston, J., Shuldiner, A.R. & Groop, L.C. (1995) Association of polymorphism in the β_3-adrenergic-receptor gene with features of the insulin-resistance syndrome in Finns. *New England Journal of Medicine* **333**, 349–351.

Woods, A.J. & Stock, M.J. (1996) Leptin activation in the hypothalamus. *Nature* **381**, 745.

Woods, S.C., Chavez, M., Riedy, C. *et al.* (1996) The evaluation of insulin as a metabolic signal influencing behavior via the brain. *Neuroscience and Biobehavioral Review* **20**, 139–144.

York, D.A. & Bray, G.A. (1996) Animal models of hyperphagia. In: Bouchard, C. & Bray, G.A. (eds) *Regulation of Body Weight: Biological and Behavioural Mechanisms*, pp. 15–31. Chichester: Wiley.

Zhang, Y., Proenca, R., Maffei, M., Barone, M., Leopold, L. & Friedman, J.M. (1994) Positional cloning of the mouse obese gene and its human homologue. *Nature* **372**, 425–431.

CHAPTER 4

Molecular Genetics of Obesity

GRAHAM A. HITMAN

Introduction

Obesity is a multifactorial disease with both genetic and environmental components. This chapter will deal solely with the genetic component and the progress in elucidating genes involved in its aetiology. At the time of writing this review, no major gene has been identified in obesity, nor has a mutation of a gene been identified which invariably leads to obesity, apart from those concerned with monogenic syndromes. A number of susceptibility gene variants have been identified which by themselves are not sufficient to lead to obesity but modulate the phenotypic expression of the disease. It seems likely that obesity will prove to be a complex disease in which several genes predispose an individual to obesity but the disease only manifests after prolonged exposure to critical environmental factors. Evidence for a genetic component to obesity is multiple and includes twin studies, adoptee studies, familial aggregation, complex segregation analysis, monogenic syndromes and gene variants which affect the obese phenotypes.

The genetic component to obesity

Amongst Danish adoptees a significant correlation exists between their weight and that of their biological but not their adoptive parents or siblings (Stunkard *et al.*, 1986; Sorenson *et al.*, 1989). Stunkard went on to study the body mass index (BMI) of identical and fraternal twins reared apart and together. The intrapair correlation coefficients of identical twins reared apart were similar to those for twins reared together (Stunkard, 1991). In other words, sharing the same childhood environment did not contribute to the similarity of the BMI of twins later on in life. They concluded that genetic influences on BMI may account for as much as 70% of variance. In a study of 12 identical twins who were deliberately over-fed, a strong intrapair correlation for increases in the amount of intra-abdominal visceral fat was found, with six times more variation between pairs than within pairs (Bouchard *et al.*, 1990). Complex segregation analysis is used to study families in which obesity is apparently segregating and test the null hypothesis that familial aggregation of obesity is due to shared environment. In obesity, the majority of studies point to a major gene effect, disease predisposition accounted for by a combination of a major gene (35–46% of total variance), polygenic loci (9–42%), and environmental factors (25–48%) (reviewed by Beales et al., 1996). It has been suggested that the major gene may define those patients with extreme obesity, whereas the polygenic effect may relate to the range from thin to fat. However, until the specific genes are identified and fitted in these models, complex segregation analysis cannot be used as hard data to infer the genetic component of obesity. Indeed, in some reports, the 'major gene' effect is reported to be non-mendelian.

Monogenic disease expressing the obese phenotype

One approach to identifying genes in obesity is to identify gene variants leading to obesity in families in which obesity is being inherited in a clear autosomal fashion. Examples of such syndromes are listed in Table 4.1. The study of Bardet–Biedl syndrome (BBS) has important lessons that point to the complexity of

Table 4.1 Genetic syndromes associated with obesity.

Syndrome	OMIN no.*
Prader–Willi	176270
Bardet–Biedl	209900, 600151, 600374
Laurence–Moon	245800
Biemond syndrome II	210350
Alstrom	203800
Schinzel	181450
Stein–Leventhal	184700
Carbohydrate-deficient glycoprotein syndrome Type 1	212065
Cohen	216550
Short stature obesity	269870
Albright hereditary osteodystrophy	300800
Borjeson	301900
Germinal cell aplasia Sertoli-cell-only syndrome	305700
Mental retardation, X-linked, syndromic-6, with gynaecomastia and obesity	309585
Simpson dysmorphia	312870

* The OMIN number refers to the index number in the Online Mendelian Inheritance in Man created by Victor McKusick and accessible via the worldwide web.

studying genes in obesity. BBS is an autosomal recessive characterized by obesity, mental retardation, renal dysplasia, retinitis pigmentosa, polydactyly, syndactyly and hypogonadism. Firstly, whilst homozygotes express the full syndrome, among the fathers (by definition heterozygotes for the BBS gene) of children with BBS just over a quarter are obese (Croft et al., 1995). Therefore, if heterozygotes are present in 1% of the general population then 2.9% of all severely overweight males may carry the BBS gene as a cause for their obesity. Several groups have performed genome searches on single large pedigrees or collections of smaller pedigrees and have now identified at least four genes in BBS leading to a similar clinical phenotype. The first pedigree to be studied was a larger inbred Bedouin family and a locus mapped to 16q21 was identified (BBS2) (Kwiteck-Black et al., 1993). Other linked loci exist on the long arm of chromosome 11 (BBS1), on chromosome 3 (BBS3) and chromosome 15 (BBS4) (Leppert et al., 1994; Sheffield et al., 1994; Beales et al., 1997). Additionally, some BBS pedigrees are not linked to any of the four above chromosomal regions, hence there must be at least one other locus yet to be identified. Therefore, what appeared to be a simple autosomal recessive disease is due to mutations in at least five different genes. At least two groups have compared clinical features of BBS according to BBS locus; there is some suggestion that onset of obesity, height and the limb distribution of the polydactyly varied between families depending on the different BBS loci (Carmi et al., 1995; Beales et al., 1997). As gene variants are identified that lead to obesity in monogenic syndromes they can then be studied in obesity itself, although it seems unlikely that they will account for the majority of obese subjects. Indeed, one group has excluded linkage of the same loci associated with BBS, Prader–Willi, Cohen, Borjeson and Wilson–Turner syndromes in 44 families (Reed et al., 1995). However, this latter study could only rule out a major effect of these loci and did not have the power to exclude smaller contributions. A parallel example from the diabetes field is the study of maturity-onset diabetes of the young (MODY). MODY is an autosomal dominant disease in which there is early-onset non-insulin-dependent type 2 diabetes (NIDDM) and a defect of insulin secretion. This can also be accounted for by several variants of genes involved in insulin secretion; glucokinase, hepatic nuclear factor 1α, hepatic nuclear factor 4α and at least one other unknown locus (Hattersley, 1992; Froguel et al., 1992; Yamagata et al., 1996a, b). Although one-third of the families with MODY type diabetes are due to mutations of the glucokinase gene, these same mutations only account for less than 1–2% of NIDDM.

Candidate genes and obesity

A number of candidate genes have been studied for either association or linkage with obesity; some of these are listed in Table 4.2. It should be pointed out,

Table 4.2 Candidate genes and obesity: peer reviewed publications.

Locus	Association (A) or linkage (L)	Phenotype studied	Independent verification
β_3-adrenergic receptor	A	Insulin resistance, visceral fat, weight gain	Yes*
Lipoprotein lipase	A	Hypertriglyceridaemia in obesity	No
Apolipoprotein D	A	Obesity, hyperinsulinaemia, NIDDM	Yes†
Apolipoprotein B	A	Visceral fat, BMI	Yes
LDL receptor	A	Obesity in hypertensives	No
Dopamine receptor D2	A	Obesity	Yes‡
Insulin gene hvr	A	Hyperinsulinaemia, visceral fat	Yes§
Tumour necrosis factor	L	Obesity	No
Glucocorticoid receptor	A	Hyperinsulinaemia	No
Uncoupling protein 1	A	Weight gain	No
Uncoupling protein 2	L	Resting metabolic rate	No
Acyl carrier protein-1	L	Obesity	No
Cell blood group	L	Body fat	No
Adenosine deaminase gene	L	Obesity	No
Ob gene	L	Extreme obesity	Yes
Insulin receptor substrate-1	A	Insulin resistance in obesity	No

* For insulin resistance only.
† For NIDDM only.
‡ Poor study design in the two publications.
§ Only one study in obesity, two other studies confirm a relationship of the insulin gene hvr and insulin levels.
Insulin gene hvr = insulin gene hypervariable region; LDL receptor = low-density lipoprotein receptor.

however, that the majority of the studies listed in Table 4.2 are of poor study design, thereby increasing the chances of a spurious positive association. Ideally, a candidate gene would be chosen as a rate-limiting step in a biochemical pathway relevant to the pathogenesis of obesity. Candidate genes can be chosen for their possible effect on body fat composition, the anatomical distribution of fat, partitioning of nutrient storage, food intake and composition, and energy expenditure (Warden *et al.*, 1996). Other clues for suitable candidate genes may come from the study of monogenic disease (as previously mentioned), gene mutations in monogenic and polygenic animal models of obesity (see Chapter 3 below) and as a result of an obesity-linked chromosomal region containing a putative candidate gene. The more recently studied candidate genes will now be reviewed, including the genes for *ob*, leptin receptor, β_3-adrenergic receptor, the uncoupling protein and insulin receptor substrate-1 (IRS-1).

The ob *and leptin receptor genes*

As previously described, the aetiology of obesity in the *ob* mouse is due to a mutation of the *ob* gene, and in the *db* mouse and *fat* rat mutations of the leptin receptor (Zhang *et al.*, 1994; Chen *et al.*, 1996; Lee *et al.*, 1996). Understanding these animal models of obesity have provided a valuable insight into the pathophysiology of obesity and, in particular, into adipocyte cell signalling (Fig. 4.1). It is now known that the *ob* gene is expressed in the adipocyte producing the protein product leptin. Expression of the *ob* gene is influenced by a change

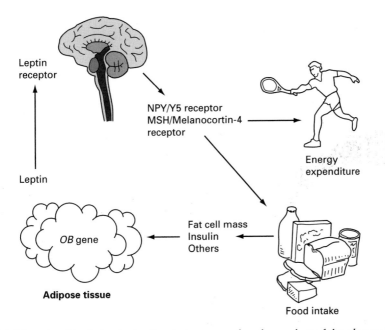

Fig. 4.1 The role of leptin in obesity. Leptin is expressed as the product of the *ob* gene in adipocytes. The diagram illustrates the action of leptin in the hypothalamus and the subsequent post-leptin receptor pathways leading to changes in energy expenditure and appetite.

in fat cell mass, insulin, glucocorticoids and other signals. Leptin then binds to the leptin receptor found in the choroid plexus and hypothalamus. Post-leptin receptor signalling is poorly understood but probably involves two pathways, one signalling the fasting state (neuropeptide Y/Y5 receptor) and the other over-nutrition (melanocyte-stimulating hormone/melanocortin-4 receptor). This then leads to changes in energy expenditure and appetite (Erickson *et al.*, 1996) in the appropriate direction. The *ob* gene and leptin receptor are therefore good candidate genes for obesity.

The regulatory region and the genomic sequence of the human *ob* gene is now known (Gong *et al.*, 1996). In the limited number of sequencing studies, only one mutation of the human *ob* gene has been found which leads to obesity (Considine *et al.*, 1996; Niki *et al.*, 1996; Montague *et al.*, 1997). In two severely obese children from the same highly consanguinous pedigree, a homozygous frameshift mutation involving a deletion of a single guanine nucleotide in codon 133 was found (Montague *et al.*, 1997). These children with an *ob* mutation had very low leptin levels with markedly elevated fat mass. It is possible that if leptin was administered then these children might lose weight. Although no variants leading to an amino acid substitution of the *ob* gene has been described in 'common' obesity, at least two groups have published weak linkage data between extreme obesity and the human *ob* gene (Clement *et al.*, 1996; Reed *et al.*, 1996). This would indicate that either regulatory variants or coding region variants of the *ob* gene may account for a small proportion of obese subjects, although they are yet to be discovered. An alternative explanation is that the linked locus is not the *ob* gene but another gene which may predispose to obesity but in the same chromosomal location as the *ob* gene. Studies on the leptin receptor gene are less advanced but at the time of writing (1997) there are no reports in linkage or association of obesity with the leptin receptor. In human obesity, leptin levels are increased and therefore it seems unlikely that variants of the *ob* gene will play a common part in the aetiology of obesity, whereas it seems more likely when more is known of the post-leptin receptor pathways that other candidate genes will come to light.

β_3-adrenergic receptor

The β_3-adrenergic receptor is the principal receptor mediating catecholamine-induced thermogenesis in brown adipose tissues (BAT) (Arner, 1995). BAT has a predominantly visceral distribution which is the fat site most strongly correlated with the insulin resistance syndrome. The β_3-adrenergic receptor is also expressed in white adipose tissue where it is involved in lipolysis and thereby may be a factor controlling fat cell size and leptin secretion. The β_3-adrenergic receptor therefore makes an attractive candidate gene for obesity.

A variant of the β_3-adrenergic receptor Trp64Arg has recently been described which has been associated with various factors of the insulin resistance syndrome (Clement *et al.*, 1995; Kadowaki *et al.*, 1995; Walston *et al.*, 1995; Widen *et al.*, 1995; Fujisawa *et al.*, 1996). Several investigators have investigated this variant, and although in one Japanese study there was an association with obesity, this was not substantiated by the other investigators. Associations of the β_3-adrenergic receptor Trp64Arg were found between the variant and an increased capacity to weight gain in morbidly obese subjects, insulin resistance and an early age of onset of NIDDM. Therefore, this variant by itself does not lead to obesity but rather modifies the phenotypic expression of those predisposed to obesity or NIDDM. It is not known whether the Trp64Arg variant has any functional consequence as would be expected if it was an aetiological mutation. At present, there is only one study expressing the mutant receptor and it was found to be pharmacologically and functionally indistinguishable from the wild-type receptor (Candelore *et al.*, 1996). Since this mutant receptor was only expressed in CHO cells, it can only be concluded that in this heterologous system there is no effect and other cell systems should be used before a direct effect of this β_3-adrenergic variant is ruled out.

Uncoupling protein genes

The uncoupling proteins (UCPs) are inner mitochondrial membrane transporters which dissipate the proton gradient, releasing stored energy as heat. Several UCPs have now been identified including UCP1 (expressed in brown fat), UCP2 (widely expressed) and UCP3 (mainly expressed in skeletal muscle). Variants of the UCP genes may be involved in the aetiology of obesity via an effect on thermogenesis.

Uncoupling protein 1. That variants of this locus lead to obesity is supported by transgenic experiments in which overexpressing UCP in genetically obese rats leads to reduction in total body-weight and subcutaneous fat (Kopecky *et al.*, 1995). A Bcl I restriction fragment length polymorphism (RFLP) located in the 5′-flanking region of the UCP1 gene has been found to be associated with increased accumulation of percentage body fat in a 12-year prospective study in 64 families from Québec (Opert *et al.*, 1994; Cassard-Doulcier *et al.*, 1996). No association was reported between the Bcl I RFLP and obesity or any other variable studied. If this study was replicated, it would point to another gene that modifies the phenotypic expression of obesity. The aetiological mutation would still need to be identified and its consequences examined by expression studies. It would be tempting to speculate that it might be found in the regulatory region since there are several important transcriptional regulation factors which bind to this region, including the peroxisome proliferator-activated receptor gamma (Sears *et al.*, 1996).

Uncoupling protein 2. UCP2 has 59% identity to UCP1 (Fleury *et al.*, 1997). UCP2 is widely expressed in humans, including tissues rich in macrophages, and it is upregulated in response to fat feeding (Fleury *et al.*, 1997). A recent linkage study in humans has found linkage between markers close to UCP2 and resting metabolic rate (Bouchard *et al.*, 1997). Within the next year, it is expected that variants of UCP2 will be described.

Uncoupling protein 3. UCP3 is preferentially expressed in skeletal muscle (Boss *et al.*, 1997; Vidal-Puig *et al.*, 1997) and has 71% homology with UCP2 and 57% homology with UCP1. At the time of writing this review, no further information is available for UCP3.

Insulin receptor substrate-1 gene

Obesity rarely occurs by itself but more commonly with other features of insulin resistance, including NIDDM, dyslipidaemia, hypertension and ischaemic heart disease. Gene variants associated with insulin resistance may therefore predispose to obesity or alter its phenotypic expression. An example of the complex inter-relationship of these disorders is afforded by recent studies of the IRS-1 gene. IRS-1 plays a central role in the generation of the insulin signal (Fig. 4.2) (Sun *et al.*, 1991). IRS-1 is a major substrate of the insulin receptor tyrosine kinase. Although it exhibits no intrinsic enzyme activity, it acts as a multisite docking protein for binding of other signal transduction molecules.

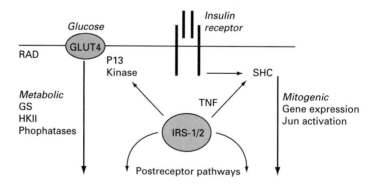

Fig. 4.2 IRS-1 and its role in insulin signalling. Insulin binds to the insulin receptor which leads to autophosphorylation of the β subunit. This in turn leads to phosphorylation of at least multisite docking proteins (IRS-1 and IRS-2) and the generation of the 'insulin signal'. RAD, ras-like protein associated with diabetes; GS, glycogen synthase; HKII, hexokinase II; TNF, tumour necrosis factor; SHC, Src-homology/collagen proteins.

Seven gene variants have been described of the IRS-1 of which the most common is at codon 972 (glycine to arginine substitution) (Almind *et al.*, 1993; Laakso *et al.*, 1994). Several, but not all, studies have found an increased frequency of the Gly972Arg variant in NIDDM (Imai *et al.*, 1994; Hitman *et al.*, 1995). However, this IRS-1 variant is also present in a high frequency in non-diabetic subjects. It was subsequently reported that in non-obese subjects there was no decreased insulin sensitivity, whether or not the variant was present. In contrast, whilst there was the expected decrease in insulin sensitivity in the obese non-carriers of the variant, in those who were both obese and had the IRS-1 variant, insulin sensitivity was further and significantly decreased (Clausen *et al.*, 1995). In other words, the Gly972Arg variant by itself does not lead to insulin resistance which is only manifested in the presence of obesity.

Strategies to identify a major gene in obesity

The tools of genetics can be used to isolate novel genes and to test the physiological function of these genes. There have been great advances in gene searching techniques in recent years such that the limiting factor for multifactorial disease is now the selection of the appropriate clinical material to maximize the chances of identifying the genetic susceptibility to the disease. With the advent of marker libraries covering the entire human genome, it is now possible to proceed to a random genome-wide search (Beales *et al.*, 1996). However, in order to implement such a stratagem, one must engage suitable clinical materials that might be drawn from:

• very large single pedigrees;
• nuclear families;
• affected pedigree members (e.g., sibling pairs, grandparent–grandchild pairs).

Linkage analysis follows segregation of a disease and DNA markers in affected families (McCarthy *et al.*, 1994). When the marker and the disease are inherited together more often than would be expected by chance alone, they are said to be linked. In general terms, the closer the marker is to the gene, the greater chance there is of their segregating. Classical linkage analysis utilizes pedigrees to calculate log of the odds (LOD) scores for linkage likelihood. The main limitations of this method are that the model of inheritance must be specified and that family collection is time consuming and costly. However, for large pedigrees characterized by a genetic syndrome in which obesity is part of the phenotype this may be the method of choice as illustrated by BBS. An alternative method of analysis for obesity is that of the affected pedigree member (sib-pair) linkage analysis. Two subtypes have been described: identity by state (IBS) and identity by descent (IBD). To perform sib-pair analysis one requires an unambiguous determination of the sib-IBD relations at the marker locus.

Such information is usually available only if parents are available for this study. In diseases such as NIDDM, the parents are more often not available and thus IBD relations are unknown. Weeks and Lange have proposed the substitution of IBS relationships as a method of circumventing this problem and thus allowing sib-pair analysis to be performed in cases in which parents are unavailable (Weeks & Lange, 1988). The IBD method, however, is likely to be the most powerful when, as is the case for obesity, both parents are alive and available for blood sampling. In order to calculate the sample size needed for analysis one can use formulae devised by Feingold *et al.* (1993) and Risch (1990). To achieve 90% power using sib pairs, we must make estimates of the risk ratio (γs) for an offspring of an affected individual compared to the general population prevalence. For obesity the relative risk is in the order of 2–4. Given that there may be a major gene contributing 40% of the total variance to the disorder, one can estimate that between 200 and 400 sib pairs and their parents will be required for IBD and approximately twice that number would be required for IBS. In order to maximize the power of the analysis, sib pairs should be sought in which it can be clearly demonstrated that one side of the family exhibits segregation of extreme obesity but the other side of the pedigree does not. Using this strategy, fewer sib pairs would be needed; this has been confirmed by simulation experiments (Price, 1995). Recently, the slightly different approach of discordant sib-pair mapping has been suggested for gene mapping in multifactorial disease with which there is early phenotypic expression of the disease (Risch & Zhang, 1996). In this approach, nuclear pedigrees are collected with pairs of sibs characterized by the extremes of the phenotype under study; thus, for obesity, two sibs characterized by the upper and lower decile for BMI in the population would be collected. The principle underlying this method is that the two discordant sibs will not share the polymorphic marker under study. Using this method, it is likely that fewer pedigrees will be required for a genome search; however, it is counterbalanced by the increased workload in order to identify the clinical material.

Summary

Progress, albeit slow, is being made to identify the genes involved in obesity. Those gene variants currently identified appear to modify the phenotypic expression of obesity. The understanding of the genetic basis of obesity will lead to a better understanding of the pathophysiology of the disorder. These advances in our understanding of obesity should lead to better primary prevention strategies and the design of effective therapeutic agents to combat a condition which affects over 10% of the world's affluent population.

References

Almind, K., Vestergaard, H., Hansen, T., Echwald, S. & Pedersen, O. (1993) Aminoacid polymorphisms of insulin receptor substrate-1 in non-insulin-dependent diabetes mellitus. *Lancet* **342**, 828–832.

Arner, P. (1995) The β_3-adrenergic receptor—a cause and cure of obesity. (1995) *New England Journal of Medicine* **333**, 382–383.

Beales, P., Kopelman, P. Vijayaraghavan, S. & Hitman, G.A. (1996) The molecular genetics of obesity. In: Bray, G. & Ryan, D.H. (eds) *Molecular and Genetic Aspects of Obesity*, Vol. V, pp. 534–545. Pennington Center Nutrition Series, Vol 5. Baton Rouge, LA: Louisiana State Press.

Beales, P.L., Warner, A.M., Hitman, G.A., Thakker, R. & Flinter, F.A. (1997) Bardet–Biedl syndrome: a molecular and phenotypic study of 18 families. *Journal of Medical Genetics* **34**, 92–98.

Boss, O., Samec, S., Paoloni-Giacobino, A. *et al.* (1997) Uncoupling protein-3: a new member of the mitochondrial carrier family with tissue-specific expression. *FEBS Letters* **408**, 39–42.

Bouchard, C., Tremblay, A., Despres, J.P. *et al.* (1990) The response to long-term overfeeding in identical twins. *New England Journal of Medicine* **322**, 1477–1482.

Bouchard, C., Perusse, L., Chagnon, Y.C., Warden, C. & Ricquier, D. (1997) Linkage between markers in the vicinity of the uncoupling protein 2 gene and resting metabolic rate in humans. *Human Molecular Genetics* **6**, 1887–1889.

Candelore, M.R., Deng, L., Tota, IM., Kelly, L.J., Cascieri, M.A. & Strader, C.D. (1996) Pharmacological characterisation of a recently described human beta 3-adrenergic receptor mutant. *Endocrinology* **137**, 2638–2641.

Carmi, R., Elbedour, K., Stone, E.M. & Sheffield, V.C. (1995) Phenotypic differences among patients with Bardet–Biedl syndrome linked to three different chromosome loci. *American Journal of Medical Genetics* **59**, 199–203.

Cassard-Doulcier, A.M. Bouillaud, F., Chagnon, M. *et al.* (1996) The Bcl I polymorphism of the human uncoupling protein (UCP) gene is due to a point mutation in the 5'-flanking region. *International Journal of Obesity* **20**, 278–279.

Chen, H., Charlat, O., Tartaglia, L.A. *et al.* (1996) Evidence that the diabetes gene encodes the leptin receptor: identification of a mutation in the leptin receptor gene in *db/db* mice. *Cell* **84**, 491–495.

Clausen, J.O., Hansen, T., Bjorbaek, C. *et al.* (1995) Insulin resistance: interactions between obesity and a common variant of insulin receptor substrate-1. *Lancet* **346**, 397–402.

Clement, K., Vaisse, C., Manning, B.S. *et al.* (1995) Genetic variation in the beta 3-adrenergic receptor and an increased capacity to gain weight in patients with morbid obesity. *New England Journal of Medicine* **333**, 352–354.

Clement, K., Garner, C., Hager, J. *et al.* (1996) Indication for linkage of the human OB gene region with extreme obesity. *Diabetes* **45**, 687–690.

Considine, R.V., Considine, E.L., Williams, C.J. *et al.* (1996) Mutation screening and identification of a sequence variation in the human OB gene coding region. *Biochemical and Biophysical Research Communications* **220**, 735–739.

Croft, J.B., Morrell, D., Chase, C.L., Swift, M. (1995) Obesity in heterozygous carriers of the gene for the Bardet–Biedl syndrome. *American Journal of Medical Genetics* **55**, 12–15.

Erickson, J.C., Hollopeter, G. & Palmiter, R.D. (1996) Attenuation of the obesity syndrome of *ob/ob* mice by the loss of neuropeptide Y. *Science* **274**, 1704–1707.

Feingold, E., Brown, P.O. & Siegmund, D. (1993) Gaussian models for genetic linkage analysis using complete high resolution maps of identity by descent. *American Journal of Human Genetics* **53**, 234–251.

Fleury, C., Neverova, M., Collins, S. *et al.* (1997) Uncoupling protein-2: a novel gene linked to obesity and hyperinsulinaemia. *Nature Genetics* **15**, 269–272.

Froguel, P.H., Vaxillaire, M., Sun, F. *et al.* (1992) Close linkage of glucokinase locus on chromosome 7p to early-onset non-insulin-dependent diabetes mellitus. *Nature* **356**, 162–165.

Fujisawa, T., Ikegami, H., Yamato, E. *et al.* (1996) Association of Trp64Arg mutation of the beta3-adrenergic-receptor with NIDDM and body weight gain. *Diabetologia* **39**, 349–352.

Gong, D.-W., Bi, S., Pratley, R.E. & Weintraub, B.D. (1996) Genomic structure and promoter analysis of the human obese gene. *Journal of Biological Chemistry* **271**, 3971–3974.

Hattersley, A.T., Turner, R.C., Permutt, M.A. *et al.* (1992) Linkage of type 2 diabetes to the glucokinse gene. *Lancet* **339**, 1307–1310.

Imai, Y., Fusco, A., Suzuki, Y. *et al.* (1994) Variant sequences of insulin receptor substrate-1 in patients with non-insulin-dependent diabetes mellitus. *Journal of Clinical Endocrinology and Metabolism* **79**, 1655–1658.

Kadowaki, H., Yasuda, K., Iwamoto, K. *et al.* (1995) A mutation in the beta 3-adrenergic receptor gene is associated with obesity and hyperinsulinaemia in Japanese subjects. *Biochemical and Biophysical Research Communications* **215**, 555–560.

Kopecky, J., Clarke, G., Enerback, S., Spiegelman, B. & Kozak, L.P. (1995) Expression of the mitochondrial uncoupling protein gene from the aP2 gene promoter prevents genetic obesity. *Journal of Clinical Investigation* **96**, 2914–2923.

Kwitek-Black, A.E., Carmi R., Duyk, G.F. *et al.* (1993) Linkage of Bardet–Biedl Sydrome is linked to DNA chromosome markers on chromosome 11q and is genetically heterogeneous. *Nature Genetics* **5**, 392–396.

Laakso, M., Malkki, M., Kekalainen, P., Kuusisto, J. & Deeb, S.S. (1994) Insulin receptor substrate-1 gene mutations in NIDDM; implications for the study of polygenic disease. *Diabetologia* **38**, 481–486.

Lee, G.-H., Proenca, R., Montez, J.M. *et al.* (1996) Abnormal splicing of the leptin receptor in diabetic mice. *Nature* **379**, 632–635.

Leppert, M., Baird, L., Anderson, K.L., Otterud, B., Lupski, J.R. & Lewis, R.A. (1994) Bardet–Biedl syndrome is linked to DNA markers on chromosome 11q and is genetically heterogeneous. *Nature Genetics* **7**, 108–112.

McCarthy, M., Froguel, P. & Hitman, G. (1994) The genetics of non-insulin-dependent diabetes mellitus: tools and aims. *Diabetologia* **37**, 959–968.

Montague, C.T., Farooqi, I.S., Whitehead, J.P. *et al.* (1997) Congenital leptin deficiency is associated with severe early-onset obesity in humans. *Nature* **387**, 903–908.

Niki, T., Mori, H., Tamori, Y. *et al.* (1996) Human obese gene; molecular screening in Japanese and Asian Indian NIDDM patients associated with obesity. *Diabetes* **45**, 675–678.

Oppert, J.M., Vohl, M.C., Chagnon, M. *et al.* (1994) DNA polymorphism in the uncoupling protein (UCP) gene and human body fat. *International Journal of Obesity and Related Metabolic Disorders* **18**, 526–531.

Price, R.A. (1995) Obesity genes in human populations. In: Bray, G.A. & Ryan, D.H. (eds) *Molecular and Genetic Aspects of Obesity*, pp. 453–461. Pennington Centre Nutrition, Vol. 5. Genes Baton Rouge, LA: Louisiana State Press.

Reed, D.R., Ding, Y, Xu, W., Cather, C. & Price, R.A. (1995) Human obesity does not segregate with the chromosomal regions of Prader–Willi, Bardet–Biedl, Cohen, Borjeson or Wilson–Turner syndromes. *International Journal of Obesity* **19**, 599–603.

Reed, D.R., Ding, Y., Xu, W. *et al.* (1996) Extreme obesity may be linked to markers flanking the human OB gene. *Diabetes* **45**, 691–694.

Risch, N. (1990) Linkage strategies for genetically complex traits II: the power of affected relative pairs. *American Journal of Human Genetics* **46**, 229–241.

Risch, N.J. & Zhang, H. (1996) Mapping quantitative trait loci with extreme discordant sib pairs: sampling conditions. *American Journal of Human Genetics* **58**, 836–843.

Sears, I.B., MacGinnitie, M.A., Kovacs, L.G. & Graves, R.A. (1996) Differentiation-dependent expression of the brown adipocyte uncoupling protein gene: regulation by peroxisome proliferator-activated receptor gamma. *Molecular and Cellular Biology* **16**, 3410–3419.

Sheffield, V.C., Carmit, C., KwitekBlack, A. *et al.* (1994) Identification of a Bardet–Biedl syndrome locus on chromosome 3 and evaluation of an efficient approach to homozygosity mapping. *Human Molecular Genetics* **3**, 1331–1335.

Sorensen, T.I., Price, R.A., Stunkard, A.J. & Schulsinger, F. (1989) Genetics of obesity in adult adoptees and their biological siblings. *British Medical Journal* **298**, 87–90.

Stunkard, A.J. (1991) Genetic contributions to human obesity. *Association for Research in Nervous and Mental Disease* **69**, 205–218.

Stunkard, A.J., Sorensen, T.I., Hanis, C. *et al.* (1986) An adoption study of human obesity. *New England Journal of Medicine* **314**, 193–198.

Sun, X.J., Rothenberg, P., Kahn, C.R. *et al.* (1991) Structure of the insulin receptor substrate IRS-1 defines a unique signal transduction protein. *Nature* **352**, 73–77.

Vidal-Puig, A., Solanes, G., Grujic, D., Flier, J.S. & Lowell, B.B. (1997) UCP3: an uncoupling protein homologue expressed preferentially and abundantly in skeletal muscle and brown adipose tissue. *Biochemical and Biophysical Research Communications* **235**, 79–82.

Walston, J., Siwer, K., Bogardus, C. *et al.* (1995) Time of onset of non-insulin-dependent diabetes mellitus and genetic variation in the β_3-adrenergic-receptor gene. *New England Journal of Medicine*, **333**, 343–347.

Warden, C.H., Bouchard, J.M., Friedman, J.M. *et al.* (1996) Group report: How can the best apply the tools of genetics to study body weight regulation. In: Bouchard, C. & Bray, G.A. (eds) *Regulation of Body Weight: Biological and Behavioural Mechanisms*, pp. 285–305. Chichester: Wiley.

Weeks, D.E. & Lange, K. (1988) The affected-pedigree-member method of linkage analysis. *American Journal of Human Genetics* **42**, 315–326.

Widen, E., Lehto, M., Kanninen, T., Walston, J., Shuldiner, A.R. & Groop, L.C. (1995) Association of a polymorphism in the beta 3-adrenergic-receptor gene with features of the insulin resistance syndrome in Finns. *New England Journal of Medicine* **333**, 348–351.

Yamagata, K., Oda, N., Kasaki, P. *et al.* (1996a) Mutations in the hepatic nuclear factor-1α gene in maturity-onset diabetes of the young (MODY3). *Nature* **384**, 455–458.

Yamagata, K., Furuta, H., Oda, N. *et al.* (1996b). Mutations in the hepatocyte nuclear factor-4α gene in maturity-onset diabetes of the young (MODY1). *Nature* **384**, 458–460.

Zhang, Y., Proenca, R., Maffei, M., Barone, M., Leopold, L. & Friedman, J.M. (1994). Positional cloning of the mouse obese gene and its human homologue. *Nature* **372**, 425–432.

CHAPTER 5

Food Intake and Eating Behaviour in Humans

ANDREW J. HILL AND PETER J. ROGERS

Introduction

Among the variety of causal explanations proposed for obesity, overeating has been one of the most obvious and yet has waxed and waned in scientific popularity. Research progress in the general areas of metabolism and appetite has tended to create a cycle of polarization in which one side is favoured and then the other. Recent methodological developments, particularly in the measurement of energy expenditure, have led to the resurrection of hyperphagia as an important mechanism in obesity. Thus, Prentice *et al.* (1989) have suggested that the 'primary defect' may be in the control of food intake and that observed changes in energy metabolism could then be secondary to alterations in body-weight. But why has it taken so long for eating behaviour to be rehabilitated in the field of obesity?

One reason is the domination of biological perspectives. These approaches carry an assumption that appetite is controlled by a homeostatic system that serves to maintain energy balance. Accordingly, attempts to identify the physiological mechanisms underlying energy homeostasis have tended to dominate research in the area, and experimental models of obesity have been studied mainly for their potential to provide insight into these mechanisms. However, the contribution of this approach to the understanding of human eating behaviour and obesity is questionable. This is not say that the study of the physiology of appetite is unimportant, but simply that these mechanisms should be integrated into a wider context. This context should include the roles played by learned and cognitive influences guiding eating behaviour, and ecological constraints and opportunities afforded by the social setting, lifestyle habits, economic climate, and culture of the society in which we eat. The resultant systems approach is integrative, providing a broad framework which acknowledges the interplay of events beneath and outside the skin (Blundell, 1984; Blundell & Hill, 1986). A central feature of the systems view is that adjustments in one domain will influence, or be influenced by, the state of components elsewhere in the system. The forces governing appetite control, therefore, are in a constantly dynamic state and encompass biological, psychological and environmental events.

This chapter will provide an overview of the control of human food intake from this perspective. A psychobiological approach to appetite will be described that shows how our biological systems have inbuilt mechanisms that help us to adapt (mostly) to our environment. In addition, self-imposed cognitive control over food intake (and its failure) will be examined. But first, the methodology of research into eating behaviour will be considered. The aim is to reveal the structure of eating behaviour via an examination of past attempts to understand and measure it. These have been varied, often ingenious, used in laboratory and real-life settings, and demonstrate the coordinated complexity of an activity that is performed so frequently that it is often taken for granted.

The measurement of food intake and eating behaviour

Food intake and eating behaviour, while related concepts, are separate parts of food consumption, one reflecting what is eaten, the other the act of eating. This distinction between 'fuel intake' and 'eating behaviour' is both conceptual and technical, and has arisen in part due to the multi-professional interest in food consumption (Blundell, 1996). Those scientists and practitioners primarily interested in fuel intake are concerned with the quantitative aspects of consumption and the energy value of food. Those interested in eating behaviour are additionally concerned with more qualitative features of eating such as food choice and preference, the subjective experiences of hunger and satiety, and the hedonics of eating. Accordingly, each group has developed their own particular research methodologies. The resultant difference in approaches creates its own problem since they are rarely integrated. So for example, what is the relationship between the pattern of meals and snacks, the feelings of hunger and satiety, the tastes and other sensory attributes of the foods consumed, and the total amount of food, and its nutrient content, consumed over a 24-hour period? As Blundell points out, it will be difficult to understand the origins of obesity without reconciling these levels of analysis.

It follows that in providing a summary of the strategies and techniques used in research into food consumption, it is useful to separate those directed at the disposition to eat, from those directed at the act of eating, and from the food that is eaten. What is detailed below is very much an overview, and the reader should consult Hill *et al.* (1995) for a more detailed methodological review.

The disposition to eat

Techniques that evaluate the disposition or willingness to eat fall into three groupings: ratings of hunger, satiety and palatability; food checklists; and measuring salivation. Of these, the self-report ratings of subjective experience have been the most frequently used.

The two most commonly used methods for assessing feelings of hunger, satiety and palatability are fixed-point rating scales and visual analogue scales. As Table 5.1 shows, there are several forms to choose from. Fixed-point scales, in particular, vary in complexity, from scales with a few labelled points (example (a), Durrant & Royston, 1979) to those with more but unlabelled points ((b), Wooley et al., 1977). In considering the appropriate number of scale points, the freedom to make a range of possible responses must be balanced against the precision and reliability of the device. Research seems to indicate that scales with an insufficient number of fixed-points can be insensitive to subtle changes in subjective experience. An additional issue is that both the fixed points and the words used to define the points are important influences on the way people use the scales and distribute their ratings.

One way of overcoming these problems is to abolish the points completely. Thus, visual analogue scales are horizontal lines (often 100 or 150 mm long), unbroken and unmarked except for word anchors at either end that describe extremes of experience (example (c)). The participant is instructed to mark the scale with a vertical line at a point that most accurately reflects the intensity of the feeling at that moment in time. The researcher measures the distance to that mark in millimetres from the negative end (e.g., no hunger), thus yielding a score of 0–100 (or 150). This is done either by hand or automatically if presented by computer screen.

While the capture and quantification of hunger and satiety is relatively straightforward there is still mistrust directed at assessments of subjective

Table 5.1 Examples of different types of scale used in the assessment of hunger. (a) Fixed-point scale with points defined; (b) 7-point scale; (c) Visual analogue scale.

(a) How hungry do you feel?				
0	1	2	3	4
Full	Indifferent	Peckish	Hungry	Starving/ ravenous

(b) How hungry do you feel?						
1	2	3	4	5	6	7
Not at all hungry						Extremely hungry

(c) How hungry do you feel?

Not at all hungry	Extremely hungry

experience. However, a good deal of this is unjustified. Certainly, hunger ratings cannot be used simply as a proxy measure of food intake (Mattes, 1990). But in many research circumstances self-report ratings of hunger, appetite, desire to eat, etc., do correlate highly and significantly with subsequent food intake (e.g., Hill *et al.*, 1987; Blundell & Rogers, 1991). One problem is that in certain circumstances hunger and food intake can be disengaged. So, for example, eating can occur when hunger is low (such as when highly palatable food is offered unexpectedly, e.g., Cornell *et al.*, 1989) and not at other times when hunger is high (when food is unavailable, or other activities have priority). A second problem is that many experimental analyses of the correlational association between hunger and food intake report the relationship only when subjects are hungry. In other words, the association is examined only for a small proportion of the relationship between the two variables.

An additional issue concerns the interpretation of differences between the fixed-points or intervals on a visual analogue scale. So, for example, it should not be assumed that the difference between 20 and 30 mm on a hunger scale is perceptually the same as that between 80 and 90 mm. Nor can a rating of 80 mm be said to represent a feeling that is twice the intensity of that rated at 40 mm. Related to this is the issue of 'end-effects'. This refers to the reluctance of a minority of participants to make ratings away from the upper or lower end-points of the scale *or* to avoid those parts of the scale completely. Despite these qualifications, data from such scales are very often analysed using parametric statistical procedures, such as analysis of variance, providing information that is both meaningful and sensitive.

The alternative procedures of food checklists and measuring salivation were developed in part to provide more 'objective' measures of the willingness to eat. However, they have both been less frequently used than the above scales and so far have not justified this optimism. Food checklists require participants to judge whether they would like to eat any or all of the listed food items at that moment in time. The degree of endorsement is then used as an index of motivation to eat. This can be quantified as the number of items selected from the list or as the number of portions of each item selected. An additional facility offered by this method is the possibility of measuring changes in selective preference. So, for example, Blundell and Rogers (1980) used a checklist of 15 high-carbohydrate and 15 high-protein foods to investigate potential nutrient-selective effects of an appetite suppressant drug. Overall, there is potential for development of this technique.

Increases in salivary flow occur in response to the taste and chewing of food. Salivation also occurs prior to eating, in response to the sight and smell of food. This anticipatory salivation was proposed as a new measure of appetite in the early 1970s by Wooley and Wooley (1973). Using dental rolls to absorb released saliva they found flow rate to vary meaningfully as a function of food deprivation and food palatability, and was positively correlated with rated hunger. The possibility that this 'involuntary' response might be a useful and improved measure of disposition to eat was reviewed in a collection of papers published in *Appetite* in 1981 (Volume 2, pp. 331–391). This remains probably the best single source comparing results obtained by different procedures and for discussion of more theoretical issues. These studies, together with a relatively modest number of later investigations, showed that anticipatory salivation is influenced by a large number of variables, some of which are only indirectly diet related. Anticipatory salivation is a partly conditioned response that is adaptable to different circumstances. Research also shows that there is at least some voluntary control over salivary flow. For these reasons salivation cannot be regarded as an 'improved' measure of the disposition to eat, although again there is potential for further development of this technique.

The act of eating

Human eating behaviour may be regarded as bouts of coordinated and synchronized movements involving the hands and mouth. Its investigation and quantification are dominated by two approaches: behavioural observation, and the use of apparatus that records specific parts of the act of eating.

Observing eating behaviour is a strategy that has its basis in the study of animal behaviour. It involves breaking the act of eating into discrete and unambiguous events that can be sampled. Operational definitions of each activity are necessary to ensure high levels of agreement between observers. Events such as taking a mouthful of food and chewing motions are amenable to accurate observation and if combined with a measurement of time produce a variety of discrete indices of the act of eating (Hill *et al.*, 1995). These include measures of eating rate which, if the meal duration is divided into segments such as meal quarters, may show changes over the course of a meal. In their study of the action of anorexic drugs, for example, Rogers and Blundell (1979) found that eating rate after placebo treatment steadily declined across the course of the meal. In contrast, one pharmacological agent (but not the other) slowed eating rate from the start of the meal.

In terms of application, a large proportion of the research using observational methodology has been directed at questioning whether there is an 'obese eating style'. If part of the reason for obesity lies in *how* a person eats, rather than (or in addition to) what is eaten and in what quantity, the behavioural structure should be amenable to modification (Mahoney, 1975; see Chapter 17). Unfortunately, the research outcome does not justify this optimism. Two reviews written at this proposal's peak of popularity concluded that there were no clear and consistent differences in the eating behaviour of obese and normal-weight people (Stunkard & Kaplan, 1977; Spitzer & Rodin, 1981). What Spitzer and Rodin noted as particularly disappointing was the lack of consistency in procedures or measures used. For example, results of several studies appeared to show a faster eating rate in obese compared with lean persons. However, this conclusion was based mainly on observations made in naturalistic settings (e.g., restaurants) where there was a lack of control in food choice. In fact, the pattern of results suggests that differences in menu choice may have influenced eating rate more than any inherent differences in eating style. Overall, the failure to establish the expected obese eating style, together with the demanding nature of observational methodology, has resulted in a decline in the popularity of this technique.

The use of mechanical apparatus in the measurement of the act of eating has a limited but interesting history. One device, the bite-indicating telemetry (BITE), included sensors in the handles of specially constructed spoons and forks to send an impulse to a remote sensor every time food was placed in the mouth (Moon, 1979). By continuously monitoring these contacts it was shown that most subjects inter-bite intervals (pauses between mouthfuls) were larger in the last quarter of the meal than the first, indicative of a slowing of eating rate. Unfortunately, while ingenious, only one publication resulted from this invention.

In contrast to the BITE, the 'edogram' (Bellisle & Le Magnen, 1980) and the 'oral sensor' (Stellar & Shrager, 1985) are targeted at other key parts of the act of eating—chewing and swallowing. In the edogram, chewing is measured by a strain gauge that monitors jaw movements, while swallowing is detected by changes in pressure in a balloon resting on the Adam's apple. The oral sensor, on the other hand, is a modified dental retainer implanted against the palate in a dental arch that is mounted on the back upper molars.

Perhaps unsurprisingly, more research has tested the external recording apparatus and studies with lean participants show chewing time and the number of chewing movements per mouthful to decrease with increased liking of food (Bellisle & Le Magnen, 1980; Bellisle et al., 1984). The effects of food deprivation were less clear and mainly apparent in the first quarter of the meal. Interestingly, similar effects were found when the eating behaviour of obese individuals was examined (Bellisle & Le Magnen, 1981).

The food consumed

Experimental investigations of eating have most frequently focused on the target of consumption, food. Several imaginative techniques have been developed that permit the measurement or eating rate of the selection from a choice of foods offered. These will be described briefly below. Little will be said about dietary recording or recall methods. The techniques are cornerstones of dietetic and nutritional practice and are described by Summerbell (see Chapter 16).

The first automated device for delivering and monitoring human food intake appeared in the literature in the 1960s. Used to help the feeding of a patient with carcinoma of the lip, it consisted of flexible tubing connecting a mouthpiece to a reservoir containing a liquid food, with a valve and pump incorporated into the circuit (Hashim & Van Itallie, 1964). When the patient pressed a button, the pump delivered a fixed amount of food through the mouthpiece. Each of these pulses of food delivery was timed and recorded, providing a continuous record of intake. Subsequent studies used variations of this type of apparatus in which liquid food was either pumped (Jordan, 1969) or sucked through a straw from a hidden reservoir (Jordan et al., 1966).

One strength of the procedure is the resulting cumulative record of food consumption. An intriguing question is whether it is possible to characterize individuals on the basis of their intake curves. Mayer and Pudel (1972) replaced one meal every day for 10 consecutive days with this apparatus, and distinguished two types of curve (Fig. 5.1). In one (Type A), 80% of the total liquid meal was consumed during the first half of the meal duration. This 'decelerated curve' was taken to reflect normal biological satiation and is in

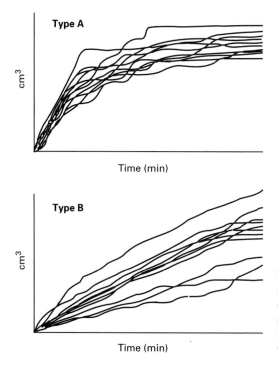

Fig. 5.1 Multiple cumulative records of food consumption obtained from two subjects showing two types of intake curves. From Mayer and Pudel (1972), with permission.

accord with the slowing of eating rate described above. The second curve was linear (Type B) with a rate of intake remaining constant over the meal. Moreover, this apparent defect of satiation was reported to be more characteristic of obese subjects. An alternative explanation, however, may be that the failure to slow the eating rate was due to the conscious restriction over eating that is typical of dieters (Westerterp-Plantagena *et al.*, 1992), and therefore also of many obese individuals (see below).

An alternative to monitoring the flow of liquid food is to monitor the weight of food as it is being eaten. This is achieved by the continuous weighing of the subject's plate with a concealed electronic balance on which the plate rests. The device has been called the universal eating monitor (UEM), and it can be used with either solid food on plates or liquid food such as soup in dishes (Kissileff *et al.*, 1980). The great advantage of this technique over food reservoirs is that food can be eaten normally from a plate or bowl instead of being sucked or pumped through a tube. An additional development has been the fitting of quadratic equations to individual intake curves providing further quantitative measures of ingestive behaviour (Kissileff *et al.*, 1982).

A rather less technical strategy developed to monitor food intake over time is to offer food in small portions or 'solid food units' (Stellar & Shrager, 1985). The preparation of sandwich meals presented in small bite-sized pieces has similarities to the food pumps delivering pulses of liquid diet. The solid food units (or sandwich pieces) are offered in abundance but typically presented on a plate hidden in a box. Access to the food is through a circular hole in the box. In a later variation, a light beam and photo-cell were placed at the box opening, with the sensor registering on a counter in the next room. By observing the subject or by monitoring the counter value at regular times it is possible to obtain a basic measure of eating rate (Spiegel & Stellar, 1990).

Related to the above technique, but actually pre-dating it, is the use of food dispensing machines. Most of those used in research are modifications of commercially available vending machines. In the earliest form, the dispenser was a four-channel refrigerated sandwich vendor (Silverstone *et al.*, 1980). Four types of sandwich were prepared, cut into quarters and individually wrapped. Every time the participant pressed a button to gain access to the food, this was registered by an event recorder. Thus, the type of sandwich chosen and the time of selection were recorded. One of the limitations, however, was that participants had to be tested individually, otherwise the dispenser output would simply reflect group ingestion. In a technically more sophisticated machine, subjects obtained food via a three-digit personal access code which unlocked all the dispenser windows (Wurtman *et al.*, 1981). A computer monitored both the access code and which of the 10 types of food items that were chosen. While it does have limitations, the food dispenser can present real food items and permits variation in the food on offer. It provides a hidden and apparently inexhaustible food supply over an extended period of observation. Moreover, the frequency, quantity and choice of foods are recorded automatically.

The final technique to mention here is the experimental test meal. Since human beings eat in bouts, the meal may be regarded as the basic unit of study in human eating behaviour research (Sunday & Halmi, 1990). And what could be simpler than offering participants a pre-weighed amount of food and re-weighing what is left? We have argued elsewhere that there are many important considerations in designing a test meal protocol (Hill *et al.*, 1995). These include the state and expectancy of the participant, the experimental setting, and the type and variety of food on offer. As an example, buffet-style, multi-item meals are now commonplace in research since by permitting choice they yield measures of food and/or nutrient selection in addition to total energy intake. Many people would regard these meals as having greater 'external validity' since they are more typical of the availability of foods in 'real-life' than more simply composed test meals. However, it is not often that people sit down to eat faced by a banquet of highly palatable foods. Indeed, this circumstance may actually prevent or mask experimental effects, rather than achieve greater accuracy. Simply offering a broad range of foods does not in itself create a more sensitive experimental test. Rather, the test meal, like all other research devices, must prove its sensitivity to known modulators of food intake and must be amenable to variables that increase as well as decrease food consumption.

The psychobiology of appetite

Set-points and settling-points

Homeostatic models of motivation use ideas derived from engineering control theory describing regulatory systems capable of maintaining relatively stable states. Commonly, these models incorporate a set point and negative feedback (Toates, 1986). A textbook analogy for such a system is the regulation of room temperature by a thermostatically controlled heater (Carlson, 1994). Set-point models can account for the maintenance of energy balance and the observation that in adulthood there is rather little long-term variation in body-weight. Unfortunately, other evidence is clearly inconsistent with the existence, in a strict sense, of a set point for body-weight or body fat.

There are, for example, some simple dietary manipulations which can markedly affect energy intake and body-weight. These studies have been carried out on animals, mainly rats, but the results appear to be highly relevant to human eating behaviour and obesity. When switched from a standard laboratory diet to a high fat diet or to a 'cafeteria diet' (consisting of a variety of foods such as bread, chocolate, cheese and breakfast cereals) rats overeat and become grossly obese (see Chapter 3). Although the degree of obesity differs according to the strain of rat (e.g., Schemmel *et al.*, 1970), implicating a significant genetic component in the control of energy balance, this dietary-induced obesity can reach impressive proportions (Rogers & Blundell, 1984).

While dietary-induced obesity contradicts a body fat set-point model, it is not inconsistent with a negative-feedback effect of body fat on appetite. Further results show that as body-weight (fatness) increases in cafeteria-fed rats there is a decline in food intake, until a point is reached at which a new stable weight is maintained. This suggests a reduction in appetite with fattening which, physiologically, could be due the increase in fat mobilization or a related signal such as leptin that changes in proportion with the accumulation of body fat (Friedman, 1991; Sorensen *et al.*, 1996). Computer models indicate that only a small background influence feeding back to suppress food intake is sufficient to provide a marked long-term stabilizing effect on body-weight and fat (Booth & Mather, 1978).

Of course, the phenomenon of dietary-induced obesity raises the question as to what factors related to the diet are responsible for the very substantial differences in energy intake and body-weight. One answer is that eating is increased because of the greater palatability of cafeteria diets and diets high in fat (e.g., Sclafani, 1980; Rogers & Blundell, 1984). Food variety, as available in cafeteria diets, also appears to play a significant role in increasing food intake, perhaps by further enhancing overall palatability. In terms of control theory models, these influences can be represented as external factors having a positive input into the system, thereby tending to stimulate eating.

Unfortunately, the statement that food palatability is a cause of obesity is not a very revealing suggestion unless there is an understanding of the basis of palatability, and this is discussed further below. For the present purposes we can use palatability as part of a model simply to illustrate how feedback control can account very well for observations on food intake (appetite) in relation to body-weight (Fig. 5.2). Sometimes the term settling-point is used to describe the behaviour of this model (Wirtshafter & Davis, 1977; Pinel, 1993), the idea being that weight appears to be regulated around a point at which the various factors that influence its level achieve equilibrium.

Unlike rats, human beings also exert a degree of deliberate control over their eating, most typically in order to lose weight or prevent weight gain. An individual's preferred weight, shape, waist size, etc., derived from cultural norms can be viewed as a 'cognitive set-point' (Booth, 1978). Deviations from this set point are detected when the person notices a change in the fit of their clothes, an increase in measured weight, or a perception of chubbiness when looking in a mirror, causing them to eat less and eventually restore weight to the desired

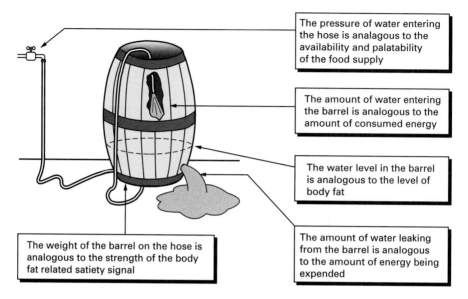

The pressure of water entering the hose is analogous to the availability and palatability of the food supply

The amount of water entering the barrel is analogous to the amount of consumed energy

The water level in the barrel is analogous to the level of body fat

The weight of the barrel on the hose is analogous to the strength of the body fat related satiety signal

The amount of water leaking from the barrel is analogous to the amount of energy being expended

Fig. 5.2 Leaky-barrel model illustrating eating and body-weight homeostasis. Adapted from Pinel (1993).

level. Actually, although cognitively restrained eating and dieting is common, it is not always successful (see below).

It is also useful to take an ecological perspective on energy balance. As discussed above, because the storage capacity of adipose tissue is very large and the feedback inhibition on appetite is rather weak, stability of body-weight and body fat can occur within a very wide range of values. These characteristics probably evolved to buffer uncertainties in food supply. In most natural habitats food supplies are unpredictable or may vary seasonally. The storage of energy in the form of body fat in times of plenty can reduce the impact of food shortages, but where food availability rarely or never limits intake, this adaptation will encourage the development of obesity. More generally, the need for precise control of nutrient intakes is avoided by sophisticated metabolic regulatory mechanisms (Frayn, 1996). At the level of behaviour, the nutritional priorities for omnivorous species like ourselves are to select a diet that meets certain minimal nutritional requirements, and in doing so avoid ingesting harmful substances. Excesses are dealt with by metabolic transformation, storage and excretion.

The physiological and learned control of eating patterns

As previously noted, eating occurs in bouts called meals, and food intake can vary according to the number and/or size of meals eaten. The ubiquitous 'snack' is probably best considered as a small meal, since this appears to be a distinction based mainly on social convention rather than any substantial differences in the processes controlling eating. The meal, therefore, can be considered the basic unit for the analysis of eating behaviour which, in turn, may be divided into three phases: namely, the initiation, maintenance, and termination of eating.

Meal initiation is identified with appetitive states such as hunger and food cravings which direct behaviour towards eating and perhaps specific foods. Internal cues related to, for example, the dynamics of blood glucose can provide a reliable stimulus for the initiation of eating (Campfield & Smith, 1990). However, the role of energy depletion in meal initiation appears to have been overemphasized compared with the effects of external cues. The idea that hunger is generated by internal physiological signals related to energy or nutrient needs fails to account for many aspects of eating, including how our appetite is stimulated by someone offering us an unexpected treat, how desire to eat may fade in the afternoon even though we were too busy to eat lunch, and why many people do not eat breakfast despite the fact that this meal follows the longest fast of the day. These and other observations indicate that eating usually occurs in anticipation of nutritional requirements rather than in direct response to low energy availability (Collier, 1986), and can be motivated by the sight and smell of food and learned contextual cues such as location and time of day. This is demonstrated in studies showing that external stimuli previously associated with food consumption can reliably motivate eating in the absence of immediate nutritional deprivation or 'need' (Weingarten, 1983).

A basic issue arising from these observations concerns the specificity of the effects of external stimuli conditioned to eating. One possibility is that exposure to such stimuli triggers certain physiological responses in preparation for eating, including salivation, insulin release and gastric acid secretion (the so-called cephalic phase of digestion), the consequences of which feed back to the brain where they are interpreted as an internal signal for hunger. Against this, though, is the finding that blockade of cephalic-phase responses (with atropine), does not disrupt the initiation of eating in response to learned cues (Weingarten, 1984). Alternatively, rather than a general state of hunger, the presentation of stimuli which have become associated with consumption of a food may elicit a desire to eat that specific food (Weingarten, 1985). An analogy is to consider visiting the cinema where in the past you have usually eaten popcorn. What is the effect of exposure to this eating-related setting? Does it trigger a general feeling of hunger, or a specific desire to eat popcorn?

Figure 5.3 depicts stimulatory and inhibitory influences controlling eating during a meal. Of course, similar cumulative intake curves can be obtained

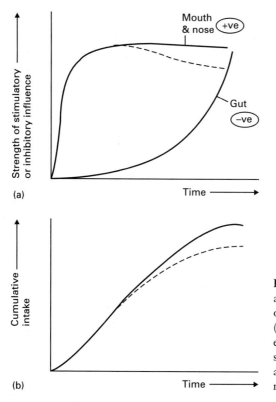

Mouth & nose (+ve)

Gut (−ve)

Strength of stimulatory or inhibitory influence

Time

(a)

Cumulative intake

Time

(b)

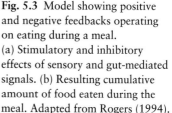

Fig. 5.3 Model showing positive and negative feedbacks operating on eating during a meal. (a) Stimulatory and inhibitory effects of sensory and gut-mediated signals. (b) Resulting cumulative amount of food eaten during the meal. Adapted from Rogers (1994).

with these influences varying in a number of different ways; so, for instance, there may be some decline in the strength of positive feedback during the meal (indicated by the dashed lines in Fig. 5.3).

The operation of negative feedback during normal eating is demonstrated by the results of studies on sham feeding. Rats fitted with a chronic gastric fistula eat (drink) vastly increased amounts when the liquid food is allowed to drain out of the open fistula, compared to when the fistula is closed (Smith *et al.*, 1974). In other words, satiety does not occur if ingested food fails to distend the stomach or enter the small intestine—thus excluding taste, other oral stimuli, pharyngeal and oesophageal movements, and the contact of food with the gastric mucosa as potent stimuli for satiety. Other evidence shows that the postingestive and postabsorptive effects of food ingestion which influence meal size and the maintenance of satiety in the post-meal interval, include filling of the gastrointestinal tract, release of regulatory hormones such as cholecystokinin and the detection of nutrients absorbed into the systemic circulation (Blundell, 1991).

Results from sham feeding experiments also indicate that learning contributes to satiety and the control of meal size. A large increase in meal size is not seen on the first occasion that rats are sham fed. Instead, there is a suppression of eating during initial sham feeds due to learned satiety (Weingarten & Kulikovsky, 1989). During normal feeding the visual and orosensory properties (appearance, smell, taste, flavour, texture, etc.) of the food become associated with the postingestive effects experienced, and this provides anticipatory control of meal size. On the first sham feed, meal size is modulated according to the 'expected' postingestive effects, but with continued sham feeding this learning extinguishes and meal size increases. The learned control of meal size has also been demonstrated in human volunteers (Booth *et al.*, 1982), although in studies not involving sham feeding!

The learned anticipatory control of meal size is a potential refinement which could help overcome the problem posed by the delay between the moment of eating and the postingestive and postabsorptive effects of food. It is not clear, however, whether this mechanism can operate effectively where meals are composed of many tastes and flavours. A further problem is that there is not always a consistent relationship between the orosensory characteristics and the energy content of foods or drinks (e.g., a food sweetened with an artificial sweetener can have a much lower energy content than the same food sweetened with sugar).

The positive feedback effect is assumed to arise from orosensory contact with food. This stimulation of eating by eating would appear to be consistent with subjective experience—*l'appétit vient en mangeant* (appetite comes with eating). Furthermore, the strength of the positive-feedback effect is influenced by food palatability, so that consumption of highly palatable foods strongly stimulates eating and increases meal size (Rogers, 1994).

Palatability: the hedonistic response to food

A dictionary definition of 'palatable' is 'agreeable to the taste'. Palatability is a term used widely but inconsistently in the scientific literature. Often its use appears to be synonymous with food intake, but in this sense palatability is merely a descriptive term which contributes little or nothing to the understanding of eating behaviour. Here we treat palatability as equivalent to liking and pleasantness, and use it to refer to an individual's hedonistic or affective response to the taste, flavour, texture, etc. of a food or drink (Rogers, 1990). As the following example shows, however, this is not the same as food preference. Consider a person choosing between margarine and butter: the person may eat more margarine because of price or perceived health benefits, but he or she may like the 'taste' of butter more than that of margarine. As measured by the amount consumed, this person would show a preference for margarine, although on a hedonic measure butter would score higher. Therefore, although preference will generally be strongly affected by palatability, it can also be influenced by a variety of other factors.

Biases towards certain tastes are present at birth. For example, the facial expressions of human newborns indicate acceptance and a postive hedonic response to sweet stimuli, while bitter stimuli evoke rejection coupled with negative expressions (Steiner, 1987). However, in contrast to our limited taste repertoire (sweet, salty, sour and bitter), the number of unique odours human beings can discern appears to be essentially unlimited, and there does not appear to be an inbuilt liking for any particular odours or indeed textures. Perceptions of 'flavour' in foods and drinks come largely from combinations of tastes together with smells arising from volatile compounds sensed retro-nasally.

Food palatability is also modified by learning, and one way in which this occurs is through the association of the orosensory and postingestive effects of eating and drinking. For example, animals rapidly learn to avoid food when consumption of that food is paired with nausea and sickness (Garcia et al., 1974). The same basic Pavlovian conditioning processes appear to underlie food aversions acquired by human beings, with the result that strong aversions are sometimes formed despite the person's awareness that the food did not cause the illness.

Similarly, the positive after-effects of food ingestion can increase liking for a food. This has been demonstrated convincingly by Sclafani and his colleagues (Sclafani, 1990), who reported that rats acquired strong preferences for flavours paired with intragastric starch infusions. Other results suggested that these changes in preference were indeed due to increased palatability of the starch-paired flavour. Studies on human volunteers have confirmed significant reinforcing effects of carbohydrate, fat and protein (e.g., Kern et al., 1993), as well as increased liking for flavours paired with the consumption of caffeine and alcohol (e.g., Rogers et al., 1995).

Palatability, therefore, plays a central role in motivating ingestive behaviour. It guides the choice of foods in relation to their biological utility and acts to stimulate and maintain consumption during a meal through a positive-feedback effect on eating.

Hunger, palatability and satiety

It is often assumed that palatability is enhanced in a state of depletion and diminishes during repletion. However, the evidence on this subject suggests that hunger, palatability and postingestive satiety may act largely independently (Rogers, 1990). For example, opioid peptides appear to play a significant role in the regulation of food and fluid intake, and specifically in the mediation of hedonistic responses to orosensory stimuli. Experiments using opioid antagonist drugs such as naloxone have generally found that these compounds have minimal effects on self-reported hunger, although they reduce the intake and pleasantness ratings of preferred foods and/or sweet and high-fat foods (Yeomans & Wright, 1991; Drewnowski *et al.*, 1992). Perception of the intensity of sensory stimuli is unaffected.

Other results confirm these dissociations. During a test meal, hunger was found to decline and fullness increase as expected, but ratings of the pleasantness of the 'taste' of the food eaten remained relatively unchanged (Rogers & Blundell, 1990). This is consistent with little or no reduction in positive feedback from eating, as depicted in Fig. 5.3. That is, sensory contact with preferred food is always stimulatory, and never itself contributes to the development of satiation and satiety as claimed by some authors (e.g., Rolls *et al.*, 1984). One source of confusion here may have been the failure to distinguish between the pleasantness of the taste of food in the mouth (influenced by palatability) and the pleasantness of eating or ingesting that food, which presumably is influenced both by palatability, and hunger and satiety (fullness of the stomach etc.). Even after a large meal, food remains palatable, but feelings of fullness prevent further eating. If there is no 'room' left the extra piece of chocolate cake will not be eaten however delicious it tastes.

The cognitive control of eating

The psychosomatic theory of obesity and beyond

Stated simply, the psychosomatic view of obesity is that obesity is due to overeating that occurs in response to emotional stimuli. While the most common response to arousal states, such as anger, fear and anxiety is the loss of appetite, it is argued that some individuals react by eating excessively. In turn, eating modifies the emotional state, e.g., by reducing anxiety. Overeating is thus a learned behaviour which can be viewed either as a coping response, or as resulting from a confusion of internal cues associated with activation and stress and 'natural' hunger cues (Kaplan & Kaplan, 1957; Robbins & Fray, 1980). Similar analyses have been suggested to explain bulimic behaviour (e.g., Mizes, 1985). These and related ideas have been investigated extensively and have received some empirical support (Slochower, 1983). However, a difficulty with much of the research testing the psychosomatic hypothesis is that it has failed to take into account the possible interaction between effects related to obesity and the effects attributable to dieting. For instance, current dieting appears to be a better predictor of the amount eaten when depressed than is obesity (Baucom & Aiken, 1981).

In the late 1960s, Schachter and his colleagues began a series of highly original and influential studies on human eating behaviour which led to the proposal of the so-called externality theory of human obesity (Schachter, 1971). This drew parallels between the behaviour of rats made obese by ventromedial lesions of the hypothalamus and the behaviour of obese people. Compared with their lean counterparts, both obese rats and people were supposedly less willing to work to obtain food, less sensitive to a food preload (i.e., they showed poor 'caloric compensation'), but were influenced more by the sight and taste (i.e., palatability) of food. Such findings were interpreted as showing that the obese are more reactive to, or more 'driven' by, external cues and at the same time are less sensitive to internal hunger and satiety cues than lean individuals. Furthermore, this was argued to be a prominent factor in the aetiology of obesity: high external responsiveness would, in the face of a highly palatable and available food supply, encourage overeating and hence the development of obesity.

These ideas were subsequently tested in a variety of further studies which, while confirming many of the original results, also indicated that the relationship between externality and overweight is more complex than originally proposed. Nonetheless, Spitzer and Rodin (1981) were able to conclude from their review that, 'palatability is the most consistent variable influencing amount eaten and *producing overweight–normal differences in amount eaten*' [our italics]. Despite this, the concept of externality has since been largely ignored in favour of related ideas concerning dietary restraint and the effects of dieting.

Dietary restraint and disinhibition

Following on directly from Schachter's influential research, a further significant advance in the study of human food intake and body-weight regulation was the recognition of the important influence of voluntary dietary restriction on human eating behaviour. This was initially highlighted by Nisbett (1972) who proposed that the obese–normal differences in eating behaviour identified by Schachter (1971) were due to the greater hunger of obese individuals. The difference in hunger was assumed to arise because of a higher prevalence of dieting in the obese population. Nisbett suggested that the obese have a high set-point for weight (fat), but because of societal and medical pressures many tend to maintain a lower weight. Paradoxically, therefore, obesity and overweight were supposed to be associated with chronic hunger.

Such a view clearly rejects the notion that eating behaviour is determined solely by physiological and sensory cues and the related sensations of hunger and satiety. Instead, it proposes that it is commonplace to resist the operation of these factors, this self-imposed resistance or restraint being motivated by the desire to suppress weight. The desire to lose weight or maintain a low weight by dieting is, however, not confined to overweight and obese people. Indeed, there are many dieters whose weight is statistically normal or below normal (Hill, 1993). Nisbett's hypothesis, therefore, suggests an examination of the eating behaviour of people classified according to their degree of dietary restraint and dieting rather than body-weight. This was first carried out in a series of studies which were based on the revised restraint scale (RRS) developed by Herman and Polivy (see Herman, 1978). The RRS is a self-report questionnaire which assesses concern with dieting and weight, and short-term weight fluctuation (Table 5.2).

In what soon became a widely quoted study, Herman and Mack (1975) gave participants preloads of either two glasses of milkshake, one glass or none, and then required them to rate the taste of various ice-creams. Whereas the intake of ice-cream was inversely related to the size of the preload in unrestrained

Table 5.2 The revised restraint scale. From Herman (1978).

---

1 How often are you dieting? Never; rarely; sometimes; often; always. (*Scored 0–4*)

2 What is the maximum amount of weight (in pounds) that you have ever lost within one month? 0–4; 5–9; 10–14; 15–19; 20+. (*Scored 0–4*)

3 What is your maximum weight gain in one week? 0–1; 1.1–2; 2.1–3; 3.1–5; 5.1+. (*Scored 0–4*)

4 In a typical week, how much does your weight fluctuate? 0–1; 1.1–2; 2.1–3; 3.1–5; 5.1+. (*Scored 0–4*)

5 Would a weight fluctuation of 5 lb affect the way you live your life? Not at all; slightly; moderately; very much. (*Scored 0–3*)

6 Do you eat sensibly in front of others and splurge alone? Never; rarely; often; always. (*Scored 0–3*)

7 Do you give too much time and thought to food? Never; rarely; often; always. (*Scored 0–3*)

8 Do you have feelings of guilt after overeating? Never; rarely; often; always. (*Scored 0–3*)

9 How conscious are you of what you are eating? Not at all; slightly; moderately; extremely. (*Scored 0–3*)

10 How many pounds over your desired weight were you at your maximum weight? 0–1; 1–5; 6–10; 11–20; 21+. (*Scored 0–4*)

In much of the research using this questionnaire, individuals displaying a high score were designated as restrained eaters or dieters and those displaying a low score as unrestrained eaters or non-dieters. However, for reasons explained in the text, these terms should now be revised. In addition, the classification is somewhat arbitrary because usually subjects were divided into groups of restrained and unrestrained eaters based on a median split of their questionnaire scores.

subjects, restrained subjects responded in a so-called 'counter-regulatory' fashion, i.e., their intake of ice-cream increased as the size of the preload increased. A similar result was obtained by manipulating subjects' beliefs about the calorie content of the preload consumed while keeping constant its actual calorie content (Spencer & Fremouw, 1979). These findings have been interpreted in terms of a process of disinhibition. The preload, by forcing the perceived intake of calories above a critical threshold or 'diet boundary', causes normally restrained eaters to suspend their self-imposed restraint, thereby releasing their underlying desire to eat (due to hunger, emotional or other reasons) (Herman & Mack, 1975; Herman & Polivy, 1984). The restrained eater's diet boundary represents his or her self-imposed quota of calories for a given occasion, and crucially is lower than the physiologically determined satiety boundary. In other words, referring to the model shown in Fig. 5.3, the diet boundary is reached before the negative-feedback effects of eating outweigh the positive-feedback effects.

The pattern of thinking identified with this disinhibition of behaviour has been characterized as follows, 'My diet has been broken (by the requirement of the experiment to consume the preload), I might as well go ahead and enjoy myself/stop feeling hungry (eat a lot of the test foods), I can always start my diet again tomorrow.' This, in turn, has sometimes been called the 'what-the-hell effect'! Other disinhibitors of eating in restrained eaters include emotional events, the consumption of alcohol, the behaviour of others and even anticipated future overeating (Ruderman, 1986).

The explanation for disinhibited eating in restrained eaters in terms of a temporary abandonment of restraint following a failure to stay within the self-imposed rules for eating is highly plausible. It does, though, suggest a simplistic all-or-nothing (or none-or-all) cognitive style which might seem to under-estimate the sophistication of many dieters, who will presumably have experienced and had the opportunity to learn from previous instances of disinhibited eating. In fact, surprisingly little is known about the thinking of restrained eaters, or their emotional responses, in this situation.

A somewhat different account of the processes underlying disinhibited eating proposes that it is the emotional distress caused by the consumption of 'forbidden foods' which undermines the restrained eater's ability to maintain restraint (Herman & Polivy, 1988; Rogers & Hill, 1989). Ogden and Greville (1993) confirmed the expected increase in anxiety in restrained eaters following consumption of a high-calorie preload. However, they also found that accompanying the anxiety these subjects experienced marked increases in feelings of rebelliousness and defiance, and a desire to challenge the limitations set by their restraint. In other words, the restrained eaters responded to preloading with an 'active state of mind', rather than passively abandoning their dietary goal.

Dietary restraint, and successful and unsuccessful dieting

The significance of the RRS is its ability to identify individuals with different eating patterns, and particularly eating in response to preloading and manipulations of, for example, mood. The items making up the RRS (see Table 5.2), though, are concerned principally with concern with dieting and weight fluctuation. None of the questions appears to capture very directly the notion of restraint as self-imposed resistance to eating (Herman, 1978). In contrast, two questionnaires developed after the RRS claim to identify a separate restraint factor.

The first of these questionnaires is the Three-Factor Eating Questionnaire (TFEQ, Stunkard & Messick, 1985) which identifies three factors named (i) cognitive restraint of eating; (ii) disinhibition; and (iii) hunger. It consists of 51 items, such as 'When I have eaten my quota of calories, I am usually good about not eating any more' (*restraint*); 'I usually eat too much at social occasions, like parties and picnics' (*disinhibition*); 'I often feel so hungry that I have to eat something' (*hunger*). A similarly narrow definition of restraint is found in the 33-item Dutch Eating Behaviour Questionnaire (DEBQ, van Strien *et al.*, 1986). Example items for the DEBQ restraint scale are: 'If you put on weight, do you eat less than you usually do?', 'Do you eat less at mealtimes than you would like to eat?', and 'Do you watch exactly what you eat?'

Although there is some overlap between the RRS and the restrained eating scales of the TFEQ and the DEBQ, the latter differ substantially from the RRS in that they have very few items on overeating and weight fluctuations, and they emphasize cognitive and behavioural strategies for limiting food and energy intake. Crucially, they also appear to identify restrained eaters who are less susceptible to disinhibited eating in laboratory tests (Lowe, 1993), leading to the suggestion that the RRS tends to identify unsuccessful dieters, whereas the TFEQ and DEBQ restraint scales largely identify successful dieters (Heatherton *et al.*, 1988). Empirical support for this includes the consistent finding that restraint measured by the TFEQ and the DEBQ, but not the RRS, is negatively related to energy intake recorded in food diaries (de Castro, 1995). In addition, total daily energy expenditure measured using the doubly labelled water method has been reported to be lower in restrained compared to unrestrained subjects (TFEQ restraint), this difference being if anything somewhat larger than the difference in self-reported energy intake (410 kcal) (Tuschl *et al.*, 1990).

The discussion above shows that the relationships between energy intake, energy expenditure, body-weight and restrained eating are complex and difficult to disentangle. A reasonable interpretation, though, is that individuals with relatively low energy requirements, perhaps inherited or perhaps acquired as a result of past dieting attempts (e.g., Heshka *et al.*, 1990), are forced to adopt a restrained eating style in order to avoid excessive weight gain.

Some consequences of dietary restraint: hunger and eating variability

Dieting and restrained eating are motivated by concern to achieve a culturally and personally acceptable weight. The concept of dietary restraint is that in order to lose weight or maintain a 'low' weight many individuals find it necessary to consciously restrict their food intake. Results from studies using the RRS led originally to the conclusion that restraint is fragile and easily disinhibited, and that consequently it tends to undermine eating and weight control, even to the extent of playing a direct role in the aetiology of binge eating and bulimia nervosa (Wardle & Beinart, 1981; Polivy & Herman, 1985). It is now clear, however, that restrained eating, as measured by the TEFQ and DEBQ, is often associated with successful dietary control. The RRS predicts unsuccessful restraint and dieting, including disinhibited eating and weight fluctuation, because this is mainly what it describes.

One possible explanation for this predictability of successful vs unsuccessful dietary control is that these outcomes are due to certain self-perpetuating patterns of eating behaviour. In this respect a crucial observation is that hunger tends to be diminished in successful weight suppressors but increased in individuals having a highly variable eating pattern. This is demonstrated by the results of a study which investigated salivary responses as a function of two extreme styles of 'dietary restraint', namely strict and unrelenting dieting exemplified by a group of restricting anorexic patients, and variable dieting exemplified by a group of bulimic patients (LeGoff et al., 1988). Compared with age-matched control subjects, anticipatory salivation to the smell of food was exaggerated among the bulimics but reduced among the anorexics. The anorexics also reported lower levels of hunger.

LeGoff et al. (1988) conclude that these different appetite responses are a direct consequence of the different eating patterns adopted by restricting anorexic and bulimic patients. The explanation for the reduced anticipatory salivation and hunger associated with the unrelenting anorexic style of dietary restriction is that these conditioned responses have been extinguished, because typically little or nothing is consumed on occasions when food-related stimuli are present (Herman et al., 1988; LeGoff et al., 1988). This implies that, despite their undernourished weight, the presence of food will have a relatively weak (stimulatory) effect on appetite for such individuals. Paradoxically, therefore, they may experience reduced rather than enhanced appetite as they continue their dietary restriction, a view which is consistent with the evidence outlined earlier suggesting that external stimuli conditioned to eating play a major role in the regulation of appetite.

Conclusion

Escalating population levels of obesity place even greater importance on our understanding of the processes that govern food intake and eating behaviour. We have argued in this chapter that appetite, and therefore eating, is a truly psychobiological phenomenon, linking biological processes, psychological events and environmental circumstance. Learning mechanisms pervade these associations enabling the complete system to be dynamic and adaptable. It follows from this perspective that the cause of human obesity is unlikely to be attributable to a specific obesity-inducing mechanism such as that occurring in certain rodent strains. Rather, obesity should be seen as a legacy of the evolutionary development of our biological system coupled with a newly encountered aggressive or 'toxic' environment, in which energy expenditure is low and food abundant (Blundell, 1996). Faced by a life circumstance that discourages routine physical effort and activity, and that offers a surfeit of highly palatable, high-energy and high-fat foods, in bewildering variety, weight gain is an understandable consequence. A challenge for the future will be to reveal, through research, ways in which the system may be rebalanced and weight gain become less of an inevitability.

References

Baucom, D.H. & Aiken, P.A. (1981) Effect of depressed mood on eating among obese and nonobese dieting and nondieting persons. *Journal of Personality and Social Psychology* **41**, 577–585.

Bellisle, F. & Le Magnen, J. (1980) The analysis of human feeding patterns: the edogram. *Appetite* **1**, 141–150.

Bellisle, F. & Le Magnen, J. (1981) The structure of meals in humans: eating and drinking patterns in lean and obese subjects. *Physiology and Behaviour* **27**, 649–658.

Bellisle, F., Lucas, F., Amrani, R. & Le Magnen, J. (1984) Deprivation, palatability, and the micro-structure of meals in human subjects. *Appetite* **5**, 85–94.

Blundell, J.E. (1984) Systems and interactions: an approach to the pharmacology of eating and hunger. In: Stunkard, A.J. & Stellar, E. (eds) *Eating and its Disorders*, pp. 39–65. New York: Raven.

Blundell, J.E. (1991) Pharmacological approaches to appetite suppression. *Trends in Pharmacological Sciences* **12**, 147–157.

Blundell, J.E. (1996) Food intake and body weight regulation. In: Bouchard, C. & Bray, G.A. (eds) *Regulation of Body Weight: Biological and Behavioural Mechanisms*, pp. 111–133. Chichester: Wiley.

Blundell, J.E. & Hill, A.J. (1986) Biopsychological interactions underlying the study and treatment of obesity. In: Christie, M.J. & Mellet, P.G. (eds) *The Psychosomatic Approach: Contemporary Practice of Whole Person Care*, pp. 113–138. Chichester: Wiley.

Blundell, J.E. & Rogers, P.J. (1980) Effects of anorexic drugs on food intake, food selection and preferences, hunger motivation and subjective experiences. *Appetite* **1**, 151–165.

Blundell, J.E. & Rogers, P.J. (1991) Hunger, hedonics, and the control of satiation and satiety. In: Friedman, M.I., Tordoff, M.G. & Kare, M.R. (eds) *Chemical senses*, Vol. 4: *Appetite and Nutrition*, pp. 127–148. New York: Marcel Dekker.

Booth, D.A. (1978) Acquired behaviour controlling energy intake and output. *Psychiatric Clinics of North America* **1**, 545–579.

Booth, D.A. & Mather, P. (1978) Prototype model of human feeding, growth and obesity. In: Booth, D.A. (ed.) *Hunger Models: Computable Theory of Feeding Control*, pp. 279–322. London: Academic Press.

Booth, D.A., Mather, P. & Fuller, J. (1982) Starch content of ordinary foods associatively conditions human appetite and satiation, indexed by intake and eating pleasantness of starch-paired flavours. *Appetite* **3**, 163–184.

Campfield, L.A. & Smith, F.J. (1990) Systemic factors in the control of food intake: Evidence for patterns as signals. In: Stricker, E.M. (ed.) *Handbook of Behavioral Neurobiology*, Vol. 10: *Neurobiology of Food and Fluid Intake*, pp. 183–206. New York: Plenum Press.

Carlson, N.R. (1994) *Physiology of Behaviour*, 5 th edn. Boston: Allyn and Bacon.

Collier, G. (1986) The dialogue on the strategy between the economist and the resident physiologist. *Appetite* **7**, 188–189.

Cornell, C.E., Rodin, J. & Weingarten, H. (1989) Stimulus-induced eating when satiated. *Physiology and Behaviour* **45**, 695–704.

de Castro, J.M. (1995) The relationship of cognitive restraint to the spontaneous food and fluid intake of free-living humans. *Physiology and Behaviour* **57**, 287–295.

Drewnowski, A., Krahn, D.D., Demitrack, M.A., Nairn, K. & Gosnell, B.A. (1992) Taste responses and preferences for sweet high-fat foods: evidence for opioid involvement. *Physiology and Behaviour* **51**, 371–379.

Durrant, M. & Royston, P. (1979) Short-term effects of energy density on salivation, hunger and appetite in obese subjects. *International Journal of Obesity* **3**, 335–347.

Frayn K.N. (1996) *Metabolic Regulation: A Human Perspective*. Portland Press: London.

Friedman, M.I. (1991) Metabolic control of food intake. In: Friedman, M.I., Tordoff, M.G. & Kare, M.R. (eds) *Chemical Senses*, Vol. 4: *Appetite and Nutrition*, pp. 19–38. New York: Marcel Dekker.

Garcia, J., Hankins, W.G. & Rusiniak, K.W. (1974) Behavioural regulation of the milieu interne in man and rat. *Science* **185**, 824–831.

Hashim, S.A. & Van Itallie, T.B. (1964) An automatically monitored food dispensing apparatus for the study of food intake in man. *Federation Proceedings* **23**, 82–84.

Heatherton, T.F., Herman, C.P., Polivy, J. King, G.A. & McGree, S.T. (1988) The (mis)measurement of restraint: An analysis of conceptual and psychometric issues. *Journal of Abnormal Psychology* **97**, 19–28.

Herman, C.P. (1978) Restrained eating. *Psychiatric Clinics of North America* **1**, 593–607.

Herman, C.P. & Mack, D. (1975) Restrained and unrestrained eating. *Journal of Personality* **43**, 647–660.

Herman, C.P. & Polivy, J. (1984) A boundary model for the regulation of eating. In: Stunkard, A.J. & Stellar, E. (eds) *Eating and Its Disorders*, pp. 141–156. New York: Raven Press.

Herman, C.P. & Polivy, J. (1988) Restraint and excess in dieters and bulimics. In: Pirke, K.M., Vandereycken, W. & Ploog, D. (eds) *The Psychobiology of Bulimia Nervosa*, pp. 18–32. Berlin: Springer-Verlag.

Herman, C.P., Polivy, J., Klajner, F. & Esses, V.M. (1988) Salivation in dieters and nondieters. *Appetite* **2**, 356–361.

Heshka, S., Yang M-U., Wang, J., Burt, P. & Pi-Sunyer, F.X. (1990) Weight loss and change in resting metabolic rate. *American Journal of Clinical Nutrition* **52**, 981–986.

Hill, A.J. (1993) Causes and consequences of dieting and anorexia. *Proceedings of the Nutrition Society* **52**, 211–218.

Hill, A.J., Leathwood, P.D. & Blundell, J.E. (1987) Some evidence for short-term caloric compensation in normal weight subjects: the effects of high and low energy meals on hunger, food preferences and food intake. *Human Nutrition: Applied Nutrition* **41**, 244–257.

Hill, A.J., Rogers, P.J. & Blundell, J.E. (1995) Techniques for the experimental measurement of human eating behaviour and food intake: a practical guide. *International Journal of Obesity* **19**, 361–375.

Jordan, H.A. (1969) Voluntary intragastric feeding: oral and gastric contributions to food intake and hunger in man. *Journal of Comparative and Physiological Psychology* **68**, 498–506.

Jordan, H.A., Wieland, W.F., Zebley, S.P., Stellar, E. & Stunkard, A.J. (1966) Direct measurement of food intake in man: a method for the objective study of eating behaviour. *Psychosomatic Medicine* **28**, 836–842.

Kaplan, H.I. & Kaplan, H.S. (1957) The psychosomatic concept of obesity. *Journal of Nervous and Mental Disorders* **125**, 181–201.

Kern, D.L., McPhee, L., Fisher, J., Johnson, S. & Birch, L.L. (1993) The postingestive consequences of fat condition preferences for flavours associated with high dietary fat. *Physiology and Behaviour* **54**, 71–76.

Kissileff, H.R., Klingsberg, G. & Van Itallie, T.B. (1980) Universal eating monitor for continuous recording of solid or liquid consumption in man. *American Journal of Physiology* **238**, 14–22.

Kissileff, H.R., Thornton, J. & Becker, E. (1982) A quadratic equation adequately describes the cumulative food intake curve in man. *Appetite* **3**, 255–272.

LeGoff, D.B., Leichner, P. & Spigelman, M.N. (1988) Salivary response to olfactory food stimuli in anorexics and bulimics. *Appetite* **11**, 15–25.

Lowe, M.R. (1993) The effects of dieting on eating behaviour: a three-factor model. *Psychological Bulletin* **114**, 100–121.

Mahoney, M.J. (1975) The obese eating style: bites, beliefs and behaviour modification. *Addictive Behaviours* **1**, 47–53.

Mayer, J.E. & Pudel, V. (1972) Experimental studies on food-intake in obese and normal weight subjects. *Journal of Psychosomatic Research* **16**, 305–308.

Mattes, R. (1990) Hunger ratings are not a valid proxy measure of reported food intake in humans. *Appetite* **15**, 103–113.

Mizes, J.S. (1985). Bulimia: A review of its symptomatology and treatment. *Advances in Behaviour Research and Therapy* **7**, 91–142.

Moon, R.D. (1979) Monitoring human eating patterns during the ingestion of non-liquid foods. *International Journal of Obesity* **3**, 281–288.

Nisbett, R.E. (1972) Hunger, obesity, and the ventromedial hypothalamus. *Psychological Review* **79**, 433–453.

Ogden, J. & Greville, L. (1993) Cognitive changes to preloading in restrained and unrestrained eaters as measured by the Stroop task. *International Journal of Eating Disorders* **14**, 185–195.

Pinel, J.P.J. (1993) *Biopsychology*, 2nd edn. Boston: Allyn and Bacon.

Polivy, J. & Herman, C.P. (1985) Dieting and binging: a causal analysis. *American Psychologist* **40**, 193–201.

Prentice, A.M., Black, A.E., Murgatroyd, P.R., Goldberg, G.R. & Coward, W.A. (1989) Metabolism or appetite: questions of energy balance with particular reference to obesity. *Journal of Human Nutrition and Dietetics* **2**, 95–104.

Robbins, T.W. & Fray, P.J. (1980) Stress-induced eating: fact, fiction or misunderstanding? *Appetite* **1**, 103–133.

Rogers, P.J. (1990) Why a palatability construct is needed. *Appetite* **14**, 167–170.

Rogers, P.J. (1994) Mechanisms of moreishness and food craving. In: Warburton, D.M. (ed.) *Pleasure: the Politics and the Reality*, pp. 38–49. Chichester: Wiley.

Rogers, P.J. & Blundell, J.E. (1979) Effect of anorexic drugs on food intake and the microstructure of eating in human subjects. *Psychopharmacology* **66**, 159–165.

Rogers, P.J. & Blundell, J.E. (1984) Meal patterns and food selection during the development of obesity in rats fed a cafeteria diet. *Neuroscience and Biobehavioral Reviews* **8**, 441–453.

Rogers, P.J. & Blundell, J.E. (1990) Psychobiological bases of food choice. *British Nutrition Foundation Nutrition Bulletin* **15** (suppl. 1), 31–40.

Rogers, P.J. & Hill, A.J. (1989) Breakdown of dietary restraint following mere exposure to food stimuli: interrelationships between restraint, hunger, salivation, and food intake. *Addictive Behaviours* **14**, 387–397.

Rogers, P.J., Richardson, N.J. & Elliman, N.A. (1995) Overnight caffeine abstinence and negative reinforcement of preference for caffeine-containing drinks. *Psychopharmacology* **120**, 457–462.

Rolls, B.A., Duijvenvoorde, P.M. & Rolls, E.T. (1984) Pleasantness changes and food intake in a varied four course meal. *Appetite* 5, 337–348.

Ruderman, A.J. (1986) Dietary restraint: A theoretical and empirical review. *Psychological Bulletin* 99, 247–262.

Schachter, S. (1971) Some extraordinary facts about obese humans and rats. *American Psychologist* 26, 129–144.

Schemmel, R., Mickelsen, O. & Gill, J.L. (1970) Dietary obesity in rats: Body weight and body fat accretion in seven strains of rats. *Journal of Nutrition* 100, 1041–1048.

Sclafani, A. (1980) Dietary obesity. In: Bray, G. (ed.) *Hunger: Basic Mechanisms and Clinical Implications*, pp. 281–295. London: Newman.

Sclafani, A. (1990) Nutritionally based learned flavour preferences in rats. In: Capaldi, E.D. & Powley, T.L. (eds) *Taste, Feeding and Experience*, pp. 139–156. Washington D.C.: American Psychological Association.

Silverstone T., Fincham, J. & Brydon, J. (1980) A new technique for the continuous measurement of food intake in man. *American Journal of Clinical Nutrition* 33, 1852–1855.

Slochower, J.A. (1983) *Excessive Eating*. New York: Human Sciences Press.

Smith, G.P., Gibbs, J. & Young, R.C. (1974) Cholecystokinin and intestinal satiety in the rat. *Federation Proceedings* 33, 1146–1149.

Sorensen, T.I., Echwald, S.M. & Holm, J-C. (1996) Leptin in obesity. *British Medical Journal* 313, 953–954.

Spencer, J.A. & Fremouw, W.J. (1979) Binge eating as a function of restraint and weight classification. *Journal of Abnormal Psychology* 88, 262–267.

Spiegel, T.A. & Stellar, E. (1990) Effects of variety on food intake of underweight, normal weight and overweight women. *Appetite* 15, 47–61.

Spitzer, L. & Rodin, J. (1981) Human eating behaviour: A critical review of studies in normal weight and overweight individuals. *Appetite* 2, 293–329.

Steiner, J.E. (1987) What the neonate can tell us about umami. In: Kawamura, Y. & Kare, M.R. (eds) *Umami: a Basic Taste*, pp. 97–123. Marcel Dekker: New York.

Stellar, E. & Shrager, E.E. (1985) Chews and swallows and the microstructure of eating. *American Journal of Clinical Nutrition* 42, 973–982.

Stunkard, A.J. & Kaplan, D. (1977) Eating in public places: a review of the direct observation of eating behaviour. *International Journal of Obesity* 1, 89–101.

Stunkard, A.J. & Messick, S. (1985) The Three-Factor Eating Questionnaire to measure dietary restraint, disinhibition and hunger. *Journal of Psychosomatic Research* 29, 71–78.

Sunday, S.R. & Halmi, K.A. (1990) The meal as the unit of study of human ingestive behaviour. *Appetite* 14, 65–67.

Toates, F. (1986) *Motivational Systems*. Cambridge: Cambridge University Press.

Tuschl, R.J., Platte, P., Laessle, R.G., Stichler, W. & Pirke, K-M. (1990) Energy expenditure and everyday eating behaviour in healthy young women. *American Journal of Clinical Nutrition* 52, 81–86.

van Strien, T., Frijters, J.E.R., Bergers, G.P.A. & Defares, P.B. (1986) The Dutch Eating Behaviour Questionnaire (DEBQ) for assessment of restrained, emotional, and external eating behaviour. *International Journal of Eating Disorders* 5, 295–315.

Wardle, J. & Beinart, H. (1981) Binge eating: a theoretical review. *British Journal of Clinical Psychology* 20, 97–109.

Weingarten, H.P. (1983) Conditioned cues elicit eating in sated rats: A role for learning in meal initiation. *Science* 220, 431–433.

Weingarten, H.P. (1984) Meal initiation controlled by learned cues: Effects of peripheral cholinergic blockade and cholecystokinin. *Physiology and Behaviour* 32, 403–408.

Weingarten, H.P. (1985) Stimulus control of eating: implications for a two-factor theory of hunger. *Appetite* 6, 387–401.

Weingarten, H.P. & Kulikovsky, O.T. (1989) Taste-to-postingestive consequence conditioning: is the rise in sham feeding with repeated experience a learned phenomenon? *Physiology and Behaviour* 45, 471–476.

Westerterp-Plantagena, M.S., Van den Heuvel, E., Wouters, L. & Ten Hoor, F. (1992) Diet-induced thermogenesis and cumulative intake curves as a function of familiarity with food and dietary restraint in humans. *Physiology and Behaviour* 51, 457–465.

Wirtshafter, D. & Davis, J.D. (1977) Set points and settling points, and the control of body weight. *Physiology and Behaviour* 19, 75–78.

Wooley, O.W., Wooley, S.C., Williams, B.S. & Nurre, C. (1977) Differential effects of amphetamine and fenfluramine on appetite for palatable food in humans. *International Journal of Obesity* 1, 293–300.

Wooley, S.C. & Wooley, O.W. (1973) Salivation to the sight and thought of food: A new measure of appetite. *Psychosomatic Medicine* 35, 136–142.

Wurtman, J.J., Wurtman, R.J., Growdon, J.H., Henry, P., Lipscomb, A. & Zeisel, S.H. (1981) Carbohydrate craving in obese people: suppression by treatments affecting serotoninergic transmission. *International Journal of Eating Disorders* 1, 2–15.

Yeomans, M.R. & Wright, P. (1991) Lower pleasantness of palatable foods in nalmafene-treated human volunteers. *Appetite* 16, 249–259.

....

CHAPTER 6

Energy Expenditure in Humans: the Influence of Activity, Diet and the Sympathetic Nervous System

IAN A. MacDONALD

....

This chapter will consider the basic components of whole-body energy metabolism, including the contributions from physical activity and diet, and the potential regulatory role of the sympathetic nervous system. The main part of the chapter will focus on non-obese individuals, aiming to describe the underlying normal physiology, but the final sections will consider the influence of obesity on energy expenditure.

Energy expenditure: definition and components

Definitions

The various chemical processes which underly the functions of the body require the continuous provision of energy. In most cases, this energy is supplied as high-energy bonds within adenosine triphosphate (ATP), with the amount of ATP available being maintained by the utilization of the major fuels, glucose and fatty acids. Whilst in the short term some fuel utilization and ATP production can occur anaerobically (e.g., by the production of lactate from glucose), the capacity and duration of such provision is limited, and for all practical purposes only the oxidation of the fuels to carbon dioxide and water is of importance. Thus, the overall processes involved in the body's energy metabolism can be summarized by first, the oxidation of fuels producing carbon dioxide, water and ATP (with approximately 60% of the food energy being released as heat during the production of ATP) and second, the utilization of the ATP in the chemical processes of the body. Thus, the energy contained within the fuels (originally the food consumed) is first converted to ATP, or lost as heat, and subsequently utilized in various metabolic processes (Fig. 6.1). This overall process is referred to as energy expenditure, and represents the utilization of food energy to maintain the functions of the body. The close relationship between energy expenditure and the metabolic processes of the body explains why the term metabolic rate is used synonomously with energy expenditure.

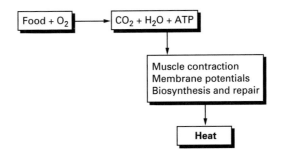

Fig. 6.1 Summary of energy exchanges in the body.

Measurements

The expenditure of energy by the body requires the consumption of oxygen, and leads to the production of carbon dioxide and release of heat (as a by-product of the chemical reactions). Thus, whole-body energy expenditure can be assessed by making calorimetric measurements, i.e., measuring heat released. To do this directly requires complex, expensive equipment (a direct calorimeter) and is only appropriate in closely defined, experimental conditions. An alternative, more widely used approach is to assess energy expenditure using indirect calorimetry, calculating energy expenditure from the rates of oxygen use and carbon dioxide production. The advantage of such measurements of respiratory gas exchange is that an assessment can also be made of which fuel (i.e., carbohydrate or fat) is being used as a substrate for energy metabolism. The disadvantage of indirect calorimetry is the need for either a respiratory valve and noseclip (for exercising subjects) or a ventilated canopy for resting subjects. A respiration chamber can be used for both resting and exercising measurements, the complexity and expense being less than for a direct calorimeter. A more extensive account of the principles of indirect calorimetry and methods of measurement can be found in Frayn and Macdonald (1997) and Murgatroyd *et al.* (1993).

An important principle in relation to energy expenditure and substrate utilization relates to the differences in oxygen utilization and energy release for the different macronutrients. Table 6.1 illustrates the major differences, showing the more than twofold difference in energy released per gram of nutrient during the oxidation of fat compared with carbohydrate or protein, and that for the *same* energy expenditure a greater oxygen uptake is needed when using fat as a fuel compared to carbohydrate. The other major difference between the substrates is the ratio of carbon dioxide produced to oxygen consumed—the respiratory quotient (RQ). Thus, measurement of respiratory gas exchange enables energy expenditure to be estimated, and the RQ value provides an indication of the principal substrate(s) being utilized.

Table 6.1 Summary of oxidation of the macronutrients. Adapted from Frayn and Macdonald (1997).

Glucose
1 g glucose + 0.747 lO_2 = 0.747 lCO_2 + 0.6 g H_2O + 15.15 kJ
RQ = 1.0
Energy content = 15.56 kJ
Energy release = 20.83 kJ/lO_2

Triglyceride
1 g fat + 2.023 lO_2 = 1.436 lCO_2 + 1.07 g H_2O + 39.63 kJ
RQ = 0.71
Energy content = 39.63 kJ/g
Energy release = 19.59 kJ/lO_2

Protein
1 g protein + 1.031 lO_2 = 0.859 lCO_2 + 0.403 g H_2O + (urea, ammonia
    and creatinine) + 19.72 kJ
RQ = 0.833
Energy content = 19.72 kJ/g
Energy release = 19.13 kJ/lO_2

The traditional approaches of using direct or indirect calorimetry techniques to determine energy expenditure can be of limited use in longer-term studies, or for measuring free-living energy expenditure. This problem can be overcome by using the doubly-labelled water technique (using the non-radioactive isotopes deuterium, and 18-oxygen) to assess total energy expenditure of a period of 10–14 days in adults (for review see Prentice, 1988). This technique is based on the principle that the metabolic processes of the body involve the incorporation of water in a number of reactions. When such reactions occur the oxygen from the water will end up as carbon dioxide (and be lost from the body in expired air) whereas the hydrogen will end up as water and be lost in sweat, urine and as respiratory water vapour. The rate of incorporation of water into these metabolic pathways is proportional to the rate of whole-body energy metabolism, so a measurement of the differential loss of oxygen and hydrogen labels from an initial, 'doubly-labelled' loading dose provides an estimate of the body's rate of carbon dioxide production, and thus oxygen consumption, over the period of measurement (see Murgatroyd *et al.*, 1993, for a more detailed account). The disadvantages of the doubly-labelled water method are the duration and cost of the measurements, and the inability of the technique to determine what fuel mix is being used. The former problems can be overcome with the 'bicarbonate–urea' method (Elia *et al.*, 1995), which produces valid estimates of total energy expenditure over a period of 2–3 days, involving the measurement of 14-carbon appearance in urinary urea. This method is relatively inexpensive, but does involve administering a radioactive substance (admittedly in very small amounts).

Components of energy expenditure

Whole-body energy expenditure can be separated into a number of components, with the major distinctions being between rest and activity (Fig. 6.2). The actual distribution of total energy expenditure between these two components obviously depends on the level of physical activity. In sedentary, non-obese individuals the energy expended in physical activity accounts for only 20–40% of total energy expenditure (Ravussin *et al.*, 1986), whilst this proportion can be even less in obese individuals.

RESTING ENERGY EXPENDITURE

Fasting, resting metabolic rate

Resting energy expenditure can be subdivided into a number of separate components, as illustrated in Fig. 6.2, and is usually referred to as resting metabolic rate (RMR). The fasting RMR, measured after an overnight fast and a period of at least 30 minutes supine rest, is a more appropriate assessment of someone's baseline level of metabolism than trying to determine their basal metabolic rate (BMR). The latter is of little value when considering energy metabolism in relation to obesity, and is an expression which should not be used. The fasting RMR includes the expenditure of energy for maintaining membrane potentials, resting cardiorespiratory function, basal rates of turnover

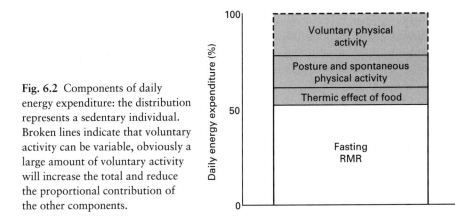

Fig. 6.2 Components of daily energy expenditure: the distribution represents a sedentary individual. Broken lines indicate that voluntary activity can be variable, obviously a large amount of voluntary activity will increase the total and reduce the proportional contribution of the other components.

of proteins, and maintenance of body temperature. The main determinants of fasting RMR are body size and composition, in particular the size of the fat-free mass (FFM) which is of course where the metabolic processes occur. Thus, the larger a person is, the greater their fasting RMR will be. Whilst the size of the FFM is the major determinant of fasting RMR, there may also be an influence of fat mass, age and sex, and these four factors can together account for approximately 80% of the variation in fasting RMR seen between individuals (Rising *et al.*, 1994). However, it is clear that FFM is the most important determinant of fasting RMR, as Segal *et al.* (1989) showed that in young men (thus, removing influences of age and gender) when differences in FFM were taken into account by analysis of covariance, there was no residual effect of fat mass, even though their subjects had a wide range of fat masses.

In general, fasting RMR is approximately 90 J/kg FFM/min. Thus, someone weighing 75 kg, with a FFM of 63 kg (i.e., 15% fat), will have a fasting RMR of approximately 5.7 kJ/min. Some variation in the metabolic activity of the FFM does occur, as a consequence of differences in the composition of the FFM (Elia, 1992). Thus, someone with a larger proportion of their FFM as muscle will tend to have a lower fasting RMR/kg FFM than someone who had a greater proportion as visceral organs, brain and heart (which have a higher metabolic activity than resting muscle).

Food ingestion

The consumption of food is associated with an increase in energy expenditure and oxygen consumption. This was first observed over 200 years ago by Lavoisier, and since then has been described by a number of terms. The most appropriate terms for this process are the thermic effect of food (TEF) and dietary (or diet-induced) thermogenesis (DIT). Thermogenesis literally means heat production, and so can be equated with energy expenditure. However, it is most appropriately used to represent conditions in which energy expenditure is stimulated above baseline. The term TEF is most appropriately used when considering the increase in metabolism associated with a single meal, and can be measured in resting subjects using indirect calorimetry with a ventilated canopy. DIT should really be used to describe the longer-term effects on total energy expenditure of a given dietary intake, i.e., it is that component of 24-hour energy expenditure associated with the amount and composition of the food consumed. Thus, DIT can be reduced during periods of under-feeding, or when consuming a high-fat diet, or increased during over-feeding, especially with a high carbohydrate intake.

The thermic effect of food: influences of meal size and composition. A major problem when trying to draw conclusions about possible differences in thermogenic responses to different-sized meals is the duration of the responses. Large meals (in excess of 4 MJ) can stimulate energy expenditure for several hours, making it very difficult to determine the total responses. There is some evidence that small meals produce smaller overall thermogenic responses than large meals, but in many cases the conclusions may not be reliable because of inappropriate study designs. For example, Tai *et al.* (1991) compared the thermogenic responses over a 5-hour period to a single, 3.1 MJ meal, or to six 0.52 MJ meals eaten at 30-minute intervals. The overall thermogenic response over the 5 hours was less with the six small meals, but this is likely to be in part due to the intermittent nature of the measurements, and the failure to measure the total response to the multiple small meals. Similarly, Vaz *et al.* (1995) found a smaller thermogenic response over 2 hours to three 1.05 MJ meals consumed in the first 60 minutes, compared to a single 3.15-MJ meal at the start of the 2 hours. However, neither responses were maximal by 2 hours, and measurements of energy expenditure were only made for 10–12 minutes in every 30. Thus, it would be unsafe to conclude that for the same total energy intake, a series of small meals are associated with a smaller thermogenic response than a single large meal.

It appears that meal type affects the TEF, with solid food producing a greater response than homogenized liquids with the same nutrient content (Brondel & Le Blanc, 1985). This has been attributed to the solid food being more palatable, producing a hedonistic response that increases the activation of the sympathetic nervous system (SNS). However, whilst we have recently confirmed this effect of solid food (compared with a liquid test meal), we did not find an accompanying enhancement of the plasma noradrenalin response (an index of the SNS) to the test meal (Habas & Macdonald, 1997).

It is widely believed that the TEF is greater when consuming a high-carbohydrate meal than after a meal high in fat. This is partly based on the demonstrations that administration of glucose (either orally or intravenously) stimulates energy expenditure by the equivalent of 7–10% of the amount of glucose stored (Thiebaud *et al.*, 1983a) but triglyceride infusion only produces an increase in energy expenditure equivalent to 2% of the fat stored (Thiebaud *et al.*, 1983b). However, these effects are not always apparent when food is ingested, as Kinabo and Durnin (1990) found no difference in the TEF over 5 hours when meals with 70% carbohydrate or 65% fat were compared.

The types of carbohydrate and fat ingested may also have significant effects on the TEF. Oral ingestion of fructose produces a greater thermogenic response than the same amount of glucose (Tappy *et al.*, 1986), but it is less clear whether similar effects occur when mixed nutrient test meals are used. Meals containing saturated fat appear to produce a lower TEF than meals containing medium-chain triglyceride (Scalfi *et al.*, 1991). It has recently been shown that substitution of 6 g visible fat by fish oil for a period of 3 weeks was accompanied by an increase in fasting energy expenditure and fat oxidation (Couet *et al.*, 1997). Further work is needed to establish the effect of diet composition on energy expenditure.

Diet-induced thermogenesis: effects on total energy expenditure. With normal diets, eaten in sufficient quantities to satisfy energy requirements, the overall stimulation of energy expenditure is equal to 8–10% of the energy intake (Schutz *et al.*, 1984). Thus, an individual with a fasting RMR of 4 kJ/min remaining supine and fasting for 24 hours would use 5.76 MJ of energy. In order to maintain energy balance, the individual would require an energy intake equivalent to 110% of this (6.34 MJ) because of the amount of energy expended in DIT. Thus, it should be obvious that a low total energy intake will be associated with a lower DIT, and thus a small total energy expenditure. This contributes to the reduction in energy expenditure seen with negative energy balance. An excessive total energy intake can lead to increased DIT and total energy expenditure, especially if carbohydrate is eaten to excess. However, this is unlikely to occur with the modest degrees of overeating which are likely to contribute to the development of obesity.

Growth

Growth in children involves numerous complex chemical processes which have a substantial energy cost. Protein synthesis and turnover alone account for approximately 25% of fasting RMR in healthy adults. The increased protein deposition occurring during growth has an additional energy cost and contributes to the elevated energy expenditure seen during growth spurts in children.

Cold

There is no doubt that in many animal species (e.g., rats), chronic exposure to the cold is associated with an increase in energy expenditure. During the early stages of cold exposure, energy expenditure increases due to shivering, but in the rat this is soon replaced by non-shivering mechanisms of increased energy expenditure (non-shivering thermogenesis).

   Exposure of human beings to the cold will produce an increase in energy expenditure due to shivering. Vigorous shivering can raise energy expenditure at least fourfold above baseline, resting values. There is some controversy over the effects of cold exposure on non-shivering energy expenditure in humans. There is some evidence of increased thyroid hormone function and sleeping energy expenditure in non-obese women exposed to mild cold (Lean *et al.*, 1988), which may represent a stimulation of non-shivering thermogenesis. In addition, Bruck *et al.* (1976) showed that 10 days of continued exposure to mild/moderate cold was associated with an increase in fasting, resting energy expenditure. However, this effect was small (10–15%) compared to the effect seen in cold-adapted rodents, and was only observed in those subjects demonstrating adaptation to the cold by a lowering of the core temperature threshold needed to elicit a shivering response.

PHYSICAL ACTIVITY

As mentioned earlier, the majority of the population is now so sedentary that physical activity only accounts for approximately 30% of total daily energy expenditure. This has undoubtedly contributed to the increased incidence of obesity in recent years, and low levels of physical activity are also a separate identified risk factor for the occurrence of cardiovascular disease. Thus, increased levels of physical activity are important for promoting health, and as part of the necessary lifestyle strategy needed to reduce the chances of developing obesity. This section will focus on the latter, considering the levels of energy expenditure associated with different types of physical activity, and also assessing the potential effects of regular physical activity on resting energy expenditure and weight control.

At the simplest level, activity-related energy expenditure can be defined as any situation which raises energy expenditure above the resting supine or seated level. Thus, maintaining an upright posture requires a higher energy expenditure than when seated, and the difference is usually 20–50% of the seated value. Any type of activity which is weight bearing (e.g., walking, running, climbing) requires an energy expenditure which is proportional to body-weight and speed of movement. By contrast, activities such as swimming, rowing and to some extent cycling, are less affected by body-weight. Table 6.2 shows approximate energy expenditures for standard activities, although the actual value for any individual is dependent on his or her body-weight, and how the exercise is performed. One of the effects of learning an activity and performing it regularly is that improvements can be made in the effectiveness (or efficiency) of movements, so that a slightly lower energy expenditure is needed for the same activity. However, this effect is fairly modest, and is unlikely to alter the energy expenditure by more than a few per cent.

Consideration of the values presented in Table 6.2 show the potential effect

Table 6.2 Energy costs of physical activities. Values are kJ/min for a non-obese 70-kg individual.

Sleeping	4.5
Sitting	5.0
Standing	6.0
Brisk walking (6.4 km/hr)	30
Running (8 km/hr)	43
Cycling (16 km/hr)	30
Swimming (25 m/min)	28

of different levels of physical activity on energy expenditure. If a 70-kg individual with an inactive total daily energy expenditure of 9 MJ, increased his or her activity levels by walking for 30 minutes every day at 6.4 km/hr, this would require the expenditure of an additional 750 kJ (i.e., 30 kJ/min for exercise – 5 kJ/min resting value) × 30 minutes. Thus, this would only increase total daily energy expenditure by 8%. Obviously if the individual walked or ran faster, for longer, uphill, or carrying a load, this would increase the energy costs.

Types of physical activity

The simplest distinction which can be made is to separate the types of activity into those which occur due to aerobic metabolic pathways, and those which require anaerobic mechanisms of energy release. The latter are the short-duration, high-intensity types of activity such as sprinting (e.g., running for a bus) or running up the stairs. These types of activity have very high rates of energy expenditure (over 100 kJ/min) but can only be sustained for a few seconds. Thus, the total amount of energy expended is small. In addition, because the immediate energy release is anaerobic (usually with the production of lactate) it takes several minutes to recover from the metabolic disturbances produced. This anaerobic type of activity is of little value in relation to the control of body-weight, although it may be of value in relation to developing and maintaining muscle mass.

Aerobic types of physical activity are of much greater importance for total daily energy expenditure, and the prevention and treatment of obesity. When describing an individual's capacity for aerobic activity, the term maximal oxygen uptake ($\dot{V}O_2$ max) is widely used. This is usually expressed as mlO_2/kg body-weight (or sometimes kg FFM)/min, and describes the maximum rate an individual can sustain for at least 1 minute. Sedentary individuals with low $\dot{V}O_2$ max will usually have values ranging from 30–40 ml/kg/min, whilst those with high levels of physical activity and a high $\dot{V}O_2$ max can have values exceeding

60 ml/kg/min. When one considers that a non-obese individual would have a fasting, resting energy expenditure of approximately 75 J/kg/min (equivalent to 3.8 ml O_2/kg/min), if his or her $\dot{V}O_2$ max was 35 ml/kg/min the individual would be exhausted when increasing energy expenditure by less than 10-fold above resting.

Physical activity at a large proportion of $\dot{V}O_2$ max (above 70%) cannot be maintained for long periods of time, except in those who are physically highly trained. However, provided someone becomes accustomed to being active, lower intensities of effort (40–60% $\dot{V}O_2$ max) can be sustained for extensive periods of time (up to several hours). Under these conditions, physical activity can make a substantial contribution to total energy expenditure, especially if the person's $\dot{V}O_2$ max is reasonably high. For example, a 75-kg individual with a $\dot{V}O_2$ max of 45 ml/kg/min would consume approximately 300 l of oxygen if exercising at 50% of this maximum for 3 hours, which is the equivalent of 6 MJ (1 litre of oxygen leading to the release of approximately 20 kJ of energy). If the individual remained at rest for those 3 hours, the energy expenditure would have been 1 MJ. Thus, sustained recreational activities such as walking or cycling can be associated with a substantial energy expenditure.

Fuel utilization during activity

It has been known for many years that high-intensity activity requires a continuous supply of carbohydrate to the exercising muscles, whilst lower-intensity exercise can be sustained through the oxidation of fatty acids (for review see Astrand & Rodahl, 1977). At exercise intensities below 50% of an individual's $\dot{V}O_2$ max, oxidation of fat is the major source of energy, whilst activity above this intensity requires a greater contribution from carbohydrate. Thus, if increased physical activity is to be used as part of a lifestyle strategy to prevent or treat obesity, it is usually of benefit to use lower-intensity activities which maximize the rates of fat oxidation. There have been some suggestions that obese individuals are characterized by an alteration in the fibre-type profile within their skeletal muscles, such that they have a reduced capacity for oxidizing fat (Wade et al., 1990), but this is a controversial topic which has not been confirmed by subsequent studies. It is clear that increasing the level of habitual physical activity (training) can improve fat utilization at a given exercise intensity, and as most obese individuals are physically inactive, this will reduce the level of fat utilization during activity.

Physical activity and resting energy expenditure

There has been substantial debate for many years as to whether the level of physical activity, or training, can affect resting energy expenditure. It is well established that prolonged, high-intensity exercise can elevate resting energy expenditure for several hours but it is less clear whether regular exercise training, or increased habitual physical activity, has a similar effect. In a cross-sectional study, Broeder *et al.* (1992a) could find no relationship between $\dot{V}O_2$ max and resting energy expenditure (per kg FFM), although it is interesting to note that the subjects with the lowest $\dot{V}O_2$ max had the highest percentage body fat content. An associated study from the same authors (Broeder *et al.*, 1992b) could find no effect of 12 weeks of increased physical activity, which increased $\dot{V}O_2$ max by 10% on resting energy expenditure of young men. However, an interesting observation from this study was that the trained subjects showed small reductions in body fat content, indicative of a slight negative energy balance over the study period. Normally, negative energy balance is associated with a reduction in resting energy expenditure, but the exercise-trained subjects did not show such a reduction. By contrast, Poehlman *et al.* (1991) found a weak relationship between resting energy expenditure and $\dot{V}O_2$ max in non-obese young women, even when body composition was taken into account.

Physical activity, energy balance and body-weight

One argument against the use of increased physical activity as a means of regulating energy balance is that it will stimulate energy intake. However, many studies have now shown that when subjects change from a sedentary lifestyle to moderate degrees of physical activity, there is no increase in energy intake. The study by Broeder *et al.* (1992b) provides an example of this, where 1 hour of exercise, 4 days per week for 12 weeks was not accompanied by any increase in voluntary food intake. Obviously, very high levels of physical activity need to be accompanied by an appropriate energy intake, with a high-carbohydrate diet being of particular importance when high-intensity exercise is performed.

The other benefit of increased physical activity is as an adjunct to dietary modification for weight loss in obesity. Obviously if increased activity is added to a certain dietary energy deficit, then theoretically a greater negative energy balance and more body fat loss should be achieved. However, of greater importance is that the combination of diet and exercise produces a greater loss of body fat (but not FFM) than diet alone (Kempen *et al.*, 1995). Furthermore, Racette *et al.* (1995) showed that increasing physical activity level improved the ability of obese subjects to comply with a dietary restriction programme.

Mechanisms and sites of thermogenesis and sympathetic nervous system

There are numerous thermogenic mechanisms, including substrate cycling, mitochondrial uncoupling in brown adipose tissue and increased sodium pump activity, the details of which are beyond the scope of this chapter. However, it is worthwhile considering which tissues and organs may be important sites of thermogenesis (i.e., increased resting energy expenditure) in adult humans, and what role the SNS may have in regulating their metabolic activity.

Thermogenic stimuli

It has been known for over 60 years that the catecholamines noradrenalin and adrenalin can stimulate resting energy expenditure in humans (Cori & Buchwald, 1930). The plasma adrenalin threshold for stimulating energy expenditure is just above normal resting adrenalin concentrations (Macdonald et al., 1985) with mild stimuli such as postural change and mental arithmetic, being capable of raising the concentrations above this threshold. Maximal stimulation of energy expenditure (25–30% above resting) occurs when adrenalin concentrations rise to five- to 10-fold above basal. It was originally thought that catecholamine-induced thermogenesis was due to a stimulation of lipolysis in adipose tissue and increased fat oxidation (Steinberg et al., 1964) but it is now clear that at steady state there is a generalized stimulation of metabolism with increased fat and carbohydrate oxidation and little change in RQ. In association with this, it is clear that many tissues of the body are involved in the thermogenic response to catecholamines, with skeletal muscle and the viscera being particularly important (for review see Webber & Macdonald, 1993).

It is possible that some of the nutrient-induced thermogenesis discussed earlier is due to a stimulatory effect of catecholamines, as in some circumstances the β-adrenoceptor antagonist propranolol can reduce the energy expenditure response to glucose (Acheson et al., 1983) or to food (Astrup et al., 1990).

However, it is of interest that not all nutrients produce thermogenic responses in the same tissues or organs. Intravenous infusion of amino acids increases whole-body energy expenditure by 19%, with half of the effect occurring in the splanchnic tissues (Aksnes et al., 1995). By contrast, the stimulation of energy expenditure due to oral ingestion of fructose or glucose has no effect on the splanchnic tissues (Brundin & Wahren, 1993).

The sympathetic nervous system

Since the demonstration by Landsberg and Young (1978) of reduction in SNS activity during fasting in rats, there has been great interest in the possibility that altered sympathoadrenal control of metabolism and thermogenesis may contribute to the development of obesity. Furthermore, sympathomimetics which stimulate energy expenditure are viewed as of potential therapeutic value for obese individuals. However, review of the literature on the assessment of sympathoadrenal activity in the obese yields conflicting information, with similar numbers of studies showing reduced, unchanged or increased SNS activity in obese compared to lean subjects (Young & Macdonald, 1992). Interestingly, this review provided clearer evidence of reduced adrenal medullary activity in the obese, and the implications of this for energy expenditure deserve further attention. A recent extension to this review (Macdonald, 1995) revealed an altered relationship between an index of SNS activity (muscle sympathetic nerve activity) and resting energy expenditure in Pima Indians, indicating that the development of obesity in this group may be associated with a defective SNS influence on metabolism.

Whilst there is some evidence of a link between SNS activation and the TEF response to a meal, especially in younger but not older subjects (Schwartz et al., 1990), the administration of a β-adrenoceptor antagonist does not always reduce the TEF response (Nacht et al., 1987). However, we have recently observed an effect of diet composition on fasting plasma noradrenalin concentrations (an index of SNS activity) and the responses to meal ingestion, such that high-sucrose diets and test meals produce larger responses than high starch or high fat (Raben et al., 1997). In addition, the high-sucrose diet was associated with a greater 24-hour energy expenditure than the other two diets. Thus, further studies are needed to examine the influence of diet composition on any SNS effect on energy expenditure.

Some caution is needed when considering the possible use of sympatho-mimetics to stimulate energy expenditure in the obese, because undesirable cardiovascular effects may occur. It is clear that catecholamine stimulation of energy expenditure in humans is mediated by β-adrenoceptors, with some debate as to the dominant receptor subtype (β_2 or β_3). However, the concern is that any generalized activation of the SNS or release of adrenalin from the adrenal medulla has the potential of producing stimulation of the heart (β_1-adrenoceptors) or of increasing blood pressure due to α-adrenoceptor effects causing arterial vasoconstriction. Thus, any pharmacological approach needs to be selective for effects on energy expenditure, in order that undesirable side-effects are avoided.

Obesity and energy expenditure

Given that obesity can only develop as a consequence of a prolonged period of positive energy balance, a reduction in energy expenditure can theoretically contribute to weight gain. For many years there was a widely held view that very low resting energy expenditures may be a cause of obesity. However, it is now clear that such low resting energy expenditures only occur in severe hypothyroidism, and that this is a negligible cause of obesity. The advent of respiration chamber and doubly-labelled water techniques for the measurement of 24-hour energy expenditure has shown that the obese do not have reduced resting or total energy expenditures compared to non-obese subjects. In fact, because the obese are larger, with a greater FFM, than the non-obese they usually have a greater total energy expenditure, expressed per person (Welle *et al.*, 1992). This higher total energy expenditure is usually accompanied, in weight-stable obese subjects, by a fasting resting energy expenditure per kg FFM which is the same as that seen in non-obese subjects.

That the development of obesity requires a prolonged period of positive energy balance is easily demonstrated by considering the amounts of energy involved. Table 6.3 compares the body composition of a non-obese 70-kg individual and a 100-kg obese person. The difference in total body fat (26.6 kg) is equivalent to 1037 MJ of stored energy. If the non-obese person's total energy expenditure was 10 MJ/day, with a positive energy balance of +10% of this (1 MJ/day) it would take at least 3 years to increase body-weight and fat content to those of the 100-kg person. In reality, most cases of obesity probably develop over a longer period of time with a smaller daily positive energy balance. The recent increased incidence of obesity in the U.K. has occurred at a time when the total energy intake of the population has fallen (Prentice & Jebb, 1995), indicating the important contribution that low energy expenditure is likely to have. Recent prospective studies in the Pima Indians (a group with a high predisposition to the development of obesity), have shown that in adults a low 24-hour energy expenditure is associated with a high weight gain over the

Table 6.3 Body composition and body energy content.

	Non-obese	Obese
Weight (kg)	70	100
Fat mass (kg)	8.4	35
% body-weight	12	35
Fat energy (MJ)	327	1365
FFM (kg)	61.6	65
Glycogen (kg)	1	1
CHO energy (MJ)	16	16
Protein (kg)	15	16
Protein energy (MJ)	255	272
Total energy (MJ)	598	1653
Fat energy as % total	55	83

next 2 years (Ravussin *et al.*, 1988). Similar observations have been made in infants (Roberts *et al.*, 1988) and children (Griffiths *et al.*, 1990), although in all cases the lower energy expenditure does not statistically account for more than 40% of the weight gain. Subsequent observations on the Pima Indians showed that in males (but not females), weight gain was associated with a lower energy expenditure associated with spontaneous physical activity (Zurlo *et al.*, 1992).

Thus, a low 24-hour energy expenditure, due at least in part to low physical activity, is a risk factor for weight gain and the development of obesity. The weight-stable obese do not have a low energy expenditure, if anything it is elevated, but physical activity makes a smaller contribution to total energy expenditure than in the non-obese. Whilst there is evidence of reduced TEF responses to meals in the obese, this is probably secondary to their insulin resistance and possibly the insulating effect of the adipose tissue (Brundin *et al.*, 1992). Weight reduction to non-obese values is almost always associated with a normalization of these reduced TEF responses (Bukkens *et al.*, 1991; Tataranni *et al.*, 1994).

References

Acheson, K.J., Jequier, E. & Wahren, J. (1983) Influence of β-adrenergic blockade on glucose induced thermogenesis in man. *Journal of Clinical Investigation* 72, 893–902.

Aksnes, A.K., Brundin, T., Hjeltnes, N. & Wahren, J. (1995) Metabolic, thermal and circulatory effects of intravenous infusion of amino acids in tetraplegic patients. *Clinical Physiology* 15, 377–396.

Astrand, P.O. & Rodahl, K. (1977) *Textbook of Work Physiology*, 2nd edn. New York: McGraw-Hill.

Astrup, A., Christensen, N.J., Simonsen, L. & Bulow, J. (1990) Effects of nutrient intake on sympathoadrenal activity and thermogenic mechanisms. *Journal of Neuroscience Methods* 34, 187–192.

Brondel, I. & Le Blanc, J. (1985) Role of palatability on meal-induced thermogenesis in human subjects. *American Journal of Physiology* 248, E333–E336.

Broeder, C.E., Burrhus, K.A., Svanevik, L.S. & Wilmore, J.H. (1992a) The effects of aerobic fitness on resting metabolic rate. *American Journal of Clinical Nutrition* 55, 795–801.

Broeder, C.E., Burrhus, K.A., Svanevik, L.S. & Wilmore, J.H. (1992b) The effects of either high-intensity resistance or endurance training on resting metabolic rate. *American Journal of Clinical Nutrition* 55, 802–810.

Bruck, K., Baum, E. & Schwennicke, H.P. (1976) Cold-adaptive modifications in man induced by repeated short-term cold exposures and during a 10-day and night cold exposure. *Pflugers Archives* 363, 125–133.

Brundin, T. & Wahren, J. (1993) Whole body and splanchnic oxygen consumption and blood flow after oral ingestion of fructose or glucose. *American Journal of Physiology* 264, E504–E513.

Brundin, T., Thörne, A. & Wahren, J. (1992) Heat leakage across the abdominal wall and meal-induced thermogenesis in normal-weight and obese subjects. *Metabolism* 41, 49–55.

Bukkens, S.G.F., McNeill, G., Smith, J.S. & Morrison, D.C. (1991) Postprandial thermogenesis in post-obese women and weight matched controls. *International Journal of Obesity* 15, 147–154.

Cori, C.F. & Buchwald, K.W. (1930) Effect of continuous injection of epinephrine on the carbohydrate metabolism, basal metabolism and vascular system of normal man. *American Journal of Physiology* **95**, 71–78.

Couet, C., Delarue, J., Ritz, P., Antoine, J-M. & Lamisse, F. (1997) Effect of dietary fish oil on body fat mass and basal fat oxidation in healthy adults. *International Journal of Obesity* **21**, 637–643.

Elia, M. (1992) Organ and tissue contribution to metabolic rate. In: Kinney, J.M. & Tucker, H.N. (eds) *Energy Metabolism: Tissue Determinants and Cellular Corollaries*, pp. 61–79. New York: Raven Press.

Elia, M., Jones, M.G., Jennings, G. *et al.* (1995) Estimating energy expenditure from the specific activity of urine urea during lengthy subcutaneous infusion of $NaH^{14}CO_3$. *American Journal of Physiology* **269**, E172–E182.

Frayn, K.N. & Macdonald, I.A. (1997) Assessment of substrate and energy metabolism *in vivo*. In: Draznin, B. & Rizza, R. (eds) *Clinical Research in Diabetes and Obesity*, Vol. 1, pp. 101–124. Totoura, NJ: Humana Press.

Griffiths, M., Payne, P.R., Stunkard, A.J., Rivers, J.P.W. & Cox, M. (1990) Metabolic rate and physical development in children at risk of obesity. *Lancet* **336**, 76–77.

Habas, E.M.M.A. & Macdonald, I.A. (1998) Metabolic and cardiovascular responses to a liquid and solid test meal. *British Journal of Nutrition*, in press.

Kempen, K.P.G., Saris, W.H.M. & Westerterp, K.R. (1995) Energy balance during an 8-wk energy restricted diet with and without exercise in obese women. *American Journal of Clinical Nutrition* **62**, 722–729.

Kinabo, J.L. & Durnin, J.V.G.A. (1990) Thermic effect of food in man: effect of meal composition and energy content. *British Journal of Nutrition* **74**, 37–44.

Landsberg, L. & Young, J.B. (1978) Fasting, feeding and the regulation of the sympathetic nervous system. *New England Journal of Medicine* **298**, 1295–1301.

Lean, M.E.J., Murgatroyd, P.R., Rothnie, I., Reid, I.W. & Harvey, R. (1988) Metabolic and thyroid responses to mild cold are abnormal in obese and diabetic women. *Clinical Endocrinology* **28**, 665–673.

Macdonald, I.A. (1995) Advances in our understanding of the role of the sympathetic nervous system in obesity. *International Journal of Obesity* **19** (suppl. 7), 52–57.

Macdonald, I.A., Bennett, T. & Fellows, I.W. (1985) Catecholamines and the control of metabolism in man. *Clinical Science* **68**, 613–619.

Murgatroyd, P.R., Shetty, P.S. & Prentice, A.M. (1993) Techniques for the measurement of human energy expenditure: a practical guide. *International Journal of Obesity* **17**, 549–568.

Nacht, C.A., Christin, L., Temler, E., Chiolero, R., Jequier, E. & Acheson, K. (1987) Thermic effect of food: possible implication of parasympathetic nervous system. *American Journal of Physiology* **253**, E481–E488.

Poehlman, E.T., Viers, H.F. & Detzer, M. (1991) Influence of physical activity and dietary restraint on resting energy expenditure in young, non-obese females. *Canadian Journal of Physiology and Pharmacology* **69**, 320–326.

Prentice, A.M. (1988) Applications of the doubly labelled water ($^2H_2^{18}O$) method in free-living adults. *Proceedings of the Nutrition Society* **47**, 259–268.

Prentice, A.M. & Jebb, S.A. (1995) Obesity in Britain, gluttony or sloth. *British Medical Journal* **311**, 437–439.

Raben, A., Macdonald, I.A. & Astrup, A. (1997) Replacement of dietary fat by sucrose or starch: Effects on 14 days' *ad libitum* energy intake, energy expenditure and body weight in formerly obese and non-obese subjects. *International Journal of Obesity* **21**, 846–859.

Racette, S.B., Schoeller, D.A., Kushner, R.F. & Neil, K.M. (1995) Exercise enhances dietary compliances during moderate energy restriction in obese women. *American Journal of Clinical Nutrition* **62**, 345–349.

Ravussin, E., Lillioja, S., Anderson, T.E., Christin, L. & Bogardus, C. (1986) Determinants of 24-hour energy expenditure in man: methods and results using a respiratory chamber. *Journal of Clinical Investigation* **78**, 1568–1578.

Ravussin, E., Lillioja, S., Knowles, W.C. *et al.* (1988) Reduced rate of energy expenditure as a risk factor for body weight gain. *New England Journal of Medicine* **318**, 467–472.

Rising, R., Harper, I.T., Fontvieille, A.M., Ferraro, R.T., Spraul, M. & Ravussin, E. (1994) Determinants of total daily energy expenditure: variability in physical activity. *American Journal of Clinical Nutrition* **59**, 800–804.

Roberts, S.B., Savage, J., Coward, W.A., Chew, B. & Lucas, A. (1988) Energy expenditure and intake in infants born to lean and overweight mothers. *New England Journal of Medicine* **318**, 461–466.

Scalfi, L., Coltorti, A. & Contaldo, F. (1991) Post-prandial thermogenesis in lean and obese subjects after meals supplemented with medium-chain and long-chain triglycerides. *American Journal of Clinical Nutrition* **53**, 1130–1133.

Schutz, Y., Bessard, T. & Jequier, E. (1984) Thermogenesis measured over a whole day in obese and non-obese women. *American Journal of Clinical Nutrition* **40**, 542–552.

Schwartz, R.S., Jaeger, L.F. & Veith, R.C. (1990) The thermic effect of feeding in older men: the importance of the sympathetic nervous system. *Metabolism* **39**, 733–737.

Segal, K.R., Lacayanga, I., Dunaif, A., Gutin, B. & Pi-Sunyer, F.X. (1989) Impact of body fat mass and percent fat on metabolic rate and thermogenesis in men. *American Journal of Physiology* **256**, E573–E579.

Steinberg, D., Nestel, P.J., Buskirk, E.R. & Thompson, R.H. (1964) Calorigenic effect of norepinephrine correlated with plasma free fatty acid turnover and oxidation. *Journal of Clinical Investigation* **43**, 167–176.

Tai, M.M., Cartillo, P. & Pi-Sunyer, F.X. (1991) Meal size and frequency: effect on the thermic effect of food. *American Journal of Clinical Nutrition* **54**, 783–787.

Tappy, L., Randin, J.P., Felber, J.P. *et al.* (1986) Comparison of thermogenic effect of fructose and glucose in normal humans. *American Journal of Physiology* **250**, E718–E724.

Tataranni, P.A., Mingrone, G., Greco, A.V. *et al.* (1994) Glucose-induced thermogenesis in post-obese women who have undergone biliopancreatic diversion. *American Journal of Clinical Nutrition* **60**, 320–326.

Thiebaud, D., Schutz, Y., Acheson, K. *et al.* (1983a) Energy cost of glucose storage in human subjects during glucose–insulin infusions. *American Journal of Physiology* **244**, E216–E221.

Thiebaud, D., Acheson, K., Schutz, Y. *et al.* (1983b) Stimulation of thermogenesis in men after combined glucose, long-chain triglyceride infusion. *American Journal of Clinical Nutrition* **37**, 603–611.

Vaz, M., Tunet, A., Kingwell, B. *et al.* (1995) Postprandial sympathoadrenal activity: its relation to metabolic and cardiovascular events and to changes in meal frequency. *Clinical Science* **89**, 349–357.

Wade, A.J., Marbut, M.M. & Round, J.M. (1990) Muscle fibre type and aetiology of obesity. *Lancet* **335**, 805–808.

Webber, J. & Macdonald, I.A. (1993) Metabolic actions of catecholamines in man. *Baillière's Clinical Endocrinology and Metabolism* **7**, 393–413.

Welle, S., Forbes, G.B., Statt, M., Barnard, R.R. & Amatruda, J.M. (1992) Energy expenditure under free-living conditions in normal weight and overweight women. *American Journal of Clinical Nutrition* **55**, 14–21.

Young, J.B. & Macdonald, I.A. (1992) Sympathoadrenal activity in human obesity: heterogeneity of findings since 1980. *International Journal of Obesity* **16**, 959–967.

Zurlo, F., Ferraro, R., Fontvieille, A.M., Rising, R., Bogardus, C. & Ravussin, E. (1992) Spontaneous physical activity and obesity: cross-sectional and longitudinal studies in Pima Indians. *American Journal of Physiology* **263**, E296–E300.

CHAPTER 7

Substrate Fluxes in Skeletal Muscle and White Adipose Tissue and their Importance in the Development of Obesity

KEITH N. FRAYN AND LUCINDA K.M. SUMMERS

Metabolic importance of skeletal muscle and white adipose tissue

Skeletal muscle makes up 40% of body-weight in 'reference man' and rather less (30%) in 'reference woman' (Snyder, 1975). In trained athletes, skeletal muscle may contribute up to 65% of body mass (Spenst *et al.*, 1993). Even at rest, skeletal muscle metabolism plays a major role in whole-body energy fluxes simply by virtue of its bulk. During exercise the metabolic flux in skeletal muscle may increase enormously and skeletal muscle metabolism dominates whole-body energy fluxes.

Skeletal muscle is the major reservoir of carbohydrate, in the form of glycogen, in the body. A typical liver glycogen content in the fed state is around 100 g, whereas whole-body skeletal muscle contains about 400 g typically, and may contain much more under certain conditions (Acheson *et al.*, 1988). It is therefore reasonable to suppose that skeletal muscle plays a major role in the regulation of the metabolic disposal of carbohydrate in the body. This role is accentuated under some conditions by the high rates of glucose oxidation in skeletal muscle. However, the role of skeletal muscle in lipid metabolism should not be underestimated. Whilst skeletal muscle does not appear to release lipids, it plays a major role in the removal from the bloodstream of non-esterified fatty acids (NEFA) both at rest (particularly in the fasting state) and during exercise. It is also an important site of the removal of plasma triacylglycerol (TAG) in the postprandial period.

Skeletal muscle plays an important role in amino acid metabolism. Intracellular concentrations of some amino acids are several-fold greater than those in plasma, and again by virtue of its mass, skeletal muscle constitutes the largest reservoir of free amino acids in the body (Bergström *et al.*, 1974). Skeletal muscle also contains the largest amount of protein of any single tissue in the body, and although its rate of protein turnover is slower than that of some smaller organs, the absolute rate of turnover is the largest in the body (Daniel *et al.*, 1977).

The oxygen consumption of skeletal muscle at rest, expressed per unit of tissue weight, is not as high as that of some other organs (e.g., liver 60 ml O_2/min/kg wet weight; resting skeletal muscle 4 ml O_2/min/kg wet weight; Frayn, 1992), but once again because of its mass it is one of the major consumers of oxygen in the whole body. Variations in skeletal muscle oxygen consumption have been shown to make a major contribution to the between-person variability in resting energy expenditure (Zurlo et al., 1990).

In comparison with skeletal muscle, white adipose tissue contributes a smaller proportion of body-weight in non-obese subjects: 20% in 'reference man' and 30% in 'reference woman' (Snyder, 1975). However, as the sole source of NEFA, one of the most important plasma energy-bearing fuels, the contribution of white adipose tissue to whole-body energy fluxes is of major importance. In trained athletes the proportion of adipose tissue is smaller than in non-athletes (typically 9–12% of body-weight in males and females; Björntorp, 1991a), but it still plays a key role in the supply of NEFA to exercising muscle. In obesity the amount of adipose tissue may, of course, increase enormously. Although this excessive adipose tissue may not be so metabolically active as in lean subjects, by virtue of its mass it exerts powerful influences on whole-body energy fluxes.

The important role of adipose tissue in regulation of delivery of NEFA into the plasma is clear, but adipose tissue also plays an important part in the regulation of plasma TAG concentrations, due both to the crucial role of NEFA delivery in determining hepatic TAG secretion rates, and to the ability of adipose tissue to extract TAG fatty acids especially during the postprandial period. In contrast, it is clear that adipose tissue plays only a small role in whole-body glucose disposal (Mårin et al., 1992). The importance of white adipose tissue in whole-body amino acid metabolism is not entirely clear, although for some amino acids it may approach that of skeletal muscle (Frayn et al., 1991).

The metabolism of brown adipose tissue is different in most respects from that of white adipose tissue and since its contribution to whole-body energy fluxes in adult humans is probably small, it will not be covered in this chapter.

Both skeletal muscle and white adipose tissue are distributed in discrete sites throughout the body. These sites are not homogeneous in their metabolic characteristics. Muscles vary in their oxidative capacity, although in humans (as opposed to rodents) all skeletal muscles are of mixed fibre type (Johnson et al., 1973). Clearly during exercise there are muscle-specific differences in metabolism since different muscles are recruited to different extents, and this implies that there is local regulation of skeletal muscle metabolism. In the case of adipose tissue, the differences between depots in their metabolic characteristics may be quite marked and may be relevant to their role in whole-body energy metabolism. These site-specific properties will be discussed later in this chapter and elsewhere in this book (see Chapter 8), but it is important at this stage to note the large body of evidence which links the accumulation of intra-abdominal adipose tissue with adverse metabolic changes in obesity (Kissebah & Krakower, 1994). Unfortunately, because the intra-abdominal fat depots are not accessible for direct study, our knowledge of them comes only from *in vitro* studies on the metabolic properties of samples removed at operation. Most of the metabolic properties of adipose tissue discussed below are therefore based on studies of subcutaneous adipose tissue, which is accessible for study *in vivo* (Arner & Bülow, 1993).

The metabolic pathways of skeletal muscle (Jones & Round, 1990; Henriksson, 1995) and adipose tissue (Crandall & DiGirolamo, 1990; Hollenberg, 1990; Frayn *et al.*, 1995b), and their regulation in different states, have been discussed in detail elsewhere. The theme of this chapter will be the main fluxes of energy-bearing fuels in these tissues, and their contributions to whole-body energy fluxes. Because our emphasis will be on energy metabolism, we will say little about amino acid and protein metabolism, although we do not wish to minimize its importance. We will outline the normal metabolic contributions of these tissues in the whole body, and then discuss whether alterations in skeletal muscle or adipose tissue metabolism may underlie the development of obesity. Since evidence on this question is weak, we will devote more space to a consideration of the consequences of obesity on skeletal muscle and adipose tissue metabolism, and show how such consequences may lead in turn to many of the adverse metabolic characteristics associated with obesity.

Role of skeletal muscle and adipose tissue in normal daily energy fluxes

Humans on a typical Western diet in which fat provides around 40% of energy eat around 300 g of carbohydrate and 100 g fat (mainly TAG) per day. (Clearly these are round figures, for illustration only.) Since we eat most of this in three main meals, a 'typical' meal might contain around 100 g carbohydrate and 30–40 g fat.

The free glucose content of the body in the postabsorptive state is around 12 g. (The plasma glucose concentration is 5 mmol/L or about 0.9 g/L, and the extracellular fluid volume about 20% of body-weight or 13 litres.) Therefore at one meal we eat enough glucose to raise the plasma glucose concentration around eightfold. In normal people, however, the rise is more like 60–80% of basal. There are powerful homeostatic mechanisms which minimize the excursions of plasma glucose concentration. These mechanisms include rapid suppression of endogenous hepatic glucose production, together with increased glucose disposal into cells. As we will show, skeletal muscle metabolism switches rapidly in the postprandial state from almost complete independence from carbohydrate, to rapid glucose uptake, such that skeletal muscle is undoubtedly the major extrahepatic tissue involved in this coordinated regulation of glucose metabolism. The contribution of white adipose tissue is very small in comparison.

A very similar argument can be made for TAG fluxes. In a normal individual the extracellular TAG is confined to the plasma volume (around 3 litres at 1 mmol/L or 0.85 g/L, i.e., 2.5–3 g extracellular TAG). We eat enough TAG in a typical meal to raise our plasma TAG concentration at least 10-fold. Again this does not happen; a typical postprandial excursion in plasma TAG concentration is more like 50–60% of the fasting concentration. This must also imply the existence of coordinated mechanisms for regulating the delivery of endogenous TAG to the circulation, and stimulating TAG clearance. These have been much less studied than those responsible for glucose homeostasis, particularly the regulation of hepatic TAG secretion in the postprandial period (because of the methodological difficulties of such experiments), but it is clear that peripheral tissues are responsible for most of the increased TAG clearance in the postprandial period. Amongst these, skeletal muscle and adipose tissue play major roles. The role of skeletal muscle appears to be very variable from person to person, and greatest in the highly endurance-trained individual. It may be much less in the habitually sedentary person. In non-athletes the role of adipose tissue appears to be larger than that of skeletal muscle, and this may be understood metabolically on the basis that insulin (released in the postprandial period) activates adipose tissue lipoprotein lipase (LPL), the key enzyme in plasma TAG clearance. Adipose tissue also plays a key role in overall lipid homeostasis since a major and dramatic effect of meal ingestion is to suppress intra-adipocyte TAG hydrolysis and thus the release of NEFA from adipose tissue. The rate of supply of NEFA to the liver is a major determinant of hepatic TAG secretion, and reduction in adipose tissue NEFA release is an important component of the suppression of hepatic TAG secretion by insulin *in vivo* (Cummings *et al.*, 1995).

It is important to realize that metabolic regulation in tissues such as skeletal muscle and adipose tissue is not simply a matter of fine-tuning metabolic pathways: even during the normal daily pattern of meal ingestion and fasting overnight, there are major and dramatic switches in the patterns of metabolism and the fluxes through pathways. This is clearly illustrated in Fig. 7.1, which also illustrates one important methodological approach to investigation of these regulatory mechanisms.

Since there can be no doubt that obesity represents a state of disturbed energy fluxes and storage, it is very reasonable to consider that disturbances in these highly regulated pathways of energy metabolism in skeletal muscle

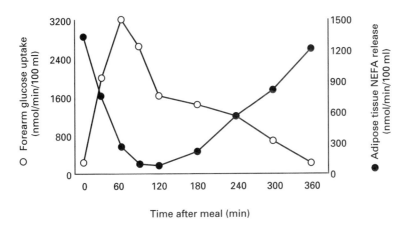

Time after meal (min)

Fig. 7.1 Major metabolic fluxes in skeletal muscle (glucose uptake) and white adipose tissue (NEFA release) in the overnight-fasted state, and their responses to ingestion of a mixed meal. Changes of several-fold are observed within 60–90 minutes of meal ingestion. Fluxes were estimated by selective venous catheterization with measurement of arteriovenous differences and blood flow. Data taken from the studies reported in Coppack *et al.* (1990, 1996) with the addition of further subjects for NEFA release.

and adipose tissue might underlie the development of obesity. It is also easy to imagine that, if such disturbances develop as a result of obesity, they might have widespread and potentially adverse metabolic consequences.

Skeletal muscle

Routes of adenosine triphosphate synthesis in skeletal muscle: outline and methodology

Skeletal muscle is a major site of adenosine triphosphate (ATP) turnover in the body, especially during exercise. During a marathon run the mass of ATP turned over in skeletal muscle alone exceeds total body mass several-fold. Clearly skeletal muscle has very efficient pathways for regeneration of ATP.

The main sources of free energy for ATP synthesis in skeletal muscle are anaerobic glycolysis, and the complete oxidation of both carbohydrate and fatty acids. Amino acid oxidation also plays an important role, especially oxidation of the branched-chain amino acids valine, leucine and isoleucine: in humans, these are largely completely oxidized within skeletal muscle. These substrates arise from the circulation (plasma glucose, NEFA, TAG-fatty acids and amino acids), from the intramuscular stores of glycogen and TAG, and from muscle protein. These sources of substrate are illustrated in Fig. 7.2. Typical muscle contents of glycogen and of TAG are difficult to define (since there is considerable

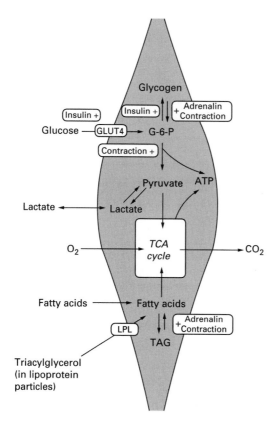

Fig. 7.2 Major routes of ATP generation in skeletal muscle. Each arrow may represent more than one step in a pathway. Glucose uptake is mainly by the insulin-regulatable transporter GLUT4 in the fed state but GLUT1 may play an important role in the fasting state. The contribution of amino acids to oxidative metabolism is not shown for simplicity. 'Contraction' refers to stimulation of muscle contraction, which is coordinated with metabolism via a number of intracellular mediators including intracellular Ca^{2+}. G-6-P, glucose 6-phosphate; LPL, lipoprotein lipase; TAG, triacylglycerol; TCA cycle, tricarboxylic acid (Krebs) cycle. Reproduced from Frayn (1996) with permission.

variability between muscles, between nutritional states and between individuals) but some representative figures are collated on Table 7.1.

The relative contributions of extramuscular and intramuscular sources of fuel have been the subject of much research although there are many methodological difficulties in such studies. For instance, the contribution of intramuscular TAG during exercise has been estimated in several studies by sequential biopsy of the muscles involved. The results are not consistent, due in part to the fact that skeletal muscle TAG concentrations are extremely variable even from site to site within a single muscle (Frayn, 1980). Recently a novel approach has been used in which the contribution of plasma NEFA to oxidative metabolism is estimated by the infusion of a labelled NEFA tracer to measure plasma NEFA turnover, while whole-body fat oxidation is measured by indirect calorimetry, and the difference is assumed to reflect oxidation of intramuscular TAG fatty acids on the basis that, during exercise, all fatty acids removed from plasma are oxidized (Romijn et al., 1993). However, this technique does not distinguish intramuscular TAG fatty acids from those arising from plasma (lipoprotein) TAG. Muscle biopsy techniques have been more informative on

Table 7.1 Typical glycogen and TAG contents of human skeletal muscle.

	Low-carbohydrate diet	Mixed diet	High-carbohydrate diet	Reference
Glycogen				
(g/kg wet wt)	10	20	30–40	Bergström et al. (1967)
(kJ/kg wet wt)	170	340	510–680	
Typical whole-body store (MJ)	4.25	8.5	15	(assumes 25 kg muscle)
TAG				
(mmol/kg wet wt)		15		Collated from a number of sources: range from Phillips et al. (1996)
		(range 1–100)		
(kJ/kg wet wt)		450		
		(range 30–3000)		
Typical whole-body store (MJ)		11		(assumes 25 kg muscle)

the utilization of muscle glycogen during exercise and a reasonably consistent picture of glycogen depletion during exercise and repletion thereafter has been built up (Coyle, 1995). Recently muscle glycogen deposition in the resting state after a meal has been studied by the technique of carbon-13 nuclear magnetic resonance (NMR) spectroscopy (Taylor *et al.*, 1993).

A technique which has provided a great deal of consistent information on skeletal muscle substrate utilization is the 'glucose clamp' (De Fronzo *et al.*, 1979). In this technique, glucose is infused intravenously, usually against a background of insulin infusion at a constant rate to raise the plasma insulin concentration to some predetermined level (hyperinsulinaemic clamp). The rate of glucose infusion is varied as necessary to keep the plasma glucose concentration, measured regularly at the bedside, constant within narrow limits: hence the plasma glucose concentration is 'clamped'. Under these conditions the rate of glucose disappearance from the plasma must equal the rate of glucose entry, which is known (since it is being infused). Any contribution from hepatic glucose release is usually small under these conditions although it may be estimated by additional infusion of a labelled glucose tracer. The technique therefore provides a means for assessing whole-body glucose utilization at controlled plasma insulin concentrations, and thus gives a measure of whole-body 'insulin sensitivity': it is usually regarded as providing the 'gold standard' assessment of this parameter. If indirect calorimetry is performed at the same time, the whole-body rate of carbohydrate oxidation can be assessed. It is usually found that under hyperinsulinaemic conditions glucose oxidation increases and accounts for around 20–30% of the total glucose disposal rate (DeFronzo *et al.*, 1981, Felber *et al.*, 1993). The remainder reflects 'non-oxidative glucose disposal', sometimes called glucose storage, although anaerobic glycolysis will also be included in this portion. This technique may be combined with selective catheterization of the venous drainage of skeletal muscle, usually that of the forearm. This allows the estimation of glucose uptake by a specific muscle, and — making assumptions about the uniformity of the muscle mass — by skeletal muscle to the whole body. Such studies show that the contribution of skeletal muscle in whole-body glucose disposal during hyperinsulinaemia is a major one (70–85%; DeFronzo *et al.*, 1981; Yki-Järvinen *et al.*, 1987). A corollary is that skeletal muscle is the tissue which predominantly 'sets' the insulin sensitivity of glucose metabolism in the whole body.

Carbohydrate metabolism in skeletal muscle at rest and during exercise

It has been known since the forearm venous catheterization experiments of Andres, Zierler and colleagues in the 1950s that the main oxidative fuel of skeletal muscle after an overnight fast at rest must be lipid: the respiratory quotient measured across the forearm is around 0.76 (Baltzan et al., 1962). Plasma glucose disposal by skeletal muscle in that state is therefore small. The rate of anaerobic glycolysis of glucosyl units from both plasma glucose and muscle glycogen also appears to be small: net release of lactate from resting skeletal muscle after an overnight fast is close to zero, and inconsistent (Jackson et al., 1987).

This picture changes rapidly, however, after a meal. In the postprandial state the increased plasma glucose and insulin concentrations lead to increased glucose uptake by muscle, mainly by the insulin-regulatable glucose transporter GLUT4, and to increased glucose disposal within the muscle cell by coordinated regulation of the pathways of glycogen deposition, glycolysis and pyruvate oxidation. Skeletal muscle rapidly begins to dominate the extrahepatic disposal of glucose in the body. The glucose taken up from the plasma by muscle is either oxidized or stored as glycogen, with some being released as lactate. Measurements made by selective venous catheterization suggest that around 25% (Elia et al., 1988; Kelley et al., 1988; Coppack et al., 1990) to 45% (Jackson et al., 1987) of an oral glucose load (whether given as a pure glucose load or as part of a mixed meal) is disposed of by resting skeletal muscle during the 4–6-hour postprandial period. Direct measurements of muscle glycogen deposition by 13-carbon-NMR spectroscopy show muscle glycogen content increasing by around 25%; net glycogen deposition in muscle during the 7 hours following a mixed meal accounted for around 20% of that ingested (Taylor et al., 1993).

In resting subjects, therefore, the role of skeletal muscle in whole-body carbohydrate metabolism in the fasted state is small, but in the fed state it is extremely important and dominates that of extrahepatic tissues.

During exercise the situation changes even more dramatically. During light exercise (25% $\dot{V}O_2$ max) there is little mobilization of muscle glycogen, but glucose uptake, oxidation and conversion to lactate are stimulated. In this condition whole-body glucose turnover increases initially about 50% and it seems likely that all this increase is directed to skeletal muscle (Romijn et al., 1993). The major point of regulation of increased glucose uptake in this condition is not clear, but muscle vasodilatation with increased glucose delivery may be a major factor. Plasma insulin concentrations do not change during light exercise, although there is some evidence for acute recruitment of additional GLUT4 transporters (Rodnick et al., 1992).

During heavier exercise (e.g., 65% $\dot{V}O_2$ max), muscle glycogen breakdown is stimulated and glucosyl residues from this source are a major fuel for anaerobic and oxidative metabolism. Plasma glucose utilization is also increased and lactate may thus be recycled via hepatic gluconeogenesis. Whole-body glucose turnover increases to more than three times its resting value after 2 hours of exercise at this intensity, and again this is largely taken up by skeletal muscle (Romijn *et al.*, 1993). Whole-body glucose oxidation measured by indirect calorimetry may increase by about 12-fold (Romijn *et al.*, 1993) and most of this must be accounted for by skeletal muscle; at 85% $\dot{V}O_2$ max glucose oxidation increases about 30-fold. Metabolic and physiological adjustments bringing about this increased carbohydrate oxidation include increased cardiac output and muscle vasodilatation, vastly increasing glucose delivery to working muscle, and the coordinated regulation, via changes in intracellular Ca^{2+} and P_i concentrations, of contraction and of glycogenolysis (reviewed in Frayn, 1996). During moderate or heavy exercise skeletal muscle is therefore by far the dominant tissue in glucose disposal in the body.

Lipid metabolism in skeletal muscle at rest and during exercise

The size of the intramuscular TAG store does not appear to fluctuate greatly during normal daily life except during exercise. Whilst it may turn over, it is not therefore a net contributor to muscle fatty acid oxidation at rest. In the overnight fasted state muscle extracts both NEFA and lipoprotein-TAG fatty acids from the plasma. As in adipose tissue, the key enzyme in plasma TAG extraction is lipoprotein lipase (LPL) bound to the skeletal muscle capillary endothelium. This enzyme is more active in oxidative compared with glycolytic muscles, and it is activated by training. Selective venous catheterization clearly demonstrates that TAG extraction does occur (Kiens & Lithell, 1989; Potts *et al.*, 1991). Nevertheless, measurements of plasma TAG extraction by muscle are difficult to make and we lack much information on the magnitude and metabolic importance of this process. In contrast, the extraction of plasma NEFA by muscle has been much studied usually by a combination of tracer infusion and selective venous catheterization (Capaldo *et al.*, 1994). At rest, in the overnight fasted state, NEFA extraction from plasma appears to provide most of the fatty acids required for oxidation. (Whether these fatty acids pass through an intramuscular TAG pool before oxidation is not clear: older evidence for such a pathway (Dagenais *et al.*, 1976) has recently been challenged (Sidossis *et al.*, 1995).) The rate of fatty acid extraction from the plasma by skeletal muscle appears under most circumstances to be limited by their delivery in plasma, i.e., by the product of muscle blood flow and the plasma NEFA concentration (Soop *et al.*, 1988).

The rate of uptake of fatty acids by skeletal muscle is also a determinant of their oxidation, since the muscle TAG pool is of relatively constant size. The oxidation of fatty acids is linked to that of glucosyl units by mechanisms described by Randle and colleagues in the 1960s (summarized in Randle *et al.*, 1963). Essentially the products of fatty acid oxidation (acetyl-CoA, citrate) exert inhibitory feedback control over the rate of glucose uptake and oxidation. This link has received most attention in pathological states although there is also evidence for it operating in normal daily life (Piatti *et al.*, 1991).

In the period following a meal, fatty acid utilization by skeletal muscle decreases rapidly as glucose uptake and oxidation become the more important processes. There is no clear mechanism whereby increased availability of glucose or insulin might reduce NEFA uptake or fatty acid oxidation. Instead it seems that control is exerted at the level of NEFA release from adipose tissue, which is rapidly reduced after a meal (see Fig. 7.1).

During exercise muscle NEFA utilization increases dramatically. Plasma NEFA are the major fuel for exercise at low intensity (25% $\dot{V}O_2$ max) (Romijn *et al.*, 1993). At greater intensities of exercise they are also important, but other fuel sources are more important at least for the first 2 hours or so. After that these other sources (e.g., muscle glycogen) are depleted, and the ultra-endurance athlete utilizes again almost entirely plasma NEFA as a fuel. Considering the size of the adipose tissue TAG store, this seems entirely sensible.

The extraction of plasma TAG-fatty acids by muscle has been little explored, as mentioned above. Again, whilst it may not occur at a high rate per unit mass of skeletal muscle, the bulk of skeletal muscle means that its contribution to whole-body plasma TAG clearance may be substantial. The activity of skeletal muscle LPL is increased considerably by training, and training is also associated with a marked improvement in fat tolerance (the increase in plasma TAG concentration following a fat load, also called postprandial lipaemia). It has been suggested that plasma TAG-fatty acids extracted by skeletal muscle serve mainly to replenish the intramuscular TAG pool (Oscai *et al.*, 1990). Skeletal muscle LPL is suppressed by insulin (Farese *et al.*, 1991), in contrast to adipose tissue in which LPL is activated by insulin. This suggests that adipose tissue plays a more important role than skeletal muscle in clearance of plasma TAG in the postprandial state. This may not be accurate, because the suppression of skeletal muscle LPL by insulin is not very marked, and the bulk of skeletal muscle — particularly in an athlete in whom muscle LPL is particularly active — may give it an equally, or even more important, role. The situation probably differs considerably between individuals.

It is usually considered that plasma TAG fatty acids make only a small contribution to oxidative fuel metabolism during exercise. This seems to be true for exercise carried out in the fasting state in which plasma TAG is mainly present as very-low-density lipoprotein (VLDL)-TAG. However, it is possible that the situation is different after a meal containing fat (Griffiths *et al.*, 1994; Henriksson, 1995). Chylomicron-TAG is a better substrate for muscle LPL than is VLDL-TAG (Potts *et al.*, 1991) and there is some evidence for marked TAG clearance from postprandial plasma by exercising muscle (Ruys *et al.*, 1989; Griffiths *et al.*, 1994). In addition, if the marked improvement in fat tolerance evident in highly trained subjects does indeed reflect improved TAG clearance by skeletal muscle, then this again suggests more than a modest contribution to muscle fatty acid delivery. However, more work is needed in this area.

Disturbances in skeletal muscle metabolism and the development of obesity

In principle, disturbances of a number of aspects of muscle metabolism might impinge upon the development of obesity. Since skeletal muscle is such an important site for the ultimate oxidation of energy-bearing substrates, any impairment of muscle oxidative metabolism will lead to the accumulation of bodily energy stores. Because skeletal muscle oxygen consumption is a major determinant of resting metabolic rate, it has been suggested that differences between individuals in muscle oxidative capacity might play a role in the pathogenesis of obesity (Zurlo et al., 1990).

In practice, evidence for specific impairments of muscle metabolism in subjects at risk of developing obesity, or in the post-obese, is slight. The impairment of fatty acid oxidation in skeletal muscle apparent in obese subjects (Blaak et al., 1994a,b; Colberg et al., 1995) might be a causal factor in the development of obesity, but until there is clear evidence for the direction of cause and effect it is difficult to interpret such findings. It is interesting, however, that this impairment was not reversed by weight reduction, whereas some other aspects of muscle metabolism were, such as glucose uptake and lactate release (Blaak et al., 1994b).

One of the marked consequences of obesity (discussed in greater detail below) is the development of insulin resistance. In skeletal muscle this is evidenced by low rates of glucose uptake during hyperinsulinaemic clamp, and most studies of obesity and of non-insulin-dependent diabetes mellitus (NIDDM) show that the main defect, under these specific conditions, is in glucose storage (i.e., glycogen synthesis) rather than glucose oxidation (Bonora et al., 1993). This finding has been extended by looking at glycogen synthetase activation in muscle biopsies and cultured fibroblasts from non-diabetic relatives of subjects with NIDDM. Although glycogen synthetase activation in such samples is indeed insulin resistant (Schalin Jantti et al., 1992; Wells et al., 1993) it is difficult to know whether this represents cause or effect, since such relatives are themselves already insulin resistant (Schalin Jantti et al., 1992).

It is even more difficult to know whether any such defect in insulin sensitivity could be a cause of obesity. In fact, in prospective studies of weight change over several years, those most at risk of gaining weight are those showing better insulin sensitivity (Swinburn et al., 1991; Hoag et al., 1995). This has been interpreted in terms of insulin resistance tending to favour fat oxidation over that of glucose, and thus helping to maintain a favourable fat balance (Eckel,

1992). Therefore, a change in skeletal muscle predisposing to the development of obesity might be more in the direction of increased sensitivity to insulin. This seems counter-intuitive and may be an over-interpretation of prospective data. Against the prospective data, and in favour of insulin resistance in muscle as a primary defect, is the demonstration that transgenic mice with targeted disruption of insulin sensitivity only in skeletal muscle accumulate body fat and display some of the dyslipidaemic characteristics of obesity (Moller *et al.*, 1996).

It is known that in obese subjects postprandial skeletal muscle blood flow is reduced (Baron *et al.*, 1990). Impaired muscle blood flow, either resting, postprandially, during exercise or in all these states might predispose to obesity. Since muscle blood flow delivers substrates such as glucose, NEFA and TAG to the muscle tissue, defects in muscle blood flow regulation might well have important effects leading to the development of insulin resistance and the laying down of adipose tissue TAG stores. However, as yet there has been no prospective work in this area so it is again difficult to determine whether reduced muscle blood flow causes obesity or whether it occurs as a result of the obese state.

Despite the difficulties of determining cause and effect, it can clearly be seen that a reduction in the oxidative capacity of skeletal muscle, whether due to some intrinsic change within the muscle or simply to lack of muscle mass, will lead to low rates of substrate oxidation and thereby to a propensity for positive energy storage. This situation is particularly evident in one situation, that of the sedentary individual. The sedentary lifestyle clearly leads to reduction in muscle mass, in muscle capillary density and thus substrate delivery, and in muscle oxidative capacity. Of course, the sedentary lifestyle also leads to positive energy balance simply on the grounds of reduced energy expenditure, but changes in skeletal muscle metabolism might be seen as the internal means by which this is mediated.

Skeletal muscle metabolism in obesity

The insulin resistance of skeletal muscle in obese subjects was noted in 1961 by Rabinowitz and Zierler (Rabinowitz & Zierler, 1961), who injected insulin into a brachial artery in obese subjects and noted a diminished stimulation of glucose uptake compared with lean controls. The impairment of insulin-stimulated glucose utilization in muscle in obesity is now well recognized (Fig. 7.3). Because of the important role of skeletal muscle in whole-body insulin-mediated glucose disposal outlined earlier, the result is reduced sensitivity to insulin in the whole body. The consequent persistent hyperinsulinaemia may, in turn, lead to down-regulation of insulin-stimulated pathways in other tissues including adipose tissue, as discussed later.

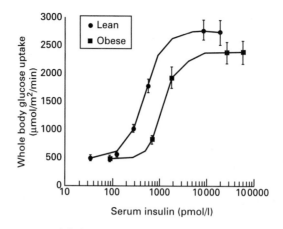

Fig. 7.3 Insulin resistance of skeletal muscle glucose uptake in obesity. Glucose uptake was measured across the leg by femoral venous catheterization and measurement of blood flow, and insulin was infused at increasing rates to construct the dose–response curves. Plasma glucose concentrations were 'clamped' at 5 mmol/L. There is a clear shift to the right of the dose–response curve of glucose uptake against serum insulin concentration in the obese group. Reproduced from Laakso *et al.* (1990a) with permission of Rockefeller University Press.

The relationship between degree of obesity and insulin resistance is not strong (Bogardus *et al.*, 1985). Some of the variability observed, however, undoubtedly reflects variations in fat distribution: it is clear that visceral or upper body fat distribution is more strongly associated with insulin resistance than is lower body fat distribution (Björntorp, 1991b; Kissebah & Krakower, 1994). The impact of NIDDM on insulin sensitivity is much greater than that of obesity (Hollenbeck *et al.*, 1984), although within subjects with NIDDM, the degree of obesity is a major determinant of insulin resistance (Campbell & Carlson, 1993). The latter observation suggests a reason why weight loss can induce marked improvement in glycaemic control in NIDDM (Campbell & Carlson, 1993).

One consistent hypothesis for the development of insulin resistance in obesity is that increased delivery of NEFA to the circulation from the expanded adipose tissue mass (discussed in more detail below) reduces the sensitivity of muscle glucose uptake to insulin by substrate competition. This hypothesis has been fully developed (Felber *et al.*, 1993). There is also evidence that skeletal muscle in obese subjects has an impaired ability to oxidize fatty acids (Blaak *et al.*, 1994a,b, Colberg *et al.*, 1995), and insulin resistance has been correlated with accumulation of intramuscular TAG (Falholt *et al.*, 1988; Phillips *et al.*, 1996). Obese women accrue more fat in their muscle and this is directly related to the degree of insulin resistance, decreased oxidative capacity, increased anaerobic and increased glycolytic capacity (Simoneau *et al.*, 1995).

The cellular mechanisms for the loss of sensitivity to insulin in obesity have been studied both in humans *in vivo* and in animal models. There has been considerable study in animal models of the cellular and molecular mechanisms which may underlie such a change (Chapter 3). In humans, there is a clear impairment of the uptake of glucose across the muscle cell membrane demonstrated by a number of means (Laakso *et al.*, 1990a; Friedman *et al.*, 1992; Kelley *et al.*, 1996). It appears that there is no deficiency in total cellular content of the insulin-regulatable glucose transporter GLUT4, but its translocation to the cell membrane in response to insulin is defective (Friedman *et al.*, 1992; Kelley *et al.*, 1996). In addition, it has been proposed that a defect in insulin-mediated vasodilatation, potentially an important aspect of the stimulation of glucose uptake by insulin, might be involved. This has been demonstrated both during infusion of insulin (Laakso *et al.*, 1990a,b) and during the endogenous hyperinsulinaemia following an oral glucose load (Baron *et al.*, 1990). The cytokine tumour necrosis factor (TNF)-α is over-expressed in adipose tissue in obesity (discussed below), and recently it has been shown that the same is true of skeletal muscle (Saghizadeh *et al.*, 1996). TNF-α expression (mRNA content) in skeletal muscle was negatively related to whole-body insulin sensitivity (Saghizadeh *et al.*, 1996).

The reduction in glucose uptake, at least during conditions of hyper-insulinaemia, reflects impairment of both oxidative and non-oxidative glucose disposal, the latter being much more affected than the former (Felber *et al.*, 1987; Bonora *et al.*, 1993). In obese subjects skeletal muscle has reduced oxidative capacity and increased anaerobic and glycolytic capacities (Simoneau *et al.*, 1995). Skeletal muscle insulin resistance in obesity has been explored in more detail in subjects with NIDDM in addition to obesity, and again it appears that multiple aspects of glucose metabolism are deranged (Kelley *et al.*, 1992).

White adipose tissue

Major metabolic pathways relevant to this chapter in white adipose tissue are outlined on Fig. 7.4.

Adipose tissue carbohydrate metabolism

The uptake of glucose by white adipocytes *in vitro* must be one of the most-studied metabolic processes. Unfortunately there is little evidence that it contributes more than a few per cent to whole-body glucose utilization, and even less that adipose tissue glucose uptake makes a significant contribution to glucose disposal in the postprandial period when it is dwarfed by the

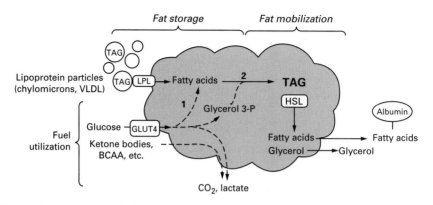

Fig. 7.4 Major routes of fuel metabolism in white adipose tissue. A distinction is made between fuel utilization and the routes of fat storage and fat mobilization. Pathways are (1) *de novo* lipogenesis (not quantitatively important in human white adipose tissue), (2) the phosphatidic acid pathway of fatty acid esterification. BCAA, branched-chain amino acids; HSL, hormone-sensitive lipase. Reproduced from Frayn *et al.* (1995b) with permission of the Nutrition Society.

contribution of skeletal muscle. Adipocytes have a small store of glycogen, whose concentration varies with feeding and fasting (Rigden *et al.*, 1990), but again this cannot be a major contributor to whole-body carbohydrate economy.

The role of glucose in adipocyte metabolism is twofold. First, glucose metabolism (mainly complete oxidation) seems to be the major route of ATP generation in white adipocytes (Frayn *et al.*, 1995b). In addition, in the postprandial period glycolysis provides glycerol 3-phosphate which is needed for esterification of the fatty acids delivered to adipocytes from LPL in the capillaries. It might therefore be expected that adipose tissue glucose uptake would increase at this time, but the proportion of glucose metabolism diverted to glycerol 3-phosphate production even under conditions of extreme stimulation of fat storage (high-fat meal followed by insulin infusion) is only around 20% (Frayn *et al.*, 1994).

Non-esterified fatty acid release from adipose tissue

The rate of release of NEFA from adipose tissue is, as outlined above, the major determinant of the systemic plasma NEFA concentration and thus of the delivery of NEFA to other tissues. As shown in Fig. 7.1, this is a highly regulated process, switching in a short time from its maximal rate in the normal daily pattern to almost zero. These rapid changes in NEFA release reflect regulation of the key enzyme in the hydrolysis of adipocyte TAG, the intracellular enzyme hormone-sensitive lipase (HSL) (see Fig. 7.4). Regulation of HSL is coordinated (inversely) with regulation of the pathway of fatty acid esterification: when HSL is suppressed by insulin, fatty acid esterification is stimulated and fatty acids are effectively trapped in adipocytes.

In normal daily life it appears that most of the regulation of NEFA delivery from adipose tissue reflects the inhibitory effect of insulin on HSL. HSL is stimulated by agents which raise the cellular cyclic adenosine monophosphate (AMP) concentration, particularly β-adrenergic agents, and in the longer term by a number of hormones including growth hormone and cortisol which may either affect enzyme expression, or may modify the sensitivity to catecholamines (e.g., by regulation of adrenoceptor expression). In normal subjects fasted overnight, local introduction of propranolol into subcutaneous adipose tissue has no effect on lipolysis, suggesting that adrenergic stimulation of lipolysis is not operative in this state (Arner *et al.*, 1990). Instead the lipolytic 'tone' against which insulin acts may be set by the normal early morning rise in cortisol (Samra *et al.*, 1996a) and perhaps by growth hormone pulses (Cersosimo *et al.*, 1996).

During exercise, however, there is a marked increase in NEFA delivery from adipose tissue, and this is undoubtedly mediated primarily by β-adrenergic stimulation (Arner *et al.*, 1990). In sustained high-intensity exercise it may be reinforced by a slight fall in the plasma insulin concentration, and by secretion of both cortisol and growth hormone (Hodgetts *et al.*, 1991). Despite these changes, the rate of NEFA delivery does not increase in proportion to the intensity of exercise (Romijn *et al.*, 1993). It seems that adipose tissue perfusion during intense exercise may be inadequate to carry away all the fatty acids released in lipolysis (Bülow, 1993). Evidence for this comes from the sudden release of NEFA which is observed when exercise stops (Hodgetts *et al.*, 1991; Romijn *et al.*, 1993): presumably a sudden relief of relative vasoconstriction allows 'flushing out' of NEFA which have been trapped within the tissue.

Triacylglycerol clearance by adipose tissue

Adipose tissue LPL is least active in the overnight-fasted state, but even in that condition there is significant removal of plasma TAG. In fact systemic plasma TAG concentrations correlate inversely with adipose tissue TAG clearance (Potts *et al.*, 1995), suggesting a role for adipose tissue in 'setting' the fasting plasma TAG concentration. Clearly the rate of hepatic VLDL-TAG secretion is also a determinant of plasma TAG concentrations, but this in turn is regulated largely by the rate of delivery of NEFA from adipose tissue. TAG clearance in skeletal muscle does not relate in such a way to the plasma TAG concentration (Potts *et al.*, 1991).

It has been suggested earlier that adipose tissue may play a particularly important role in TAG clearance in the postprandial period when its LPL is activated by insulin, and possibly by other hormones including those released from the gut in response to feeding (Oben *et al.*, 1992). Adipose tissue extraction of chylomicron-TAG is avid, averaging around 30% of the arterial concentration in a single passage through the tissue (Potts *et al.*, 1991), although we find that this varies considerably from person to person. The quantitative role of adipose tissue in removal of plasma TAG in the postprandial period has been estimated by a number of means. Mårin *et al.* (1990) fed a meal containing 120 g fat labelled with carbon-14-oleic acid and assessed deposition by sequential adipose tissue biopsies. After 24 hours 60 g of this had been deposited in adipose tissue (in a group who had eaten a carbohydrate-rich breakfast), and the figure increased slowly over the next month. Studies with selective venous catheterization suggest that in normal subjects about 35% of the fat load given in a mixed meal is stored in adipose tissue over the subsequent 6 hours (Coppack *et al.*, 1990). The magnitude of postprandial lipaemia is inversely related to the LPL activity measured in plasma following injection of heparin, which releases LPL from its endothelial binding sites (Jeppesen *et al.*, 1995), although this does not distinguish between LPL released from different tissues. Defective activation of adipose tissue LPL is associated with increased postprandial lipaemia (Katzel *et al.*, 1994).

It is important to understand differences in the action of LPL in different tissues. In skeletal muscle it appears that the fatty acids released by the action of LPL on plasma TAG are quantitatively extracted by the muscle: no net 'overspill' of fatty acids is seen during the postprandial period, for instance, when skeletal muscle LPL is active against chylomicron-TAG (Coppack *et al.*, 1990). The fate of these fatty acids is, as outlined earlier, either esterification to replenish the intramuscular TAG pool (ultimately a source for fatty acid oxidation), or direct oxidation. In adipose tissue plasma, TAG extraction by LPL potentially provides the source of fatty acids for deposition as intracellular TAG, the ultimate energy store of the body. This process must be highly regulated, since the body's fat store is so closely related to whole-body energy balance. It is not therefore surprising to find an additional level of control in adipose tissue. LPL-derived fatty acids in adipose tissue are not all taken up by adipocytes for esterification and storage. A proportion appear always to be released into the venous plasma in the form of NEFA (Frayn *et al.*, 1994). So far as is known at present, this role of LPL in delivery of NEFA into the plasma is specific to white adipose tissue. However, regulation of the fate of LPL-derived fatty acids is a key process in regulation of fat storage. In the fasted state there would seem little 'sense' in storage of plasma TAG-derived fatty acids, when the adipocyte itself is liberating fatty acids at a high rate into the plasma. Accordingly, in that state there is almost complete release of LPL-derived fatty acids as NEFA into the plasma

(Frayn *et al.*, 1994). Adipose tissue LPL in the fasted state acts as a generator of plasma NEFA additional to the intracellular HSL, except that the source of fatty acids is hepatic TAG, secreted as VLDL-TAG, rather than adipocyte TAG. In the postprandial period, however, this changes dramatically, with much greater 'capture' of LPL-derived fatty acids for esterification within the adipocytes (although never complete, at least after the relatively normal meals which we have studied) (Frayn *et al.*, 1994; Frayn *et al.*, 1995a). Regulation of fat storage in white adipose tissue therefore primarily involves regulation of LPL, but the fine-tuning is provided by regulation of the pathway of fatty acid uptake and esterification in adipocytes. The regulation of this pathway is becoming clearer. First, it depends upon simultaneous suppression of HSL activity, generating a concentration gradient so that fatty acids flow into, rather than out from, adipocytes. It is stimulated in a positive sense by insulin (Frayn *et al.*, 1994) and by a protein known as acylation-stimulating protein (ASP). ASP is the most potent known stimulator of fatty acid esterification in adipocytes (Sniderman *et al.*, 1997). It is produced locally within adipose tissue by the interaction of three components of the alternate complement pathway (D or adipsin, B and C3), themselves secreted from adipocytes, and this interaction is markedly stimulated by the presence of chylomicrons (Maslowska *et al.*, 1997). Regulation of the fate of LPL-derived fatty acids in adipose tissue is the subject of intense study at present, not least because of the potentially adverse consequences of disturbed regulation of this pathway (Sniderman *et al.*, 1997).

Disturbances in adipose tissue metabolism and the development of obesity

The question has often been posed as to whether alterations in adipose tissue metabolism might lead to a predisposition to obesity. This simple question is extraordinarily difficult to answer, not least because adipose tissue metabolism is so profoundly altered by obesity *per se*, and potentially by a previous history of obesity, that it is virtually impossible to distinguish cause and effect. Nevertheless, there are some very plausible mechanisms whereby particular characteristics of adipose tissue might predispose to obesity.

The theory, once prevalent, that the number of fat cells is determined in infancy and invariant thereafter, suggests that an overweight child may become an overweight adult because the capacity is there, whereas a lean child could not so easily become obese in adulthood. Attractive as this idea is, there is no evidence for it (Ashwell, 1992): in fact, even octagenarians have adipocyte precursors which can differentiate into mature adipocytes (Hauner *et al.*, 1989).

Much attention has centred upon adipose tissue LPL. The idea that over-expression of LPL might provide a stimulus to fat storage has found some favour, not least because many studies show adipose tissue LPL activity to be increased in established obesity (Eckel, 1989). However, it is again extremely difficult to distinguish cause and effect. Because of the complex regulation of fat storage discussed above, it seems unlikely that over-activity of LPL in itself could cause excessive storage. The possibility that disturbed regulation of other components of the fat-storage system, e.g., of the enzymes of fatty acid esterification or of ASP, could lead to excessive fat deposition has not been explored extensively, although it is known that ASP concentrations are increased in obese subjects (Cianflone *et al.*, 1995). It is clear that insulin has a fat-storage promoting effect. Weight gain is a notable feature in insulin-dependent diabetic subjects intensively treated with insulin (DCCT Research Group, 1988). It can easily be seen how insulin could promote fat storage through stimulation of adipose tissue LPL and of the esterification pathway. However, this is difficult to reconcile with the demonstration in prospective studies (discussed earlier) that insulin resistance is associated with protection against weight gain, since hyperinsulinaemia is a marker for such insulin resistance. It may be that the effect of intensive insulin treatment is mediated more via increased energy intake in response to hypoglycaemia. Alternatively, there may be differences between acute and chronic effects of insulin.

In contrast, there is some direct evidence for a role of HSL in susceptibility to obesity. Net fat deposition reflects the balance between two processes: fat mobilization and fat storage. If HSL activity is reduced, then there will be an increase in net fat deposition. This possibility was examined by measurement of HSL activity in adipose tissue biopsies in non-obese first-degree relatives of obese subjects (Hellström *et al.*, 1996); it was found that maximal HSL activity was reduced by about 50% in the relatives, compared to controls with no immediate family history of obesity. In the more physiological setting of responses *in vivo* to a mixed meal or to insulin infusion, there is evidence that in post-obese women (formerly obese women who have reduced their weight to the normal range, and are considered a model of the genetically 'at risk') the ability of insulin to suppress plasma NEFA concentrations is enhanced (Raben *et al.*, 1994; Toubro *et al.*, 1994). Thus, the tendency towards net fat storage would again be enhanced.

Again, it is possible that blood flow plays a part in the development of obesity. Fasting adipose tissue blood flow is decreased in obese subjects as is the postprandial rise (Summers *et al.*, 1996). The mechanism by which reduced blood flow could lead to obesity is not clear and other factors, such as increased ASP production, seem much more likely to predispose to an increase in adipose tissue mass.

In animal models more direct roles for changes in adipose tissue metabolism may be observed. For instance, in the model of rodent obesity produced by lesion of the ventromedial hypothalamus, adipose tissue metabolism remains normally sensitive to insulin (at least as judged by glucose uptake) whilst muscle metabolism becomes insulin resistant, and fuels are diverted to adipose tissue where they are stored as TAG (Pénicaud et al., 1987). The obese (ob/ob) mouse fails to produce the signal molecule leptin in adipose tissue, and since leptin is thought to signal to the hypothalamus both to increase energy expenditure and to decrease food intake, obesity follows (Rohner-Jeanrenaud & Jeanrenaud, 1996). However, it appears that human obesity is characterized more by 'leptin resistance' (elevated plasma leptin concentrations) than by hypoleptinaemia (Considine et al., 1996).

Adipose tissue metabolism in obesity

Obesity involves a disproportionate increase in the amount of adipose tissue relative to other tissues. A notable feature of established obesity is an elevation of the plasma NEFA concentration (Opie & Walfish, 1963). This has been attributed to the increased adipose tissue mass (Flatt, 1972). In fact NEFA release per unit mass of adipose tissue is reduced in obese compared with lean subjects (Lillioja et al., 1986), and a truer picture is probably that fat mass, responsible for NEFA release, expands more than lean body mass, responsible for NEFA clearance. The reduction in NEFA release per unit mass of adipose tissue may be explained in part by the presence of larger adipocytes, the increased volume representing mainly inert TAG in the intracellular droplet. A similar explanation may also apply to the reduction in blood flow per unit mass of adipose tissue which is observed in obesity (Coppack et al., 1992; Blaak et al., 1995; Summers et al., 1996).

In established obesity, adipose tissue acquires many characteristics which could be described as insulin resistance. HSL is not suppressed normally by insulin (Jensen et al., 1989; Coppack et al., 1992), and adipose tissue LPL is not activated normally by insulin (Eckel, 1987; Coppack et al., 1992) (Fig. 7.5). The net effect is that there is a resistance to net fat storage even in the presence of elevated insulin concentrations (Frayn et al., 1996a). Thus, it has been speculated that insulin resistance is an adaptive phenomenon in obesity, which tends to limit further weight gain (Eckel, 1992). This is probably no different from saying that energy requirements in the whole body increase in obesity (Prentice et al., 1986); thus, larger meals are needed to generate fat storage equivalent to that seen in leaner subjects. Insulin resistance of adipose tissue metabolism might then be seen as the metabolic mechanism for readjustment of body fat content (Frayn et al., 1996a).

There are many reasons, however, for supposing that the 'insulin resistance' of adipose tissue metabolism is a major factor underlying the cardiovascular risk of established obesity (Kissebah et al., 1976; Frayn & Coppack, 1992;

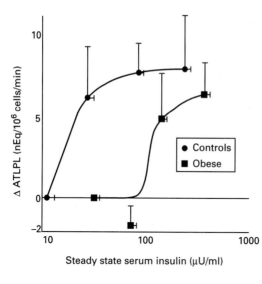

Fig. 7.5 Insulin resistance of the activation of white adipose tissue LPL (ATLPL) in obesity. Dose–response curves were constructed by infusing insulin at different rates in different occasions for 6 hours, and activation of adipose tissue LPL measured as the difference in LPL activity in biopsies taken before and after insulin infusion. Reproduced from Eckel (1987) with permission.

Frayn, 1993). Insulin resistance appears to affect multiple metabolic processes in adipose tissue. Of these, the most studied but perhaps least physiologically relevant is glucose transport: in fact, there is no clear evidence for insulin resistance of glucose utilization in adipose tissue *in vivo* in obesity (Coppack *et al.*, 1996). Other metabolic processes which are responsive to insulin in adipose tissue include suppression of fat mobilization by HSL, activation of LPL and stimulation of the pathway of fatty acid esterification. There is evidence that each of these may become 'insulin resistant' in obesity (reviewed above for HSL and LPL). The net effect may be increased delivery of fatty acids to the circulation, especially in the postprandial period due to failure to entrap fatty acids in adipose tissue. The normal postprandial suppression of systemic plasma NEFA concentrations is attenuated in proportion to the degree of obesity (Summers *et al.*, 1997). The adverse consequences of inappropriate fatty acid delivery in the postprandial period have been reviewed recently (Frayn *et al.*, 1996b; Frayn *et al.*, 1997). In addition there may be impaired clearance of circulating TAG in the postprandial period, due both to failure to activate LPL (Coppack *et al.*, 1992; Potts *et al.*, 1995) and to impaired postprandial vasodilatation in adipose tissue (Summers *et al.*, 1996): substrate delivery is an important component of LPL action (Samra *et al.*, 1996b).

Obesity is characterized by widespread insulin resistance. Since the foremost change in obesity is an accumulation of TAG in adipocytes, it is reasonable to suggest that some factor associated with increased adipose tissue mass leads to the development of insulin resistance in other tissues. One obvious candidate, discussed above, is increased delivery of NEFA to the circulation, since inappropriately elevated NEFA concentrations may induce insulin resistance (Frayn *et al.*, 1996b, 1997). Other candidates have, however, been suggested.

An interesting one is the cytokine, TNF-α. TNF-α is expressed in adipose tissue, and its expression is increased in obesity (Hotamisligil *et al.*, 1995). TNF-α is a powerful inducer of insulin resistance in other tissues including skeletal muscle (Hotamisligil *et al.*, 1994). In animal models of obesity, neutralization of TNF-α with a specific antiserum markedly improves sensitivity to insulin (Hotamisligil *et al.*, 1993). The idea that excessive TNF-α liberation from an expanded adipose tissue mass might explain the widespread insulin resistance of obesity (Hotamisligil & Spiegelman, 1994) is an attractive one, but not yet proven in humans.

Alterations in adipose tissue metabolism in obesity may therefore have profound effects throughout the body. It can certainly be argued that adipose tissue is a key site of the pathogenesis of the diverse metabolic consequences of obesity.

Acknowledgements

We thank our colleagues, past and present, in the Oxford Lipid Metabolism Group for their stimulating discussions of metabolism and obesity and for their contributions to our own experimental work in this area.

References

Acheson, K.J., Schutz, Y., Bessard, T., Anantharaman, K., Flatt, J-P. & Jéquier, E. (1988) Glycogen storage capacity and *de novo* lipogenesis during massive carbohydrate overfeeding in man. *American Journal of Clinical Nutrition* 48, 240–247.

Arner, P. & Bülow, J. (1993) Assessment of adipose tissue metabolism in man: comparison of Fick and microdialysis techniques. *Clinical Science* 85, 247–256.

Arner, P., Kriegholm, E., Engfeldt, P. & Bolinder, J. (1990) Adrenergic regulation of lipolysis *in situ* at rest and during exercise. *Journal of Clinical Investigation* 85, 893–898.

Ashwell, M. (1992) Why do people get fat: is adipose tissue guilty? *Proceedings of the Nutrition Society* 51, 353–365.

Baltzan, M.A., Andres, R., Cader, G. & Zierler, K.L. (1962) Heterogeneity of forearm metabolism with special reference to free fatty acids. *Journal of Clinical Investigation* 41, 116–125.

Baron, A.D., Laakso, M., Brechtel, G., Hoit, B., Watt, C. & Edelman, S.V. (1990) Reduced postprandial skeletal muscle blood flow contributes to glucose intolerance in human obesity. *Journal of Clinical Endocrinology and Metabolism* 70, 1525–1533.

Bergström, J., Hermansen, E., Hultman, E. & Saltin, B. (1967) Diet, muscle glycogen and physical performance. *Acta Physiologica Scandinavica* 71, 140–150.

Bergström, J., Fürst, P., Norée, L-O. & Vinnars, E. (1974) Intracellular free amino acid concentration in human muscle tissue. *Journal of Applied Physiology* 36, 693–697.

Björntorp, P. (1991a) Importance of fat as a support nutrient for energy: metabolism of athletes. *Journal of Sports Sciences* 9, 71–76.

Björntorp, P. (1991b) Metabolic implications of body fat distribution. *Diabetes Care* 14, 1132–1143.

Blaak, E.E., van Baak, M.A., Kemerink, G.J., Pakbiers, M.T., Heidendal, G.A. & Saris, W.H. (1994a) β-adrenergic stimulation of energy expenditure and forearm skeletal muscle metabolism in lean and obese men. *American Journal of Physiology* 267, E306–E315.

Blaak, E.E., van Baak, M.A., Kemerink, G.J., Pakbiers, M.T., Heidendal, G.A. & Saris, W.H. (1994b) β-Adrenergic stimulation of skeletal muscle metabolism in relation to weight reduction in obese men. *American Journal of Physiology* 267, E316–322.

Blaak, E.E., van Baak, M.A., Kemerink, G.J., Pakbiers, M.T.W., Heidendal, G.A.K. & Saris, W.H.M. (1995) β-adrenergic stimulation and abdominal subcutaneous fat blood flow in lean, obese, and reduced-obese subjects. *Metabolism* 44, 183–187.

Bogardus, C., Lillioja, S., Mott, D.M., Hollenbeck, C. & Reaven, G. (1985) Relationship between degree of obesity and *in vivo* insulin action in man. *American Journal of Physiology* 248, E286–E291.

Bonora, E., Bonadonna, R.C., Del Prato, S. *et al.* (1993) *In vivo* glucose metabolism in obese and type II diabetic subjects with or without hypertension. *Diabetes* 42, 764–772.

Bülow, J. (1993) Lipid mobilization and utilization. *Medicine and Sport Science* 38, 158–185.

Campbell, P.J. & Carlson, M.G. (1993) Impact of obesity on insulin action in NIDDM. *Diabetes* 42, 405–410.

Capaldo, B., Napoli, R., Di Marino, L., Guida, R., Pardo, F. & Saccá, L. (1994) Role of insulin and free fatty acid (FFA) availability on regional FFA kinetics in the human forearm. *Journal of Clinical Endocrinology and Metabolism* 79, 879–882.

Cersosimo, E., Danou, F., Persson, M. & Miles, J.M. (1996) Effects of pulsatile delivery of basal growth hormone on lipolysis in humans. *American Journal of Physiology* 271, E123–E126.

Cianflone, K., Kalant, D., Marliss, E.B., Gougeon, R. & Sniderman, A.D. (1995) Response of plasma ASP to a prolonged fast. *International Journal of Obesity* 19, 604–609.

Colberg, S.R., Simoneau, J-A., Thaete, F.L. & Kelley, D.E. (1995) Skeletal muscle utilization of free fatty acids in women with visceral obesity. *Journal of Clinical Investigation* 95, 1846–1853.

Considine, R.V., Sinha, M.K., Heiman, M.L. *et al.* (1996) Serum immunoreactive-leptin concentrations in normal-weight and obese humans. *New England Journal of Medicine* 334, 292–295.

Coppack, S.W., Fisher, R.M., Gibbons, G.F. *et al.* (1990) Postprandial substrate deposition in human forearm and adipose tissues *in vivo*. *Clinical Science* 79, 339–348.

Coppack, S.W., Evans, R.D., Fisher, R.M. *et al.* (1992) Adipose tissue metabolism in obesity: lipase action *in vivo* before and after a mixed meal. *Metabolism* 41, 264–272.

Coppack, S.W., Fisher, R.M., Humphreys, S.M., Clark, M.L., Pointon, J.J. & Frayn, K.N. (1996) Carbohydrate metabolism in insulin resistance: glucose uptake and lactate production by adipose and forearm tissues *in vivo* before and after a mixed meal. *Clinical Science* 90, 409–415.

Coyle, E.F. (1995) Substrate utilization during exercise in active people. *American Journal of Clinical Nutrition* 61 (suppl.), 968S–979S.

Crandall, D.L. & DiGirolamo, M. (1990) Hemodynamic and metabolic correlates in adipose tissue: pathophysiologic considerations. *FASEB Journal* 4, 141–147.

Cummings, M.H., Watts, G.F., Umpleby, A.M. *et al.* (1995) Acute hyperinsulinemia decreases the hepatic secretion of very-low-density lipoprotein apolipoprotein B-100 in NIDDM. *Diabetes* 44, 1059–1065.

Dagenais, G.R., Tancredi, R.G. & Zierler, K.L. (1976) Free fatty acid oxidation by forearm muscle at rest, and evidence for an intramuscular lipid pool in the human forearm. *Journal of Clinical Investigation* 58, 421–431.

Daniel, P.M., Pratt, O.E. & Spargo, E. (1997) The metabolic homoeostatic role of muscle and its function as a store of protein. *Lancet* ii, 446–448.

The DCCT Research Group (1988) Weight gain associated with intensive therapy in the diabetes control and complications trial. *Diabetes Care* 11, 567–573.

DeFronzo, R.A., Tobin, J. & Andres, R. (1979) Glucose clamp technique: a method for quantifying insulin secretion and resistance. *American Journal of Physiology* 237, E214–E223.

DeFronzo, R.A., Jacot, E., Jequier, E., Maeder, J., Wahren, J. & Felber, J.P. (1981) The effect of insulin on the disposal of intravenous glucose. Results from indirect calorimetry and hepatic and femoral venous catheterization. *Diabetes* 30, 1000–1007.

Eckel, R.H. (1987) Adipose tissue lipoprotein lipase. In: Borensztajn, J. (ed.) *Lipoprotein Lipase*, pp. 79–132. Chicago: Evener.

Eckel, R.H. (1989) Lipoprotein lipase. A multifunctional enzyme relevant to common metabolic diseases. *New England Journal of Medicine* 320, 1060–1068.

Eckel, R.H. (1992) Insulin resistance: an adaptation for weight maintenance. *Lancet* 340, 1452–1453.

Elia, M., Folmer, P., Schlatmann, A., Goren, A. & Austin, S. (1988) Carbohydrate, fat, and protein metabolism in muscle and in the whole body after mixed meal ingestion. *Metabolism* 37, 542–551.

Falholt, K., Jensen, I., Lindkaer, J. *et al.* (1988) Carbohydrate and lipid metabolism of skeletal muscle in type 2 diabetic patients. *Diabetic Medicine* 5, 27–31.

Farese, R.V., Yost, T.J. & Eckel, R.H. (1991) Tissue-specific regulation of lipoprotein lipase activity by insulin/glucose in normal-weight humans. *Metabolism* 40, 214–216.

Felber, J-P., Ferrannini, E., Golay, A. *et al.* (1987) Role of lipid oxidation in pathogenesis of insulin resistance of obesity and type II diabetes. *Diabetes* 36, 1341–1350.

Felber, J-P., Acheson, K.J. & Tappy, L. (1993) *From Obesity to Diabetes*. Chichester: John Wiley.

Flatt, J-P. (1972) Role of the increased adipose tissue mass in the apparent insulin insensitivity of obesity. *American Journal of Clinical Nutrition* 25, 1189–1192.

Frayn, K.N. (1980) Skeletal muscle triacylglycerol in the rat: methods for sampling and measurement, and studies of biological variability. *Journal of Lipid Research* 21, 139–144.

Frayn, K.N. (1992) Studies of human adipose tissue *in vivo*. In: Kinney, J.M., Tucker, H.N. (eds) *Energy Metabolism: Tissue Determinants and Cellular Corollaries*, pp. 267–295. New York: Raven Press.

Frayn, K.N. (1993) Insulin resistance and lipid metabolism. *Current Opinion in Lipidology* 4, 197–204.

Frayn, K.N. (1996) *Metabolic Regulation: A Human Perspective*. London: Portland Press.

Frayn, K.N. & Coppack, S.W. (1992) Insulin resistance, adipose tissue and coronary heart disease. *Clinical Science* 82, 1–8.

Frayn, K.N., Khan, K., Coppack, S.W. & Elia, M. (1991) Amino acid metabolism in human subcutaneous adipose tissue *in vivo*. *Clinical Science* 80, 471–474.

Frayn, K.N., Shadid, S., Hamlani, R. *et al.* (1994) Regulation of fatty acid movement in human adipose tissue in the postabsorptive-to-postprandial transition. *American Journal of Physiology* 266, E308–E317.

Frayn, K.N., Coppack, S.W., Fielding, B.A. & Humphreys, S.M. (1995a) Coordinated regulation of hormone-sensitive lipase and lipoprotein lipase in human adipose tissue *in vivo*: implications for the control of fat storage and fat mobilization. *Advances in Enzyme Regulation* 35, 163–178.

Frayn, K.N., Humphreys, S.M. & Coppack, S.W. (1995b) Fuel selection in white adipose tissue. *Proceedings of the Nutrition Society* 54, 177–189.

Frayn, K.N., Humphreys, S.M. & Coppack, S.W. (1996a) Net carbon flux across subcutaneous adipose tissue after a standard meal in normal-weight and insulin-resistant obese subjects. *International Journal of Obesity* 20, 795–800.

Frayn, K.N., Williams, C.M. & Arner, P. (1996b) Are increased plasma non-esterified fatty acid concentrations a risk marker for coronary heart disease and other chronic diseases? *Clinical Science* 90, 243–253.

Frayn, K.N., Summers, L.K.M. & Fielding, B.A. (1997) Regulation of the plasma non-esterified fatty acid concentration in the postprandial state. *Proceedings of the Nutrition Society* 56, 713–721.

Friedman, J.E., Dohm, G.L., Leggett Frazier, N. *et al.* (1992) Restoration of insulin responsiveness in skeletal muscle of morbidly obese patients after weight loss. Effect on muscle glucose transport and glucose transporter GLUT4. *Journal of Clinical Investigation* 89, 701–705.

Griffiths, A.J., Humphreys, S.M., Clark, M.L. & Frayn, K.N. (1994) Forearm substrate utilization during exercise after a meal containing both fat and carbohydrate. *Clinical Science* 86, 169–175.

Hauner, H., Entenmann, G., Wabitsch, M. *et al.* (1989) Promoting effect of glucocorticoids on the differentiation of human adipocyte precursor cells cultured in a chemically defined medium. *Journal of Clinical Investigation* 84, 1663–1670.

Hellström, L., Langin, D., Reynisdottir, S., Dauzats, M. & Arner, P. (1996) Adipocyte lipolysis in normal weight subjects with obesity among first-degree relatives. *Diabetologia* **39**, 921–928.

Henriksson, J. (1995) Muscle fuel selection: effect of exercise and training. *Proceedings of the Nutrition Society* **54**, 125–138.

Hoag, S., Marshall, J.A., Jones, R.H. & Hamman, R.F. (1995) High fasting insulin levels associated with lower rates of weight gain in persons with normal glucose tolerance: The San Luis Valley Diabetes Study. *International Journal of Obesity* **19**, 175–180.

Hodgetts, V., Coppack, S.W., Frayn, K.N. & Hockaday, T.D.R. (1991) Factors controlling fat mobilization from human subcutaneous adipose tissue during exercise. *Journal of Applied Physiology* **71**, 445–451.

Hollenbeck, C.B., Chen, Y-I. & Reaven, G.M. (1984) A comparison of the relative effects of obesity and non-insulin-dependent diabetes mellitus on *in vivo* insulin-stimulated glucose utilization. *Diabetes* **33**, 622–626.

Hollenberg, C.H. (1990) Perspectives in adipose tissue physiology. *International Journal of Obesity* **14** (suppl. 3), 135–152.

Hotamisligil, G.S. & Spiegelman, B.M. (1994) Tumor necrosis factor alpha: a key component of the obesity-diabetes link. *Diabetes* **43**, 1271–1278.

Hotamisligil, G.S., Shargill, N.S. & Spiegelman, B.M. (1993) Adipose expression of tumor necrosis factor-alpha: direct role in obesity-linked insulin resistance. *Science* **259**, 87–91.

Hotamisligil, G.S., Murray, D.L., Choy, L.N. & Spiegelman, B.M. (1994) Tumor necrosis factor alpha inhibits signalling from the insulin receptor. *Proceedings of the National Academy of Sciences of the USA* **91**, 4854–4858.

Hotamisligil, G.S., Arner, P., Caro, J.F., Atkinson, R.L. & Spiegelman, B.M. (1995) Increased adipose tissue expression of tumor necrosis factor-α in human obesity and insulin resistance. *Journal of Clinical Investigation* **95**, 2409–2415.

Jackson, R.A., Hamling, J.B., Sim, B.M., Hawa, M.I., Blix, P.M. & Nabarro, J.D. (1987) Peripheral lactate and oxygen metabolism in man: the influence of oral glucose loading. *Metabolism* **36**, 144–150.

Jensen, M.D., Haymond, M.W., Rizza, R.A., Cryer, P.E. & Miles, J.M. (1989) Influence of body fat distribution on free fatty acid metabolism in obesity. *Journal of Clinical Investigation* **83**, 1168–1173.

Jeppesen, J., Hollenbeck, C.B. & Zhou, M-Y. *et al.* (1995) Relation between insulin resistance, hyperinsulinemia, postheparin plasma lipoprotein lipase activity, and postprandial lipemia. *Arteriosclerosis, Thrombosis, and Vascular Biology* **15**, 320–324.

Johnson, M.A., Polgar, J., Weightman, D. & Appleton, D. (1973) Data on the distribution of fibre types in thirty-six human muscles. An autopsy study. *Journal of the Neurological Sciences* **18**, 111–129.

Jones, D.A. & Round, J.M. (1990) *Skeletal Muscle in Health and Disease. A Textbook of Muscle Physiology.* Manchester: Manchester University Press.

Katzel, L.I., Busby-Whitehead, M.J., Rogus, E.M., Krauss, R.M. & Goldberg, A.P. (1994) Reduced adipose tissue lipoprotein lipase responses, postprandial lipemia, and low high-density lipoprotein-2 subspecies levels in older athletes with silent myocardial ischemia. *Metabolism* **43**, 190–198.

Kelley, D., Mitrakou, A., Marsh, H. *et al.* (1988) Skeletal muscle glycolysis, oxidation, and storage of an oral glucose load. *Journal of Clinical Investigation* **81**, 1563–1571.

Kelley, D.E., Mokan, M. & Mandarino, L.J. (1992) Intracellular defects in glucose metabolism in obese patients with NIDDM. *Diabetes* **41**, 698–706.

Kelley, D.E., Mintun, M.A., Watkins, S.C. *et al.* (1996) The effect of non-insulin-dependent diabetes mellitus and obesity on glucose transport and phosphorylation in skeletal muscle. *Journal of Clinical Investigation* **97**, 2705–2713.

Kiens, B. & Lithell, H. (1989) Lipoprotein metabolism influenced by training-induced changes in human skeletal muscle. *Journal of Clinical Investigation* **83**, 558–564.

Kissebah, A.H. & Krakower, G.R. (1994) Regional adiposity and morbidity. *Physiological Reviews* **74**, 761–811.

Kissebah, A.H., Alfarsi, S., Adams, P.W. & Wynn, V. (1976) Role of insulin resistance in adipose tissue and liver in the pathogenesis of endogenous hypertriglyceridaemia in man. *Diabetologia* **12**, 563–571.

Laakso, M., Edelman, S.V., Brechtel, G. & Baron, A.D. (1990a) Decreased effect of insulin to stimulate skeletal muscle blood flow in obese man. A novel mechanism for insulin resistance. *Journal of Clinical Investigation* **85**, 1844–1852.

Laakso, M., Edelman, S.V., Olefsky, J.M., Brechtel, G., Wallace, P. & Baron, A.D. (1990b) Kinetics of *in vivo* muscle insulin-mediated glucose uptake in human obesity. *Diabetes* **39**, 965–974.

Lillioja, S., Foley, J., Bogardus, C., Mott, D. & Howard, B.V. (1986) Free fatty acid metabolism and obesity in man: *in vivo* and *in vitro* comparisons. *Metabolism* **35**, 505–514.

Mårin, P., Rebuffé-Scrive, M. & Björntorp, P. (1990) Uptake of triglyceride fatty acids in adipose tissue *in vivo* in man. *European Journal of Clinical Investigation* **20**, 158–165.

Mårin, P., Högh-Kristiansen, I., Jansson, S., Krotkiewski, M., Holm, G. & Björntorp, P. (1992) Uptake of glucose carbon in muscle glycogen and adipose tissue triglycerides *in vivo* in humans. *American Journal of Physiology* **263**, E473–E480.

Maslowska, M., Scantlebury, T., Germinario, R. & Cianflone, K. (1997) Acute in vitro production of acylation stimulating protein in differentiated human adipocytes. *Journal of Lipid Research* **38**, 1–11.

Moller, D.E., Chang, P-Y., Yaspelkis, B.B.I., Flier, J.S., Wallberg-Henriksson, H. & Ivy, J.L. (1996) Transgenic mice with muscle-specific insulin resistance develop increased adiposity, impaired glucose tolerance, and dyslipidemia. *Endocrinology* **137**, 2397–2405.

Oben, J., Elliott, R., Morgan, L., Fletcher, J. & Marks, V. (1992) The role of gut hormones in the adipose tissue metabolism of lean and genetically obese (*ob/ob*) mice. In: Ailhaud, G., Guy-Grand, B., Lafontan, M. & Ricquier, D. (eds) *Obesity in Europe 91. Proceedings of the 3rd European Congress on Obesity*, pp. 269–272. London: Libbey.

Opie, L.H. & Walfish, P.G. (1963) Plasma free fatty acid concentrations in obesity. *New England Journal of Medicine* **268**, 757–760.

Oscai, L.B., Essig, D.A. & Palmer, W.K. (1990) Lipase regulation of muscle triglyceride hydrolysis. *Journal of Applied Physiology* **69**, 1571–1577.

Pénicaud, L., Ferré, P., Terrataz, J. *et al.* (1987) Development of obesity in Zucker rats. Early insulin resistance in muscles but normal sensitivity in white adipose tissue. *Diabetes* **36**, 626–631.

Phillips, D.I.W., Caddy, S., Ilic, V. *et al.* (1996) Intramuscular triglyceride and muscle insulin sensitivity: evidence for a relationship in non-diabetic subjects. *Metabolism* **45**, 947–950.

Piatti, P.M., Monti, L.D., Pacchioni, M., Pontiroli, A.E. & Pozza, G. (1991) Forearm insulin- and non-insulin-mediated glucose uptake and muscle metabolism in man: role of free fatty acids and blood glucose levels. *Metabolism* **40**, 926–933.

Potts, J.L., Fisher, R.M., Humphreys, S.M., Coppack, S.W., Gibbons, G.F. & Frayn, K.N. (1991) Peripheral triacylglycerol extraction in the fasting and post-prandial states. *Clinical Science* **81**, 621–626.

Potts, J.L., Coppack, S.W., Fisher, R.M., Humphreys, S.M., Gibbons, G.F. & Frayn, K.N. (1995) Impaired postprandial clearance of triacylglycerol-rich lipoproteins in adipose tissue in obese subjects. *American Journal of Physiology* **268**, E588–E594.

Prentice, A.M., Black, A.E., Coward, W.A. *et al.* (1986) High levels of energy expenditure in obese women. *British Medical Journal* **292**, 983–987.

Raben, A., Andersen, H.B., Christensen, N.J., Madsen, J., Holst, J.J. & Astrup, A. (1994) Evidence for an abnormal postprandial response to a high-fat meal in women predisposed to obesity. *American Journal of Physiology* **267**, E549–E559.

Rabinowitz, D., Zierler, K.L. (1961) Forearm metabolism in obesity and its response to intra-arterial insulin. Evidence for adaptive hyperinsulinism. *Lancet* **i**, 690–692.

Randle, P.J., Garland, P.B., Hales, C.N. & Newsholme, E.A. (1963) The glucose fatty-acid cycle. Its role in insulin sensitivity and the metabolic disturbances of diabetes mellitus. *Lancet* **i**, 785–789.

Rigden, D.J., Jellyman, A.E., Frayn, K.N. & Coppack, S.W. (1990) Human adipose tissue glycogen levels and responses to carbohydrate feeding. *European Journal of Clinical Nutrition* **44**, 689–692.

Rodnick, K.J., Slot, J.W., Studelska, D.R. *et al.* (1992) Immunocytochemical and biochemical studies of GLUT4 in rat skeletal muscle. *Journal of Biological Chemistry* **267**, 6278–6285.

Rohner-Jeanrenaud, F. & Jeanrenaud, B. (1996) Obesity, leptin and the brain. *New England Journal of Medicine* **334**, 324–325.

Romijn, J.A., Coyle, E.F., Sidossis, L.S. *et al.* (1993) Regulation of endogenous fat and carbohydrate metabolism in relation to exercise intensity and duration. *American Journal of Physiology* **265**, E380–E391.

Ruys, T., Sturgess, I., Shaikh, M., Watts, G.F., Nordestgaard, B.G. & Lewis, B. (1989) Effects of exercise and fat ingestion on high density lipoprotein production by peripheral tissues. *Lancet* **ii**, 1119–1122.

Saghizadeh, M., Ong, J.M., Garvey, W.T., Henry, R.R. & Kern, P.A. (1996) The expression of TNFα by human muscle. Relationship to insulin resistance. *Journal of Clinical Investigation* **97**, 1111–1116.

Samra, J.S., Clark, M.L., Humphreys, S.M., Macdonald, I.A., Matthews, D.R. & Frayn, K.N. (1996a) Effects of morning rise in cortisol concentration on regulation of lipolysis in subcutaneous adipose tissue. *American Journal of Physiology* **271** E996–E1002.

Samra, J.S., Simpson, E.J. & Clark, M.L. *et al.* (1996b) Effects of epinephrine infusion on adipose tissue: interactions between blood flow and lipid metabolism. *American Journal of Physiology* **271**, E834–E839.

Schalin Jantti, C., Harkonen, M. & Groop, L.C. (1992) Impaired activation of glycogen synthase in people at increased risk for developing NIDDM. *Diabetes* **41**, 598–604.

Sidossis, L.S., Coggan, A.R., Gastaldelli, A. & Wolfe, R.R. (1995) Pathway of free fatty acid oxidation in human subjects. Implications for tracer studies. *Journal of Clinical Investigation* **95**, 278–284.

Simoneau, J.A., Colberg, S.R., Thaete, F.L. & Kelley, D.E. (1995) Skeletal muscle glycolytic and oxidative enzyme capacities are determinants of insulin sensitivity and muscle composition in obese women. *FASEB Journal* **9**, 273–278.

Sniderman, A.D., Cianflone, K., Summers, L.K.M., Fielding, B.A. & Frayn, K.N. (1997) The acylation-stimulating protein pathway and regulation of postprandial metabolism. *Proceedings of the Nutrition Society* **56**, 703–712.

Snyder, W.S. (1975) *Report of the Task Force on reference man*. Oxford: Pergamon Press, for the International Commission on Radiological Protection. International Commission on Radiological Protection No. 23.

Soop, M., Björkman, O., Cederblad, G., Hagenfeldt, L. & Wahren, J. (1988) Influence of carnitine supplementation on muscle substrate and carnitine metabolism during exercise. *Journal of Applied Physiology* **64**, 2394–2399.

Spenst, L.F., Martin, A.D. & Drinkwater, D.T. (1993) Muscle mass of competitive male athletes. *Journal of Sports Sciences* **11**, 3–8.

Summers, L.K.M., Fielding, B.A., Ilic, V. & Frayn, K.N. (1997) The effect of body mass index on postprandial non-esterified fatty acid suppression. *Proceedings of the Nutrition Society* **56**, 95A.

Summers, L.K.M., Samra, J.S., Humphreys, S.M., Morris, R.J. & Frayn, K.N. (1996) Subcutaneous abdominal adipose tissue blood flow: variation within and between subjects and relationship to obesity. *Clinical Science* **91**, 679–683.

Swinburn, B.A., Nyomba, B.L., Saad, M.F. *et al.* (1991) Insulin resistance associated with lower rates of weight gain in Pima Indians. *Journal of Clinical Investigation* **88**, 168–173.

Taylor, R., Price, T.B., Katz, L.D., Shulman, R.G. & Shulman, G.I. (1993) Direct measurement of change in muscle glycogen concentration after a mixed meal in normal subjects. *American Journal of Physiology* **265**, E224–E229.

Toubro, S., Western, P., Bülow, J. *et al.* (1994) Insulin sensitivity in post-obese women. *Clinical Science* **87**, 407–413.

Wells, A.M., Sutcliffe, I.C., Johnson, A.B. & Taylor, R. (1993) Abnormal activation of glycogen synthesis in fibroblasts from NIDDM subjects. Evidence for an abnormality specific to glucose metabolism. *Diabetes* **42**, 583–589.

Yki-Järvinen, H., Young, A.A., Lamkin, C. & Foley, J.E. (1987) Kinetics of glucose disposal in whole body and across the forearm in man. *Journal of Clinical Investigation* **79**, 1713–1719.

Zurlo, F., Larson, K., Bogardus, C. & Ravussin, E. (1990) Skeletal muscle metabolism is a major determinant of resting energy expenditure. *Journal of Clinical Investigation* **86**, 1423–1427.

....

CHAPTER 8

Effects of Obesity on Fat Topography: Metabolic and Endocrine Determinants

PETER G. KOPELMAN

....

This chapter will review the evidence for the adipocyte acting as an endocrine organ and describe the influence of the regional localization of adipose tissue on the action of specific hormones. The resulting alterations in action of these hormones appear to be additive and contribute to the metabolic derangements which so frequently accompany obesity.

Normal adipocyte function

The normal function of white adipose tissue has been discussed in detail in Chapter 7. In summary, the process of fat mobilization consists of hydrolysis of the stored triacylglycerol (TAG) to release non-esterified fatty acids (NEFA) into the circulation. The key enzyme is the intracellular TAG-lipase, hormone-sensitive lipase (HSL). The major form of regulation of HSL is reversible phosphorylation by a cyclic adenosine monophosphate (AMP)-dependent protein kinase. Lipolysis is therefore stimulated by effectors which increase the activity of adenylate cyclase in adipocytes leading to the formation of cyclic AMP from adenosine triphosphate (ATP). Adenylate cyclase is stimulated by hormones acting via the cell surface receptors and G-proteins, especially catecholamines acting via β-adrenoceptors (β_1-, β_2-, β_3-) (Burns $et\ al.$, 1970; Wahrenberg $et\ al.$, 1989; Lafontan $et\ al.$, 1993). Dephosphorylation of HSL occurs when cyclic AMP concentrations fall. The main hormonal regulator of this is insulin, which lowers adipocyte cyclic AMP concentrations (Smith $et\ al.$, 1991). The suppression of fat mobilization occurs in normal circumstances at very low insulin concentrations. Catecholamines acting on α_2-adrenoceptors will also inhibit lipolysis (Lafontan $et\ al.$, 1993; Castan $et\ al.$, 1994). Thus, catecholamines have dual effects on the lipolysis rates, both accelerating through β-adrenoceptors and retarding through α_2-adrenoceptors. HSL activity is suppressed after meals when the physiological drive is towards fat storage rather than mobilization. In the postprandial state the enzyme lipoprotein lipase (LPL) in adipose tissue is activated by insulin and possibly also by some gastrointestinal peptide hormones (Ong $et\ al.$, 1989). This enzyme is synthesized within adipocytes but exported to the capillary endothelial cells, where it is attached to the luminal side of the capillary wall and acts on circulating TAG in the TAG-rich lipoproteins (chylomicrons and very-low-density lipoproteins, VLDL). LPL releases fatty acids which may be taken up into the tissue for esterification and storage as TAG. The fatty acids released by LPL action are not all taken up by adipose tissue for storage with approximately 50% entering the systemic circulation (Eaton et al., 1969). This release of LPL-derived fatty acids is dependent upon the insulin response to the meal and the sensitivity of LPL activation to insulin and other hormones.

There is considerable evidence for LPL playing a controlling rate in the regional distribution of fat. There are significant gender and regional differences in LPL activity that largely parallel variations in fat size. Premenopausal women have higher LPL activities in gluteal and femoral regions than men but the differences disappear after the menopause (Rebuffe-Scrive & Björntorp, 1985). In addition, women have quantitatively more LPL in gluteal and femoral tissue, which contain larger fat cells than they do in abdominal adipose tissue. In contrast, men show minimal regional variations in LPL activity or fat cell size. These differences in fat distribution between men and women may explain the tendency for premenopausal women to deposit fat preferentially in lower body fat depots.

Adipocyte function in obesity

The potential differences in free fatty acid (FFA) metabolism between lean and obese subjects may reflect the anti-lipolytic effectiveness of insulin in obesity, the relationship of FFA release to the amount of body fat and the lipolytic responsiveness of obese individuals to catecholamines. It is relevant that adipocytes from various body regions differ from one another in many respects; fat cell size and basal lipolysis vary in adipocytes from omental, abdominal subcutaneous and gluteal-thigh depots (Martin et al., 1991). The basal release of FFA from adipose tissue to meet lean body mass energy needs is greater in upper body obese women than obese women with lower body fat distribution and non-obese women. Differences in the ability of insulin to suppress lipolysis and of catecholamines to stimulate lipolysis also varies according to fat distribution (Reynisdottir et al., 1994). In both men and women, the lipolytic response to noradrenalin, which acts via α_2-β-adrenoceptors, is more marked in abdominal than gluteal or femoral tissues (Krotkiewski et al., 1983). A detailed analysis has suggested that the usual pattern of male fat distribution (greater abdominal fat accumulation) results from a greater α_2-adrenoceptor activity in the abdominal tissue of men (Lafontan et al., 1979). The findings from studies looking at radioligand binding of β-adrenergic antagonists have uniformly shown twice as many β-adrenergic binding sites in abdominal adipocytes as in femoral adipocytes. Lonnqvist and colleagues (1995a) have elucidated the pathogenic role of visceral β_3-adrenoceptors in obesity. These authors studied the responsiveness of isolated omental fat cells from obese and non-obese subjects to adrenergic-subtype receptor antagonists by measuring the rate of FFA and glycerol response. They found that the visceral fat cells from the obese subjects were highly responsive to noradrenalin stimulation. This appeared mainly

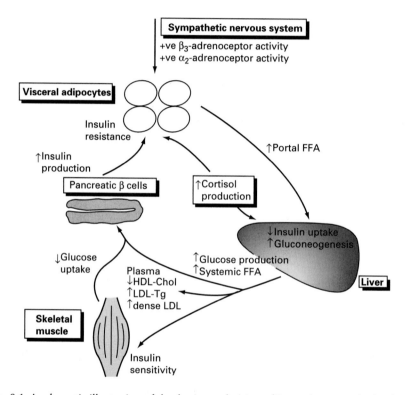

Fig. 8.1 A schematic illustration of the detrimental action of increasing upper body obesity on whole-body sensitivity to insulin and glucose tolerance. Elevated rates of lipolysis in visceral adipocytes resulting from increased β_3- and α_2-adrenoceptor activity and insulin insensitivity (enhanced by increased cortisol production) lead to elevated FFA being released into the portal system. This has a detrimental action on hepatic insulin uptake with an enhancement of gluconeogenesis. This, in turn, results in increased hepatic glucose production, increased systemic concentrations of NEFA and alterations in plasma lipid profile (decreased high-density lipoprotein (HDL)-cholesterol, increased low-density lipoprotein (LDL)-triglyceride and increased small density LDL-cholesterol). All of these factors contribute to the prevailing systemic hyperinsulinaemia and decreased skeletal muscle insulin sensitivity. The pancreatic β cells respond with a compensatory increase in insulin production to maintain normoglycaemia and thereby creating a vicious cycle of events. In time the insulin resistant individual cannot maintain this state of compensatory hyperinsulinaemia and hyperglycaemia will then prevail.

due to an enhanced lipolytic response and not to FFA re-utilization. The main finding was the markedly augmented β_3-adrenoceptors sensitivity and coupling efficiency; the authors suggested that this enhanced β_3-adrenoceptor activity was due to an increased receptor number in obese subjects. In contrast, the net lipolytic response to adrenalin is reduced in upper body obese women compared with lower body obese and non-obese women. In order for lower body obese women to maintain appropriate FFA availability despite increasing fatness, there must be down-regulation of lipolysis to prevent FFA release (Reynisdottir et al., 1994). Martin and colleagues (1991) measured FFA release from the leg, non-leg and splanchnic adipose tissue in obese women of differing body fat distribution. The most significant observation was the contrasting differences in lipolytic activity of splanchnic fat between those obese women with predominantly upper body fat and those lower body obese women. This difference was emphasized by the finding of similar FFA release from leg fat in the two groups. The important metabolic interpretation of these data is the apparently elevated rate of lipolysis in visceral fat cells due largely to increased β_3-adrenoceptor activity and partly to α_2-adrenoceptor activity. As a consequence more FFA is released into the portal system (Fig. 8.1).

Hormonal influences on adipocyte function

The hormonal mechanisms regulating adipose tissue LPL activity are not completely understood. Insulin is permissive for LPL synthesis and glucocorticoids enhance the activity of LPL when added with insulin in vitro (Cigolini & Smith, 1979). Sex steroids have been implicated in the regional distribution of body fat and gender differences are seen in LPL activity most particularly during pregnancy and lactation (Rebuffe-Scrive, 1985a). Regional variation in receptors for glucocorticoids or sex steroids could play a role in determining regional differences in adipose tissue. The reverse situation may also be true—adipose tissue having an effect on the production of sex hormones.

Insulin secretion in obesity

Obesity is characterized by an elevated fasting plasma insulin and an exaggerated insulin response to an oral glucose load (Kolterman et al., 1980). However, obesity and body fat distribution influence glucose metabolism through independent but additive mechanisms. Kissebah and colleagues (1982) have demonstrated that increasing upper body obesity is accompanied by a progressive increase in the glucose and insulin response to an oral glucose challenge. The in vivo insulin sensitivity in individuals was assessed further by determining the steady state plasma glucose (SSPG) and insulin (SSPI) attained during a simultaneous intravenous infusion of somatostatin, insulin and dextrose. Since endogenous insulin production was suppressed by somatostatin and the SSPI was comparable in each situation, SSPG directly measured the subjects' ability to dispose of an intravenous glucose load under the same insulin stimulus; SSPG can be taken as an index of insulin resistance. The results showed a positive correlation between increasing upper body obesity and SSPG. After adjustment for the effects of overall fatness (percentage ideal body-weight), upper body obesity remained independently correlated with SSPG suggesting that the location of body fat is an independent factor influencing the degree of insulin sensitivity and, in turn, metabolic profile.

Measurement of portal plasma insulin levels (as an index of insulin secretion) show similar levels in upper body and lower body obesity but hepatic insulin extraction, both basely and during stimulation by intravenous or oral glucose, is reduced in upper body obesity (Peiris *et al.*, 1986). As a consequence, posthepatic insulin delivery is increased in upper body obesity leading to more marked peripheral insulin concentrations. Studies of insulin sensitivity and responsiveness of skeletal muscle and the relationship to overall glucose disposal in premenopausal women, with varying body fat distribution, have revealed a significant decline as upper body fatness increases (Evans *et al.*, 1984). Insulin-stimulated activity of the glucose-6-phosphate-independent form of glycogen synthase (GSI) has been measured in quadricep muscle biopsies taken during a somatostatin–insulin–dextrose infusion. Despite comparable degrees of SSPI in all women, significant reductions in percentage GSI were seen as the degree of upper body fatness increased and this was accompanied by decreased efficiency in insulin-stimulated glucose disposal (reflected by increasing SSPG at similar SSPI levels). Further, a significant trend was reported for a decreased number of cellular insulin receptors associated with increasing upper body fatness, which was associated in some subjects with reduced glucose disposal during supramaximal insulin stimulation. Such findings suggest a defect at both the level of the insulin receptor and in postreceptor events.

Abdominal visceral adipose tissue is more sensitive to lipolytic stimuli than subcutaneous fat while it is less sensitive to the inhibitory action of insulin; this appears to be associated with a low density of insulin receptors. Hyperinsulinaemia of obesity mainly inhibits lipolysis of insulin-sensitive subcutaneous adipocytes and thus may accentuate the fraction of systemic FFA originating from visceral fat (Rebuffe-Scrive *et al.*, 1988, 1989). In addition, elevated portal concentrations of FFA, produced by active visceral adipocytes, results in the liver being exposed to excessive FFA concentrations. The excessive visceral fat lipolysis may create a vicious chain of events with insulin resistance in liver and skeletal muscle resulting in additional systemic insulin resistance (Fig. 8.1).

Steroid hormones

Obese subjects have a normal circulating plasma cortisol concentration with a normal circadian rhythm and normal urinary free cortisol but an accelerated degradation of cortisol which is compensated by an increased cortisol production rate (Migeon *et al.*, 1963; Galvao-Tales *et al.*, 1976). It is likely that the increase in metabolic clearance of cortisol is secondary to a decrease in cortisol-binding globulin plasma concentrations. Slavnov and colleagues (1977) have reported a moderate elevation in plasma corticotrophin (ACTH) levels in obesity to explain the increased cortisol production. The increased peripheral clearance rate of cortisol is probably mediated by binding to the glucocorticoid receptor present in glucocorticoid-responding tissue (Rebuffe-Scrive *et al.*, 1990). An increased peripheral density of this receptor will be followed by an increased metabolic clearance rate. Cortisol has effects on both lipid accumulation and mobilization. Cortisol inhibits the anti-lipolytic effect of insulin in human adipocytes and this may be particularly pronounced in visceral abdominal fat (Cigolini & Smith, 1979). It also has a permissive effect on lipid mobilization stimulated by catecholamine. Enlarged visceral adipocytes, as found in abdominal obesity, could be the site where this occurs because such tissue appears to have a higher density of glucocorticoid receptors compared to adipose tissue (Bronnegard *et al.*, 1980; Rebuffe-Scrive *et al.*, 1985b). Abdominal subcutaneous adipose tissue demonstrates a higher expression of cortisol-induced LPL as well as a higher density of glucocorticoid receptors than femoral subcutaneous adipose tissue. Furthermore, there is a higher LPL activity in visceral compared to subcutaneous adipose tissue in both men and women (Björntrop *et al.*, 1990). This could be an explanation for the functional hypercortisolism associated with abdominal obesity in subjects who are only moderately overweight. There is a close analogy between upper body obesity and Cushing's syndrome because both conditions are characterized by hypercortisolism and excessive visceral fat accumulation (Mayo-Smith *et al.*, 1989). Moreover, both have similar consequences—increasing plasma cortisol leading to insulin insensitivity and glucose intolerance, an increase in hepatic gluconeogenesis, reduced hepatic insulin uptake and insulin resistance in skeletal muscle.

The increased peripheral clearance and the obesity-associated acceleration in overall adrenocortical function lead also to an increase in adrenal androgen production. Urinary 17-ketosteroids (17-KS), which measure various androgen metabolites including etiocholananolone, androsterone, dehydroepiandrosterone (DHEA) and its sulphate conjugate (DHEAS), are elevated in obese subjects (Simkin, 1961). The changes in adrenal androgen production may simply occur in compensation for an increasing metabolic clearance but there is additional evidence to suggest alterations in adrenocortical dynamics. Kurtz and colleagues

(1987) noted an increased turnover of DHEA in obese women. These authors demonstrated a significant correlation between upper body obesity and the metabolic clearance of DHEA and androstenedione which suggests that the androgenic effects of DHEA may have a role in fat distribution. In premenopausal women serum DHEA concentration correlates positively with trunk fat and negatively with leg fat accumulation whereas no such effect is seen in men (Usiskin *et al.*, 1990; Williams *et al.*, 1993). A shift in fat accumulation in women towards abdominal obesity may be an androgenic effect of DHEA. In healthy postmenopausal women androgen levels are inversely related to fasting plasma glucose levels and are predictive of central obesity 10–15 years later (Khaw & Barret-Connor, 1991). Brody *et al.* (1987) have reported a positive correlation between body-weight and changes in DHEA and the DHEA/ 17-hydroxy progesterone ratio after exogenous administration of ACTH. This is suggestive of hyper-responsiveness of adrenal androgens in obesity. Weaver and colleagues (1993) have also provided evidence for increased ACTH release in obesity by reporting an association between the ACTH response to insulin-induced hypoglycaemia and increasing body-weight. Moreover, alterations in adrenocortical production of adrenal androgens probably reflects the influence of other factors including adrenal androgens themselves. *In vitro* studies have suggested a lesser degree of inhibition of human 17-hydroxylase activity by DHEA as compared to the inhibition of human 17,20-desmolase activity (Couch *et al.*, 1986). The increased adipose tissue breakdown and the higher urinary excretion of DHEA in such circumstances could lead to decreased intra-adrenal concentrations of the steroid. As a consequence, the inhibition of 17,20-desmolase will be further diminished and a selective increase in the production of DHEA and its metabolites occur.

DHEA may therefore contribute to a spiral of events — the greater androgenic action of DHEA contributing to abdominal fat cell accumulation with resulting hyperglycaemia and hyperinsulinaemia. Androgens have a clear effect on adipose tissue metabolism; this includes enhancement of lipolytic sensitivity by expression of lipolytic β-adrenergic receptors via an androgenic receptor, which is positively autoregulated by testosterone (Xu *et al.*, 1990a, 1991).

The density of androgen receptors, which are specific for androgens, varies in different adipose tissue regions with a higher density in intra-abdominal than subcutaneous depots in rats (Sjogren *et al.*, 1995). Indirect evidence suggests a higher density in central visceral fat in humans compared to peripheral adipose tissue (Rebuffe-Scrive *et al.*, 1989). Testosterone, in the presence of growth hormone (GH), exerts a dramatic effect on the regulation of lipolysis by increasing the number of β-adrenoceptors through an action at the level of adenylate cyclase and protein kinase A and/or HSL (Evans & Hughes, 1985; Xu *et al.*, 1990a, 1991).

Sex steroid secretion

There appears to be contrasting situations between men and women in relation to the influence of sex steroids on adipose tissue function. Men with excessive abdominal fat often have relatively low serum testosterone concentrations despite reduced levels of sex hormone binding globulin (SHBG) (Björntorp, 1996). Marin and colleagues (1992) have demonstrated a significant decrease in visceral fat mass and abdominal sagittal diameter in middle-aged abdominally obese men treated for 8 months with oral testosterone supplements. This reduction occurred without a detectable change in subcutaneous fat. In addition, there was an improvement in plasma glucose disposal and increased insulin sensitivity. The authors concluded that such men have a relative hypogonadism and associated metabolic abnormalities, which are partly corrected by testosterone supplementation. Calculations of lipid uptake and LPL activity, using isotope labelling techniques, suggested diminished activity in abdominal adipose tissue but no change in femoral fat (Marin et al., 1995). The effects of testosterone were much more marked in visceral fat compared to subcutaneous abdominal fat because the uptake of lipid was inhibited by approximately 50% in the intra-abdominal tissues. This has been confirmed by studies of lipid turnover in visceral adipose tissue from rats. Thus, testosterone supplementation in obese men decreases uptake of lipid particularly in visceral fat and increases the rate of fat mobilization.

Obese women are also characterized by distinct alterations in circulating sex hormone levels (Kopelman, 1994). Obese women demonstrate lower circulating SHBG levels and thereby an increased fraction of circulating oestradiol. In postmenopausal obese women, serum levels of oestrone and oestradiol are correlated with the degree of obesity and fat mass (Meldrum et al., 1981). The plasma ratio of oestrone to oestradiol is also increased in obesity. Interestingly, a similar pattern of changes of sex steroid concentrations and binding are found in women with the polycystic ovary syndrome (Baird, 1978). Longcope and colleagues (1986a) have reported significant associations between body-weight and conversion of testosterone to oestradiol. The interconversion of oestrone to oestradiol has been observed in vivo and in vitro in adipose tissue with a greater conversion being found in omental fat than subcutaneous fat (Longcope et al., 1986b; Deslypere et al., 1987). Adipose tissue 17-β-hydroxysteroid dehydrogenase activity, measured by the conversion of oestrone to oestradiol, is higher in premenopausal than in postmenopausal women and all women have a higher activity compared to men (Roncari & Van, 1997).

The androgen receptor in adipose tissue from women seems to have the same specificity and affinity as in men suggesting the receptor is identical. 17-β oestradiol appears to decrease androgen receptor density because oöphorectomy is necessary for testosterone to result in an increase in visceral fat mass in a woman (Elbers *et al.*, 1995). It seems possible that oestrogen protects adipocytes from the androgen effects by down-regulation of androgen receptors (Haarbo *et al.*, 1991). The centralization of body fat after the menopause, leading to a male type of adipose tissue, could be due to the loss of this protective effects of oestrogen from androgens by allowing the expression of more androgen receptors. It is of interest that hyperandrogenic women have body fat distribution which resembles males (Haffner *et al.*, 1988). Oestrogen replacement in postmenopausal women leads to a marked elevation of LPL activity specifically in the gluteo-femoral region, which results in a similar metabolic pattern of activity of adipose tissue from this region compared to that seen in premenopausal women (Rebuffe-Scrive *et al.*, 1987; Haarbo *et al.*, 1991). No specific hormonal receptors have been identified for oestrogen and progesterone and these effects may be mediated through competition with glucocorticoid receptors thereby protecting against the effects of cortisol, possibly by down-regulation of the receptor (Xu *et al.*, 1990b).

Sex steroid binding in obesity

SHBG is a circulating globulin produced by the liver which binds in high affinity, but low capacity, to many of the circulating sex hormones (Anderson, 1974). Alterations in SHBG levels have a profound impact on the metabolism and action of bound steroids. A decrease of SHBG concentration is associated with an increase in metabolic clearance and free fraction of testosterone and oestradiol. The hypothesis that insulin may regulate the hepatic production of SHBG is supported by the finding of a direct inhibitory action of insulin on SHBG secretion by cultured human hepatoma cells (Plymate *et al.*, 1988). Peiris and colleagues (1987) have shown upper body obesity in women to be associated with increased pancreatic insulin production and decreased hepatic insulin clearance. Thus, increasing splanchnic insulin concentrations may account for decreased hepatic SHBG production in this type of obesity. These authors also showed the severity of the peripheral insulin resistance to be positively correlated with the magnitude of free testosterone — the greater the free testosterone level, the greater the degree of insulin resistance. The changes in circulating androgens do not appear to influence plasma insulin levels but, conversely, increasing plasma insulin may increase androgen secretion by a number of mechanisms which include direct stimulation of androgen production by the ovary (Barbieri & Hornstein, 1988). There is recent evidence to suggest that both insulin and insulin-like growth factor-1 (IGF-1) may be important regulators of ovarian thecal and stromal androgen production with an interaction at receptor level on the ovarian stroma of these two hormones (Barbieri *et al.*, 1986).

Leptin

Leptin is a 16-kDa protein secreted almost exclusively by adipocytes in proportion to body fat with a potent inhibitory action on food intake. In rodent models of obesity leptin plays a key regulatory role in energy balance via the hypothalamus with its actions mediated through specific leptin receptors (see Chapters 3 and 4). Alterations in hypothalamic–pituitary function are features of human obesity and, unsurprisingly, it is questioned whether leptin plays a role in the development of excessive adiposity. However, in humans the precise role of leptin remains uncertain — leptin receptors are present in brain, haemopoetic stem cells, early fetal liver and placenta (Cioffi *et al.*, 1996). Recently, two severely obese children from a consanguinous pedigree have been reported with very low levels of serum leptin despite a markedly elevated fat mass. In both children, a homozygous frame-shift mutation involving the deletion of a single guanine nucleotide in codon 133 of the gene for leptin was found (Montague *et al.*, 1997a). The severe obesity found in these congenitally leptin-deficient subjects does provide genetic evidence that leptin may contribute to the regulation of energy balance in humans. However, the evidence to date about leptin in humans with 'spontaneous' obesity suggests that it is a fat 'messenger' rather than a fat 'controller'. Circulating leptin levels are positively correlated with measures of obesity including body mass index (BMI) and percentage body fat and are elevated in obesity (Considine *et al.*, 1996). Serum leptin in women suffering from various forms of eating disorders (anorexia nervosa, bulimia nervosa and non-specific types) are reduced, the level being unrelated to the specific pathology but correlated with the individual BMI (Ferron *et al.*, 1997). Progressive weight loss during hypocaloric dieting is accompanied by a decline in circulating leptin levels and adipose tissue messenger RNA (mRNA); plasma levels then increase once isocaloric diets are initiated to maintain reduced body-weight (Maffei *et al.*, 1995). In addition, expression of leptin mRNA in adipose tissue is greater in obese than in lean individuals (Lonnqvist *et al.*, 1995b). It has been proposed that human obesity results, as in the *db/db* mouse, from leptin resistance which becomes more pronounced with progressive degrees of obesity. Caro and colleagues (1996) propose that this leptin resistance results from reduced levels of leptin transport into the cerebrospinal fluid (CSF).

Recent studies have demonstrated higher expression of leptin mRNA subcutaneous rather than omental adipocytes and this finding is exaggerated in female subjects (Montague *et al.*, 1997b). A site-specific difference in adipocyte exposure to neural, endocrine or paracrine regulators could be the explanation. This raises questions about the different biological function of subcutaneous and intra-abdominal fat depots and a possible role for leptin in determining regional fat distribution.

A number of possible modulating factors of leptin secretion have been examined in human subjects in order to define more closely possible physiological functions—these include insulin, glucocorticoids and sex hormones. A close association between hyperinsulinaemia and hyperleptinaemia suggests that *ob* gene expression may be mediated by insulin in humans as in the mouse models (Cusin *et al.*, 1995). Both insulin and leptin are suppressed during fasting and increase with re-feeding. Leptin levels do not increase acutely with insulin stimulation but do so if the acute hyperinsulinaemia is extended beyond 48 hours (Kolaczynski *et al.*, 1996). Diabetes does not alter the relationship between leptin and body-weight in either men or women but leptin levels are negatively correlated with maximally stimulated glucose uptake (Haffner *et al.*, 1996). Although the role of glucocorticoids in regulating leptin in humans remains uncertain, a clearer picture is emerging for sex hormones and androgens (Butte *et al.*, 1997; Kennedy *et al.*, 1997). The higher serum leptin levels over a range of body-weights in women may explain abnormalities of sex hormones and hpothalamic function seen at extremes of body-weight and this, in turn, provide an explanation for the gender-based differences in leptin. Moreover, the physiological effects of sex hormones, in particular androgens, may contribute to leptin resistance at the leptin receptor. In this respect the findings in pregnancy are of interest. Serum leptin concentrations are positively correlated with weight, BMI, percentage fat and changes in weight, and women who gain most weight have higher leptin levels (Butte *et al.*, 1997). A similar relationship is also seen in women who fail to lose weight postpartum. Pregnancy is characterized by insulin resistance with advancing gestation. Thus, it appears likely that in both obese men and women, an additive effect of sex hormones combined with prevailing hyperinsulinaemia contribute to leptin resistance. Such an action is further compounded by gender with the possible influence of androgens on lean body mass being instrumental in determining elevated leptin levels in female subjects (Kennedy *et al.*, 1997).

In summary, current evidence from human studies of subjects with 'spontaneous' obesity points to leptin as an important messenger of adipocyte function. More studies of leptin's molecular basis and physiological interactions are required before it will be possible to determine whether leptin is additionally important in the regulation of overall fatness in humans.

Growth hormone secretion

GH is an important regulator of body mass throughout life: subcutaneous fat is markedly increased in GH-deficient children as well as in GH-deficient adults (Tanner & Whitehouse, 1967). Interestingly, in these subjects fat deposition occurs predominantly on the trunk. Moreover, hypopituitary patients have abnormally high amounts of intra-abdominal fat which may be decreased by 30% after 6 month's treatment with GH (Bengtsson *et al.*, 1994). Such evidence suggests that relative GH deficiency or insensitivity could play a role in the perpetuation of the obesity.

An impaired GH response to insulin-induced hypoglycaemia is found in association with obesity but this seems likely to be a consequence rather than a cause of extreme obesity (Kopelman, 1988). Sims and colleagues (1973) have confirmed that weight gain decreases the GH response to all types of provocative stimuli whereas the GH response to hypoglycaemia significantly increases in obese subjects following weight loss. An input of food in excess of energy expenditure appears to be important because impaired GH responsiveness is not a characteristic of subjects who are overweight as the result of increased musculature induced by vigorous exercise (Kalkhoff & Ferrow, 1971). In this situation, energy expenditure is balanced by an increase in appropriate protein and energy intake whereas 10 days of over-feeding with carbohydrate can produce impaired GH responsiveness without an increase in body-weight (Merimee & Fineberg, 1973). The explanation for the decreased output of GH in obesity has not been fully elucidated. It has been suggested that the altered GH secretion results from alterations in IGF-1 and its binding proteins (Glass *et al.*, 1981). Synthesis of IGF-1 is stimulated by insulin and the hyperinsulinaemia of obesity could directly enhance IGF-1 production and suppress the production of GH from the pituitary by a negative-feedback mechanism. A negative-feedback effect of IGF-1 has been demonstrated in pituitary cells in culture (Glass, 1989). However, several authors have reported that IGF-1 circulating levels in obese adults are normal (Rasmussen *et al.*, 1995b). By contrast, IGF binding proteins 1 and 3 (IGFBP-1, IGFBP-3) are both reduced in obesity with decreased plasma concentrations of IGFBP-1 being inversely related to fasting plasma insulin and waist/hip ratio (Weaver *et al.*, 1990; Bang *et al.*, 1994). A reduced level of IGFBP-1 suggests enhanced biological activity of IGF-1 which, in turn, may feedback on the hypothalamic–pituitary axis to suppress GH release. It is of interest that IGF-1, GH and insulin have all been shown to promote the conversion of pre-adipocytes to adipocytes and may, therefore, play a role in upper body fat deposition (Ailhaud *et al.*, 1992). Moreover, substantial weight reduction will reverse the documented alterations in insulin, GH, IGF-1 and its binding proteins (Rasmussen *et al.*, 1995a).

From obesity to non-insulin-dependent diabetes mellitus

The deleterious metabolic effects of altered regulation of adipocyte function, observed particularly in visceral obesity, frequently leads to the development of impaired glucose tolerance and non-insulin-dependent diabetes mellitus (NIDDM).

In obesity the rate of NEFA turnover/unit lean body mass is increased (Campbell *et al.*, 1994). The ability of insulin to suppress NEFA release *in vivo* is diminished in obese subjects as a result of alterations in insulin sensitivity of both lipolytic processes and fatty acid re-esterification. It is therefore unsurprising that plasma NEFA increases when insulin action is deficient (as in NIDDM) (Coppack *et al.*, 1992). A cycle of events is thereby entered with increasing insulin resistance resulting in increasing NEFA plasma concentration which, in turn, contributes to diminishing insulin sensitivity. The defect in insulin sensitivity observed in skeletal muscle may accentuate the defects in the regulation of lipolysis.

A number of mechanisms link NEFA supply and impairment of glucose utilization with the supply of NEFA to the liver being an important determinant of the rate of hepatic glucose production. The elevation in plasma NEFA concentration, particularly postprandially when they are usually suppressed, will lead to an inappropriate maintenance of glucose production and an impairment of glucose utilization (impaired glucose tolerance). These mechanisms may be critical links leading from obesity to the development of NIDDM. The progression to NIDDM may be enhanced by the suppressive effects of high NEFA concentrations on insulin secretion or even by potentially 'toxic' effects of NEFA on pancreatic β cells (Unger, 1995). A further mechanism linking increased plasma NEFA concentrations to insulin resistance is the reduced hepatic clearance of insulin—increasing delivery of NEFA to the liver reduces insulin binding to the hepatocytes. In normal circumstances, the liver removes 40% of insulin secreted from the pancreas; an impairment of this process will have a significant effect on peripheral (systemic) insulin concentrations, which contributes to hyperinsulinaemia, and leads to further down-regulation of insulin receptors and increasing insulin resistance (Svedberg *et al.*, 1990). As has been described, intra-abdominal fat accentuates this process and explains the close relationship between upper body obesity and the development of NIDDM (Fig. 8.1).

In the initial phases of this process, the pancreas can respond by maintaining a state of compensatory hyperinsulinaemia with gross decompensation of glucose tolerance being prevented. With ever-increasing plasma concentrations of NEFA, the insulin-resistant individual cannot continue to maintain this state of compensatory hyperinsulinaemia, and hyperglycaemia prevails in time. Thus, increasing NEFA concentrations, associated with a small decline in insulin secretion, will further decrease glucose uptake by muscle, increase hepatic NEFA oxidation and stimulate gluconeogenesis. This has an additive effect on plasma elevations of NEFA and glucose which, in turn, further compromise β-cell function (Reaven, 1995).

The effect of weight reduction

The beneficial action of weight reduction suggests that many, if not all, of the deleterious events associated with upper body obesity are a consequence, rather than a cause, of excessive visceral adipose tissue.

Weight reduction in women with upper body obesity has a marked effect on the regulation of lipolysis. There is approximately a fivefold increase in the sensitivity to noradrenalin with a specific effect on adrenoceptor subtype — there is increased sensitivity to β_2-receptors but no change in β_1 or α_2. However, no change occurs in the numbers of β_2-receptor binding sites which suggests possible facilitation of G protein coupling (Reynisdottir $et\ al.$, 1995). More recently a similar pattern of increased sensitivity has been reported for β_3-adrenoceptors (Lonnqvist $et\ al.$, 1995a). Weight loss is accompanied by a decrease in circulating insulin levels and a fall in plasma noradrenalin. The beneficial effects of these changes are a decrease in basal lipolysis (with decreased HSL function) and an increase in sensitivity to catecholamine stimulation of lipolysis. Thus, weight reduction appears to restore a more efficient regulation of lipolysis, with less FFA being released at rest and lower catecholamine levels required for lipolysis activation.

References

Ailhaud, G., Grimaldi, P. & Negrel, R. (1992) A molecular view of adipose tissue. *International Journal of Obesity* **16** (suppl. 2), 517–521.

Anderson, D.C. (1976) Sex hormone binding globulin. *Clinical Endocrinology* **3**, 69–96.

Baird, D.T. (1978) Polycystic ovary syndrome. In: Jacobs, H.S. (ed.) Advances in gynaecological endocrinology. *Proceedings of the Sixth Study Group of the Royal College of Obstetricians and Gynaecologists*, pp. 289–300. London: Royal College of Obstetricians and Gynaecologists.

Bang, P., Brismar, K., Rosenfeld, R.G. & Hall, K. (1994) Fasting affects serum insulin-like growth factors (IGFs) and IGF-binding proteins differently in patients with non-insulin-dependent diabetes versus healthy non-obese and obese subjects. *Journal of Clinical Endocrinology and Metabolism* **78**, 960–967.

Barbieri, R.L. & Hornstein, M.D. (1988) Hyperinsulinaemia and ovarian hyperandrogenism: cause and effect. *Endocrinology and Metabolism Clinics of North America* **17**, 685–703.

Barbieri, R.L., Makris, A., Randall, R.W. *et al.* (1986) Insulin stimulates androgen accumulation in incubations of ovarian stroma obtained from women with hyperandrogenism. *Journal of Clinical Endocrinology and Metabolism* **62**, 904–910.

Bengtsson, B.A., Eden, Lonn, L. *et al.* (1994) Treatment of adults with growth hormone deficiency with recombinant human GH. *Journal of Clinical Endocrinology and Metabolism* **78**, 960–967.

Björntorp, P. (1996) The regulation of adipose tissue distribution in humans. *International Journal of Obesity* **20**, 291–302.

Björntorp, P., Ottosson, M., Rebuffe-Scrive, M., Xu, X. (1990) Regional obesity and steroid hormone interactions in human adipose tissue. *UCLA Symposium on Cell Biology* **132**, 147–158.

Brody, S., Carlstrom, K., Lagrelius, A. *et al.* (1987) Adrenal steroids in post-menopausal women: relation to obesity and bone mineral content. *Maturitas* **9**, 25–32.

Bronnegard, M., Arner, P., Hellstrom, L. *et al.* (1990) Glucocorticoid receptor messenger ribonucleic acid in different regions of human adipose tissue. *Endocrinology* **127**, 1689–1696.

Burns, T.W. & Langley, P.E. (1970) Lipolysis by human adipose tissue: the role of cyclic 3′,5′-adenosine monophosphate and adrenergic receptors. *Journal of Laboratory and Clinical Medicine* **75**, 983–987.

Butte, N.F., Hopkinson, J.M. & Nicolson, M.A. (1997) Leptin in human reproduction: Serum leptin levels in pregnant and lactating women. *Journal of Clinical Endocrinology and Metabolism* **82**, 585–589.

Campbell, P.J., Carlson, M.G. & Nurjhan, N. (1994) Fat metabolism in human obesity. *American Journal of Physiology* **266**, E600–605.

Caro, J.F., Kolaczynski, J.W., Nyce, M.R. *et al.* (1996) Decreased cerebrospinal-fluid/serum leptin ratio in obesity: a possible mechanism for leptin resistance. *Lancet* **348**, 159–161.

Castan, I., Valet, P., Quideau, N. *et al.* (1994) Antilipolytic effects of α$_2$-agonists, neuropeptide Y, adenosine, and PGE$_1$ in mammal adipocytes. *American Journal of Physiology* **266**, R1141–1147.

Cigolini, M. & Smith, U. (1979) Human adipose tissue in culture. VIII. Studies on the insulin-antagonistic effect of glucocorticoids. *Metabolism* **28**, 502–510.

Cioffi, J.A., Shafer, A.W., Zupancic, T.J. *et al.* (1996) Novel B219/OB receptor isoforms: possible role of leptin in hematopoiesis and reproduction. *Nature Medicine* **2**, 585–588.

Considine, R.V., Sinha, M.K., Heiman, M.L. *et al.* (1996) Serum immunoreactive-leptin concentrations in normal-weight and obese humans. *New England Journal of Medicine* **334**, 292–295.

Coppack, S.W., Evans, R.D., Fisher, R.M. *et al.* (1992) Adipose tissue metabolism in obesity: lipase action *in vivo* before and after a mixed meal. *Metabolism* **41**, 264–272.

Couch, R.M., Muller, J. & Winter, J.S.D. (1986) Regulation of the activities of 17-hydroxylase and 17,20 desmolase in the human adrenal cortex: genetic analysis and inhibition by endogenous steroids. *Journal of Clinical Endocrinology and Metabolism* **63**, 613–618.

Cusin, I., Dryden, S., Wang, Q., Rohner-Jeanrenaud, F., Jeanrenaud, B. & Williams, G. (1995) Effect of sustained physiological hyperinsulinaemia on hypothalamic neuropeptide Y and NPY mRNA levels in the rat. *Journal of Neuroendocrinology* **7** (3), 193–197.

Deslypere, J.P., Verdonck, L. & Vermuulen, A. (1987) Fat tissue: a steroid reservoir and site of steroid metabolism. *Journal of Clinical Endocrinology and Metabolism* **61**, 564–570.

Eaton, R.P., Berman, M. & Steinberg, D. (1969) Kinetic studies of plasma free fatty acid and triglyceride metabolism in man. *Journal of Clinical Investigation* **48**, 1560–1579.

Elbers, J.M.H., Asscheman, H., Seidell, J.C. & Gooren, L.J.G. (1995) Increased accumulation of visceral fat after long term androgen administration in women. *International Journal of Obesity* **19** (suppl. 2), 25 (abstract).

Evans, B.A. & Hughes, I.A. (1985) Augmentation of androgen-receptor binding *in vitro*: studies in normals and patients with androgen insensitivity. *Clinical Endocrinology* **23**, 567–577.

Evans, D.J., Murray, R. & Kissebah, A.H. (1984) Relationship between skeletal muscle insulin resistance, insulin-mediated glucose disposal and insulin binding effects of obesity and body fat topography. *Journal of Clinical Investigation* **74**, 1515–1525.

Ferron, F., Considine, R.V., Peiono, R., Lado, I.G., Dieguez, C. & Casanueva, F.F. (1997) Serum leptin concentrations in patients with anorexia nervosa, bulimia nervosa and non-specific eating disorders correlate with body mass index but are independent of the respective disease. *Clinical Endocrinology* **46**, 289–293.

Galvao-Tales, A., Graves, L., Burke, C.W. *et al.* (1976) Free cortisol in obesity: effect of fasting. *Acta Endocrinology* **81**, 321–329.

Glass, A.R. (1989) Endocrine aspects of obesity. *Medical Clinics of North America* **73**, 139–160.

Glass, A.R., Burman, K.D., Dahms, W.T. & Boehm, T.M. (1981) Endocrine function in human obesity. *Metabolism* **30**, 89–104.

Haarbo, J., Marslew, U., Gottfredsen, A. & Christiansen, C. (1991) Postmenopausal hormone replacement therapy prevents central distribution of body fat after the menopause. *Metabolism* **40**, 323–326.

Haffner, S.M., Katz, M.S., Stern, M.P., & Dunn, J.F. (1988) The relationship of sex hormones to hyperinsulinaemia and hyperglycaemia. *Metabolism* **37**, 683–688.

Haffner, S.M., Stern, M.P., Miettinen, H., Wei, M. & Gingerich, R.L. (1996). Leptin concentrations in diabetic and nondiabetic Mexican-Americans. *Diabetes* **45**, 822–824.

Kalkhoff, R. & Ferrow, C. (1971) Metabolic differences between obese overweight and muscular overweight men. *New England Journal of Medicine* **284**, 1236–1239.

Kennedy, A., Gettys, T.W., Watson, P. *et al.* (1997) The metabolic significance of leptin in humans: Gender-based differences in relationship to adiposity, insulin sensitivity, and energy expenditure. *Journal of Clinical Endocrinology and Metabolism* **82**, 1293–1300.

Khaw, K-T. & Barret-Connor, E. (1991) Fasting plasma glucose levels and endogenous androgens in non-diabetic postmenopausal women. *Clinical Science* **80**, 199–203.

Kissebah, A.H., Vydelingum, N. & Murray, R. (1982) Relation of body fat distribution to metabolic complications of obesity. *Journal of Clinical Investigation* **54**, 254–260.

Kolaczynski, J.W., Nyce, M.R., Considine, R.V. *et al.* (1996) Acute and chronic effects of insulin on leptin production in humans: Studies *in vivo* and *in vitro*. *Diabetes* **45**, 699–701.

Kolterman, O.G., Insel, J., Sackow, M. & Olefsky, M. (1980) Mechanisms of insulin resistance in human obesity. *Journal of Clinical Investigation* **65**, 1272–1284.

Kopelman, P.G. (1994) Hormones and obesity. *Baillière's Clinical Endocrinology and Metabolism* **8**, 549–575.

Kopelman, P.G. (1988) Neuroendocrine function in obesity. *Clinical Endocrinology* **28**, 675–689.

Krotkiewski, M., Bjorntorp, P., Sjostrom, L. & Smith, U. (1983) Impact of obesity on metabolism in men and women: importance of regional adipose tissue distribution. *Journal of Clinical Investigation* **72**, 1150–1162.

Kurtz, B.R., Givens, J.R., Kominder, S. *et al.* (1987) Maintenance of normal circulating levels of androstenedione and dehydroepiandrosterone in simple obesity despite increased metabolic clearance rates: evidence for a servo-controlled mechanism. *Journal of Clinical Endocrinology and Metabolism* **64**, 1261–1267.

Lafontan, M., Dang-Tran, L. & Berlan, M. (1979) Alpha-adrenergic antipolytic effect of adrenaline in human fat cells of the thigh: comparison with adrenal responsiveness of different fat deposits. *European Journal of Clinical Investigation* **9**, 261–266.

Lafontan, M. & Berlan, M. (1993) Fat cell adrenergic receptors and the control of white and brown fat cell function. *Journal of Lipid Research* **34**, 1057–1091.

Longcope, C., Baker, R. & Johnston, C.C. Jr (1986a) Androgen and oestrogen metabolism: relationship to obesity. *Metabolism* **35**, 235–237.

Longcope, C., Layne, D.S. & Tait, J.F. (1986b) Metabolic clearance rates and interconversions of oestrone and 17-B-oestradiol in normal males and females. *Journal of Clinical Investigation* **47**, 93–106.

Lonnqvist, F., Thorne, A., Nilsell, K., Hoffstedt, J. & Arner, P. (1995a) A pathogenic role of visceral fat β_3-adrenoceptors in obesity. *Journal of Clinical Investigation* **95**, 1109–1116.

Lonnqvist, F., Arner, P., Nordfors, L. & Schalling, M. (1995b) Overexpression of the obese (*ob*) gene in adipose tissue of human obese subjects. *Nature Medicine* **1**, 950–953.

Maffei, M., Halaas, J., Ravussin, E. *et al.* (1995) Leptin levels in human and rodent: measurement of plasma leptin and *ob* RNA in obese and weight-reduced subjects. *Nature Medicine* **1**, 1155–1161.

Marin, P., Holmang, S., Jonsson, L. *et al.* (1992) The effects of testosterone treatment on body composition and metabolism in middle-aged obese men. *International Journal of Obesity* **16**, 991–997.

Marin, P., Lonn, L., Andersson, B. *et al.* (1995) Assimilation and mobilisation of triglycerides in subcutaneous and intraabdominal adipose tissue *in vivo* in men: effects of testosterone. *Journal of Clinical Endocrinology and Metabolism* **80**, 239–243.

Martin, M.L. & Jensen, M.D. (1991) Effects of body fat distribution on regional lipolysis in obesity. *Journal of Clinical Investigation* **88**, 609–613.

Mayo-Smith, W., Hayes, C.W. & Biller, B.M.K. (1989) Body fat distribution measured with CT: correlations in healthy subjects, anorexia nervosa and patients with Cushing's syndrome. *Radiology* **170**, 515–518.

Meldrum, D.R., Davidson, B.J., Tatryn, I.V. & Judd, H.L. (1981) Changes in circulating steroids with aging in post-menopausal women. *Obstetrics and Gynaecology* **57**, 624–628.

Merimee, T.J. & Fineberg, S.E. (1973) Dietary regulation of human growth hormone secretion. *Metabolism* **22**, 1491–1497.

Migeon, C.J., Green, O.C. & Eckert, J.P. (1963) Study of adrenocortical function in obesity. *Metabolism* **12**, 718–730.

Montague C.T., Farooqi, I.S., Whitehead, J.P. *et al.* (1997a) Congenital leptin deficiency is associated with severe early-onset obesity in humans. *Nature* **387**, 903–908.

Montague, C.T., Prins, J.B., Sanders, L., Digby, J.E. & O'Rahilly, S. (1997b). Depot- and sex-specific differences in human leptin mRNA expression: Implications for the control of regional fat distribution. *Diabetes* **46**, 342–347.

Ong, J.M. & Kern, P.A. (1989) Effect of feeding and obesity on lipoprotein lipase activity, immunoreactive protein and messenger RNA levels in human adipose tissue. *Journal of Clinical Investigation* **84**, 305–311.

Peiris, A.N., Mueller, R.A. & Smith, G.A. (1986) Splanchnic insulin metabolism in obesity: influence of body fat distribution. *Journal of Clinical Investigation* **78**, 1648–1657.

Peiris, A.N., Mueller, R.A., Strieve, M.F. *et al.* (1987) Relationship of androgenic activity to splanchnic insulin metabolism and peripheral glucose utilisation in premenopausal women. *Journal of Clinical Endocrinology and Metabolism* **64**, 162–169.

Plymate, S.R., Matej, L.A., Jones, R.A. & Friedl, K.E. (1988) Inhibition of sex hormone binding globulin production in human hepatoma (hep G2) cell line by insulin and prolactin. *Journal of Clinical Endocrinology and Metabolism* **67**, 460–464.

Rasmussen, M.H., Juul, A., Kjems, L.L. *et al.* (1995a) Lack of stimulation of 24 hour growth hormone release by hypocaloric diets in obesity. *Journal of Clinical Endocrinology and Metabolism* **80**, 796–801.

Rasmussen, M.H., Hvidberg, A., Juul, A. *et al.* (1995b) Massive weight loss restores 24 hour growth hormone release profiles and serum insulin-like growth factor 1 levels in obese subjects. *Journal of Clinical Endocrinology and Metabolism* **80**, 1407–1415.

Reaven, G.M. (1995) The fourth musketeer—from Alexander Dumas to Claude Bernard. *Diabetologia* **38**, 3–13.

Rebuffe-Scrive, M. & Bjorntorp, P. (1985) Regional adipose tissue metabolism in man. In: Vague, J., Bjorntorp, P. & Guy-Grand, B. (eds) *Metabolic Complications of Human Obesities*, pp. 149–159. Amsterdam: Excerpta Medica.

Rebuffe-Scrive, M., Enk, L., Crona, N. *et al.* (1985a) Fat cell metabolism in different regions in women. Effects of menstrual cycle, pregnancy and lactation. *Journal of Clinical Investigation* **75**, 1973–1976.

Rebuffe-Scrive, M., Lundholm, K. & Bjorntorp, P. (1985b) Glucocorticoid hormone binding to human adipose tissue. *European Journal of Clinical Investigation* **15**, 267–271.

Rebuffe-Scrive, M., Lonnroth, P. Marin, P., Wesslau, C., Bjorntorp, P. & Smith, U. (1987) Regional adipose tissue metabolism in men and postmenopausal women. *International Journal of Obesity* **11**, 347–355.

Rebuffe-Scrive, M., Krotkiewski, M., Elfverson, J. & Bjorntorp, P. (1988) Muscle and adipose tissue morphology and metabolism in Cushing's syndrome. *Journal of Clinical Endocrinology Metabolism* **67**, 1122–1128.

Rebuffe-Scrive, M., Andersson, B., Olbe, L. & Bjorntorp, P. (1989) Metabolism of adipose tissue in intraabdominal depots of non-obese men and women. *Metabolism* **38**, 453–461.

Rebuffe-Scrive, M., Bronnegard, M., Nilsso, A. *et al.* (1990) Steroid hormone receptors in human adipose tissues. *Journal of Clinical Endocrinology and Metabolism* **71**, 1215–1219.

Reynisdottir, S., Ellerfeldt, K., Wahrenberg, H., Lithell, H. & Arner, P. (1994) Multiple lipolysis defects in insulin resistance (metabolic) syndrome. *Journal of Clinical Investigation* **93**, 2590–2599.

Reynisdottir, S., Langin, D., Carlstrom, K., Holm, C., Rossner, S. & Arner, P. (1995) Effects of weight reduction on the regulation of lipolysis in adipocytes of women with upper-body obesity. *Clinical Science* **89**, 421–429.

Roncari, D.A.K. & Van, R.L.R. (1997) Promotion of human adipocyte precursor replication in 17-β-oestradiol in culture. *Journal of Clinical Investigation* **62**, 502–508.

Simkin, V. (1961) Urinary 17-ketosteroid and 17-ketogenic steroid excretion in obese patients. *New England Journal of Medicine* **264**, 974–977.

Sims, E.A.H., Danforth, E.H., Horton, E.S. *et al.* (1973) Endocrine and metabolic effects of experimental obesity in man. *Recent Progress in Hormone Research* **29**, 457–487.

Sjögren, J., Li, M. & Björntorp, P. (1995) Androgen hormone binding to adipose tissue in rats. *Biochimica et Biophysica Acta* **1244**, 117–120.

Slavnov, V.N. & Epshtein, E.V. (1977) Somatotrophic, thyrotrophic and adrenotrophic functions of the anterior pituitary in obesity. *Endocrinologie* **15**, 213–218.

Smith, C.J., Vasta, V., Degerman, E., Belfrage, P. & Manganiello, V.C. (1991) Hormone-sensitive cyclic GMP-inhibited cyclic AMP phosphodiesterase in rat adipocytes. Regulation of insulin- and cAMP-dependent activation by phosphorylation. *Journal of Biological Chemistry* **266**, 13385–13390.

Svedberg, J., Björntorp, P., Smith, U. & Lonnroth, P. (1990) Free fatty acids inhibition of insulin binding, degradation and action in isolated ra hepatocytes. *Diabetes* **39**, 570–574.

Tanner, J.M. & Whitehouse, R.H. (1967) The effect of human growth hormone on subcutaneous fat thickness in hyposomatrophic and hypopituitary dwarfs. *Journal of Endocrinology* **39**, 263–275.

Unger, R.H. (1995) Lipotoxicity in the pathogenesis of obesity-dependent NIDDM. Genetic and clinical implications. *Diabetes* **44**, 863–870.

Usiskin, K.S., Butterworth, S., Clore, J.N. *et al.* (1990) Lack of effect of dehydroepiandrosterone suphate in obese men. *International Journal of Obesity* **14**, 457–463.

Wahrenberg, H., Lonnqvist, F. & Arner, P. (1989) Mechanisms underlying regional differences in lipolysis in human adipose tissue. *Journal of Clinical Investigation* **84**, 458–467.

Weaver, J.U., Kopelman, P.G., Holly, J.M.P. *et al.* (1990) Decreased sex hormone binding globulin (SHBG) and insulin-like growth factor binding protein (IGFBP-1) in extreme obesity. *Clinical Endocrinology* **32**, 641–646.

Weaver, J.U., Kopelman, P.G., McLoughlin, L. *et al.* (1993) Hyperactivity of the hypothalamo-pituitary-adrenal axis in obesity: a study of ACTH, AVP, B-lipoprotein and cortisol responses to insulin-induced hypoglycaemia. *Clinical Endocrinology* **39**, 345–350.

Williams, D.P., Boyden, T.W., Pamenter, R.W. *et al.* (1993) Relationship of body fat percentage and fat distribution with dehydroepeiandrosterone sulphate in premenopausal females. *Journal of Clinical Endocrinology and Metaolism* **77**, 80–85.

Xu, X., De Pergola, G. & Björntorp, P. (1990a) The effects of androgens on the regulation of lipolysis in adipose precursor cells. *Endocrinology* **126**, 1229–1234.

Xu, X., Hoebeke, J. & Björntorp, P. (1990b) Progestin binds to the glucocorticoid receptor and mediates antiglucocorticoid effect in rat adipose precursor cells. *Journal of Steroid Biochemistry* **36**, 465–471.

Xu, X., De Pergola, G. & Björntorp, P. (1991) Testosterone increases lipolysis and the number of β-adrenoceptors in male rat adipocytes. *Endocrinology* **128**, 379–382.

....

CHAPTER 9

Obesity and Lipoprotein Metabolism

ANDRÉ TCHERNOF AND JEAN-PIERRE DESPRÉS

....

Dyslipidaemic states and the risk of coronary heart disease

Coronary heart disease (CHD) is recognized as a major cause of mortality and morbidity in affluent societies. In this regard, it is widely accepted that high plasma cholesterol concentrations are associated with an increased risk of CHD (Gotto et al., 1990; NIH Conference, 1985). This association has been found in several epidemiological studies, including, among others, the Framingham Heart Study (Kannel et al., 1971; Castelli, 1984) and the Multiple Risk Factor Intervention Trial (Multiple Risk Factor Intervention Trial Research Group, 1982; Stamler et al., 1986). However, the clinician only has a limited ability to identify patients at high risk of cardiovascular disease on the basis of plasma cholesterol alone. Indeed, a study from Genest and colleagues (Genest et al., 1991) has shown that there is considerable overlap in plasma cholesterol concentration among subjects with and without CHD as almost 50% of patients with the disease had relatively normal plasma cholesterol levels (Genest et al., 1991). Accordingly, Sniderman and Silberberg (1990) have suggested that although mean plasma cholesterol levels may be higher in patients with CHD compared to healthy subjects, the overlap of cholesterol values in these two groups of individuals is such that the ability of cholesterol alone to discriminate subjects at risk of CHD is quite weak (Sniderman & Silberberg, 1990). A more complete assessment of the plasma lipid–lipoprotein profile has therefore been recommended to provide further information on the risk of CHD.

Cholesterol and triglycerides are hydrophobic compounds which are transported in the blood by lipoproteins. On the basis of their density and composition, four major subclasses of lipoproteins have been identified: chylomicrons, very-low-density lipoproteins (VLDL), low-density lipoproteins (LDL) and high-density lipoproteins (HDL) (Fig. 9.1). Chylomicrons are the largest lipoproteins and they are very rich in triglycerides. They are synthesized in the intestine shortly after a meal and they represent the form by which most of the dietary fatty acids are transported in the plasma. VLDLs are responsible for the transport of endogeneous triglycerides synthesized by the liver while

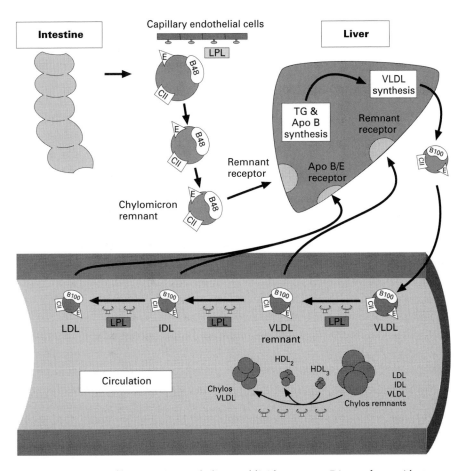

Fig. 9.1 Overview of lipoprotein metabolism and lipid transport. Dietary fatty acids are incorporated in the form of triglycerides into chylomicrons also containing Apo B48, CII and E in the intestine. Endothelial lipoprotein lipase (LPL) is responsible for the hydrolysis of the triglyceride content of chylomicrons. The resulting chylomicron remnants are taken up by the remnant receptor in the liver. VLDL particles containing Apo B100 are synthesized by the liver. These particles are submitted to the catabolic activity of endothelial LPL in the circulation, leading to the formation of VLDL remnants, IDL and LDL particles, which are depleted in triglycerides and enriched in cholesterol. VLDL remnants are taken up by the remnant receptor in the liver, whereas IDL and LDL bind to the hepatic Apo B/E receptor (LDL receptor). HDL particles are generated by aggregation of excess surface components resulting from the hydrolysis of Apo B-containing particles by LPL. The cholesterol ester content of HDL is also increased during this process (HDL$_2$ subfraction).

LDLs are the catabolic products of VLDLs, resulting from the hydrolysis of the triglyceride content of VLDL particles by the enzyme lipoprotein lipase (LPL). These LDL particles are the main carriers of cholesterol in the blood. Apolipoprotein (Apo) B100 synthesized in the liver is the main protein constituent of LDL and only one molecule of Apo B is found per LDL particle. The formation of HDL particles results from the hydrolysis of VLDL to LDL, a process during which excess surface components aggregate to form nascent HDL particles. The major apolipoproteins of HDL particles are Apo AI and Apo AII (see Fig. 9.1).

Epidemiological studies have now clearly established that low plasma HDL-cholesterol (HDL-C) concentrations are associated with an increased risk of CHD (Austin, 1991). As there is a well-established negative relationship between plasma HDL-C and triglyceride concentrations (Gordon *et al.*, 1977; Albrink, *et al.*, 1980; Davis *et al.*, 1980; Petersson *et al.*, 1984), patients characterized by low HDL-C levels also frequently have high plasma triglyceride concentrations. The contribution of plasma triglycerides as a risk factor for CHD remains equivocal. Indeed, several studies have shown that high plasma triglyceride levels were no longer a risk factor for CHD after statistical adjustment for HDL-C concentration (Austin, 1991). On the other hand, prospective data from the PROCAM Study have shown that a low HDL-C concentration was an independent predictor of an increased CHD risk (Assmann & Schulte, 1992). It appears that current statistical models cannot adequately consider the pathophysiological aspects of low HDL-C levels in association with elevated triglyceride concentrations, an issue that has been frequently raised (Lamarche *et al.*, 1996a).

The study of apolipoprotein concentrations is also likely to provide some important information on the risk of CHD as these variables could be indicative of the concentrations of lipoproteins which promote or protect against premature atherosclerosis. Cross-sectional studies have indicated that patients with CHD have higher plasma Apo B and lower Apo AI levels (Sniderman, 1992; Rader *et al.*, 1994). Further studies will be needed to determine the optimal lipoprotein predictors of CHD risk but it is now clear that the clinician needs to go beyond the measurement of plasma cholesterol and LDL cholesterol levels in the assessment of risk.

Obesity and dyslipidaemias: importance of visceral adipose tissue

Obesity is commonly associated with chronic diseases such as hypertension, diabetes and cardiovascular disease (Sims & Berchtold, 1982; Bray, 1985; Garrison *et al.*, 1987; Kissebah *et al.*, 1989). Excess body fatness has also been frequently associated with dyslipidaemic states and alterations in other cardiovascular disease risk factors (Kissebah *et al.*, 1989b; Després, 1991b, 1994b). Some prospective studies have found that obesity was a significant predictor of cardiovascular disease related mortality, although this association appears to be of lower magnitude than the relationships of cardiovascular disease mortality to well-known risk factors such as smoking, hypertension and dyslipidaemia (Bray *et al.*, 1972; Barrett-Connor, 1985; Kissebah *et al.*, 1989; Manson *et al.*, 1995). Thus, whether excess body-weight is an independent predictor of cardiovascular disease and related mortality is an issue that has not been fully resolved.

It is now also well accepted that obesity represents a heterogeneous condition from a metabolic standpoint. Vague (1947) was the first to observe that the gender-related difference in body fat distribution was a better correlate of the complications of obesity than excess body-weight *per se*. He defined the accumulation of upper body fat mostly found in men as *android* obesity, this type of obesity being more frequently associated with diabetes, hypertension, and cardiovascular disease. He also referred to *gynoid* obesity to describe a condition where body fat was preferentially accumulated in the gluteo-femoral region. He suggested that this pattern of fat distribution, mostly found in women, was not associated with the expected complications of obesity (Vague, 1947)

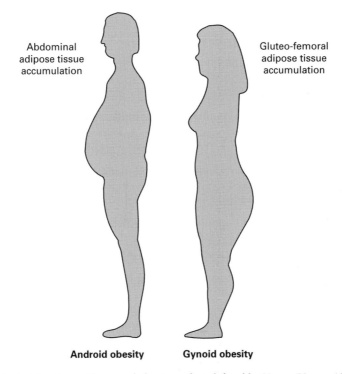

Abdominal adipose tissue accumulation

Gluteo-femoral adipose tissue accumulation

Android obesity   **Gynoid obesity**

Fig. 9.2 Android and gynoid types of obesity as first defined by Vague (Vague, 1947), with preferential accumulation of adipose tissue in the abdominal and gluteo-femoral region, respectively. The android pattern of adipose tissue distribution is more closely associated with the metabolic complications of obesity.

(Fig. 9.2). Several prospective studies which have used the ratio of the waist to hip circumferences (the widely used waist/hip ratio) have now confirmed that the android type of obesity, now referred to as abdominal obesity, is more closely associated with metabolic complications such as dyslipidaemias, hyper-insulinaemia and a higher risk of diabetes and cardiovascular diseases than an excess of total body fatness (Kissebah *et al.*, 1982; Björntorp, 1984; Lapidus *et al.*, 1984; Larsson *et al.*, 1984; Ohlson *et al.*, 1985; Ducimetière *et al.*, 1986; Donahue *et al.*, 1987).

Measurement of visceral adipose tissue: age and gender differences

As mentioned above, the most widely used measurement of body fat distribution has been the waist/hip ratio. The rationale for using this index is that the higher the accumulation of abdominal fat, the higher the ratio of waist/hip circumferences is. However, this measurement does not distinguish the amount of adipose tissue located in the abdominal cavity (the intra-abdominal or visceral adipose tissue) from the subcutaneous abdominal adipose tissue. With the development of imaging techniques such as computed tomography it has become possible to accurately evaluate the amount of fat located in the visceral compartment (Sjöström *et al.*, 1986; Ferland *et al.*, 1989; Després *et al.*, 1991). On the basis of the differences in the density of tissues, adipose tissue can be distinguished from bone and muscle tissue and areas of visceral adipose tissue can be obtained by performing a single scan at the abdominal level, usually at L4–L5 vertebrate (Sjöström *et al.*, 1986; Ferland *et al.*, 1989; Després *et al.*, 1991) (Fig. 9.3). By using this methodology, age and gender differences in visceral adipose tissue accumulation have been reported. Indeed, Lemieux and colleagues have noted that for any given body fat mass, men had on average twice the amount of visceral adipose tissue found in premenopausal women (Lemieux *et al.*, 1993) (Fig. 9.4). Whether such a gender difference in visceral adipose tissue accumulation could account for the well-known average difference in cardiovascular risk factors between men and women has also been examined (Lemieux *et al.*, 1994). It was found in a cross-sectional comparison of subgroups of men and women matched for the level of visceral adipose tissue that this procedure largely eliminated most of the differences in plasma lipoprotein levels with the exception of plasma HDL-C concentrations, which remained higher in women than in men (Lemieux *et al.*, 1994).

The prevalence of obesity increases with age (Reeder *et al.*, 1992). Furthermore, total body fat mass and visceral adipose tissue accumulation are also significant positive correlates of age (Enzi *et al.*, 1986; Seidell *et al.*, 1988; Schwartz *et al.*, 1990; Kotani *et al.*, 1994). Globally, the cardiovascular disease risk profile also deteriorates with age, and it has been shown that the

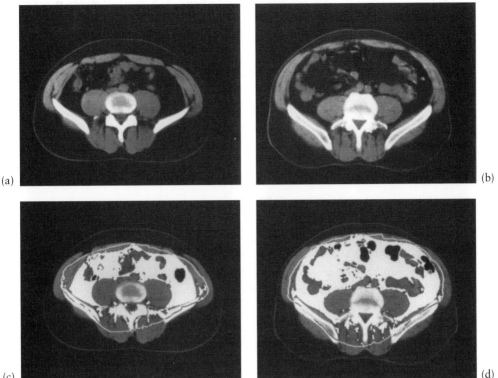

(a)   (b)

(c)   (d)

Fig. 9.3 (a, b) Cross-sectional abdominal adipose tissue area measured by computed tomography at the L4–L5 vertebrae level in a young man and a middle-aged man with comparable levels of total body fat in kilograms. (c, d) The visceral cavity was delineated with a graph pen and adipose tissue was highlighted with an attenuation range of −190 to −30 hounsfield units.

Fig. 9.4 Relationships between visceral adipose tissue area and percentage body fat in men and women ($r = 0.71$, $P < 0.0001$ in men and $r = 0.76$, $P < 0.0001$ in women). Adapted from Lemieux et al. (1993).

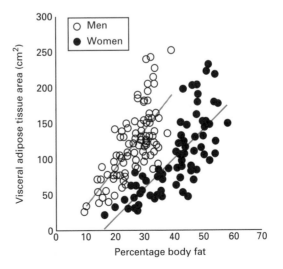

concomitant increase in visceral adipose tissue was one of the important factors associated with the development of a more atherogenic metabolic profile (Lemieux et al., 1995). However, it also appears that other age-related processes that are independent of the variation in total adiposity and visceral adipose tissue deposition contribute to the alterations in plasma lipid and lipoprotein concentrations, particularly for LDL-C concentrations (Lemieux et al., 1995). Thus, age and gender variation in the metabolic risk profile predictive of the risk of non-insulin-dependent diabetes mellitus (NIDDM) and cardiovascular disease could be partly attributed to the concomitant variation in visceral adipose tissue accumulation.

Visceral obesity and dyslipidaemias: contribution of insulin resistance

It is now well established that visceral obesity is a critical correlate of several metabolic complications found in obesity (Kissebah et al., 1989; Kissebah & Krakower, 1994). In order to sort out the relative contribution of total body fatness vs visceral adipose tissue accumulation as correlates of metabolic alterations, we have used a simple approach in which we compared two subgroups of obese subjects matched for total body fat but with either low or high levels of visceral adipose tissue measured by computed tomography. These two groups were then compared with lean controls (Fig. 9.5). As shown in Fig. 9.5, only men with high levels of visceral adipose tissue displayed significantly higher plasma triglyceride levels, lower HDL-C concentrations as well as a reduced HDL_2-C/HDL_3-C ratio compared to the two other subgroups. Comparable results were obtained when similar analyses were conducted in women (not shown).

It is also important to point out that plasma total cholesterol levels are often within the normal range in subjects with visceral obesity. However, we have reported that visceral obese subjects were characterized by significant increases in Apo B as well as in LDL-Apo B concentrations (Fig. 9.6) (Pouliot et al., 1992). Thus, visceral obesity is associated with an increased LDL-Apo B/ LDL-C ratio, which is suggestive of alterations in the composition of LDL particles. Recent studies from our group (Tchernof et al., 1996b) in which a 2–16% polyacrylamide gradient gel electrophoretic procedure was used to assess the proportion of small, dense LDL particles as well as LDL particle size have indicated that visceral obesity is indeed associated with the predominance of small, dense LDL particles in the plasma (Tchernof et al., 1996b). Furthermore, as reported in several other studies, the presence of small, dense LDL particles is closely associated with high triglyceride and low HDL-C levels (McNamara et al., 1987; Austin, 1992; Zhao et al., 1993). Indeed, we found that after including triglyceride and HDL-C concentrations in a multivariate model, visceral

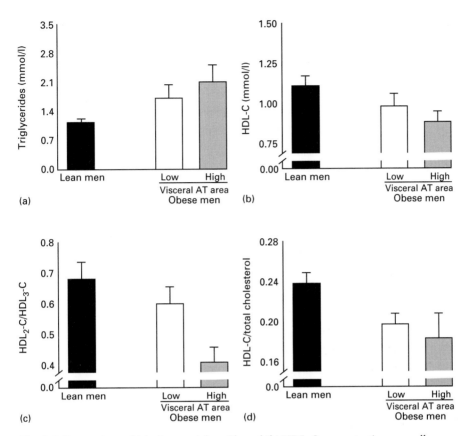

Fig. 9.5 Comparison of (a) plasma triglyceride and (b) HDL-C concentrations as well as (c) HDL_2-C/HDL_3-C and (d) HDL-C/total cholesterol ratios among a subgroup of lean men and two subgroups of obese men with the same amount of total fat but with either low or high levels of visceral adipose tissue (AT). 1: significantly different from lean controls. Adapted from Pouliot *et al.* (1992).

obesity was no longer a significant correlate of the proportion of small, dense LDL or LDL particle size, suggesting that the dense LDL phenotype is only found in visceral obesity because of the related high triglyceride–low HDL-C dyslipidaemic state (Tchernof *et al.*, 1996b).

Visceral obesity is, therefore, associated with a dyslipidaemic state which includes hypertriglyceridaemia, hypoalphalipoproteinaemia, a reduced HDL_2-C/HDL_3-C ratio, elevated Apo B concentration, a greater proportion of small, dense LDL particles and an increased cholesterol/HDL-C ratio. This dyslipidaemic phenotype has been suggested to substantially increase the risk of CHD (Després, 1994b).

By using the approach described above to compare obese subjects with either low or high levels of visceral adipose tissue to lean controls, we have observed

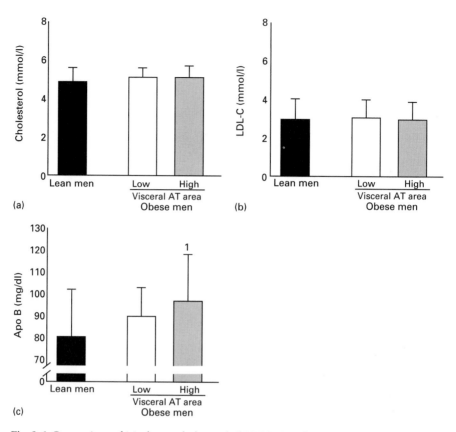

Fig. 9.6 Comparison of (a) plasma cholesterol, (b) LDL-C and (c) Apo B levels among a subgroup of lean men vs two subgroups of obese men with the same amount of total fat but with either low or high levels of visceral adipose tissue (AT). 1: significantly different from lean controls. Adapted from Lemieux and Després (1994).

that obese men and women with high levels of visceral adipose tissue were also characterized by significantly higher fasting plasma insulin concentrations and by higher insulinaemic and glycaemic responses to a standard oral glucose load (Després *et al.*, 1989b; Pouliot *et al.*, 1992b) (Fig. 9.7). These results suggest that individuals with visceral obesity are characterized by hyperinsulinaemia resulting from an insulin-resistant state. As prospective studies have shown that visceral obesity is associated with an increased risk of developing type II diabetes (Bergstrom *et al.*, 1990), this condition may evolve to glucose intolerance and even to NIDDM in the presence of genetic susceptibility factors which remain poorly understood.

Reaven (1988) was the first to suggest the term 'insulin resistance syndrome' (or syndrome X) to describe a cluster of metabolic abnormalities including: hypoalphalipoproteinaemia, hypertriglyceridaemia, hyperinsulinaemia

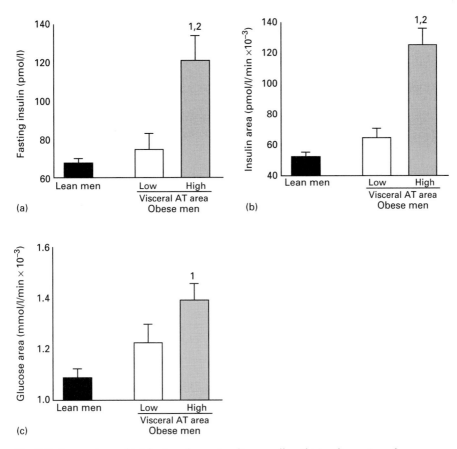

Fig. 9.7 Comparison of (a) fasting plasma insulin as well as (b) insulinaemic and (c) glycaemic responses to a 75-g oral glucose load (areas under the curves) among a subgroup of lean men and two subgroups of obese men with the same amount of total fat but with either low or high levels of visceral adipose tissue (AT). 1: significantly different from lean controls; 2: significantly different from obese men with low levels of visceral adipose tissue, $P < 0.05$. Adapted from Pouliot *et al.* (1992).

and increased blood pressure. As visceral obesity is associated with this cluster of metabolic abnormalities contributing to increase the risk of type II diabetes and cardiovascular diseases, we have suggested that excess visceral adipose tissue accumulation was an important additional component of the insulin resistance syndrome (Després, 1993; Després, 1994; Lemieux & Després, 1994). Although there is currently no prospective study having identified visceral obesity as an independent risk factor for cardiovascular disease and related mortality, several studies have suggested that the cluster of metabolic abnormalities found in visceral obesity, namely hyperinsulinaemia, insulin resistance, hyper-triglyceridaemia, hypoalphalipoproteinaemia, hyper-Apo B and the dense LDL phenotype, substantially increases the risk of cardiovascular disease (Fig. 9.8).

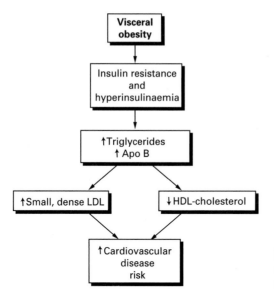

Fig. 9.8 Cluster of metabolic abnormalities found in visceral obesity.

The insulin resistant-dyslipidaemic syndrome of visceral obesity: an important cause of coronary heart disease

As mentioned earlier, a low plasma HDL-C concentration appears to be an independent risk factor for CHD. On the other hand, high plasma triglyceride levels are not considered an independent risk factor, although this issue cannot be adequately dealt with by the current statistical models used in epidemiology. These fail to recognize the contribution of alterations in the metabolism of triglyceride-rich lipoproteins to the pathophysiology of atherogenic dyslipidaemia (Austin, 1991). Few prospective studies examined the contribution of the various components of the metabolic cluster found in visceral obesity to CHD risk. In this regard, the Québec Cardiovascular Study gave us the opportunity to examine this issue in a prospective design. In 1985, we evaluated the cardiovascular disease risk profile of a random sample of 2443 middle-aged men living in the metropolitan area of Québec City (Dagenais et al., 1990). This evaluation included the measurement of fasting plasma lipid and lipoprotein levels. After exclusion of men who showed clinical signs of ischaemic heart disease (IHD) (exertional angina, coronary insufficiency, non-fatal myocardial infarction and coronary death) and of men with triglyceride concentrations above 4.5 mmol/L, we studied the 5-year incidence of IHD in a sample of 2103 men initially free from disease.

Over the 5-year follow-up, 114 men developed clinical signs of IHD. When comparing the risk profile of these 114 men with the 1989 men who remained healthy over the 5 years, it was found that men with IHD had an elevated systolic blood pressure and a much higher prevalence of diabetes (Lamarche *et al.*, 1995). Body fatness, at least as crudely assessed by the body mass index (BMI), was not significantly different among these groups. Significant differences were also found in the plasma lipoprotein and lipid profile between men with IHD and men who remained healthy. Plasma total cholesterol and triglyceride levels were significantly higher in men who developed IHD compared to those who remained event-free. The mean Apo B concentration was also 12% higher in men who developed IHD. In accordance with previous prospective data, plasma HDL-C concentrations were lower and the cholesterol/HDL-C ratio was substantially higher (by 16%) in men who developed IHD compared to men who remained healthy over the 5-year follow-up (Lamarche *et al.*, 1995).

By using an algorithm to classify subjects according to various dyslipidaemic phenotypes, Lamarche and colleagues (Lamarche *et al.*, 1995) found that, while 51% of the 1989 men who remained healthy over the follow-up were normolipidaemic, less than one-third of men who developed IHD were initially characterized by a normal lipoprotein–lipid profile (Fig. 9.9), emphasizing the importance of alterations in plasma lipoprotein–lipid levels as risk factors for the development of IHD. Moreover, an elevated Apo B concentration was found in 42% of men who developed IHD. Quantification of the relative risk of IHD associated with each dyslipidaemic phenotype indicated that, in accordance with previous studies, elevated LDL cholesterol levels were associated with an increased risk of IHD. However, men with hypertriglyceridaemia but with normal Apo B levels were not characterized by a higher risk of IHD, while men with hyper-Apo B with or without high triglyceride concentrations had a 2.5–3-fold increase in IHD risk (Fig. 9.10). Multiple regression analyses revealed that after including Apo B level in a model to predict IHD risk, this variable was found as the best metabolic predictor of IHD (Lamarche *et al.*, 1996b). These results emphasize that elevated plasma Apo B levels, which are commonly found in visceral obesity, are associated with an increased IHD risk even in the absence of marked elevation in cholesterol and LDL cholesterol levels.

Since hyperinsulinaemia is frequently found with insulin resistance, the fasting insulin concentration is often used as a crude measurement of *in vivo* insulin resistance. This assumption is especially valid in non-diabetic subjects with no impairment in glucose tolerance (Laakso, 1997). Some prospective studies had reported a significant association between fasting hyperinsulinaemia and mortality from CHD, although this relationship did not appear to be independent from other factors (Pyörälä, 1979; Welborn & Wearne, 1979; Eschwège *et al.*, 1985; Yarnell *et al.*, 1994). We have measured fasting insulin levels in the plasma of men who then developed IHD and in matched controls of the 1985 Québec Cardiovascular Study cohort. Diabetic patients were excluded from the analyses

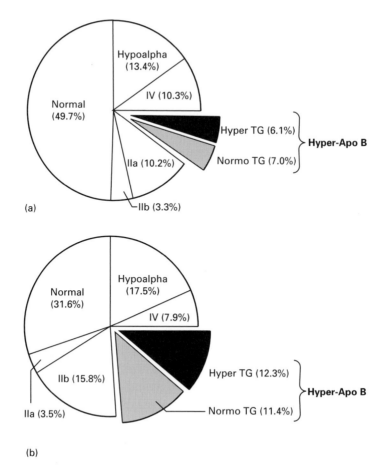

Fig. 9.9 Comparison of the prevalence of the various dyslipidaemic phenotypes among subjects of the Québec Cardiovascular Study: (a) men without IHD, (b) men with IHD. Hyper-Apo B, hyperapolipoprotein B; Hyper TG, hypertriglyceridaemia; Hypoalpha, hypoalphalipoproteinaemia; Normo TG, normal triglyceride levels; IIa, IIb, IV, type IIa, IIb and IV dyslipidaemias. Reproduced by permission from Lamarche *et al.* (1995).

and IHD subjects were matched with controls for smoking habits, BMI, alcohol consumption and age. Fasting plasma insulin levels were 18% higher in men who developed IHD compared to men who remained healthy. Furthermore, fasting plasma insulin concentration was found to be an independent IHD risk factor even after control for other risk variables, including plasma lipid and lipoprotein concentrations (Després *et al.*, 1996). By performing stratified analyses, we have also found that the combination of both hyperinsulinaemia (upper tertile of fasting insulin values distribution) and elevated Apo B levels (above the 50th percentile of Apo B distribution) was associated with more than a 10-fold increase in IHD risk (Fig. 9.11) (Després *et al.*, 1996). It is

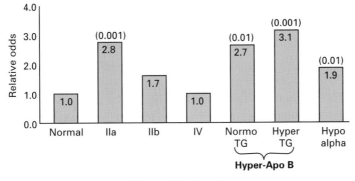

Fig. 9.10 Odds ratios for IHD in men of the Québec Cardiovascular Study characterized by various dyslipidaemic phenotypes. Odds ratios are adjusted for age, systolic blood pressure, diabetes mellitus, alcohol consumption, tobacco use and hypertension-related medication use. Abbreviations as in Fig. 9.9. *P* values are given in parentheses above bars when significant. Adapted from Lamarche *et al.* (1995).

Fig. 9.11 Odds ratios for IHD according to plasma insulin and Apo B levels in the case–control prospective design of the Québec Cardiovascular Study. The cut-off point for low or high Apo B was the 50th percentile of Apo B distribution (119 mg/dl). *P* values are given in parentheses. Reproduced by permission from Després *et al.* (1996).

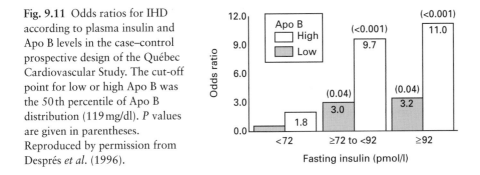

important to emphasize that this combination of hyperinsulinaemia and hyper-Apo B is frequently found in visceral obese patients even in the absence of glucose intolerance or type II diabetes. Therefore, this combination of metabolic abnormalities substantially increase the risk of IHD in these individuals.

The predominance of small, dense LDL particles in the plasma is another condition which has also been associated with an increase in the risk of IHD. Indeed, the predominance of small, dense LDL particles have been reported to be more prevalent in CHD patients than in healthy controls (Fisher, 1983; Crouse *et al.*, 1985; Austin *et al.*, 1988; Griffin *et al.*, 1990, 1994; Tornvall *et al.*, 1991; Campos *et al.*, 1992; Coresh *et al.*, 1993; Jaakkola *et al.*, 1993). There is also evidence suggesting that these particles have atherogenic properties, which could be mediated by an increased filtration rate in the subendothelial space of the artery wall (Packard, 1994; Rajman *et al.*, 1994), an increased susceptibility to oxidation (Chait *et al.*, 1993; de Graaf *et al.*, 1993; Dejager *et al.*, 1993), a reduced affinity for the LDL receptor (longer residence time in the plasma) (Nigon *et al.*, 1991), and an increased capacity to bind to intimal proteoglycans (La Belle & Krauss, 1990). Recent prospective results from the Québec Cardiovascular Study have also shown that dense LDL particles are indeed associated with a significant increase in the risk of IHD over 5 years and that this association is, at least partly, independent from the concomitant variation in the plasma lipid–lipoprotein profile. Furthermore, the simultaneous combination of small, dense LDL particles with elevated Apo B concentrations was associated with a sixfold increase in the risk of IHD (Lamarche *et al.*, 1997).

In this regard, the hypertriglyceridaemic–low HDL–cholesterol dyslipidaemic state of visceral obesity is closely associated with the predominance of small, dense LDL particles (Campos *et al.*, 1991; Katzel *et al.*, 1994; Tchernof *et al.*, 1996b). These results, combined with our recent observations on the Québec Cardiovascular Study, provide further support to the notion that small, dense LDL particles represent another component of the dyslipidaemic profile of visceral obesity which increases the risk of IHD in these patients.

Visceral adipose tissue and the insulin-resistant–dyslipidaemic syndrome: is there a cause and effect relationship?

Evidence is available to suggest that visceral adipose cells have a high lipolytic activity, which is poorly inhibited by insulin (Kissebah & Peiris, 1989; Kissebah *et al.*, 1989; Björntorp, 1990). This excess release of free fatty acids through the portal system to the liver is associated with a reduced hepatic insulin extraction (Hennes *et al.*, 1990; Svedberg *et al.*, 1990). Furthermore, the increased availability of lipids in the liver is likely to be associated with a reduced degradation of Apo B, contributing to the increased hepatic production of Apo B-containing lipoproteins (VLDL) (Björntorp, 1990; Després, 1991). Finally, this hyperlipolytic state is also associated with an increased gluconeogenesis, leading to an elevated hepatic glucose production. This phenomenon explains the deterioration in glucose tolerance frequently found in visceral obese patients (Björntorp, 1992; Després & Marette, 1994). High free fatty acid (FFA) levels released by visceral adipocytes are, therefore, likely to represent a contributing factor to insulin resistance, exacerbating the hyperinsulinaemia required to regulate plasma glucose homeostasis and increasing the secretion of Apo B-containing lipoproteins.

The activity of the enzyme LPL is responsible for the catabolism of triglyceride-rich lipoproteins such as chylomicrons and VLDL. Its activity measured in post-heparin plasma has been reported to be lower in visceral obese patients

(Després *et al.*, 1989a), which contributes to the reduction in the catabolism of triglyceride-rich particles and to elevated plasma triglyceride concentrations. These high concentrations of triglyceride-rich lipoproteins found in visceral obesity also favour an increased lipid transfer by the cholesterol ester transfer protein (CETP) between VLDL particles and LDL as well as HDL particles. HDL particles then become relatively depleted in cholesterol esters and enriched in triglycerides. Triglycerides can also be transferred to LDL by CETP and this phenomenon also reduces the cholesterol to triglyceride ratio in LDL particles. Since hepatic triglyceride lipase (HL) activity has been reported to be increased in visceral obesity (Després *et al.*, 1989; Després & Marette, 1994), triglyceride-rich HDL and LDL particles are then submitted to hydrolysis by this enzyme, generating on the one hand small, dense LDL particles and on the other reduced HDL cholesterol levels, especially in the HDL_2 subfraction (resulting in a reduced HDL_2-C/HDL_3-C ratio) (Fig. 9.12).

Therefore it appears that the increased free fatty acid flux from the adipocytes of the abdominal cavity to the liver, along with the reduced LPL activity, the increased hydrolysis of triglyceride-enriched LDL and HDL by HL and the increased insulin resistance could all be considered as contributing agents in the aetiology of the dyslipidaemic state of visceral obesity, which in turn increases the risk of cardiovascular disease.

Visceral obesity has also been associated with alterations in steroid hormone levels (Tchernof *et al.*, 1996a). In this regard, it remains to be clearly established whether visceral adipose tissue accumulation is the result or the cause of these hormonal abnormalities. One example of hormonal alterations leading to visceral obesity is the Cushing's syndrome, in which cortisol rates are very high (Beaulieu & Kelly, 1990). These patients are characterized by an important accumulation of visceral adipose tissue, which is substantially mobilized with successful treatment of the disease (Baxter & Rousseau, 1979; Björntorp, 1992). It has been hypothesized that the activation of the cortisol axis leading to hypercortisolism, which may also be present among individuals showing a maladaptive response to stress, could be causally associated with the development of visceral obesity (Björntorp, 1991, 1995). In this regard, it has been shown that the density of glucocorticoid receptors is higher in omental adipocytes compared to other subcutaneous fat depots (Rebuffé-Scrive *et al.*, 1985; Miller *et al.*, 1988). It has thus been suggested that the high LPL activity found in omental adipocytes may perhaps result from the hyperinsulinaemia of visceral obesity as well as from the action of cortisol on these adipose cells, increasing fat deposition in visceral adipocytes (Björntorp, 1991). According to this hypothesis, the activation of the hypothalamic–pituitary–adrenal axis would also lead to a reduction in gonadal steroid hormone levels, a finding also reported in visceral obese patients (Björntorp, 1995).

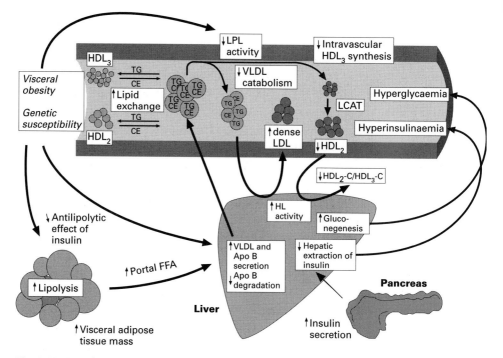

Fig. 9.12 Complex metabolic interactions that presumably occur in the insulin-resistant–dyslipidaemic syndrome of visceral obesity. The liver is exposed to high concentrations of FFA generated by the highly lipolytic activity of the enlarged visceral adipose tissue mass resulting from the reduced inhibition of lipolysis by insulin. This phenomenon stimulates VLDL synthesis and secretion as well as gluconeogenesis in the liver and inhibits hepatic extraction of insulin. The activity of LPL is low, which leads to increased plasma concentrations of triglycerides (TG), low HDL$_3$ intravascular synthesis and reduced HDL$_2$-C levels by lecithin cholesterol acyl transferase (LCAT). Increased lipid exchange between VLDL particles and HDL particles by the cholesteryl ester transfer protein combined with the increased hepatic lipase (HL) activity contribute to the reduced HDL-C concentrations and to the reduced HDL$_2$-C/HDL$_3$-C ratio noted in this condition. TG-enriched and cholesterol ester-depleted LDL particles are also generated by the increased lipid exchange between VLDL and LDL. These LDL particles have a low affinity for the hepatic Apo B/E receptor and therefore have an increased residence time in the plasma. Hydrolysis of the TG content of these particles by HL increases the formation of small, dense LDL. Adapted from Després and Marette (1994).

Visceral obesity is associated with a number of additional hormonal alterations including changes in plasma sex steroid concentrations. Studies in women have demonstrated that an hyperandrogenic state reflected by high testosterone, high free testosterone and low sex hormone binding globulin (SHBG) levels, was associated with abdominal obesity (Evans *et al.*, 1983, 1988). These alterations in SHBG and testosterone levels were also found to be independent correlates of the metabolic complications of abdominal obesity in women (Shoupe & Lobo, 1984; Peiris *et al.*, 1987; Smith *et al.*, 1987; Dunaif *et al.*, 1989).

Recent evidence obtained in men has suggested that an excess visceral adipose tissue accumulation was negatively associated with plasma SHBG and testosterone levels, a finding which is slightly at variance with previous observations in women (Seidell *et al.*, 1990; Pasquali *et al.*, 1991). The association between free testosterone levels and visceral obesity in men remains controversial, although Seidell and colleagues have reported a significant negative correlation between this variable and the amount of visceral adipose tissue measured by computed tomography (Seidell *et al.*, 1990). We have also examined these associations in a sample of men for whom we had measured visceral adipose tissue accumulation by computed tomography and we reported negative correlations between plasma testosterone and SHBG levels vs visceral adipose tissue accumulation (Tchernof *et al.*, 1995a). We also found that plasma levels of adrenal steroids such as androstenedione, androstenediol and de-hydroepiandrosterone were negatively associated with visceral adipose tissue accumulation in men. Thus, visceral obesity in men is not only associated with reductions in gonadal steroid levels but also with lower adrenal C_{19} steroid concentrations. Multiple regression analyses revealed that the adrenal steroid androstenediol was the unconjugated steroid which showed the best associations with visceral obesity in men (Tchernof *et al.*, 1995a).

Regarding the issue of causality, studies conducted by Mårin and colleagues have shown that treatment of men with visceral obesity and low plasma testosterone levels with exogenous but physiological doses of testosterone induced a 10% reduction in visceral adipose tissue mass over a period of 9 months (Mårin *et al.*, 1993). Other studies from this group have shown that testosterone treatment was also associated with an inhibition of LPL activity in abdominal adipocytes (Rebuffé-Scrive *et al.*, 1991; Mårin *et al.*, 1992, 1996). Recent data have also indicated that testosterone treatment could lead to a reduction in triglyceride mobilization in visceral adipose cells (Mårin *et al.*, 1995). The reduction in visceral adipose tissue mass noted in these studies was also associated with improvements of several risk factors for cardiovascular disease and diabetes (Mårin *et al.*, 1992, 1993). It is, therefore, likely that the reduced testosterone and perhaps other C_{19} steroid levels observed in visceral obesity could be causally involved in the aetiology of the metabolic alterations found in this condition. On the other hand, adipose tissue has been suggested to act as a steroid reservoir and also as an important site of steroid interconversion, as significant activities and mRNA levels of steroid converting enzymes have been found in adipose tissue (Deslypere *et al.*, 1985; Lueprasitsakul *et al.*, 1990; Labrie *et al.*, 1991). Therefore it is also likely that the enlarged adipose tissue mass observed in obesity may contribute significantly to alterations in steroid metabolism. This thesis is supported by findings of some studies which reported significant modifications in plasma steroid hormone levels after weight reduction in obese subjects (Stanick *et al.*, 1981; Zumoff & Strain, 1994; Leenen *et al.*, 1994).

We have also examined the associations between alterations in C_{19} steroid levels and indices of plasma glucose and insulin homeostasis in men. In accordance with previous results, we found significant negative associations between levels of these steroid hormones and fasting insulin as well as glycaemic and insulinaemic responses to a 75-g oral glucose load (Tchernof *et al.*, 1995b). However, after statistical adjustment for concomitant variation in visceral adipose tissue accumulation or total body fat mass, these associations were no longer significant, suggesting that the relationships of visceral obesity to indices of plasma glucose and insulin homeostasis could be, at least to a large extent, independent from the concomitant variation in plasma steroid hormone levels (Tchernof *et al.*, 1995b). These results also suggest that the potential associations between plasma steroid hormone levels and glucose and insulin homeostasis indices are 'overpowered' by the impact of excess visceral adipose tissue mass (Tchernof *et al.*, 1995b).

Regarding the associations between steroid hormone levels and plasma lipoprotein concentrations, there has been no general consensus. Indeed, some studies have found testosterone to be significantly associated with variables of the plasma lipid lipoprotein profile, while others failed to report such significant relationships (Barrett-Connor, 1995). However, numerous studies have now reported that low HDL cholesterol levels are generally associated with low testosterone concentrations in men (Bagatell & Bremmer, 1995; Barrett-Connor, 1995). We have reached similar conclusions when studying these associations in men as low testosterone levels were associated with an altered lipid–lipoprotein profile predictive of an increased risk of cardiovascular disease (Tchernof *et al.*, 1997). We also studied plasma levels of adrenal C_{19} steroid levels and reported that low levels of these hormones are also associated with an altered lipoprotein–lipid profile. However, after control for concomitant variation in other metabolic variables including visceral adipose tissue accumulation, most of these associations were no longer significant (Tchernof *et al.*, 1997). Low plasma concentrations of SHBG were also associated with an altered lipoprotein–lipid profile in our sample of men and these associations remained significant even after adjustment for the concomitant variation of other variables including visceral adipose tissue accumulation. These results suggest that as opposed to steroid hormone levels, SHBG concentration is independently associated with variations in the plasma lipid–lipoprotein profile. Thus, variations in steroid hormones could not fully account for the altered plasma lipid–lipoprotein profile found in visceral obese men. Our results rather suggest that visceral obesity could have represented an important confounding factor in previous studies on steroid hormone levels and alterations in glucose tolerance/insulin sensitivity as well as in lipoprotein metabolism in which body fat distribution was not considered, especially visceral adipose tissue accumulation.

Controversial results have also been generated by the study of the relationships of plasma steroid hormone levels to the incidence of cardiovascular disease. Indeed, no general consensus has been obtained on whether testosterone or other steroid hormone levels are independent correlates of the risk of cardiovascular disease (Kalin & Zumoff, 1990; Phillips, 1993). It has been suggested that differences in the methodology used, in populations studied or in the definition of the cardiovascular events could account for such equivocal results (Phillips, 1993). Barrett-Connor has also suggested that a single testosterone measurement may not necessarily provide good information on the androgenic status in prospective studies conducted over several years (Barrett-Connor, 1995). Further prospective studies are therefore clearly needed in order to sort out the relative importance of alterations in the steroid hormone profile in the pathophysiology of the insulin-resistant–dyslipidaemic syndrome of visceral obesity and related cardiovascular disease risk.

Genetic susceptibility to dyslipidaemic states in visceral obesity

Visceral obesity is a complex phenotype with a multifactorial aetiology. Although environmental factors obviously contribute to the development of obesity, it is clear that genetic factors modulate the susceptibility to this condition (Bouchard, 1991). Similarly, some visceral obese patients will be more prone to the development of the expected insulin-resistant–dyslipidaemic syndrome that others. Thus, the magnitude of the metabolic complications found in a given visceral obese patient largely depends upon the genetic predisposition of this patient. In this regard, several candidate genes could be responsible for such variability observed in the dyslipidaemic phenotype of visceral obesity. For example, genes coding for apolipoproteins, lipoprotein receptors as well as enzymes responsible for lipoprotein metabolism could be involved (Després et al., 1992).

The Apo E gene is obviously one of these candidate genes. By studying isoforms of Apo E, we found that excess visceral adipose tissue accumulation and hyperinsulinaemia were associated with hypertriglyceridaemia only in carriers of the Apo E_2 allele or in Apo E_3 homozygotes (Pouliot et al., 1990; Després et al., 1993), while Apo E_4 carriers did not show these associations. Thus, the Apo E polymorphism altered the expected relationship of visceral obesity and hyperinsulinaemia to hypertriglyceridaemia.

We have also examined the potential contribution of an Apo B100 gene *Eco*RI polymorphism in men (Pouliot *et al.*, 1994a). Our results indicated that among subjects who were heterozygous for the absence of the *Eco*RI restriction site, visceral obesity was associated with elevated Apo B concentrations. However, this relationship could not be found among homozygotes for the presence of this *Eco*RI restriction site. We have also shown that heterozygous men for the absence of the restriction site and with visceral obesity were more likely to develop the dense LDL phenotype (Vohl *et al.*, 1996). Our group has also studied a *Hind*III polymorphism in the LPL gene and homozygous carriers of this polymorphism with visceral obesity were found to be more susceptible to hypertriglyceridaemia than heterozygous visceral obese patients (Vohl *et al.*, 1995). Other candidate genes are currently examined in our laboratory but it should be pointed out that some of these polymorphisms have not necessarily been associated with altered protein levels or enzyme activities such as for the *Eco*RI polymorphism of the Apo B100 gene or the *Hind*III polymorphism of the LPL gene (Pouliot *et al.*, 1994a; Vohl *et al.*, 1995, 1996). Thus, these associations could be resulting from a linkage disequilibrium between these polymorphisms and other unknown genes significantly modulating genetic susceptibility to the dyslipidaemia in visceral obesity.

Future cross-sectional studies and more importantly prospective investigations in larger cohorts will be clearly warranted to better clarify potential gene–gene and gene–environment interactions.

Therapeutic implications

As stated above, visceral obesity is associated with a cluster of metabolic abnormalities contributing to the increased risk of NIDDM and IHD. The proper identification of patients with visceral obesity has important public health implications. The use of computed tomography represents a precise and reliable procedure but this expensive methodology is not readily available to most clinicians. In this regard, several studies have used the waist/hip ratio as a measurement of abdominal obesity and, until recently, this variable had been considered as very useful and relevant in the assessment of abdominal fat accumulation (Kissebah & Peiris, 1989). However, we have suggested that the waist circumference by itself may even be a better correlate of visceral adipose tissue accumulation than the waist/hip ratio (Pouliot *et al.*, 1994b). Sjöström has also suggested that the sagittal diameter could represent another potentially interesting anthropometric variable in the prediction of visceral adipose tissue accumulation (Sjöström *et al.*, 1986). We propose that these two anthropometric measurements are superior to the waist/hip ratio in their ability to predict the absolute amount of visceral adipose tissue. In this regard, we have suggested that a waist circumference above 1 m in both men and women was associated with an increased likelihood of finding the cluster of metabolic abnormalities of visceral obesity (Després & Lamarche, 1993). This cut-off point has been found to be altered by age and the critical waist circumference for men and women between 40 and 60 years of age appears to be above a value of 90 cm only. It should also be emphasized that these threshold values are not definite cut-off points and that they have been derived from the study of a Caucasian sample. These studies will also have to be conducted in other populations and ethnic groups in order to verify whether population-specific reference values are needed, a conclusion which is likely to be reached.

As discussed earlier, an excess accumulation of adipose tissue in the abdominal cavity plays a significant role in the pathophysiology of the dyslipidaemic state found in abdominal obese patients. Accordingly, it has been shown that weight loss leading to a reduction in the visceral adipose tissue mass was associated with improvements in the metabolic risk profile (Després & Lamarche, 1993). In this regard, it has also been shown that individuals with an important accumulation of visceral adipose tissue generally preferentially mobilize this depot when exposed to a hypocaloric diet (Fujioka et al., 1991a, b). Thus, it appears that a negative energy balance is likely to produce a significant mobilization of visceral adipose tissue in visceral obese patients, contributing to reduce the risk of NIDDM and cardiovascular disease, even when normalization of body-weight is far from being achieved.

Endurance exercise training is another relevant approach which may increase energy expenditure, contributing to induce a negative energy balance (Després & Lamarche, 1993). However, exercise training programmes have not always led to substantial weight reductions, although significant improvements of the metabolic risk profile were noted (Lamarche et al., 1992). It appears that when the associated increase in energy expenditure is substantial, endurance exercise training may induce a mobilization of visceral adipose tissue and also produce rather remarkable changes in the metabolic profile, even in the absence of major weight loss. Thus, regular endurance exercise may be helpful for the treatment of the metabolic complications of visceral obesity, particularly as a critical adjunct to a low-fat–high-complex-carbohydrate diet (Després & Lamarche, 1993).

Conclusions

Excess visceral adipose tissue deposition appears to represent the critical correlate of the metabolic complications of obesity. When present, this condition is associated, in both men and women, with a cluster of metabolic abnormalities such as insulin resistance, compensatory hyperinsulinaemia, glucose intolerance, and with a dyslipidaemic state including high plasma triglycerides, low HDL-C, an increased cholesterol/HDL-C ratio, hyper-Apo B and an increased proportion of small, dense LDL particles. Evidence from prospective studies including the recent observations on the Québec Cardiovascular Study have indicated that this cluster of metabolic abnormalities clearly increases the risk of IHD in men. It is therefore clinically relevant to identify and treat these patients, who would otherwise not always be identified on the basis of anthropometric correlates of body composition currently used by clinicians and health professionals such as weight/height indices. On the basis of its high prevalence in affluent societies, it is proposed that visceral obesity may represent the most important cause of NIDDM and CHD in these populations.

References

Albrink, M.J., Krauss, R.M., Lindgren, F.T., Von der Groeben, V.D. & Wood, P.D. (1980) Intercorrelation among high density lipoprotein, obesity, and triglycerides in a normal population. *Lipids* 15, 668–678.

Assmann, G. & Schulte, H. (1992) Relation of high-density lipoprotein cholesterol and triglycerides to incidence of atherosclerotic coronary artery disease (The PROCAM Experience). *American Journal of Cardiology* 70, 733–737.

Austin, M.A. (1991) Plasma triglyceride and coronary heart disease. *Arteriosclerosis and Thrombosis* 11, 2–14.

Austin, M.A. (1992) Genetic epidemiology of low-density lipoprotein subclass phenotypes. *Annals of Medicine* 24, 447–481.

Austin, M.A., Breslow, J.L., Hennekens, C.H., Buring, J.E., Willet, W.C. & Krauss, R.M. (1988) Low-density lipoprotein subclass patterns and risk of myocardial infarction. *Journal of the American Medical Association* 260, 1917–1921.

Bagatell, C.J. & Bremner, W.J. (1995) Androgen and progestagen effects on plasma lipids. *Progress in Cardiovascular Diseases* 38, 255–271.

Barrett-Connor, E. (1985) Obesity, atherosclerosis, and coronary artery disease. *Annals of Internal Medicine* 103, 1010–1019.

Barrett-Connor, E.L. (1995) Testosterone and risk factors for cardiovascular disease in men. *Diabète et Mètabolisme* 21, 156–161.

Baxter, J.D. & Rousseau, G.G. (1979) Glucocorticoid hormone action: an overview. In: Baxter, J.D. & Rousseau, G.G. (eds) *Glucocorticoid Hormone Action*, pp. 1–24. Berlin: Springer.

Beaulieu, E.E. & Kelly, P.A. (1990) *Hormones: From Molecules to Disease.* New York and London: Hermann Publishers in Arts and Science; New York and London: Chapman and Hall.

Bergstrom, R.W., Newell-Morris, L.L., Leonetti, D.L., Shuman, W.P., Wahl, P.W. & Fujimoto, W.Y. (1990) Association of elevated fasting C-peptide level and increased intra-abdominal fat distribution with development of NIDDM in Japanese-American men. *Diabetes* 39, 104–111.

Björntorp, P. (1984) Hazards in subgroups of human obesity. *European Journal of Clinical Investigation* 14, 239–241.

Björntorp, P. (1990) 'Portal' adipose tissue as a generator of risk factors for cardiovascular disease and diabetes. *Arteriosclerosis and Thrombosis* 10, 493–496.

Björntorp, P. (1991) Adipose tissue distribution and function. *International Journal of Obesity* 15, 67–81.

Björntorp, P. (1992) Metabolic abnormalities in visceral obesity. *Annals of Medicine* 24, 3–5.

Björntorp, P. (1995) Endocrine abnormalities of obesity. *Metabolism* 44 (suppl. 3), 21–23.

Bouchard, C. (1991) Current understanding of the etiology of obesity: genetic and nongenetic factors. *American Journal of Clinical Nutrition* 53, 1561S–1565S.

Bray, G.A. (1985) Complications of obesity. *Annals of Internal Medicine* 103, 1052–1062.

Bray, G.A., Davidson, M.B. & Drenick, E.J. (1972) Obesity: A serious symptom. *Annals of Internal Medicine* 77, 797–805.

Campos, H., Bailey, S.M., Gussak, L.S., Siles, X., Ordovas, J.M. & Schaefer, E.J. (1991) Relations of body habitus, fitness level, and cardiovascular risk factors including lipoproteins in a rural and urban Costa Rican population. *Arteriosclerosis and Thrombosis* 11, 1077–1088.

Campos, H., Genest, J.J., Blijlevens, E. *et al.* (1992) Low density lipoprotein particle size and coronary artery disease. *Arteriosclerosis and Thrombosis* 12, 187–195.

Castelli, W.P. (1984) Epidemiology of coronary heart disease: The Framingham Study. *American Journal of Medicine* 76, 4–12.

Chait, A., Brazg, R.L., Tribble, D.L. & Krauss, R.M. (1993) Susceptibility of small, dense, low-density lipoproteins to oxidative modification in subjects with the atherogenic lipoprotein phenotype, pattern B. *American Journal of Medicine* 94, 350–356.

Coresh, J., Kwiterovich, P.O. Jr, Smith, H.H. & Bachorik, P.S. (1993) Association of plasma triglyceride concentration and LDL particle diameter, density, and chemical composition with premature coronary artery disease in men and women. *Journal of Lipid Research* 34, 1687–1697.

Crouse, J.R., Parks, J.S. & Schey, H.M. (1985) Studies of low density lipoprotein molecular weight in human beings with coronary artery disease. *Journal of Lipid Research* 26, 566–574.

Dagenais, G.R., Robitaille, N.M., Lupien, P.J. *et al.* (1990) First coronary heart disease event rates in relation to major risk factors: Québec Cardiovascular Study. *Canadian Journal of Cardiology* 6, 274–280.

Davis, C.E., Gordon, D., LaRosa, J.C., Wood, P.D. & Halperin, M. (1980) Correlation of plasma high density lipoprotein cholesterol levels with other plasma lipid and lipoprotein concentrations. *Circulation* 62 (suppl. IV), IV-24–IV-30.

de Graaf, J., Hendriks, J.C., Demacker, P.N. & Stalenhoef, A.F. (1993) Identification of multiple dense LDL subfractions with enhanced susceptibility to *in vitro* oxidation among hypertriglyceridemic subjects. Normalization after clofibrate treatment. *Arteriosclerosis and Thrombosis* 13, 712–719.

Dejager, S., Bruckert, E. & Chapman, M.J. (1993) Dense low density lipoprotein subspecies with diminished oxidative resistance predominate in combined hyperlipidemia. *Journal of Lipid Research* 34, 295–308.

Deslypere, J.P., Verdonck, L. & Vermeulen, A. (1985) Fat tissue: a steroid reservoir and site of steroid metabolism. *Journal of Clinical Endocrinology and Metabolism* 61, 564–570.

Després, J.P. (1991) Obesity and lipid metabolism: relevance of body fat distribution. *Current Opinion in Lipidology* 2, 5–15.

Després, J.P. (1993) Abdominal obesity as important component of insulin-resistance syndrome. *Nutrition* 9, 452–459.

Després, J.P. (1994a) Visceral Obesity: a component of the insulin resistance-dyslipidemic syndrome. *Canadian Journal of Cardiology* 10 (suppl. B), 17B–22B.

Després, J.P. (1994b) Dyslipidaemia and obesity. *Baillière's Clinical Endocrinology and Metabolism* 8, 629–660.

Després, J.P. & Lamarche, B. (1993) Effects of diet and physical activity on adiposity and body fat distribution: implications for the prevention of cardiovascular disease. *Nutr Res Rev* 6, 137–159.

Després, J.P. & Marette, A. (1994) Relation of components of insulin resistance syndrome to coronary disease risk. *Current Opinion in Lipidology* 5, 274–289.

Després, J.P., Ferland, M., Moorjani, S. *et al.* (1989a) Role of hepatic-triglyceride lipase activity in the association between intra-abdominal fat and plasma HDL-cholesterol in obese women. *Arteriosclerosis* 9, 485–492.

Després, J.P., Nadeau, A., Tremblay, A. *et al.* (1989b) Role of deep abdominal fat in the association between regional adipose tissue distribution and glucose tolerance in obese women. *Diabetes* 38, 304–309.

Després, J.P., Prud'homme, D., Pouliot, M.C., Tremblay, A. & Bouchard, C. (1991) Estimation of deep abdominal adipose-tissue accumulation from simple anthropometric measurements in men. *American Journal of Clinical Nutrition* **54**, 471–477.

Després, J.P., Moorjani, S., Lupien, P.J., Tremblay, A., Nadeau, A. & Bouchard, C. (1992) Genetic aspects of susceptibility to obesity and related dyslipidemias. *Molecular and Cellular Biochemistry* **113**, 151–169.

Després, J.P., Verdon, M.F., Moorjani, S. *et al.* (1993) Apolipoprotein E polymorphism modifies relation of hyperinsulinemia to hypertriglyceridemia. *Diabetes* **42**, 1474–1481.

Després, J.P., Lamarche, B., Mauriège, P. *et al.* (1996) Hyperinsulinemia as an independent risk factor for ischemic heart disease. *New England Journal of Medicine* **334**, 952–957.

Donahue, R.P., Abbot, R.D., Bloom, E., Reed, D.M. & Yano, K. (1987) Central obesity and coronary heart disease in men. *Lancet* **1**, 821–824.

Ducimetière, P., Richard, J. & Cambien, F. (1986) The pattern of subcutaneous fat distribution in middle-aged men and the risk of coronary heart disease: the Paris prospective study. *International Journal of Obesity* **10**, 229–240.

Dunaif, A., Segal, K.R., Futterweit, W. & Dobrjansky, A. (1989) Profound peripheral insulin resistance, independent of obesity, in polycystic ovary syndrome. *Diabetes* **38**, 1165–1174.

Enzi, G., Gasparo, M., Biondetti, P.R., Fiore, D., Semisa, M. & Zurlo, F. (1986) Subcutaneous and visceral fat distribution according to sex, age and overweight, evaluated by computed tomography. *American Journal of Clinical Nutrition* **44**, 739–746.

Eschwège, E., Richard, J.L., Thibult, N., Ducimetière, P., Warnet, J.M. & Rosselin, G. (1985) Coronary heart disease mortality in relation with diabetes, blood glucose and plasma insulin levels: The Paris Prospective study, ten years later. *Hormone and Metabolic Research* **15** (suppl.), 41–46.

Evans, D.J., Hoffmann, R.G., Kalkhoff, R.K. & Kissebah, A.H. (1983) Relationship of androgenic activity to body fat topography, fat cell morphology, and metabolic aberrations in premenopausal women. *Journal of Clinical Endocrinology and Metabolism* **57**, 304–310.

Evans, D.J., Barth, J.H. & Burke, C.W. (1988) Body fat topography in women with androgen excess. *International Journal of Obesity* **12**, 157–162.

Ferland, M., Després, J.P., Tremblay, A. *et al.* (1989) Assessment of adipose tissue distribution by computed axial tomography in obese women: association with body density and anthropometric measurements. *British Journal of Nutrition* **61**, 139–148.

Fisher, W.R. (1983) Heterogeneity of plasma low density lipoprotein manifestations of the physiologic phenomenon in man. *Metabolism* **32**, 283–291.

Fujioka, S., Matsuzawa, Y., Tokunaga, K. *et al.* (1991a) Improvement of glucose and lipid metabolism associated with selective reduction of intra-abdominal visceral fat in premenopausal women with visceral fat obesity. *International Journal of Obesity* **15**, 853–859.

Fujioka, S., Matsuzawa, Y., Tokinaga, K., Kano, Y., Kobatake, T. & Tarui, S. (1991b) Treatment of visceral obesity. *International Journal of Obesity* **15**, 59–65.

Garrison, R.J., Kannel, W.B., Stokes III, J. & Castelli, W.P. (1987) Incidence and precursors of hypertension in young adults: The Framingham Offspring Study. *Preventive Medicine* **16**, 235–251.

Genest, J.J., McNamara, J.R., Salem, D.N. & Schaefer, E.J. (1991) Prevalence of risk factors in men with premature coronary heart disease. *American Journal of Cardiology* **67**, 1185–1189.

Gordon, T., Castelli, W.P., Hjortland, M.C., Kannel, W.B. & Dawber, T.R. (1977) High density lipoprotein as a protective factor against coronary heart disease: The Framingham Study. *American Journal of Medicine* **62**, 707–714.

Gotto, A.M., LaRosa, J.C., Hunninghake, D. *et al.* (1990) The cholesterol facts: A summary of the evidence relating dietary fats, serum cholesterol and coronary heart disease. *Circulation* **81**, 1721–1733.

Griffin, B.A., Caslake, M.J., Yip, B., Tait, G.W., Packard, C.J. & Shepherd, J. (1990) Rapid isolation of low density lipoprotein (LDL) subfractions from plasma by density gradient ultracentrifugation. *Atherosclerosis* **83**, 59–67.

Griffin, B.A., Freeman, D.J., Tait, G.W. *et al.* (1994) Role of plasma triglyceride in the regulation of plasma low density lipoprotein (LDL) subfractions: relative contribution of small dense LDL to coronary heart disease risk. *Atherosclerosis* **106**, 241–253.

Hennes, M., Shrago, E. & Kissebah, A.H. (1990) Receptor and post receptor effects of FFA on hepatocyte insulin dynamics. *International Journal of Obesity* 14, 831–841.

Jaakkola, O., Solakivi, T., Tertov, V.V., Orekhof, A.N., Miettinen, T.A. & Nikkari, T. (1993) Characteristics of low-density lipoprotein subfractions from patients with coronary artery disease. *Coronary Artery Disease* 4, 379–385.

Kalin, M.F. & Zumoff, B. (1990) Sex hormones and coronary disease: a review of the clinical studies. *Steroids* 55, 330–352.

Kannel, W.B., Castelli, W.P., Gordon, T. & McNamara, P.M. (1971) Serum cholesterol, lipoproteins, and the risk of coronary heart disease. The Framingham Study. *Annals of Internal Medicine* 74, 1–12.

Katzel, L.I., Krauss, R.M. & Goldberg, A.P. (1994) Relations of plasma TG and HDL-C concentrations to body composition and plasma insulin levels are altered in men with small LDL particles. *Arteriosclerosis and Thrombosis* 14, 1121–1128.

Kissebah, A.H. & Peiris, A.N. (1989) Biology of regional body fat distribution. Relationship to non-insulin-dependent diabetes mellitus. *Diabetes/Metabolism Reviews* 5, 83–109.

Kissebah, A.H. & Krakower, G.R. (1994) Regional adiposity and morbidity. *Physiological Reviews* 74, 761–811.

Kissebah, A.H., Vydelingum, N. & Murray, R. (1982) Relation of body fat distribution to metabolic complications of obesity. *Journal of Clinical Endocrinology and Metabolism* 54, 254–260.

Kissebah, A.H., Freedman, D.S. & Peiris, A.N. (1989) Health risks of obesity. *Medical Clinics of North America* 73, 111–138.

Kotani, K., Tokunaga, K., Fujioka, S. et al. (1994) Sexual dimorphism of age-related changes in whole-body fat distribution in the obese. *International Journal of Obesity* 18, 207–212.

La Belle, M. & Krauss, R.M. (1990) Differences in carbohydrate content of low density lipoproteins associated with low-density lipoprotein subclass patterns. *Journal of Lipid Research* 31, 1577–1588.

Laakso, M. (1997) How good a marker is insulin level for insulin resistance? *American Journal of Epidemiology* 137, 959–965.

Labrie, F., Simard, J. & Luu-The, V. et al. (1991) Expression of 3β-hydroxysteroid dehydrogenase/Δ5-Δ4 isomerase (3β-HSD) and 17β-hydroxysteroid dehydrogenase (17β-HSD) in adipose tissue. *International Journal of Obesity* 15, 91–99.

Lamarche, B., Després, J.P., Pouliot, M.C. et al. (1992) Is body fat loss a determinant factor in the improvement of carbohydrate and lipid metabolism following aerobic exercise training in obese women? *Metabolism* 41, 1249–1256.

Lamarche, B., Després, J.P., Moorjani, S., Cantin, B., Dagenais, G.R. & Lupien, P.J. (1995) Prevalence of dyslipidemic phenotypes in ischemic heart disease; prospective results from the Quebec Cardiovascular Study. *American Journal of Cardiology* 75, 1189–1195.

Lamarche, B., Després, J.P., Moorjani, S., Cantin, B., Dagenais, G.R. & Lupien, P.J. (1996a) Triglycerides and HDL-cholesterol as risk factors for ischemic heart disease. Results from the Québec Cardiovascular Study. *Atherosclerosis* 119, 235–245.

Lamarche, B., Moorjani, S., Lupien, P.J., Cantin, B., Dagenais, G.R. & Després, J.P. (1996b) Apolipoprotein A-I and B levels and the risk of ischemic heart disease during a five-year follow-up of men in the Québec Cardiovascular Study. *Circulation* 94, 273–278.

Lamarche, B., Tchernof, A., Moorjani, S. et al. (1997) Small, dense low-density lipoprotein particles as a predictor of the risk of ischemic heart disease in men. Prospective results from the Québec Cardiovascular Study. *Circulation* 95, 69–75.

Lapidus, L., Bengtsson, C., Larsson, B., Pennert, K., Rybo, E. & Sjöström, L. (1984) Distribution of adipose tissue and risk of cardiovascular disease and death: a 12 year follow up of participants in the population study of women in Gothenburg, Sweden. *British Medical Journal* 289, 1261–1263.

Larsson, B., Svardsudd, K., Welin, L., Wilhemsen, L., Björntorp, P. & Tibblin, G. (1984) Abdominal adipose tissue distribution, obesity and risk of cardiovascular disease and death: 13-year follow-up of participants in the study of men born in 1913. *British Medical Journal* 288, 1401–1404.

Leenen, R., van der Kooy, K., Seidell, J.C., Deurenberg, P. & Koppeschaar, H.P. (1994) Visceral fat accumulation in relation to sex hormones in obese men and women undergoing weight loss therapy. *Journal of Clinical Endocrinology and Metabolism* 78, 1515–1520.

Lemieux, S. & Després, J.P. (1994) Metabolic complications of visceral obesity: contribution to the aetiology of type 2 diabetes and implications for prevention and treatment. *Diabète et Mètabolisme* 20, 375–393.

Lemieux, S., Prud'homme, D., Bouchard, C., Tremblay, A. & Després, J.P. (1993) Sex differences in the relation of visceral adipose tissue accumulation to total body fatness. *American Journal of Clinical Nutrition* 58, 463–467.

Lemieux, S., Després, J.P., Moorjani, S. *et al.* (1994) Are gender differences in cardiovascular disease risk factors explained by the level of visceral adipose tissue? *Diabetologia* 37, 757–764.

Lemieux, S., Prud'homme, D., Moorjani, S. *et al.* (1995) Do elevated levels of abdominal visceral adipose tissue contribute to age-related differences in plasma lipoprotein concentrations in men? *Atherosclerosis* 118, 155–164.

Lueprasitsakul, P., Latour, D. & Longcope, C. (1990) Aromatase activity in human adipose tissue stromal cells: effect of growth factors. *Steroids* 55, 540–544.

Manson, J.E., Willet, W.C., Stampfer, M.J. *et al.* (1995) Body weight and mortality among women. *New England Journal of Medicine* 333, 677–685.

Mårin, P., Holmäng, S., Jönsson, L. *et al.* (1992) The effects of testosterone treatment on body composition and metabolism in middle-aged and obese men. *International Journal of Obesity* 16, 991–997.

Mårin, P., Holmäng, S., Gustafsson, C., Holm, G. & Björntorp, P. (1993) Androgen treatment of abdominally obese men. *Obesity Research* 1, 245–251.

Mårin, P., Odén, B. & Björntorp, P. (1995) Assimilation and mobilization of triglycerides in subcutaneous abdominal and femoral adipose tissue *in vivo* in men: effects of androgens. *Journal of Clinical Endocrinology and Metabolism* 80, 239–243.

Mårin, P., Lönn, L., Andersson, B. *et al.* (1996) Assimilation of triglycerides in subcutaneous and intraabdominal adipose tissues *in vivo* in men: effects of testosterone. *Journal of Clinical Endocrinology and Metabolism* 81, 1018–1022.

McNamara, J.R., Campos, H., Ordovas, J.M., Peterson, J., Wilson, P.W.F. & Schaefer, E.J. (1987) Effect of gender, age, and lipid status on low density lipoprotein subfraction distribution. Results of the Framingham Offspring Study. *Arteriosclerosis and Thrombosis* 7, 483–490.

Miller, L.K., Kral, J.G., Strain, G.W. & Zumoff, B. (1988) Differential binding of dexamethasone to ammonium sulphate precipitates of human adipose tissue cytosols. *Steroids* 49, 507–522.

Multiple Risk Factor Intervention Trial Research Group (1982) Multiple risk factor Intervention Trial: Risk factor changes and mortality results. *Journal of the American Medical Association* 248, 1465–1477.

Nigon, F., Lesnik, P., Rouis, M. & Chapman, M.J. (1991) Discrete subspecies of human low density lipoproteins are heterogeneous in their interaction with the cellular LDL receptor. *Journal of Lipid Research* 32, 1741–1753.

NIH Consensus Conference (1985) Lowering blood cholesterol to prevent heart disease. *Journal of the American Medical Association* 253, 2080–2086.

Ohlson, L.O., Larsson, B., Svardsudd, K. *et al.* (1985) The influence of body fat distribution on the incidence of diabetes mellitus 13.5 years of follow-up of the participants in the study of men born in 1913. *Diabetes* 34, 1055–1058.

Packard, C.J. (1994) Plasma triglycerides, LDL heterogeneity and atherogenesis. *Ther Exp* 85, 1–6.

Pasquali, R., Casimirri, F., Cantobelli, S. *et al.* (1991) Effect of obesity and body fat distribution on sex hormones and insulin in men. *Metabolism* 40, 101–104.

Peiris, A.N., Mueller, R.A., Struve, M.F., Smith, G.A. & Kissebah, A.H. (1987) Relationship of androgenic activity to splanchnic insulin metabolism and peripheral glucose utilization in premenopausal women. *Journal of Clinical Endocrinology and Metabolism* 64, 162–169.

Petersson, B., Trell, E. & Hood, B. (1984) Premature death and associated risk factors in urban middle-aged men. *American Journal of Medicine* 77, 418–426.

Phillips, G.B. (1993) Relationship of serum sex hormones to coronary heart disease. *Steroids* 58, 286–290.

Pouliot, M.C., Després, J.P., Moorjani, S., Lupien, P.J., Tremblay, A. & Bouchard, C. (1990) Apolipoprotein E polymorphism alters the association between body fatness and plasma lipoprotein in women. *Journal of Lipid Research* 31, 1023–1029.

Pouliot, M.C., Després, J.P., Nadeau, A. *et al.* (1992) Visceral obesity in men: associations with glucose tolerance, plasma insulin, and lipoprotein levels. *Diabetes* 41, 826–834.

Pouliot, M.C., Després, J.P., Dionne, F.T. *et al.* (1994a) Apolipoprotein B-100 gene *Eco*RI polymorphism: relations to the plasma lipoprotein changes associated with abdominal visceral obesity. *Arteriosclerosis and Thrombosis* 14, 527–533.

Pouliot, M.C., Després, J.P., Lemieux, S. *et al.* (1994b) Waist circumference and abdominal sagittal diameter: best simple anthropometric indexes of abdominal visceral adipose tissue accumulation and related cardiovascular risk in men and women. *American Journal of Cardiology* 73, 460–468.

Pyörälä, K. (1979) Relationship of glucose tolerance and plasma insulin to the incidence of coronary heart disease: Results from the two population studies in Finland. *Diabetes Care* 2, 131–141.

Rader, D.J., Hoeg, J.M. & Brewer, H.M. (1994) Quantification of plasma apolipoproteins in the primary and secondary prevention of coronary artery disease. *Annals of Internal Medicine* 120, 1012–1025.

Rajman, I., Maxwell, S., Cramb, R. & Kendall, M. (1994) Particle size: the key to the atherogenic lipoprotein? *Quarterly Journal of Medicine* 87, 709–720.

Reaven, G.M. (1988) Role of insulin resistance in human disease. *Diabetes* 37, 1595–1607.

Rebuffé-Scrive, M., Lundholm, K. & Björntorp, P. (1985) Glucocorticoid hormone binding to human adipose tissue. *European Journal of Clinical Investigation* 15, 267–271.

Rebuffé-Scrive, M., Mårin, P. & Björntorp, P. (1991) Effect of testosterone on abdominal adipose tissue in men. *International Journal of Obesity* 15, 791–795.

Reeder, B.A., Angel, A., Ledoux, M., Rabkin, S.W., Young, T.K. & Sweet, L.E. (1992) Obesity and its relation to cardiovascular disease risk factors in Canadian adults. Canadian Heart Health Surveys Research Group. *Canadian Medical Association Journal* 146, 2009–2019.

Schwartz, R.S., Shuman, W.P., Bradbury, V.L. *et al.* (1990) Body fat distribution in healthy young and older men. *Journal of Gerontology* 45, M181–M185.

Seidell, J.C., Oosterlee, A., Deurenberg, P., Hautvast, J.G.A. & Ruijs, J.H. (1988) Abdominal fat depots measured with computed tomography: Effects of degree of obesity, sex, and age. *European Journal of Clinical Nutrition* 42, 805–815.

Seidell, J.C., Björntorp, P., Sjöström, L., Kvist, H. & Sannrstedt, R. (1990) Visceral fat accumulation in men is positively associated with insulin, glucose, and C-peptide levels, but negatively with testosterone levels. *Metabolism* 39, 897–901.

Shoupe, D. & Lobo, R.A. (1984) The influence of androgens on insulin resistance. *Fertility and Sterility* 41, 385–388.

Sims, E.A.H. & Berchtold, P. (1982) Obesity and hypertension: mechanisms and implications for management. *Journal of the American Medical Association* 247, 49–52.

Sjöström, L., Kvist, H., Cederblad, A. & Tylen, U. (1986) Determination of total adipose tissue and body fat in women by computed tomography, 40K, and tritium. *American Journal of Physiology* 250, E736–E745.

Smith, S., Ravnikar, V.A. & Barbieri, R.L. (1987) Androgen and insulin response to an oral glucose challenge in hyperandrogenic women. *Fertility and Sterility* 48, 72–77.

Sniderman, A.D. (1992) The measurement of apolipoprotein B should replace the conventional lipid profile in screening for cardiovascular risk. *Canadian Journal of Cardiology* 8, 133–138.

Sniderman, A.D. & Silberberg, J. (1990) Is it time to measure apolipoprotein B? *Arteriosclerosis* 10, 665–667.

Stamler, J., Wentworth, D. & Neaton, J.D. (1986) Is relationship between serum cholesterol and risk of premature death from coronary heart disease continuous and graded? Findings in 356 222 primary screenees of the Multiple Risk Factor Intervention Trial (MRFIT). *Journal of the American Medical Association* 256, 2823–2828.

Stanick, S., Dornfeld, L.P., Maxwell, M.H., Viosca, S.P. & Korenman, S.G. (1981) The effect of weight loss on reproductive hormones in obese men. *Journal of Clinical Endocrinology and Metabolism* 53, 828–832.

Svedberg, J., Björntorp, P., Smith, V. & Lonnroth, P. (1990) FFA inhibition of insulin binding, degradation, and action in isolated hepatocytes. *Diabetes* **39**, 570–574.

Swinkels, D.W., Demacker, P.N., Hendriks, J.C. & van 't Laar, A. (1989) Low density lipoprotein subfractions and relationship to other risk factors for coronary artery disease in healthy individuals. *Atherosclerosis* **9**, 604–613.

Tchernof, A., Després, J.P., Bélanger, A. *et al.* (1995a) Reduced testosterone and adrenal C19 steroid levels in obese men. *Metabolism* **44**, 513–519.

Tchernof, A., Després, J.P., Dupont, A. *et al.* (1995b) Relation of steroid hormones to glucose tolerance and plasma insulin levels in men. *Diabetes Care* **18**, 292–299.

Tchernof, A., Labrie, F., Bélanger, A. & Després, J.P. (1996a) Obesity and metabolic complications: contribution of dehydroepiandrosterone and other steroid hormones. *Journal of Endocrinology* **150**, S155–S164.

Tchernof, A., Lamarche, B., Prud'homme, D. *et al.* (1996b) The dense LDL phenotype: association with plasma lipoprotein levels, visceral obesity, and hyperinsulinemia in men. *Diabetes Care* **19**, 629–637.

Tchernof, A. Labrie, F., Bélanger, A. *et al.* (1997) Relationships between endogenous steroid hormone, sex hormone-binding globulin and lipoprotein levels in men: contribution of visceral obesity, insulin levels and other metabolic variables. *Atherosclerosis* **133**, 235–244.

Tornvall, P., Karpe, F., Carlson, L.A. & Hamsten, A. (1991) Relationships of low density lipoprotein subfractions to angiographically defined coronary artery disease in young survivors of myocardial infarction. *Atherosclerosis* **90**, 67–80.

Vague, J. (1947) La différenciation sexuelle, facteur déterminant des formes de l'obésité. *Presse Medicale* **30**, 339–340.

Vohl, M.C., Lamarche, B., Moorjani, S. *et al.* (1995) The lipoprotein lipase *Hind*III polymorphism modulates plasma triglyceride levels in visceral obesity. *Arteriosclerosis, Thrombosis, and Vascular Biology* **15**, 714–720.

Vohl, M.C., Tchernof, A., Dionne, F.T. *et al.* (1996) The ApoB-100 Gene *Eco*RI polymorphism influences the relationship between features on the insulin resistance syndrome and the hyper-ApoB and dense LDL phenotype in men. *Diabetes* **45**, 1405–1411.

Welborn, T.A. & Wearne, K. (1979) Coronary heart disease incidence and cardiovascular mortality in Busselton with reference to glucose and insulin concentrations. *Diabetes Care* **2**, 154–160.

Yarnell, J.W.G., Sweetnam, P.M., Marks, V., Teale, J.D. & Bolton, C.H. (1994) Insulin in ischaemic heart disease: Are associations explained by triglyceride concentrations? The Caerphilly Prospective Study. *British Heart Journal* **171**, 293–296.

Zhao, S.P., Verhoven, M.H., Vink, J. *et al.* (1993) Relationship between apolipoprotein E and low density lipoprotein particle size. *Atherosclerosis* **102**, 147–154.

Zumoff, B. & Strain, G.W. (1994) A perspective on the hormonal abnormalities of obesity: are they cause or effect? *Obesity Research* **2**, 56–67.

CHAPTER 10

Effects of Obesity on Cardiovascular System and Blood Pressure Control, Digestive Disease and Cancer

LUC F. VAN GAAL AND ILSE L. MERTENS

Cardiovascular system

Several authors have proposed different (but not mutually exclusive) explanations for the difficulty in demonstrating a relationship between obesity and all-cause mortality (Simopoulos & Van Italie, 1984; Manson *et al.*, 1987; Sjöström, 1992; Pi-Sunyer, 1993). First, cigarette smoking is an important confounder of the relationship between obesity and mortality (Garrison *et al.*, 1983). Smokers tend to have a lower body-weight (Albanes *et al.*, 1987), but smoking also increases morbidity and mortality risk (Garfinkel & Stellman, 1988). In the Nurses Health Study (Manson *et al.*, 1995) a separate group of women who had never smoked were studied and a more direct relationship emerged between body mass index (BMI) and mortality, instead of a J-shaped or U-shaped association. Second, it is inappropriate to control for the direct physiological and metabolic consequences of obesity such as hypertension and hyperglycaemia because these are not confounders but intermediate risk factors (Manson *et al.*, 1987; Sjöström, 1992). Third, a clinical or subclinical disease present at baseline, may underestimate the risk of being overweight and overstate the risk of being underweight (Manson *et al.*, 1987; Pi-Sunyer, 1993). Fourth, the definition of obesity is often imprecise or indirect (Pi-Sunyer, 1993). BMI does not always accurately differentiate between obesity and overweight (Garn *et al.*, 1986) and estimates of fat distribution have not been taken into account in older studies. Finally, the relationship between obesity and mortality often is not seen in short-term studies. The more recent reports of the Framingham Heart Study, with a follow-up of more than 20 years, showed a stronger association between body-weight and coronary heart disease (CHD) when compared to the earlier reports (Feinleb, 1985).

Cardiovascular disease (CVD) appears to be a major cause of morbidity and mortality among obese individuals. In the prospective Nurses Health Study (Manson *et al.*, 1995) of 115 195 U.S. women during 16 years of follow-up, death-rates from CVD among the obese (BMI$\geq$29 kg/m^2) were fourfold compared to the leanest women. Nevertheless, it is still unclear whether obesity has an independent effect on CVD or whether its effect is only mediated through the effect of obesity on other cardiovascular risk factors.

Evidence for a connection between obesity and CVD is derived from epidemiological studies. The Framingham Study (Hubert *et al.*, 1983), which used multivariate analysis to control for other cardiovascular risk factors, confirmed, after 26 years of follow-up, the independent relationship between severe and even mild to moderate overweight and increased risk of CVD (Hubert *et al.*, 1983). Also, left ventricular hypertrophy, considered to be a less common but ominous risk factor for coronary disease, stroke and cardiac failure, seems to increase with greater BMI at any age. Body-weight is one of the most powerful determinants of left ventricular size and wall thickness (Lavie *et al.*, 1992).

Weight gain after the age of 25 years appears to have the greatest impact on cardiovascular risk (Hubert *et al.*, 1983; Manson *et al.*, 1995). The Framingham data (Hubert *et al.*, 1983) showed that weight gain after the young adult years increased the risk of CVD in both sexes in a manner that could not be attributed to the initial weight or to the level of the risk factors that may have resulted from weight gain. In the Nurses Health Study cohort (Manson *et al.*, 1995), weight gain after adulthood approximately doubled the coronary risk after controlling for the initial relative weight level.

As previously mentioned, obesity mediates its risk on CVD partly through its effect on cardiovascular risk factors. Cardiovascular risk factors tradition-ally have been divided into two categories: modifiable risk factors such as smoking habits, dyslipidaemia (high total cholesterol and low high-density lipoprotein (HDL) fraction), and diabetes control and non-modifiable risk factors such as increased age, male gender, and hereditary factors (Genest & Cohen, 1995).

The traditional risk factors do not fully account for the increased prevalence of vascular disease in obesity. In recent years, studies of subjects with central obesity (upper body obesity) have identified new risk factors which include increased waist/hip ratio (WHR), insulin resistance, hypertriglyceridaemia, lipid oxidation, hypercoagulability and hypofibrinolysis. (Kannel *et al.*, 1992; Ditschuneit *et al.*, 1995; Van Gaal *et al.*, 1995; Cushman *et al.*, 1996).

A number of studies have shown a strong relationship between obesity and a number of these cardiovascular risk factors: hypertension, hypercholes-terolaemia, low HDL-cholesterol, hypertriglyceridaemia, glucose intolerance, hyperinsulinaemia (Folsom *et al.*, 1989a), non-insulin-dependent diabetes mellitus (NIDDM) (Wilson *et al.*, 1981), haemostatic factors; elevated fibrinogen (Rillaerts *et al.*, 1989; Kannel *et al.*, 1992; Ditschuneit *et al.*, 1995); blood viscosity (Rillaerts *et al.*, 1989) and factor VII and VIIIc (Meade *et al.*, 1980); increased plasma activator inhibitor 1 (PAI-1) (Vague *et al.*, 1986; Van Gaal, 1990; Lundgren *et al.*, 1996); hyperuricaemia (Folsom *et al.*, 1989a; Bonora *et al.*, 1996); and left ventrical hypertrophy as measured by electrocardiography (Lauer *et al.*, 1991).

Fat distribution

During the last 15 years, important new knowledge concerning obesity and CVD has emerged. Most of the research done in this period of time focused on the influence of body fat distribution, and the role of visceral fat in particular. It became apparent that many risk factors cluster in individuals prone to develop CVD (Fig. 10.1). In his Banting lecture, Reaven (1988) proposed the name of syndrome X to refer to the clustering of (abdominal) obesity, hypertension, hypertriglyceridaemia, reduced levels of HDL, hyperinsulinaemia, glucose intolerance and NIDDM. Syndrome X has also been referred to as the 'insulin-resistance syndrome' (Haffner *et al.*, 1992), the 'metabolic syndrome' (Van Gaal *et al.*, 1993) and 'the deadly quartet' (Kaplan, 1989). Recently, hyperuricaemia (Bonora *et al.*, 1996), elevated PAI-1 levels (Van Gaal *et al.*, 1993) and the atherogenic small, dense low-density lipoprotein (LDL) particles (Desprès &

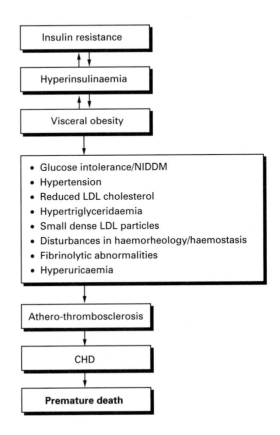

Fig. 10.1 Syndrome X.

Marette, 1994) have been suggested as new elements of this syndrome. The latter may in turn lead to the increased *in vitro* oxidizability of non-HDL particles in obese subjects and subsequent increased risk of atheromatous plaque formation and endothelial damage (Van Gaal *et al.*, 1995).

About 40 years ago, Vague (1956) suggested that body fat distribution is important in determining health risk. Several cohort studies have examined fat patterning as a predictor of morbidity and mortality due to CVD over substantial time periods (Lapidus *et al.*, 1984; Larsson *et al.*, 1984; Ducimetière *et al.*, 1986; Donahue *et al.*, 1987). From the results obtained in these prospective studies it became apparent that central (visceral) body fat distribution is associated with a greater cardiovascular morbidity and mortality than obesity itself. In the study of men born in 1913 (Larsson *et al.*, 1984) significant correlations were found between WHR and the three end points studied: stroke, ischaemic heart disease (IHD) and death from all causes (Fig. 10.2). Another study from Gothenburg (Lapidus *et al.*, 1984) showed a similar significant positive association between the WHR and the 12-year incidence of myocardial infarction, angina pectoris, stroke and death in a large cohort of (apparently healthy) women. Even in near to normal weight subjects, the WHR seems to be associated with stroke, IHD and death from all causes (Larsson *et al.*, 1984) (Fig. 10.2).

The amount of visceral abdominal fat appears to be particularly associated with metabolic disorders, such as glucose intolerance and hyperinsulinism

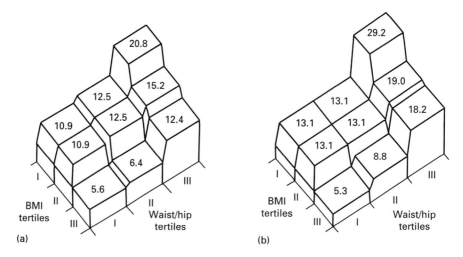

Fig. 10.2 Body fat distribution is important in determining health risk. Significant correlations were found between the WHR and (a) IHD and (b) death from all causes. Even in near to normal weight subjects, the WHR seems to be associated with cardiovascular end points. Adapted from Larsson *et al.* (1984).

(Pouliot *et al.*, 1992). Fujioka *et al.* (1987) proposed two types of obesity: a visceral type, characterized by an accumulation of fat in the abdominal cavity, and a subcutaneous type, characterized by an accumulation mainly in the subcutis.

Large-scale epidemiological studies often have used the WHR for classifying different types of fat distribution (Lapidus *et al.*, 1984; Larsson *et al.*, 1984). Fujioka *et al.* (1987) revealed a close and significant correlation between the intra-abdominal fat/subcutaneous fat area ratio and the WHR.

Fat distribution is correlated with several CVD risk factors. Central obesity increases the risk of hypertension (Krotkiewski *et al.*, 1983; Hartz *et al.*, 1984; Baumgartner *et al.*, 1987; Wing *et al.*, 1991), hypertriglyceridaemia (Krotkiewski *et al.*, 1983; Lapidus *et al.*, 1984; Baumgartner *et al.*, 1987; Wing *et al.*, 1991), hypercholesterolaemia (Wing *et al.*, 1991), hyperglycaemia (Krotkiewski *et al.*, 1983), hyperinsulinaemia (Krotkiewski *et al.*, 1983), low levels of HDL (Ostlund *et al.*, 1990), NIDDM (Hartz *et al.*, 1984), elevated fibrinogen and PAI-1 (Vague *et al.*, 1989; Ditschuneit *et al.*, 1995) and hyperuricaemia (Bonora *et al.*, 1996) in normal and obese subjects and in subjects with NIDDM (Van Gaal *et al.*, 1988b).

Next to physiological risk factors, central body fat seems to be related to a number of behavioural and psychosocial risk factors. An association with a high WHR was found for smoking (Laws *et al.*, 1990; Wing *et al.*, 1991), physical inactivity (Tremblay *et al.*, 1990; Wing *et al.*, 1991), high caloric intake (Wing *et al.*, 1991) and alcohol use and abuse (Laws *et al.*, 1990). Wing *et al.* (1991) found an association of WHR with higher levels of anger, anxiety and depression and lower levels of perceived social support. Björntorp (1991) hypothesized that those individuals who experience a great deal of stress or who have difficulty coping with stress may experience higher cortisol levels and consequently may deposit more body fat in the abdominal area (Björntorp, 1991).

Several mechanisms by which central body fat distribution may predispose to increased CVD risk have been postulated. Little is known about the mechanism by which obesity *per se* can increase the cardiovascular risk. Several risk factors for CVD seem to cluster in the individual as seen in the metabolic syndrome. Insulin resistance and compensatory hyperinsulinaemia are seen as the underlying cause of this syndrome (Reaven, 1988). Proposed pathogenic mechanisms related to insulin resistance have been summarized previously (Després & Marette, 1994; Taskinen, 1995).

One of the possible mechanisms of the insulin-resistance syndrome is clearly described by Björntorp (1990). In this pathogenic model, free fatty acids (FFA) seem to play the key role. The abdominal obese have an enlarged portal adipose tissue depot, which is very sensitive to lipolytic stimuli. This leads to high FFA concentrations in the portal vein. This in turn inhibits hepatic insulin clearance and might be followed by insulin resistance. Exposure of the liver to elevated concentrations of portal FFA also leads to hyperlipidaemia (Björntorp, 1990) (see Chapter 9).

The Québec Family Study (Bouchard *et al.*, 1996; Pérusse *et al.*, 1996) investigated in 100 French-Canadian families the importance of familial aggregation in abdominal visceral fat as assessed by computed tomography (CT). The results suggest that genetic factors are important determinants of the familial aggregation observed in the amount of visceral fat (Pérusse *et al.*, 1996). The authors suggest that this could be accounted for by a major gene on an autosomal recessive locus, accounting for 51% of the phenotypic variance and affecting 10% of the sample (Bouchard *et al.*, 1996).

Weight reduction

In the inter-relation between abdominal obesity, hyperinsulinaemia/insulin resistance, NIDDM, hypertension and lipid abnormalities, the most natural target of intervention is obesity. Since the independent effect of obesity on CVD risk is well established (Hubert *et al.*, 1983; Manson *et al.*, 1995), weight loss not only directly reduces risk but also indirectly decreases it through favourable changes in serum lipoproteins and blood pressure (Datillo & Kris-Etherton, 1992). In the Framingham Study (Hubert *et al.*, 1983), it was shown that those who throughout 26 years of follow-up lost greater than 10% of their weight had a moderately reduced risk for CHD than those whose weight remained unchanged. In contrast, the study of Walker *et al.* (1995) showed no reduction in the risk for heart attack with weight loss in the obese or overweight middle-aged men.

Studies show that even a moderate amount of weight loss has a beneficial effect on cardiovascular morbidity and mortality. In the Lifestyle Heart trial (Ornish *et al.*, 1990), 1 year of comprehensive lifestyle changes (low-fat vegetarian diet, stopping smoking, stress management training and moderate exercise) led to a weight loss of approximately 10 kg. At the same time 82% of this group of patients showed some regression of coronary arterial lesions as assessed by quantitative angiography. In the control group, however, a progression of the lesions was observed. A study by Singh *et al.* (1992), also showed the effect of moderate weight loss on CVD. A fat-reduced diet, with the addition of soluble dietary fibre and vitamins, was prescribed to patients with a previous history of myocardial infarction. After 1 year it was shown that when weight loss reached 7.1 kg there was a significant reduction of cardiac events, total cardiac mortality and total mortality.

For patients who are unable to attain and maintain substantial weight reduction, modest weight loss should be recommended (Goldstein, 1992; Van Gaal *et al.*, 1997).

In the light of the recent interest in the possible detrimental effects of weight cycling, the impact of weight cycling on cardiovascular risk has been investigated. At the end of a follow-up period of 1 year of a very-low-calorie diet (VLCD) treatment, Hainer *et al.* (1992) could not demonstrate any significant difference in serum lipids between weight regainers and weight losers. The authors suggest that some kind of adherence to a weight reduction regimen including physical exercise may explain these results. In the study of Rodin *et al.* (1990), a higher WHR was significantly associated with a higher degree of weight cycling, controlling for age and parity.

Obesity and blood pressure

Hypertension as defined by a systolic/diastolic blood pressure of greater than 140/90 mmHg is one of the major risk factors for CHD and the most important risk factor for cerebrovascular disease (Joint National Committee on detection and evaluation and treatment of higher blood pressure, 1993).

The association between hypertension and obesity is well documented. Results of several, mostly epidemiological studies, indicate that obesity is a strong (independent) risk factor for hypertension (Stamler *et al.*, 1978; Modan *et al.*, 1985; Friedman *et al.*, 1988). In the study of Stamler *et al.* (1978), the prevalence of hypertension in the obese was estimated to be 50–300% higher than in the lean subjects. Body-weight also correlates with blood pressure within the so-called normotensive range of blood pressure (Hypertension Prevention Trial 1990; Pi-Sunyer, 1993). In the longitudinal study of Friedman *et al.* (1988), weight gain was independently related to increased blood pressure. The magnitude of the association between blood pressure and weight may vary according to gender, ethnicity and age (Hsueh & Buchanan, 1994).

Several studies have also demonstrated a positive association between body fat distribution and blood pressure (Blair *et al.*, 1984; Baumgartner *et al.*, 1987; Troisi *et al.*, 1990). Body fat distribution, once again, appears to be a more powerful determinant of blood pressure than overall measures of obesity (Blair *et al.*, 1984). This is also true in NIDDM patients (Van Gaal *et al.*, 1988a).

The body fat distribution–blood pressure relationship may be affected by smoking or the intake of alcohol. Troisi *et al.* (1990) showed that the relationship between body fat distribution and blood pressure was no longer statistically significant, after adjustment for alcohol intake.

Hypertension is generally seen as an essential part of the insulin-resistance syndrome (Ferrannini *et al.*, 1987). Correlations have been identified between blood pressure and plasma insulin (Modan *et al.*, 1985) and hypertension and hyperinsulinaemia (Feskens *et al.*, 1995). Assessments of insulin sensitivity also correlate with blood pressure: hypertensive individuals appear to be more insulin resistant than normotensive controls (Ferrannini *et al.*, 1987). In addition, it should be noted that not all hypertensive subjects are insulin resistant and not all insulin-resistant subjects are hypertensive (Reaven, 1996).

Mechanism(s)

The pathogenesis of increased blood pressure in the obese is poorly understood. Several mechanisms, linking obesity to hypertension, have been proposed: hypervolaemia causing increased cardiac output with failure of an appropriate reduction in systemic vascular resistance (Reisin *et al.*, 1983), stimulation of the renin–angiotensin–aldosterone system (Tuck *et al.*, 1981) and increased salt intake due to increased caloric intake (Tuck, 1991). The FFA composition of cell membranes also seems to play an important role in the pathogenesis of hypertension: the membrane polyunsaturated FFA content, which is to a great extent dependent on dietary intake, seems to be decreased in essential hypertension (Sinclair, 1984; Simopoulos, 1991).

Recent research has focused on the possible role of insulin resistance and hyperinsulinaemia in hypertension (DeFronzo & Ferrannini, 1991). Hypertension in insulin-resistant states is generally attributed to selective insulin resistance mainly in skeletal muscle with preservation of the renal and sympathetic nervous system (SNS) sensitivity to insulin (Rocchini, 1991). A comprehensive review of the association between insulin and hypertension has been published by DeFronzo and Ferrannini (1991). In this paper the authors give an overview of the different mechanisms by which insulin resistance can lead to hypertension through increased SNS activity, enhanced renal sodium/water reabsorption, and alterations in Na^+/K^+ adenosine triphosphatase (ATPase) pump activity (DeFronzo & Ferrannini, 1991).

Weight reduction

Although the mechanisms linking obesity to hypertension are not completely understood, clinical intervention trials have consistently shown the blood pressure-lowering effect of weight loss (Reisin *et al.*, 1978; Fagerberg *et al.*, 1984; Imai *et al.*, 1986; Rocchini *et al.*, 1989; Schotte & Stunkard, 1990; Davis *et al.*, 1993; Su *et al.*, 1995).

Weight reduction is the single most effective non-pharmacological approach to the control of blood pressure in humans (Davis *et al.*, 1993; McCarron & Reusser, 1996), and even modest reductions in weight have been shown to improve blood pressure (Schotte & Stunkard, 1990). In the Trial of Antihypertensive Interventions, both short-term (Langeford *et al.*, 1991) and long-term interventions (Wassertheil-Smoller *et al.*, 1992), with weight reductions of as little as 3–5 kg, resulted in normalization of blood pressure among people with slightly increased blood pressure (borderline hypertension). Modest weight loss has a blood pressure-lowering effect in lean hypertensive (Imai *et al.*, 1986), obese hypertensive and normotensive obese persons (Su *et al.*, 1995).

The reduction in blood pressure is related to the amount of weight lost, rather than to the method of treatment (Schotte & Stunkard, 1990). VLCD (Ikeda *et al.*, 1996), moderate calorie restriction (Rocchini *et al.*, 1989), behavioural therapy (Schotte & Stunkard, 1990) and moderate caloric restriction combined with light exercise (Su *et al.*, 1995) all resulted in a significant reduction in blood pressure.

Although the efficacy of weight reduction in hypertensives have been well established, the effectiveness of additional sodium restriction has been more controversial. In the study of Reisin *et al.* (1978), weight loss lead to a reduction in blood pressure, independently of salt intake. In the study of Fagerberg *et al.* (1984), a reduction of blood pressure in hypertensive obese men was only possible when the moderate weight loss was combined with a restriction in sodium intake. It is possible that the difference in caloric restriction (VLCD vs moderate caloric restriction) may account for these conflicting results. More recently, the INTERSALT Study (Dyer *et al.*, 1994) showed that for most populations with a high average salt intake, effects of dietary sodium reduction and weight loss on blood pressure are independent and additive. Rocchini *et al.* (1989) showed that the blood pressure of untreated obese adolescents is sensitive to dietary sodium intake, whereas the blood pressure of non-obese adolescents was not; this sensitivity was altered by weight loss (Rocchini *et al.*, 1989).

Significant weight reduction can lead to a reduction of chronic antihypertensive medication requirements, in normal-weight hypertensive patients (Imai *et al.*, 1986) as well as in overweight hypertensive patients (Fagerberg *et al.*, 1984; Davis *et al.*, 1993).

In two studies (Rocchini *et al.*, 1989; Su *et al.*, 1995), weight loss was associated with the normalization of blood pressure, even though the patients in both studies did not achieve their ideal body-weight. In addition, Cohen and Flamenbaum (1986) postulated that there is a 'floor effect': a degree of weight loss beyond which further decrements in blood pressure will not occur. These findings may be important in the light of the disappointing long-term results of weight reduction in obesity (Brownell & Wadden, 1992). It is not necessary to achieve the ideal body-weight in order to have an important lowering or even normalizing effect on blood pressure (McCarron & Reusser, 1996). The problem with the non-pharmacological treatment of hypertension is that it is very difficult to motivate asymptomatic mild hypertensive patients to change their diet and lifestyle. The attrition rate in the non-pharmacological treatment study of Krzesinski *et al.* (1993) was 47%.

Digestive diseases

Gastrointestinal function

A number of studies have investigated the relationship between obesity and gastrointestinal function.

In a prospective study of 1224 patients referred for upper alimentary endoscopy, Stene-Larsen *et al.* (1988) found reflux oesophagitis in 195 (16%) of the patients and hiatus hernia in 249 (20%). In patients with reflux oesophagitis a coexisting hiatus hernia was found in 68%. In patients with mild to moderate oesophagitis (grades 1 and 2) the overweight was most pronounced, whereas in patients with severe oesophagitis (grade 3) body-weight was normal. The results support the view that adiposity is associated with both sliding hiatus hernia and reflux oesophagitis and that hiatus hernia plays a role in the development of reflux oesophagitis (Stene-Larsen *et al.*, 1988). These results are not in accordance with the results obtained in the study of Lundell *et al.* (1995). In this study of morbidly obese subjects, no significant correlations could be found between body-weight, BMI or WHR and a number of reflux variables.

Studies on the relationship between gastric emptying and obesity have yielded conflicting results. Some found gastric emptying to be accelerated in the obese (Wright *et al.*, 1983), others found it to be delayed (Maddox *et al.*, 1989) or even unchanged (Glasbrenner *et al.*, 1993). Maddox *et al.* (1989) suggest that the differences probably reflect methodological discrepancies and variations in subject selection.

A more rapid gastric emptying in obesity might result in a reduced feeling of satiety and an increase in food intake resulting in obesity (Wisén & Hellström, 1995). If gastric emptying is delayed in obese persons, disordered gastric emptying cannot be seen as a factor in the pathogenesis of obesity (Maddox *et al.*, 1989).

In one study (Wisén & Johansson, 1992) obesity was associated with an elevated rate of nutrient uptake in the proximal jejunum. The authors speculated that rapid absorption in obese subjects results in less prominent activation of satiety signals from the intestine, and can be of pathophysiological importance for the development of obesity.

Gallstones

Gallbladder disease is a well-recognized complication of obesity (Barbara *et al.*, 1987; Jørgenson, 1989). About 50% of morbidly obese patients seeking treatment have gallstones or a history of gallbladder disease, as reported by Amaral and Thompson (1985). The Nurses Health Study (Stampfer *et al.*, 1992), which followed nearly 90 000 women for 8 years, found a substantial increase in the incidence of clinically recognized gallstone disease with increasing BMI. Women with a BMI > 45 kg/m² had a sevenfold excess risk compared to those, whose BMI was < 24 kg/m².

There is some controversy concerning the association of gallstone disease and obesity in men. Jørgenson (1989) found no relationship between BMI and gallstone disease in men. In contrast Barbara *et al.* (1987) reported an association between obesity and gallstone prevalence in males. It is possible that some studies may not have adequate statistical power to detect any effect of obesity in men, because gallstone disease is less common among men than women (Everhart, 1993). Comparing BMI *per se*, weight gain and WHR indicated that among more than 800 men the relative risk for gallstone was clearly related to the presence of abdominal fat, rather than body-weight or weight gain (Heaton *et al.*, 1991).

Most gallstones are thought to be cholesterol gallstones (Busch & Matern, 1991; Everhart, 1993). It is generally accepted that at least three primary defects must be present simultaneously for the formation of gallstone disease: a solubility defect, leading to supersaturation of gallbladder bile; a kinetic factor, the presence of nucleating factors; and a residence time effect caused by gallbladder hypomobility (Busch & Matern, 1991). The higher risk of gallstone disease in the obese appears to be mainly the result of the first factor.

The risk for gallstone formation in the obese seems to increase during weight loss. Liddle *et al.* (1989) reported a higher risk for lithogenesis in women with a rapid weight loss due to VLCD. In the prospective Nurses Health Study (Stampfer *et al.*, 1992), recent weight loss was associated with a modest increased risk of gallstone formation after adjustment for pretreatment BMI. Some authors (Jørgenson, 1989; Stampfer, *et al.*, 1992) suggested that the underlying obesity, rather than weight changes, is the most important factor in the risk of gallstone formation. This hypothesis is in accordance with the results of the study of Thijs *et al.* (1992), which demonstrated that controlling for dieting did not affect the association between BMI and gallstone disease.

Steatosis and steatohepatitis

The association of liver disease with obesity is well documented and can be divided into four histological groups: fatty liver, fatty hepatitis, fatty fibrosis and fatty cirrhosis (Braillon *et al.*, 1985; Clain & Lefkowitch, 1987). Most patients show only fatty change and despite the high percentage of morbidly obese patients who show histological abnormalities of the liver, most patients remain asymptomatic (Klain *et al.*, 1989; Powell *et al.*, 1990) and may even present with normal liver tests (Klain *et al.*, 1989). Non-alcoholic steatohepatitis

(NASH), or fatty liver hepatitis or steatohepatitis, is histologically identical to alcoholic hepatitis (Van Steenbergen & Lanckmans, 1995).

In a recent study, Luyckx *et al.* (1998) studied liver biopsies of 528 obese patients undergoing bariatric surgery and found fatty change in 74% of the patients. In some studies the degree of overweight correlates with the severity of liver disease (Braillon *et al.*, 1985; Klain *et al.*, 1989; Luyckx *et al.*, 1998), while in other studies no correlation could be observed (Powell *et al.*, 1990; Andersen *et al.*, 1991).

Controversy still exists concerning obesity as a single risk factor for progression of NASH to severe liver disease (Clain & Lefkowitch, 1987). In the study of Powell *et al.* (1990), 42 patients with NASH, of whom 40 were obese, were followed for a median of 4.5 years (range 1.5–21.5 years). The authors concluded that NASH is a cause of hepatic inflammation, but usually slowly progressive and of low-grade severity. However, the disorder may ultimately result in cirrhosis (Powell *et al.*, 1990).

Recently, it has been suggested that steatohepatitis in the obese is another feature of the insulin-resistance syndrome and independently related to body fat topography (Kral *et al.*, 1993). An increased amount of deep abdominal fat, as seen in central obesity, may lead to an increased delivery of fatty acids to the liver, followed by an increased synthesis and secretion rate of triglycerides and very-low-density lipoproteins (VLDL), and by the development of liver steatosis which is further potentiated by the hyperinsulinaemic situation (Van Steenbergen & Lanckmans, 1995). A comprehensive review of Van Steenbergen and Lanckmans (1995) addresses in detail the pathogenesis of liver disturbances in obesity.

Major weight loss as seen after gastroplasty (Luyckx *et al.*, 1998) or VLCD (Andersen *et al.*, 1991), improves fatty liver changes, but also seems to increase inflammatory hepatitis. Therefore a large and rapid weight loss may, in itself, represent a risk factor for the development of hepatic fibrosis.

Cancer

Obesity is associated with the development of different forms of cancer. Most of the research on this subject focused on the relationship between obesity and breast and endometrial cancer.

Breast cancer

Numerous studies have examined the relationship between body-weight and breast cancer. There appears to be an important difference between pre- and postmenopausal women. Most studies found lean women to be at increased risk of developing premenopausal breast cancer (London *et al.*, 1989; Swanson *et al.*, 1989; Vatten & Kvinnsland, 1992; Swanson *et al.*, 1996). In postmenopausal women, however, breast cancer seems to be related to obesity (Le Marchand *et al.*, 1988; Swanson *et al.*, 1989). However, this positive relationship was not found in all studies (London *et al.*, 1989; Ballard-Barbash *et al.*, 1990).

It was initially hypothesized that higher relative weight led to poorer detection of tumours, because the apparent protective effect of obesity on breast cancer risk was limited to women with small tumours (Swanson *et al.*, 1989). Vatten and Kvinnsland (1992) demonstrated that this was not a sufficient explanation. Weight gain during adult life might influence the risk of breast cancer and can be a possible explanation for the discrepancy in results found in postmenopausal women. Some authors did report a correlation between the risk of postmenopausal breast cancer and weight gain occurring during adult life (Le Marchand *et al.*, 1988; London *et al.*, 1989).

In addition to body-weight the relationship between fat distribution and breast cancer risk in both pre- and postmenopausal women has yielded conflicting results. In premenopausal women some authors found a correlation between body fat distribution and breast cancer risk (Ballard-Barbash *et al.*, 1990), while others did not (Bruning *et al.*, 1992a; Petrek *et al.*, 1993; Swanson *et al.*, 1996). An association between central adiposity and breast cancer in postmenopausal women has been reported (Ballard-Barbash *et al.*, 1990; Folsom *et al.*, 1990; Bruning *et al.*, 1992a; Sellers *et al.*, 1992). In one study, however, no association was found (Petrek *et al.*, 1993). The Iowa Women's Health Study (Sellers *et al.*, 1992) demonstrated that the increase in risk of breast cancer associated with a high WHR was more pronounced among women with a family history of breast cancer.

A number of mechanisms for the association between body-weight or fat distribution, breast cancer and menopausal status have been proposed (Stoll, 1994). Most of the tentative hypotheses focus on hormonal metabolism. Hulka *et al.* (1994) summarized the epidemiological literature on this subject. Initially most of the attention was drawn on oestrogen metabolism (Kirschner *et al.*, 1981) with a current focus on the effects of oestrogen augmented by progesterone (Key & Pike, 1988; Hulka *et al.*, 1994).

Different factors have been put forward to increase the bioavailability of oestradiol and its metabolites and hereby increasing the risk of tumour growth:
- conversion of androgens to oestrogens in adipose tissue (tissue specific);
- low values of sex hormone binding globulin (SHBG);
- high values of FFA;
- insulin resistance and hyperinsulinaemia.

Adipose tissue contains high levels of aromatase, the enzyme that converts androgens into oestrogen; accumulation of adipose tissue can lead directly to a rise in oestrogen levels. This modulation could be a possible explanation for the difference in results between pre- and postmenopausal women. Before menopause ovarian oestrogen production rates overwhelm changes in oestrogen metabolism in adipose tissue (Hulka *et al.*, 1994).

The bioavailability of oestradiol is dependent on the degree and strength of its binding to several protein carriers. SHBG is the predominant protein carrier of oestradiol and the percentage of free oestradiol is generally inversely related to the level of SHBG (Enriori *et al.*, 1986). Abdominal fat has been shown to be related with lower concentrations of SHBG (Bruning *et al.*, 1992a; Van Gaal *et al.*, 1994) and a concomitant increase in bioavailable oestrogen.

Increases in FFA have been reported to increase the level of free oestradiol by displacing oestradiol from SHBG (where it is tightly bound) to albumin (where it is less tightly bound). This results in a greater availability of oestradiol for target cells (Bruning *et al.*, 1992a). Bruning *et al.* (1992a) found a positive correlation between WHR and serum levels of triglycerides and available oestradiol.

Research exploring the metabolic factors mediating the influence of body size on breast cancer has focused on the influence of hyperandrogenaemia (Secreto *et al.*, 1991) and hyperinsulinaemia (Bruning *et al.*, 1992b), found among women with central adiposity before and after menopause. Bruning *et al.* (1992b) observed that C-peptide levels and an apparent insulin insensitivity are significantly related to breast cancer risk, independent of general adiposity or body fat distribution. In this study SHBG was inversely related to C-peptide levels while triglycerides and available oestradiol were positively related to C-peptide. Insulin resistance and concomitant high serum levels of insulin suppress circulating concentrations of SHBG rendering a larger fraction of the total circulating pool of oestradiol available for activity at tissue level. Insulin resistance may also result in the amplification of insulin-like growth factor-1 (IGF-1) action at the tissue level by altering serum concentrations of IGF-1 binding proteins (Kazer, 1995). Young obese women may have reduced risk of breast cancer because they have more anovulatory cycles and thus lower exposure to oestrogen and progesterone (Swanson, 1996).

Endometrial cancer

Consistent and positive associations have been shown between obesity and the incidence of endometrial cancer (Folsom *et al.*, 1989b; Austin *et al.*, 1991). Results of studies investigating the association between fat distribution and the incidence of endometrial cancer are not as consistent, with some authors finding an association between WHR and endometrial cancer risk (Lapidus *et al.*, 1988) and others who do not (Austin *et al.*, 1991).

Methodological differences could account for the discrepancy in results. In the study of Folsom *et al.* (1989b) WHR was self-reported. Surprisingly Austin *et al.* (1991) did not find an association between endometrial cancer and the WHR but they did find a positive association for the subscapular/triceps skinfold ratio, a measure of central vs peripheral obesity on endometrial cancer risk.

The mechanism by which obesity is thought to increase the risk of endometrial cancer is the same as in breast cancer: increased levels of serum oestrogen unopposed by progesterone (Austin *et al.*, 1991).

Prostate cancer

Information on the impact of body-weight on prostate hypertrophy and cancer is scarce. A preliminary report by Demark-Wahnefield (1992) in 28 men, 60–70 years of age, suggested that the waist/thigh ratio rather than BMI or WHR was significantly higher in men with prostate cancer. On the contrary, a better prognosis for such men with prostate cancer has recently been suggested, based on findings of increased endogenous oestrogen and decreased testosterone (Daniell, 1996).

More recent data from the Health Professionals follow-up study (Giovanucci *et al.*, 1994), showed that abdominal obese men (expressed as a waist circumference of ≥ 109 cm), have a higher risk of benign prostatic hyperplasia. Whether this hyperplasia can be considered as a precancer state still remains unclear. Also, the restricted data of one single study on cancer are not enough to accept prostatic cancer as being an evident consequence of obesity.

References

Albanes, D., Jones, Y., Micozzi, M. & Mattson, M. (1987) Associations between smoking and body weight in the US population: analysis of NHANES II. *American Journal of Public Health* **77**, 439–444.

Amaral, J. & Thompson, W. (1985) Gallbladder disease in the morbidly obese. *American Journal of Surgery* **149**, 551–557.

Andersen, T., Gluud, C., Franzmann, M. & Christoffersen, P. (1991) Hepatic effects of dietary weight loss in morbidly obese subjects. *Journal of Hepatology* **12**, 224–229.

Austin, H., Austin, J., Partridge, E., Hatch, K. & Shingleton, H. (1991) Endometrial cancer, obesity and body fat distribution. *Cancer Research* **51**, 568–572.

Ballard-Barbash, R., Schatzkin, A., Carter, C. *et al.* (1990) Body fat distribution and breast cancer in the Framingham study. *Journal of the National Cancer Institute* **82**, 286–290.

Barbara, L., Sama, C., Labate, A.M.M. *et al.* (1987) A population study on the prevalence of gallstone disease: the Sirmione study. *Hepatology* **7**, 913–917.

Baumgartner, R., Roche, A., Chumlea, W., Siervogel, R. & Glueck, C. (1987) Fatness and fat patterns: association with plasma lipids and blood pressures in adults 18 to 57 years of age. *American Journal of Epidemiology* **126**, 614–628.

Björntorp, P. (1990) 'Portal' adipose tissue as a generator of risk factors for cardiovascular disease and diabetes. *Arteriosclerosis* 10, 493–496.

Björntorp, P. (1991) Hypothesis. Visceral fat accumulation: the missing link between psychosocial factors and cardiovascular disease? *Journal of Internal Medicine* 230, 195–201.

Blair, D., Habicht, J.P., Sims, E., Sylwester, D. & Abraham, S. (1984) Evidence for an increased risk for hypertension with centrally located body fat and the effect of race and sex on this risk. *American Journal of Epidemiology* 119, 526–540.

Bonora, E., Targher, G., Zenere, M. *et al.* (1996) Relationship of uric acid concentration to cardiovascular risk factors in young men. Role of obesity and central fat distribution. The Verona Young Men Atherosclerosis Risk Factors Study. *International Journal of Obesity* 20, 975–980.

Bouchard, C., Rice, T., Lemieux, S., Després, J.P., Pérusse, L. & Rao, D.C. (1996) Major gene for abdominal visceral fat area in the Québec Family Study. *International Journal of Obesity* 20, 420–427.

Braillon, A., Capron, J.P., Hervé, M., Degott, C. & Quenum, C. (1985) Liver in obesity. *Gut* 26, 133–139.

Brownell, K. & Wadden, T. (1992) Etiology and treatment of obesity: understanding a serious, prevalent and refractory disorder. *Journal of Consulting and Clinical Psychology* 60, 505–517.

Bruning, P., Bonfrèr, J., Hart, A. *et al.* (1992a) Body measurement, oestrogen availability and the risk of human breast cancer: a case–control study. *International Journal of Cancer* 51, 14–19.

Bruning, P., Bonfrèr, J., Van Noord, P., Hart, A., De Jong-Bakker, M. & Nooijen, W. (1992b) Insulin resistance and breast-cancer risk. *International Journal of Cancer* 52, 511–516.

Busch, N. & Matern, S. (1991) Currents concepts in cholesterol gallstone pathogenesis. *European Journal of Clinical Investigation* 21, 453–460.

Clain, D. & Lefkowitch, J. (1987) Fatty liver disease in morbid obesity. *Gastroenterology Clinics of North America* 16, 239–252.

Cohen, N. & Flamenbaum, W. (1986) Obesity and hypertension. Demonstration of a 'floor effect'. *American Journal of Medicine* 80, 177–181.

Cushman, M., Yanez, D., Psaty, B. *et al.* (1996) Association of fibrinogen and coagulation factors VII and VIII with cardiovascular risk factors in the elderly. *American Journal of Epidemiology* 143, 665–676.

Daniell, H.W. (1996) A better prognosis for obese men with prostate cancer. *Journal of Urology* 155; 220–225.

Dattilo, A. & Kris-Etherton, P. (1992) Effects of weight reduction on blood lipids and lipoproteins: a meta-analysis. *American Journal of Clinical Nutrition* 56, 320–328.

Davis, B., Blaufox, M.D., Oberman, A. *et al.* (1993) Reduction in long-term antihypertensive medication requirements. *Archives of Internal Medicine* 153, 1773–1782.

DeFronzo, R. & Ferrannini, E. (1991) Insulin resistance: a multifaceted syndrome responsible for NIDDM, obesity, hypertension, dyslipidemia and atherosclerotic cardiovascular disease. *Diabetes Care* 14, 173–194.

Demark-Wahnefried, W., Paulson, D., Robertson, C., Anderson, E., Conaway, M. & Rimer, B. (1992) Body dimension differences in men with or without prostate cancer. *Journal of the National Cancer Institute* 84, 1363–1364.

Després, J.P. & Marette, A. (1994) Relation of components of insulin resistance syndrome to coronary disease risk. *Current Opinion in Lipidology* 5, 274–289.

Ditschuneit, H., Flechtner-Mors, M. & Adler, G. (1995) Fibrinogen in obesity before and after weight reduction. *Obesity Research* 3, 43–48.

Donahue, R., Abbott, R., Bloom, E., Reed, D. & Yano, K. (1987) Central obesity and coronary heart disease in men. *Lancet* 11, 821–824.

Ducimetière, P., Richard, J. & Cambien, F. (1986) The pattern of subcutaneous fat distribution in middle-aged men and the risk of coronary heart disease: the Paris Prospective Study. *International Journal of Obesity* 10, 229–240.

Dyer, A., Elliot, P., Shipley, M., Stamler, R. & Stamler, J. (1994) Body mass index and associations of sodium and potassium with blood pressure in INTERSALT. *Hypertension* 23, 729–736.

Enriori, C., Orsini, W., Del Carmen Cremona, M. *et al.* (1986) Decrease of circulating level of

SHBG in postmenopausal obese women as a risk factor in breast cancer, reversible effect of weight loss. *Gynecologic Oncology* **23**, 77–86.

Everhart, J. (1993) Contributions of obesity and weight loss to gallstone disease. *Annals of Internal Medicine* **119**, 1029–1035.

Faberberg, B., Andersson, O., Isaksson, B. & Björntorp, P. (1984) Blood pressure control during weight reduction in obese hypertensive men: separate effects of sodium and energy restriction. *British Medical Journal* **288**, 11–14.

Feinleb, M. (1985) Epidemiology of obesity in relation to health hazards. *Annals of Internal Medicine* **103**, 1019–1024.

Ferrannini, E., Buzzigoli, G., Bonadonna, R. *et al.* (1987) Insulin resistance in essential hypertension. *New England Journal of Medicine* **317**, 350–357.

Feskens, E., Tuomilehto, J., Stengard, J., Pekkanen, J., Nissinen, A. & Kromhout, D. (1995) Hypertension and overweight associated with hyperinsulinemia and glucose tolerance: a longitudinal study of the Finnish and Dutch cohorts of the Seven Countries Study. *Diabetologia* **38**, 839–847.

Folsom, A., Burke, G., Ballew, C. *et al.* (1989a) Relation of body fatness and its distribution to cardiovascular risk factors in young blacks and whites. The role of insulin. *American Journal of Epidemiology* **130**, 911–924.

Folsom, A., Kaye, S., Potter, J. & Prineas, R. (1989b) Association of incident carcinoma of the endometrium with body weight and fat distribution in older women: early findings of the Iowa Women's Health Study. *Cancer Research* **49**, 6828–6831.

Folsom, A., Kaye, S., Prineas, R., Potter, J., Gapstur, S. & Wallace, R. (1990) Increased incidence of carcinoma of the breast associated with abdominal adiposity in postmenopausal women. *American Journal of Epidemiology* **131**, 794–803.

Friedman, G., Selby, J., Quesenberry, C., Armstrong, M. & Klatsky, A. (1988) Precursors of essential hypertension: body weight, alcohol and salt use, and parental history of hypertension. *Preventive Medicine* **17**, 387–402.

Fujioka, S., Matsuzawa, Y., Tokunaga, K. & Tarui, S. (1987) Contribution of intra-abdominal fat accumulation to the impairement of glucose and lipid metabolism in human obesity. *Metabolism* **36**, 54–59.

Garfinkel, L. & Stellman, S. (1988) Smoking and lung cancer in women: findings in a prospective study. *Cancer Research* **48**, 6951–6955.

Garn, S., Leonard, W. & Hawthorne, V. (1986) Three limitations of the body mass index. *American Journal of Clinical Nutrition* **44**, 996–997.

Garrison, R., Feinleb, M., Castelli, W. & McNamara, P. (1983) Cigarette smoking as a confounder of the relationship between relative weight and long-term mortality. *Journal of the American Medical Association* **249**, 2199–2203.

Genest, J. & Cohn, J.S. (1995) Clustering of cardiovascular risk factors: targetting high-risk individuals. *American Journal of Cardiology* **76**, 8A–20A.

Giovanucci, E., Rimm, E., Chute, C. *et al.* (1994) Obesity and benign prostatic hyperplasia. *American Journal of Epidemiology* **140**, 989–1002.

Glasbrenner, B., Pieramico, O., Brecht-Krauss, D., Baur, M. & Malfertheiner, P. (1983) Gastric emptying of solids and liquids in obesity. *Clinical Investigation* **71**, 542–546.

Goldstein, D. (1992) Beneficial health effects of modest weight loss. *International Journal of Obesity* **16**, 397–415.

Haffner, S., Valdez, R., Hazuda, H., Mitchell, B., Morales, P. & Stern, M. (1992) Prospective analysis of the insulin-resistance syndrome (Syndrome X). *Diabetes* **41**, 715–722.

Hainer, V., Kunesova, M., Stich, V. *et al.* (1992) Body fat distribution and serum lipids during long-term follow-up of obese patients treated initially with a very-low-calorie diet. *American Journal of Clinical Nutrition* **56**, 283S–285S.

Hartz, A., Rupley, D. & Rimm, A. (1984) The association of girth measurements with disease in 32 586 women. *American Journal of Epidemiology* **119**, 71–80.

Heaton, K., Braddon, F., Emmett, P. *et al.* (1991) Why do men get gallstones? Roles of abdominal fat and hyperinsulinemia. *European Journal of Gastroenterology and Hepatitis* **3**, 745–751.

Hsueh, W. & Buchanan, T. (1994) Obesity and hypertension. *Endocrinology and Metabolism Clinics of North America* **23**, 405–427.

Hubert, H., Feinleb, M., McNamara, P. & Castelli, W. (1983) Obesity as an independent risk factor for cardiovascular disease: a 26-year follow-up of participants in the Framingham study. *Circulation* **67**, 968–977.

Hulka, B., Liu, E. & Lininger, R. (1994) Steroid hormones and risk of breast cancer. *Cancer* **74**, 1111–1124.

Hypertension Prevention Trial Research Group (1990) The Hypertensive Prevention Trial: Three-year effects of dietary changes on blood pressure. *Archives of Internal Medicine* **150**, 153–162.

Ikeda, T., Gomi, T., Hirawa, N., Sakurai, J. & Yoshikawa, N. (1996) Improvement of insulin sensitivity contributes to blood pressure reduction after weight loss in hypertensive subjects with obesity. *Hypertension* **27**, 1180–1186.

Imai, Y., Sato, K., Abe, K. *et al.* (1986) Effect of weight loss on blood pressure and drug consumption in normal weight patients. *Hypertension* **8**, 223–228.

The Joint National Committee on detection, evaluation and treatment of high blood pressure. (1993) The fifth report of the joint National committee on detection, evaluation and treatment of high blood pressure. *Archives of Internal Medicine* **153**, 154–183.

Jørgenson, T. (1989) Gall stones in a Danish population. Relation to weight, physical activity, smoking, coffee consumption, and diabetes mellitus. *Gut* **30**, 528–534.

Kannel, W., D'Agostino, R. & Belanger, A. (1992) Update on fibronigen as a cardiovascular risk factor. *Annals of Epidemiology* **2**, 457–466.

Kaplan, N. (1989) The deadly quartet: upper-body obesity, glucose intolerance, hypertriglyceridemia and hypertension. *Archives of Internal Medicine* **149**, 1514–1520.

Kazer, R. (1995) Insulin resistance, insulin-like growth factor 1 and breast cancer: a hypothesis. *International Journal of Cancer* **62**, 403–406.

Key, T. & Pike, M. (1988) The role of oestrogens and progestagens in the epidemiology and prevention of breast cancer. *European Journal of Cancer and Clinical Oncology* **24**, 29–43.

Kirschner, M., Ertel, N. & Schneidel, G. (1981) Obesity, hormones and cancer. *Cancer Research* **41**, 3711–3717.

Klain, J., Fraser, D., Goldstein, J. *et al.* (1989) Liver histology abnormalities in the morbidly obese. *Hepatology* **10**, 873–876.

Kral, J., Schaffner, F., Pierson, R. & Wang, J. (1993) Body fat topography as an independent predictor of fatty liver. *Metabolism* **42**, 548–551.

Krotkiewski, M., Björntorp, P., Sjöström, L. & Smith, U. (1983) Impact of obesity on metabolism in men and women. Importance of regional adipose tissue distribution. *Journal of Clinical Investigation* **72**, 1150–1162.

Krzesinski, J., Janssens, M., Vanderspeeten, F. & Rorive, G. (1993) Importance of weight loss and sodium restriction in the treatment of mild and moderate essential hypertension. *Acta Clinica Belgica* **48**, 234–235.

Langeford, H., Davis, B., Blaufox, D. *et al.* (1991) Effect of drug and diet treatment of mild hypertension on diastolic blood pressure. The TAIM Research Group. *Hypertension* **17**, 210–217.

Lapidus, L., Bengtsson, C., Larsson, B., Pennert, K., Rybo, E. & Sjöström, L. (1984) Distribution of adipose tissue and risk of cardiovascular disease and death: a 12 year follow up of participants in the population study of women in Gothenburg, Sweden. *British Medical Journal* **289**, 1257–1261.

Lapidus, L., Helgesson, O., Merck, C. & Björntorp, P. (1988) Adipose tissue distribution and female carcinomas. A 12 year follow-up, of participants in the population study of women in Gothenburg, Sweden. *International Journal of Obesity* **12**, 361–368.

Larsson, B., Svärdsudd, K., Welin, L., Wilhelmsen, L., Björntorp, P. & Tibblin, G. (1984) Abdominal adipose tissue distribution, obesity and risk of cardiovascular disease and death: 13 year follow up of participants in the study of men born in 1913. *British Medical Journal* **288**, 1401–1404.

Lavie, C., Ventura, H. & Messerli, F. (1992) Left ventricular hypertrophy. Its relationship to obesity and hypertension. *Postgraduate Medicine* **91**, 131–143.

Lauer, M., Anderson, K., Kannel, W. & Levy, D. (1991) The impact of obesity and left ventrical mass and geometry: the Framingham Study. *Journal of the American Medical Association* **266**, 231–236.

Laws, A., Terry, R. & Barrett-Connor, E. (1990) Behavioural covariates of waist-to-hip-ratio in Rancho Bernardo. *American Journal of Public Health* **80**, 1358–1362.

Le Marchand, L., Kolonel, L., Earle, M. & Mi, M. (1988) Body size at different periods of life and breast cancer risk. *American Journal of Epidemiology* **1287**, 137–152.

Liddle, R., Goldstein, R. & Saxton, J. (1989) Gallstone formation during weight reduction dieting. *Archives of Internal Medicine* **149**, 1750–1753.

London, S., Colditz, G., Stampfer, M., Willett, W., Rosner, B. & Speizer, F. (1989) Prospective study of relative weight, height, and risk of breast cancer. *Journal of the American Medical Association* **262**, 2853–2858.

Lundell, L., Ruth, M., Sandberg, N. & Bove-Nielsen, M. (1995) Does massive obesity promote abnormal gastroesophageal reflux? *Digestive Diseases and Sciences* **40**, 1632–1635.

Lundgren, C., Brown, S., Nordt, T., Sobel, B. & Fujii, S. (1996) Elaboration of type-1 plasminogen activator inhibitor from adipocytes. A potential pathogenic link between obesity and cardiovascular disease. *Circulation* **93**, 106–110.

Luyckx, F., Desaive, C., Thiry, A. *et al.* (1998) Liver abnormalities in severely obese subjects: effect of drastic weight loss after gastroplasty. *International Journal of Obesity* **22**, 222–226.

Maddox, A., Horowitz, M., Wishart, J. & Collins, P. (1989) Gastric and oesophagal emptying in obesity. *Scandinavian Journal of Gastroenterology* **24**, 593–598.

Manson, J., Stampfer, M., Hennekens, C. & Willett, W. (1987) Body weight and longevity. A reassessment. *Journal of the American Medical Association* **257**, 353–358.

Manson, J., Willett, W., Stampfer, M. *et al.* (1995) Body weight and mortality among women. *New England Journal of Medicine* **333**, 677–685.

McCarron, D. & Reusser, M. (1996) Body weight and blood pressure regulation. *American Journal of Clinical Nutrition* **63** (suppl.), 423S–425S.

Meade, T., North, W., Chakrabarti, R., Stirling, Y., Haines, A. & Thompson, S. (1980) Hemostatic function and cardiovascular death: early results of a prospective study. *Lancet* **17**, 1050–1053.

Modan, M., Halkin, H., Almog, S. *et al.* (1985) Hyperinsulinemia. A link between hypertension obesity and glucose intolerance. *Journal of Clinical Investigation* **75**, 809–816.

Ornish, D., Brown, S., Scherwitz, L. *et al.* (1990) Can lifestyle changes reverse coronary heart disease? *Lancet* **336**, 129–133.

Ostlund, R., Staten, M., Kohrt, W.M., Schultz, J. & Malley, M. (1990) The ratio of waist-to-hip circumference, plasma insulin level and glucose intolerance as independent predictors of HDL_2 chol in older adults. *New England Journal of Medicine* **322**, 229–234.

Pérusse, L., Després, J.P., Lemieux, S., Rice, T., Rao, D.C. & Bouchard, C. (1996) Familial aggregation of abdominal visceral fat level: results from the Quebec Family Study. *Metabolism* **45**, 378–382.

Petrek, J., Peters, M., Cirrincione, C., Rhodes, D. & Bajorunas, D. (1993) Is body fat topography a risk factor for breast cancer? *Annals of Internal Medicine* **118**, 356–362.

Pi-Sunyer, F. (1993) Medical hazards of obesity. *Annals of Internal Medicine* **199** (7Pt 2), 655–660.

Pouliot, M., Després, J., Nadeau, A. *et al.* (1992) Visceral obesity in men. Associations with glucose tolerance, plasma insulin and lipoprotein levels. *Diabetes* **41**, 826–834.

Powell, E., Cooksley, G., Hanson, R., Searle, J., Halliday, J. & Powell, L. (1990) The natural history of nonalcoholic steatohepatitis: a follow-up study of forty-two patients up to 21 years. *Hepatology* **11**, 74–80.

Reaven, G. (1988) Role of insulin resistance in human disease. *Diabetes* **37**, 1595–1607.

Reaven, G., Lithell, H. & Landsberg, L. (1996) Hypertension and associated metabolic abnormalities: the role of insulin resistance and the sympathoadrenal system. *New England Journal of Medicine* **334**, 374–381.

Reisin, E., Abel, R., Modan, M., Silverberg, D., Eliahou, H. & Modan, B. (1978) Effect of weight loss without salt restriction on the reduction of blood pressure in overweight hypertensive patients. *New England Journal of Medicine* **298**, 1–6.

Reisin, E., Frohlich, E., Messerli, F.H. *et al.* (1983) Cardiovascular changes after weight reduction in obesity hypertension. *Annals of Internal Medicine* **98**, 315–319.

Rillaerts, E., Van Gaal, L., Xiang, D., Vansant, G. & De Leeuw, I. (1989) Blood viscosity in human obesity: relation to glucose tolerance and insulin status. *International Journal of Obesity* **13**, 739–745.

Rocchini, A. (1991) Insulin resistance and blood pressure regulation in obese and nonobese subjects. Special lecture. *Hypertension* **17**, 837–842.

Rocchini, A., Key, J., Bondie, D. *et al.* (1989) The effect of weight loss on the sensitivity of blood pressure to sodium in obese adolescents. *New England Journal of Medicine* **321**, 580–585.

Rodin, J., Radke-Sharpe, N., Rebuffé-Scrive, M. & Greenwood, M. (1990) Weight cycling and fat distribution. *International Journal of Obesity* **14**, 303–310.

Schotte, D. & Stunkard, A. (1990) The effect of weight reduction on blood pressure in 301 obese patients. *Archives of Internal Medicine* **150**, 1701–1704.

Secreto, G., Toniolo, P., Berrino, F. *et al.* (1991) Serum and urinary androgens and risk of breast cancer in postmenopausal women. *Cancer Research* **51**, 2572–2576.

Sellers, T., Kushi, L., Potter, J. *et al.* (1992) Effect of family history, body-fat distribution and reproductive factors on the risk of postmenopausal breast cancer. *New England Journal of Medicine* **326**, 1323–1329.

Simopoulos, A. (1991) Omega-3 fatty acids in health and disease and in growth and development. *American Journal of Clinical Nutrition* **54**, 438–463.

Simopoulos, A. & Van Italie, T. (1984) Body weight, health and longevity. *Annals of Internal Medicine* **100**, 285–295.

Sinclair, H. (1984) Essential fatty acid in perspective. *Human Nutrition: Clinical Nutrition* **38**, 245–260.

Singh, R., Rastogi, S., Verma, R. *et al.* (1992) Randomised controlled trial of cardioprotective diet in patients with recent acute myocardial infarction: results of one year follow up. *British Medical Journal* **304**, 1015–1019.

Sjöström, L. (1992) Mortality of severely obese subjects. *American Journal of Clinical Nutrition* **55**, 516S–523S.

Stamler, R., Stamler, J., Riedlinger, W., Algera, G. & Robers, R. (1978) Weight and blood pressure. Findings in hypertension screening of 1 million Americans. *Journal of the American* **240**, 1607–1610.

Stampfer, M., Maclure, K., Colditz, G., Manson, J. & Willett, W. (1992) Risk of symptomatic gallstones in women with severe obesity. *American Journal of Clinical Nutrition* **55**, 652–658.

Stene-Larsen, G., Weberg, R., Larsen, I., Bjørtuft, O., Hoel, B. & Berstad, A. (1988) Relationship of overweight to hiatus hernia and reflux oesophagitis. *Scandinavian Journal of Gastroenterology* **23**, 427–432.

Stoll, B. (1994) Breast cancer: the obesity connection. *British Journal of Cancer* **69**, 799–801.

Su, H., Sheu, W., Chin, H., Jeng, C., Chen, Y. & Reaven, G. (1995) Effect of weight loss on blood pressure and insulin resistance in normotensive and hypertensive obese individuals. *American Journal of Hypertension* **8**, 1067–1071.

Swanson, C., Brinton, L., Taylor, P., Licitra, L., Ziegler, R. & Schairer, C. (1989) Body size and breast cancer risk assessed in women participating in the breast cancer detection demonstration project. *American Journal of Epidemiology* **130**, 1133–1141.

Swanson, C., Coates, R., Schoenberg, J. *et al.* (1996) Body size and breast cancer risk among women under age 45 years. *American Journal of Epidemiology* **143**, 698–706.

Taskinen, M. (1995) Insulin resistance and lipoprotein metabolism. *Current Opinion in Lipidology* **6**, 153–160.

Thijs, C., Knipschild, P. & Leffers, P. (1992) Is gallstone disease caused by obesity or dieting? *American Journal of Epidemiology* **135**, 274–280.

Tremblay, A., Després, J.P., Leblanc, C. *et al.* (1990) Effect of intensity of physical activity on body fatness and fat distribution. *American Journal of Clinical Nutrition* **51**, 153–157.

Troisi, R., Weiss, S., Segal, M., Cassano, P., Vokonas, S. & Landsberg, L. (1990) The relationship of body fat distribution to blood pressure in normotensive men: the normative ageing study. *International Journal of Obesity* **14**, 515–525.

Tuck, M. (1991) Role of salt in the control of blood pressure in obesity and diabetes mellitus. *Hypertension* **17** (suppl. 1), I135–I142.

Tuck, M., Sowers, J., Dornfeld, L., Kledzik, G. & Maxwell, M. (1981) The effect of weight reduction on blood pressure, plasma renin activity, and plasma aldosterone levels in obese patients. *New England Journal of Medicine* **304**, 930–933.

Vague, J. (1956) The degree of masculine differentiation of obesities, a factor determining predisposition to diabetes, atherosclerosis, gout and uric calculous disease. *American Journal of Clinical Nutrition* **4**, 20–34.

Vague, P., Juhan-Vague, I., Aillaud, M. *et al.* (1986) Correlation between blood fibrinolytic activity, plasminogen activator inhibitor level, plasma insulin level and relative body weight in normal and obese subjects. *Metabolism* **35**, 250–253.

Vague, P., Juhan-Vague, I., Chabert, V., Alessi, M. & Atlan, C. (1989) Fat distribution and plasminogen activator inhibitor activity in non-diabetic obese women. *Metabolism* **38**, 913–915.

Van Gaal, L. (1990) *Body fat distribution: endocrine, metabolic and therapeutic aspects.* PhD Thesis, University of Antwerp.

Van Gaal, L., Nobels, F., Rillaerts, E., Creten, W. & De Leeuw, I. (1988a) Hypertension in obese and non-obese non-insulin dependent diabetics. A matter of regional adiposity? *Diabete et Metabolisme* **14**, 289–293.

Van Gaal, L., Rillaerts, E., Creten, W. & De Leeuw, I. (1988b) Relationship of body fat distribution pattern to atherogenic risk factors in NIDDM. Preliminary results. *Diabetes Care* **11**, 103–106.

Van Gaal, L., Steijaert, M., Rillaerts, E. & De Leeuw, I. (1993) The plurimetabolic syndrome and the haemocoagulation system. In: Crepaldi, G., Tiengo, A. & Manzato, E. (eds) *Diabetes, Obesity and Hyperlipidemia*, pp. 229–237. Amsterdam: Elsevier Science Publishers.

Van Gaal, L., Vanuytsel, J., Vansant, G. & De Leeuw, I. (1994) Sex hormones, body fat distribution, resting metabolic rate and glucose-induced thermogenesis in premenopausal obese women. *International Journal of Obesity* **18**, 333–338.

Van Gaal, L., Zhang, A., Steijaert, M. & De Leeuw, I. (1995) Human obesity: from lipid abnormalities to lipid oxidation. *International Journal of Obesity* **19** (suppl. 3), S21–S26.

Van Gaal, L., Wauters, M. & De Leeuw, I. (1997) The beneficial effects of modest weight loss on cardiovascular risk factors. *International Journal of Obesity* **21** (suppl. 1), S5–S9.

Van Steenbergen, W. & Lanckmans, S. (1995) Liver disturbances in obesity and diabetes mellitus. *International Journal of Obesity* **19** (suppl. 3), S27–S37.

Vatten, L. & Kvinnsland, S. (1992) Prospective study of height, body mass index and risk of breast cancer. *Acta Oncologica* **31** (2), 195–200.

Walker, M. & Wannamethee, G., Whincup, P.H. & Shaper, A.G. (1995) Weight change and risk of heart attack in middle-aged British men. *International Journal of Epidemiology* **24**, 694–703.

Wassertheil-Smoller, S., Blaufox, D., Oberman, A., Langford, H., Davis, B. & Wylie-Rosett, J. (1992) The Trial of Antihypertensive Interventions and Management (TAIM) Study. Adequate weight loss, alone and combined with drug therapy in the treatment of mild hypertension. *Archives of Internal Medicine* **152**, 131–136.

Wilson, P., Mc Gee, D. & Kannel, W. (1981) Obesity, VLDL, and glucose intolerance over 14 years—The Framingham study. *American Journal of Epidemiology* **114**, 697–704.

Wing, R., Matthews, K., Kuller, L., Meilahn, E. & Plantinga, P. (1991) Waist to hip ratio in middle-aged women. Associations with behavioral and psychosocial factors and with changes in cardiovascular risk factors. *Arteriosclerosis and Thrombosis* **11**, 1250–1257.

Wisén, O. & Johansson, C. (1992) Gastrointestinal function in obesity: motility, secretion, and absorption following a liquid test meal. *Metabolism* **41**, 390–395.

Wisén, O. & Hellström, P.M. (1995) Gastrointestinal motility in obesity. *Journal of Internal Medicine* **237**, 411–418.

Wright, R., Krinsky, S., Fleeman, C., Trujillo, J. & Teague, E. (1983) Gastric emptying and obesity. *Gastroenterology* **84**, 747–751.

....

CHAPTER 11

Obesity, Infertility, Contraception and Pregnancy

STEPHEN ROBINSON AND STEVEN FRANKS

....

Introduction

In the U.K. obesity is highly prevalent in women of reproductive age. Morbid obesity (body mass index (BMI) > 30) has a prevalence of 5% at the age of 20 years increasing to 8% at the age of 44 years (Millar & Stephens 1987). In the North West Thames area, 27.0% of women were moderately obese (BMI 25–30) and 9.9% were very obese (BMI > 30). There are considerable differences between countries. In Western World the prevalence of obesity is increasing and women are having their children older when they are more likely to be obese. Fertility and the general health of women are compromised by obesity. Maternal obesity carries implications for the course of the pregnancy with increased maternal morbidity, fetal morbidity and mortality.

Obesity and fertility

Nutrition and ovarian function

Nutritional status has a considerable influence on female reproduction. In most mammals this is a means of ensuring that the pregnant mother and her newborn have access to enough food to maximize the chances of survival. Not only is being underweight associated with amenorrhoea as with anorexia nervosa through hypothalamic mechanisms, but obesity is also associated with anovulation. In obesity the mechanisms of ovulation are complex involving both peripheral and central pathways.

Body fat and body fat as a percentage of total weight are important to ovulation; however, polycystic ovaries have an effect additional to that of obesity. The term polycystic ovaries refers to the typical ovarian morphology — enlarged ovaries with increased stroma and increased follicle number. Polycystic ovary *syndrome* (PCOS) is conventionally defined as the combination of hyper-androgenism (hirsutism and acne) and anovulation (oligomenorrhoea, infertility and dysfunctional uterine bleeding) with polycystic ovaries on ultrasound scanning

(Franks, 1989). The aetiology of PCO and PCOS remains unclear and appears to be a genetic and environmental predisposition with environmental precipitants.

Obesity is a common feature, occurring in 35–40% of cases of PCOS (Goldzieher & Green 1962; Conway et al., 1989; Franks, 1989). It is not clear whether obesity acts to amplify the effects of PCOS or whether the mechanisms of the obesity and aetiology of PCOS are linked. Obese women presenting with PCOS were more likely to have menstrual disturbance and more likely to be hirsute than lean PCOS women. Total testosterone and luteinizing hormone (LH) are similar in the two groups (Kiddy et al., 1990), but sex hormone binding globulin (SHBG) concentrations were lower in obese women. SHBG levels were inversely correlated with BMI in PCOS women and controls, the values being lower in PCOS women. Insulin may be the factor which links SHBG and obesity, and hyperinsulinaemia may be related to the anovulation in these women. Indeed hyperinsulinaemia and insulin resistance may be the final common pathway by which anovulation occurs in women with obesity or in women with PCOS.

Hyperinsulinaemia and insulin insensitivity are well-recognized features of uncomplicated obesity (see Chapter 8), although it is not clear whether the insulin resistance precedes the obesity or is a complication of the obesity. Women with polycystic ovaries are hyperinsulinaemic (Burghen et al., 1980; Pasquali et al., 1982; Chang et al., 1983; Shoupe et al., 1983; Dunaif et al., 1987; Jialal et al., 1987; Mahabeer et al., 1989) but, unlike type II diabetes, this is associated with normal proportion of split pro-insulin and concentrations of specific insulin are significantly elevated (Conway et al., 1993; Robinson et al., 1994). Women with polycystic ovaries are more insulin resistant than weight-matched control women, the obese PCOS women having a degree of insulin insensitivity similar to that found in non-insulin-dependent diabetes mellitus (NIDDM) (Dunaif et al., 1989). The hyperinsulinaemia is associated with insulin resistance in terms of glucose and lipid metabolism (Robinson et al., 1996). Oligomenorrhoeic PCOS women but not PCOS women with regular menstrual cycles are more insulin resistant than weight-matched control women (Robinson et al., 1993b). Menstrual dysfunction does not appear to affect insulin sensitivity. Amenorrhoea due to suppression of the pituitary ovarian axis does not alter insulin levels or action (Geffner et al., 1986; Dunaif et al., 1990). It seems more likely that hyperinsulinaemia and/or insulin resistance contributes to menstrual disturbance. Weight loss following calorie restriction in obese PCOS subjects is associated with improvement in ovulatory function and a reduction in insulin concentrations (Kiddy et al., 1990). Reduced hyperinsulinaemia precedes improved ovulatory function (Kiddy et al., 1992).

The clinical relationship of insulin and ovarian action would seem to be in accord with in vitro experiments demonstrating that insulin augments LH-driven oestrogen secretion from granulosa cells (Willis *et al.*, 1996). How does hyperinsulinaemia have a biological effect in the face of insulin resistance? Insulin resistance is usually measured in terms of glucose effect. The possibility exists therefore that insulin action on ovarian function is not influenced by insulin insensitivity in other tissues.

Total energy expenditure can be considered to have three main contributors, resting energy expenditure (REE), exercise and thermogenic activities such as postprandial thermogenesis (PPT) (Chapter 6). PPT is believed to have an obligate and facultative component and the latter may be reduced in obese and pre-obese subjects, although there is considerable debate about this point. PPT and REE have been measured in women with PCOS and compared with weight-matched controls (Robinson *et al.*, 1992a). REE was similar in PCOS subjects and controls but PPT was reduced in women with PCOS. PPT correlated negatively with insulin sensitivity in the women with PCOS but not in the control group. This association has not been demonstrated by other workers (Segal & Dunaif, 1990). Reduced PPT may predispose to obesity although the obese women clearly had an increased energy intake compared to the lean women by virtue of increased lean body mass. Reduced PPT may be a marker for an associated reduction of satiety, acting at a hypothalamic level.

Pregnancy

Maternal body composition

The weight gain of the materno-fetal unit is a function of the accumulated energy stores and the energy required to maintain these stores (Hytten & Leitch, 1971). Protein and fat are accumulated through pregnancy, whilst the increased lean body mass demands an increase resting energy expenditure (Table 11.1). There is also an increase in PPT associated with the increased energy intake. In order to measure the fat stores and to facilitate assessment of basal metabolic rate (BMR) per unit lean body mass, body composition must been measured. This may be achieved by assessing body density, total body water, total body potassium or skinfold thickness. The measurement of body composition should allow for the increase in water content of lean tissue during pregnancy, from 72.5% at 10 weeks' to 75.0% at 40 weeks' gestation (van Raaij. *et al.*, 1988). Two whole-body methods combined give the best estimate of fat gained during pregnancy (Prentice *et al.*, 1996), with an average total fat gain of 3.0 kg by late pregnancy and a gain in maternal fat stores of 2.6 kg.

Table 11.1 also shows the total energy needs of pregnancy amounting to 360 MJ or about 1.2 MJ/day (Hytten & Chamberlain, 1980). This was later modified (Hytten, 1991) and gives values for a 2.7-kg increase in fat stores for a

Table 11.1 The theoretical energy cost of pregnancy. The four time periods are shown, with the cumulative total in the last column. The increased lean body mass of the mother and fetus increase resting energy expenditure. The additional energy intake also is associated with increased postprandial thermogenesis (assumed to be 10%). It is assumed that protein contains 23.5 kJ/g and fat 39 kJ/g energy. From Hytten and Leitch (1971) with permission.

	0–10 weeks (kJ/day) [g/day])	10–20 weeks (kJ/day) [g/day])	20–30 weeks (kJ/day) [g/day])	30–40 weeks (kJ/day) [g/day])	Cumulative total (kJ/day) [kg/pregnancy])
Protein	15 [0.64]	43 [1.8]	112 [4.8]	144 [6.1]	21 800 [0.93]
Fat	234 [5.9]	1065 [26.8]	872 [22.0]	132 [3.3]	157 900 [3.96]
Resting energy expenditure	188	416	622	954	150 000
Total net additional energy	437	1522	1606	1229	329 500
Total net + 10%	481	1677	1767	1352	362 400

pregnancy where the weight gain was 12.4 kg with a baby delivered of 3.3 kg. The extra requirements of energy through pregnancy are not equal to the increased energy intake of normal pregnancy and there is a large field of work on why this should be the case.

BMR or resting metabolic rate has been measured in several longitudinal studies. There were differences in the developed compared to the developing world; this review will concentrate on the 'developed' world. In a serial study using 24-hour calorimetry it was concluded there were highly characteristic changes with each subject and large intersubject differences (Prentice *et al.*, 1989). Lean women tended to have a decrease in BMR early in pregnancy before the rise beyond 20 weeks' gestation, whereas women with an increased BMI and increased fat mass showed an increased BMR from the beginning of gestation. The energy maintenance costs of pregnancy were strongly correlated with the degree of fat mass of the women before they became pregnant ($R = 0.72$) and the weight gained during pregnancy ($R = 0.79$) (Prentice *et al.*, 1996).

Diet-induced thermogenesis (DIT) and PPT have been studied in pregnancy. This is the increment in energy expenditure after consumption of a meal. Two studies have demonstrated no change in DIT during pregnancy (Nagy & King, 1984; Spaaij *et al.*, 1994). Two other studies have demonstrated decreased PPT during pregnancy (Illingworth *et al.*, 1987; Robinson *et al.*, 1993c). The latter study also demonstrated the reduction in PPT to correlate with the degree of insulin insensitivity during normal pregnancy. There has been no specific study of obesity and PPT in pregnancy, but obese women are more insulin resistant. The thermogenic response to weight- or non-weight-bearing exercise appears to change little during pregnancy.

Energy intake is difficult to establish, although there is little evidence for increased error in longitudinal studies through pregnancy. Prentice (Prentice *et al.*, 1996) concludes that there is an energy intake increment between 0.3 and 0.5 MJ/day, representing 84–140 MJ through pregnancy. The increased intake does not meet the increased energy needs.

Metabolism during normal and obese pregnancy

Normal pregnancy is characterized by significant changes to intermediary metabolism wherein insulin resistance appears to play a central role. Fasting blood glucose levels are decreased in normal pregnancy, reaching a nadir at 12 weeks' gestation and remaining at this level until term. The mechanism for this is uncertain. It does not appear to be related to fetal demand (the fetus weighs 16 g at 12 weeks) nor to changes in insulin concentration. Plasma glucose fluctuations around the fasting level are not great after food until the third trimester and cumulative glucose concentrations over 24 hours have been reported to be slightly increased (Cousins *et al.*, 1980) or decreased (Gillmer *et al.*, 1975) compared to non-pregnant levels.

After a glucose load peripheral glucose uptake is enhanced in insulin-sensitive tissues (largely skeletal muscle), whilst hepatic glucose production is suppressed. During pregnancy, compared to the same postpartum women, the peak glucose concentration is increased by approximately 0.5 mmol/l and delayed, from 30 to 60 minutes (Lind, 1975). No data are available for obese pregnant women. In the non-pregnant state, however, obesity is associated with similar post-glucose load plasma glucose concentrations to lean subjects, but insulin concentrations are increased.

Fasting plasma insulin levels increase through pregnancy but these changes do not occur at the same stage of pregnancy as the decrease in glucose concentrations. This would seem to preclude any cause and effect relationship between the two unless insulin sensitivity is also changing and the pancreatic β cell glucostat is set at a different level (Lind *et al.*, 1973; Kuhl & Holst, 1976). For a given glucose challenge the pregnant woman is stimulated to produce more insulin so that plasma insulin concentrations may be double that observed in the non-pregnant state (Lind, 1975; Freinkel, 1980). A cohort of obese women (>150% ideal body weight (IBW) roughly equivalent to a BMI of 33 kg/m^2) have been studied through pregnancy (Kalkhoff *et al.*, 1988), the same pattern of changes in plasma glucose and hyperinsulinaemia were seen when compared to a non-obese control group.

Obese premenopausal women are insulin resistant compared to non-obese control women (Ludvik *et al.*, 1995). Insulin action in normal pregnancy has been studied with the hyperinsulinaemic euglycaemic clamp technique. Ryan *et al.*(1985) demonstrated resistance to exogenous insulin in non-diabetic women during the third trimester. Glucose and insulin dynamics can be studied following glucose injection; the minimal model method uses the mathematical representation of glucose disappearance. Endogenous insulin sensitivity and β-cell responsiveness were studied in pregnancy using this method (Buchanan *et al.*, 1990). They found insulin sensitivity during the third trimester to be one-third that of non-pregnant controls. In addition the first-phase and second-phase insulin responses to glucose were three times greater than in non-pregnant women but there were no data to suggest whether this represented intact insulin or only immunoreactive insulin. Insulin resistance has been demonstrated in normal pregnancy as early as the second trimester compared to non-pregnant control women (Robinson *et al.*, 1993c). In this study the insulin resistance was correlated with the degree of obesity. Normal pregnant women are hyperinsulinaemic and insulin resistant state compared with non-pregnant women; the insulin resistance is found as early as the second trimester. This insulin resistance has far-reaching effects on intermediary metabolism. The insulin resistance is more marked in obese women before and during otherwise uncomplicated pregnancy but the effects of the increased insulin resistance are unknown.

Glucose turnover in pregnant women has been assessed with non-radioactive stable isotopes (Kalhan *et al.*, 1979). The isotopic enrichment of a glucose tracer primed infusion method allows the calculation of systemic glucose production or hepatic glucose output. Systemic glucose production (hepatic glucose output) in five control women was similar to five pregnant women when referenced to their non-pregnant weights. Using a similar method no difference in glucose turnover was demonstrated between nine pregnant women and five non-pregnant controls, when referenced to body-weight (pregnant weight), but absolute values were higher in the pregnant women (Cowett *et al.*, 1983). Fasting hepatic glucose production was similar in 10 pregnant women compared to control non-pregnant women and there was no association with obesity or insulin resistance (Robinson *et al.*, 1992b). Although one would expect hepatic glucose output to be similar in obese and lean pregnant women there are no data regarding this. Hepatic glucose output is not elevated in subjects with NIDDM until the fasting plasma glucose is greater than 8 mmol/L (DeFronzo, 1988).

Non-esterified fatty acid (NEFA) concentrations are variable in non-pregnant normal subjects and the length of fasting has a major influence. There is no agreement in the literature as to whether postabsorptive NEFA concentrations are altered in normal pregnancy. NEFA levels rise more quickly in pregnant women fasting from 12 to 18 hours compared to non-pregnant controls (Metzger *et al.*, 1982). Triglyceride (TG) levels fall in early pregnancy and then rise to term; by the third trimester of pregnancy there is a two- to threefold increase in plasma TG (Herrera *et al.*, 1987). There is less of an increase in cholesterol concentration. Very-low-density lipoprotein (VLDL), low-density lipoprotein (LDL) and high-density lipoprotein (HDL) all show increased concentrations in normal pregnancy. VLDL and intermediate-density lipoprotein (IDL) levels are increased but compositionally unchanged (Warth *et al.*, 1975). TG rises more than cholesterol and phospholipid in LDL and HDL. Cholesterol levels rise through pregnancy mainly as LDL-C. HDL-C levels peak in mid-pregnancy, then fall towards term. The hypertriglyceridaemia probably results from three factors: (i) increased adipose tissue lipolysis, related to insulin insensitivity enhances NEFA delivery to the liver and contributes to the increased VLDL (Kissebah *et al.*, 1982), (ii) maternal hyperphagia and unmodified lipid absorption from the gut lead to increased chylomicron concentrations; and (iii) reduced lipoprotein lipase activity, especially in adipose tissue, means there is reduced capacity for TG removal (Herrera *et al.*, 1987). Maternal hypertriglyceridaemia is present in the second and third trimester of normal pregnancy, and is associated with the degree of maternal insulin resistance

(Robinson *et al.*, 1993a). Maternal BMI correlates with TG concentrations ($r = 0.58$, $P < 0.01$) in the second trimester but this association is lost in the third trimester.

Obese pregnant women had increased concentrations of branched-chain amino acids compared to lean pregnant control women (Felig *et al.*, 1969). During normal pregnancy total plasma amino acid concentrations decrease compared to non-pregnant women (Kalkhoff *et al.*, 1988). During the second trimester of non-diabetic pregnancy total amino acid concentrations were reduced in obese women compared to the lean group. There was no significant difference in total amino acid concentrations during the third trimester, but histidine concentrations were increased in the obese women.

Although there are several studies of protein turnover in normal pregnancy using stable non-radioactive tracers, there are no specific studies of the effects of obesity (de Benoist *et al.*, 1985; Fitch & King, 1987; Denne *et al.*, 1991; Thompson & Halliday, 1992). One would predict that the insulin resistance of normal pregnancy would be associated with increased amino acid turnover and this would be further elevated in insulin-resistant obese women. Other factors such as substrate concentrations and sex steroid alterations may play a role in pregnancy.

Fetal growth

Glucose has been believed to be the main fuel for fetal growth (Ginsberg & Cramp, 1977). Although other fuels are now believed to be important, the relative caloric load to the fetus from glucose, fat and protein is unknown (Sheath *et al.*, 1972; Kalkhoff *et al.*, 1988; Knopp *et al.*, 1992). Increased serum TG concentrations in the mother were thought to be an indicator of the increased importance of maternal lipid oxidation, sparing carbohydrate and protein for fetal use (Warth *et al.*, 1975). Furthermore, the propensity for ketosis is more rapid and profound in the postabsorptive state than in non-pregnant women and the term 'accelerated starvation' was coined to described these changes (Metzger & Frienkel, 1987). It was suggested that the increased ketone body and free fatty acid concentrations in the postabsorptive state represent increased oxidation by the mother of these metabolites and that this more rapid adjustment to fat catabolism allows glucose to be spared for transplacental transfer. The other side of this process was said to be 'facilitated anabolism'. The increased postprandial rise in glucose and other fetal fuels was hypothesized to be a mechanism for promoting fetal growth.

In the placenta of the guinea pig, which is haemochorial and therefore similar to the human, hydrolysis of maternal TG in VLDL liberates NEFA in the placental bed and is potentially a major fetal fuel (Thomas, 1987). In support of this hypothesis is the observation that maternal TG concentrations measured in the second trimester correlate better with fetal birth-weight than does maternal glucose (Knopp *et al.*, 1992; Nolan *et al.*, 1995).

Fetal macrosomia has been defined by a variety of methods, the relative importance of each may depend on the outcome of interest. For example a fetal weight greater than 4 kg will have 'mechanical' implications for safe delivery and beyond. Centile for gestational age birth-weight, or a more sophisticated birth-weight ratio based on gestation, maternal weight, maternal height, parity and ethnic group has more predictive power (Sanderson *et al.*, 1994). Macrosomia could also be defined in terms of relative obesity (for example skinfold thickness or magnetic resonance imaging of abdominal fat) and one could hypothesize the long-term outcome for the infant is more dependant on relative obesity.

The main risk factors for fetal macrosomia are maternal diabetes and maternal obesity. The original Pederson hypothesis (Pederson *et al.*, 1954) suggested that the increased glucose concentrations in the diabetic mother led to fetal hyperglycaemia. The fetal pancreas, able to respond to hyperglycaemia from the 20th week of gestation, produced fetal hyperinsulinaemia. The fetus then used the glucose to increase fat stores. The hyperinsulinaemia was to an

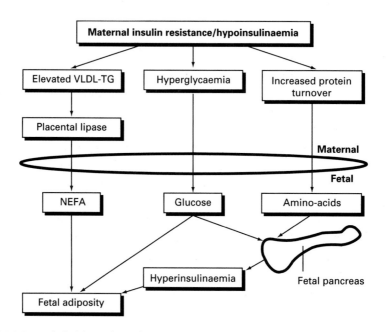

Fig. 11.1 Extended Pedersen hypothesis to explain macrosomia in the normoglycaemic mother with a macrosomic fetus. Increased proteolysis with amino acid delivery to the fetus, in addition to mild increase in glucose delivery to the fetus, stimulates fetal hyperinsulinaemia. The glucose and NEFA are stored in the fetus under the control of fetal hyperinsulinaemia.

extent autonomous and this led to neonatal hypoglycaemia. However, fetal macrosomia is more common in the obese non-diabetic mother compared to the lean mother with gestational diabetes (Maresh *et al.*, 1989). Maternal obesity may have a role in fetal macrosomia, but by what mechanism if the mother's glucose concentrations are normal? Maternal obesity is associated with fetal hyperinsulinaemia even in the absence of maternal diabetes (Hoegsburg *et al.*, 1993). Fetal macrosomia may involve glucose protein and lipid metabolism (Fig. 11.1). Maternal insulin resistance would be associated with elevated VLDL-TG and increased energy delivery to the fetus. The insulin resistance could also lead to increased protein turnover, which would lead to fetal hyperinsulinaemia.

The effect of obesity on pregnancy

Carbohydrate metabolism

Maternal diabetes is associated with an increased incidence of fetal macrosomia, polycythaemia, intra-uterine death, birth trauma and neonatal hypoglycaemia. The mothers have an increased risk of birth trauma due to the macrosomic infant and most importantly have an increased chance of developing NIDDM in later life. In the medium term the infant may have developmental delay (Rizzo *et al.*, 1991). In the long term there may be metabolic complications for the offspring of the diabetic mother as adults in terms of obesity or early diabetes (Pettitt *et al.*, 1983, 1988).

Gestational diabetes mellitus (GDM) can be defined as diabetes first discovered during pregnancy. It usually remits after pregnancy but this is not required to make the diagnosis. The increased incidence of GDM in obese pregnant women has been ascribed to increased insulin resistance combined with an insulin secretory deficit (Table 11.2). Increasing BMI is associated with insulin insensitivity in normal pregnancy (BMI vs insulin sensitivity second trimester $r = 0.71$), (Robinson *et al.*, 1993). As there is considerable evidence that GDM precedes NIDDM (O'Sullivan, 1984; Metzger *et al.*, 1985; Stowers *et al.*, 1985; Dornhorst *et al.*, 1990) these women probably represent a subset of insulin-resistant women who have inadequate insulin secretion in the face of insulin resistance. That being the case, the increased prevalence of obesity in women with GDM may represent a combined predisposition to both obesity and NIDDM rather than obesity *per se* increasing the risk of NIDDM.

The prevalence of diabetes in pregnancy, mostly GDM, with maternal obesity was found to be 10.6% compared to 2.8% in lean women (Edwards *et al.*, 1978). When obesity is defined as 135% or more of IBW the relative risk for GDM is 6.57 (Abrams & Parker, 1988).

Table 11.2 Prevalence of some antepartum complications in under- and overweight pregnant women (all $P < 0.05$). From Garbaciak *et al.* (1985).

	Underweight (<85% IBW)	Normal (85–120% IBW)	Obese (120–150% IBW)	Severe obesity (>150% IBW)
n	607	7170	1445	444
Hypertensive(%)	0.9	1.9	7.0	17.2
PET(%)	3.8	4.4	6.6	6.9
Diabetes(%)	1.2	1.4	3.9	10.4
Anaemia(%)	5.4	4.3	3.2	2.4
Thrombo-phlebitis(%)	0.3	0.1	0.4	0.4
UTI(%)	5.9	5.8	8.0	9.4

PET, pre-eclampsia or eclampsia; UTI, urinary tract infection.

The logical treatment of GDM complicating maternal obesity is not clear, not least because of the differing diagnostic criteria for diabetes in pregnancy. Maternal obesity and excessive weight gain in pregnancy are associated with fetal macrosomia and treatment should be directed to avoid this (Boyd *et al.*, 1983), although the long-term outcome of such treatment is unknown. The U.S. Institute of Sciences made recommendations for weight gain in pregnancy including obese women (BMI > 26–29) to gain 7.0–11.5 kg during pregnancy although that would not be our practice and many U.K. units observe good outcome with mothers gaining less than 6.8 kg (Pimblett, 1996).

Total energy intake is crucial in pregnancy complicated by diabetes or obesity. Women with GDM are often treated with energy restriction. In a trial of hypocaloric diets for women with GDM, women gained a mean of 2 kg from 28 weeks' gestation (Dornhorst *et al.*, 1991). The incidence of macrosomia was reduced to that of the general population whilst no infant was small for gestational age. Maternal ketosis should be avoided as this may be detrimental to the fetus (Rizzo *et al.*, 1991). When the maternal energy intake was restricted to 5.02 MJ/day, improved glycaemic control was accompanied by increased maternal ketonaemia (Magee *et al.*, 1990). When energy is restricted to 6.92 MJ/day there was improved glycaemic control and reduced TG levels more than women treated with insulin without increased maternal ketonaemia (Knopp *et al.*, 1991). Excercise is a useful adjunct to dietary management of GDM and has been shown to improve glycaemic control (Jovanovic-Peterson & Peterson, 1991). Women with pre-existing insulin-dependent diabetes or NIDDM (most of whom will need insulin before and during the pregnancy) will have dietary prescriptions on the basis of their weight. Hypoglycaemia can be a problem, especially in the first trimester, and the dietary prescription should take this into account.

Generally a diet high in complex carbohydrate is recommended, around 50% of the total energy intake. This should also be combined with an effort to reduce refined carbohydrate although moderate amounts of sucrose are not harmful. Soluble fibre reduces glucose and TG although this has not specifically tested in obese women with diabetes. Most women in the U.K. consume more than the recommended 51 g of protein a day prior to pregnancy. There is a theoretical concern that excessive protein restriction could lead to an increased likelihood of adult diabetes by programming insulin secretion in the infant (Hales & Barker, 1992). Protein restriction should therefore be avoided.

Hypertensive disorders of pregnancy

The relationship between essential hypertension and obesity in non-pregnant subjects is well recognized (Kannel *et al.*, 1967). Hypertension during pregnancy may be pre-existing or pregnancy associated, the two conditions are not entirely separate and the studies do not always differentiate them. The prevalence of hypertension in severely obese pregnant women varies between 5 and 66% (Edwards *et al.*, 1978; Gross *et al.*, 1980; Garbaciak *et al.*, 1985; Abrams & Parker, 1988). The relative risk of hypertension (compared to a lean control group) is 4.49 when obesity is defined as >135% IBW (Abrams & Parker, 1988), and 8.70 (Garbaciak *et al.*, 1985) and 2.42 (Edwards *et al.*, 1978) when obesity is defined as >150% IBW (Table 11.2).

The prevalence of pregnancy-associated hypertension was 9.1% (Garbaciak *et al.*, 1985), 6.9% (Abrams & Parker, 1988) and 14.0% (Edwards *et al.*, 1978). The relative risk of pregnancy-induced hypertension is 1.9 for the woman with an IBW >135% (Abrams & Parker, 1988). There are no data on energy restriction in the management of hypertension during pregnancy in obese women.

Infections including urinary tract infections

Urinary tract infections (UTI) include urethritis, cystitis and pyelonephritis. The relative risk of UTI in mild obesity is 1.42 (Abrams & Parker, 1988). Some (Garbaciak *et al.*, 1985; Abrams & Parker, 1988) but not all (Edwards *et al.*, 1978) workers have found a further increase in the incidence of UTI in the severely obese during pregnancy.

Anaemia

Anaemia is less common in obese non-pregnant women compared to lean women (Rimm *et al.*, 1975). This may be related to oligomenorrhoea and therefore reduced menstrual blood loss prior to conception. Obese pregnant women also have a reduced prevalence of anaemia; it is not clear whether this relates to obese women starting pregnancy with more iron stores than lean women (Edwards *et al.*, 1978; Garbaciak *et al.*, 1985; Abrams & Parker, 1988). The relative risk for anaemia in severely obese pregnant women is between 0.56 and 0.72.

Weight gain of pregnancy

Normal pregnant women gain between 10 and 12 kg during their pregnancy. Women with severe obesity (>150% ideal pre-pregnancy weight) had a higher prevalence of low weight gain (5.5 kg) during pregnancy (31.2%) compared to a non-obese control group (4.3%) (Edwards *et al.*, 1978). Women weighing over 90 kg were more likely to have low weight gain compared to those mothers weighing less than 90 kg (Gross *et al.*, 1980). However, it is not clear whether this low weight gain can be labelled inadequate. Whilst many would treat maternal obesity with GDM by energy restriction, formal randomized controlled trials of maternal calorie restriction on maternal and fetal outcome are required. Certainly the meals should be spread through the day to avoid ketosis.

Thromboembolic disease

Thromboembolic disease is rare in pregnancy, therefore large studies are required to have the power necessary to demonstrate any increase in prevalence. In a study of the North-West Thames Area, the prevalence of thromboembolism was 0.05% in normal weight population compared to 0.06% in the moderately obese but 0.12% in the very obese group (odds ratio 1.60, 1.01–2.56, $P < 0.001$) with smoking included in the regression model (Sebire, 1996).

Delivery

Caesarian section is more commonly performed in the obese pregnant woman. In three American studies the nonobese Caesarian section rate was between 8.6 and 13.3% (Edwards *et al.*, 1978; Garbaciak *et al.*, 1985; Abrams & Parker, 1988). In the moderately obese the Caesarian section rate was 12.4–16.9% rising to 11.0–21.5% in the very obese groups. The reasons for the increased Caesarian section rate are difficult to evaluate in these epidemiological studies. Infection is more likely to complicate emergency (as opposed to elective) Caesarian section in obese women.

Effect of obesity on the fetus

Macrosomia

The definition and mechanisms of fetal macrosomia are discussed above. When macrosomia is defined in terms of birth-weight greater than 4000 g the prevalence is 1.3–1.7% and mothers are more likely to be obese. Mothers are also more likely to be older, have greater parity, have a greater prevalence of maternal diabetes and more likely to be postmature (>42 weeks' gestation) (Spellacy et al., 1985).

The association of maternal obesity and fetal macrosomia is independent of maternal diabetes mellitus but the effects are additive. Indeed the risk of fetal macrosomia is greater for the infant of the non-diabetic obese mother compared to the infant of a lean mother with GDM.

There is a relationship between maternal weight gain and birth weight for mothers who are underweight, normal weight and mildly obese (Abrams & Laros, 1986). However, very obese mothers (greater than 135% IBW) demonstrate no correlation between weight gain during pregnancy and fetal weight.

Clinical methods or special investigations poorly predict fetal macrosomia. Ultrasound prediction of birth weight is particularly poor for macrosomic infants (Grandjean et al., 1980). Macrosomia is a major cause of obstructed labour (Boyd et al., 1983). There is a higher rate of induction of labour and a higher rate of operative delivery. A macrosomic infant is more likely to have low apgar scores at 1 and 5 minutes. Other complications include birth asphyxia, fractured clavicle and brachial cord injuries.

Perinatal mortality

Perinatal mortality is defined as the number of stillbirths and deaths within the first week of life, per 1000 births. Although all studies using a non-obese control group have demonstrated an increased perinatal mortality rate, this was only significant in the larger studies (Table 11.3). The overall perinatal mortality was increased and related to the degree of obesity. The presence of other antenatal complications was additive to the perinatal mortality.

In a study of preterm delivery survival in 771 infants, the number of deaths from 48 hours to 18 months was increased in obese mothers. Maternal obesity and gestational age at delivery were associated with an increased death rate.

Long-term consequences for the fetus of maternal obesity

Both environmental and genetic factors are important in the development of

Table 11.3 Perinatal outcome in the three largest studies of maternal obesity. These studies used percentage IBW to define obesity.

n		Non-obese	Moderate obesity	Very obese	Authors
208	Percentage	1.9		2.4	Edwards *et al.* (1978)
16858	No antenatal complications	0.5	0.93	1.16	Garbaciak *et al.*
	With antental complications	1.19	3.15	3.76*	(1985)
	Perinatal mortality	0.67	1.66	2.25*	
4100	Percentage	1.8	1.7	2.3	Abrams & Parker (1987)

* Significant across the three groups.

obesity. The intra-uterine environment may be an important non-genetic factor in the development of adult obesity. Low birth-weight is associated with increased prevalence of several adult conditions, including diabetes, although the relative contribution of maternal energy intake and genetic factors to birth-weight are not clear (Hales & Barker, 1992). Birth-weight is a crude measure of the effect of the intra-uterine environment of metabolic programming and the relative increase in fat mass with low lean body mass of the macrosomic infant may turn out to be as important.

The doubly labelled water method has been used to examine energy expenditure in infants, lean and obese mothers (Roberts *et al.*, 1988). Infants who became obese after 6 months of age were studied; energy intake was said to be similar in both groups. Obese infants had a lower total daily energy expenditure than lean infants. These data would suggest that low energy expenditure rather than increased energy intake was responsible for the obesity in this group.

Maternal diabetes during pregnancy is associated with an increase in the delivery of calories to the fetus. The offspring are more likely to be obese as children, adolescents and as young adults (Pettitt *et al.*, 1983). Diabetes during pregnancy in Pima Indian women results in a higher prevalence of NIDDM (45%) in the offspring at the age 20–24 years than in those of non-diabetic women (1.4%) or prediabetic women (8.6%) (Pettitt *et al.*, 1988). It is not possible to attribute the increased risk to maternal diabetes or the resulting fetal macrosomia.

The effect of the pregnancy on maternal obesity

Many women attribute long-term weight gain to a previous pregnancy. In a study of 7000 women who had two pregnancies within 6 years, a weight gain of 9 kg in the first pregnancy had a significant effect on weight prior to the second pregnancy. Therefore weight gain in excess of 9 kg during pregnancy is more likely to be retained when not pregnant (Greene et al., 1988). A weight gain of 10 kg is statistically associated with best fetal outcome, but those data are based on the whole population, lean and obese. The ideal weight gain for the mother may not be the same as the ideal weight gain for the fetus.

Contraception

Pregnancy carries higher risks for the obese mother compared to the lean mother, and it would therefore be prudent for a mother to conceive at a time when these risks can be minimized and, if possible, not conceive when overweight. Ten women per 100 000 die from complications of pregnancy, whereas 1.3 women non-smokers per 100 000 may die of circulatory disease taking combined oral contraception (Guillebaud, 1995). It should be emphasized that any risk to the woman from the side-effects of contraceptive methods are minimal compared to her, and her infants', risk from pregnancy.

Combined (oestrogen and progestagen-containing) oral contraceptives increase the blood pressure (within the normotensive range) and increase venous thromboembolic disease risk. These risks are greater in obesity. However, the same precautions regarding advice for contraceptive measures should be applied to obese women as non-obese women. Therefore previous venous thromboembolic disease, present hypertension and present smoking should be taken into account when prescribing oestrogen-containing contraception. (Vessey et al., 1977). Although there are large epidemiological studies regarding the use of combined oral contraception and their relative effects of obesity, randomized studies for obese women are lacking. A woman without previous thromboembolic disease, hypertension or smoking can use standard combined oral contraception (containing ethynyloestradiol 30 or 35 mg). Desogestrel and gestodene are associated with around a twofold increase in risk of thromboembolic disease compared to those containing the other progestagens. It is advised that obese women (BMI > 30 kg/m^2) would not use combined oral contraception containing gestodene or desogestrel, but can use levonorgestrel, norethisterone or ethynodiol. Using the latter three, the excess risk of thromboembolic disease is about 5–10 cases per 100 000 women per annum.

Depoprovera is equally effective in obese and non-obese women. In the overall population the progestagen-only pill has a higher failure rate than the combined oral contraceptive: 3.1 compared to 0.38 user failure rates per 100 woman years (Vessey et al., 1982). A non-significant increase in failure rate was found in overweight users of the progestagen-only pill compared to non-obese. If no other form of contraception is suitable it is recommended that overweight women take two progestagen-only pills per day especially in the under-30-year-old group (Guillebaud, 1995). Both progestagen ring and Norplant have increased failure rate in obese compared to lean women. Therefore one can appreciate that the decreased effectiveness of progestagen-only contraception in obese women is dependent on the general failure rate of the method of delivery.

The risk of deep vein thrombosis is high in obese subjects having surgery or following leg immobilization. Contraception should be stopped prior to surgery and heparin prophyalaxis considered.

Summary

Obesity is highly prevalent in women of reproductive age and becoming more so. Female nutrition and obesity are associated with considerable changes to the reproductive system. The mechanisms for these alterations are unknown, but are associated with increased insulin resistance. This is best described for women with PCOS. Treatment of the obesity with diet is associated with increased fertility in obese women with PCOS.

Normal pregnancy is associated with maternal weight gain. There is considerable discussion regarding any energy-saving mechanisms in normal pregnancy. It is unclear whether these are exacerbated with maternal obesity. Maternal obesity is associated with increased maternal and fetal complications and an adverse fetal outcome. There have been no randomized controlled studies of the use of dieting in treating maternal obesity.

Combined oral contraceptives increase blood pressure and increase venous thromboembolic disease risk. Both these risks are increased with female obesity. However, smoking is a far greater risk and contraceptive advice for obese women is similar to that of non-obese women.

References

Abrams, B.F. & Laros, R.K. (1986) Prepregnancy weight, weight gain, and birth weight. *American Journal of Obstetrics and Gynecology* **154**, 503–509.

Abrams, B. & Parker, J. (1988) Overweight and pregnancy complications. *International Journal of Obesity* **12**, 293–303.

Boyd, M.E., Usher, R.H. & McLean, F.H. (1983). Fetal macrosomia: prediction, risks, proposed management. *Obstetrics and Gynecology* **61**, 715–722.

Buchanan, T.A., Metzger, B.E., Frienkel, N. & Bergman, R.N. (1990) Insulin sensitivity and B-cell responsiveness to glucose during late pregnancy in lean and moderately obese women with normal glucose tolerance or mild gestational diabetes. *American Journal of Obstetrics and Gynecology* **162**, 1008–1014.

Burghen, G.A., Givens, J.R. & Kitabchi, A.E. (1980) Correlation of hyperandrogenism with hyperinsulinism in polycystic ovarian disease. *Journal of Clinical Endocrinology and Metabolism* **50**, 113–116.

Chang, R.J., Nakamura, R.M., Judd, H.L. & Kaplan, S.L. (1983) Insulin resistance in nonobese patients with polycystic ovarian disease. *Journal of Clinical Endocrinology and Metabolism* **57**, 356–359.

Conway, G.S., Honour, J.W. & Jacobs, H.S. (1989) Heterogeneity of the polycystic ovary syndrome: clinical, endocrine and ultrasound features in 556 patients. *Clinical Endocrinology* **32**, 213–220.

Conway, G.S., Clark, P.M.S. & Wong, D. (1993) Hyperinsulinaemia in the polycystic ovary syndrome confirmed with a specific immunoradiometric assay for insulin. *Clinical Endocrinology* **38**, 219–222.

Cousins, L., Rigg, L., Hollingsworth, D., Brink, G., Aurand, J. & Yen, S.S.C. (1980) The 24-hour excursion and diurnal rhythm of glucose, insulin, and C-peptide in normal pregnancy. *American Journal of Obstetrics and Gynecology* **136**, 483–488.

Cowett, R.M., Susa, J.B., Kahn, C.B., Gilleti, B., Oh, W. & Schwartz, R. (1983) Glucose kinetics in nondiabetic and diabetic women during the third trimester of pregnancy. *American Journal of Obstetrics and Gynecology* **146**, 773–780.

de Benoist, B., Jackson, A.A., Hall, S.E. & Persaud, C. (1985) Whole-body protein turnover in Jamaican women during normal pregnancy. *Human Nutrition: Clinical Nutrition* **39C**, 167–179.

DeFronzo, R. (1988) The triumvirate, B cell, muscle and liver: A collusion responsible for NIDDM. *Diabetes* **37**, 667–875.

Denne, S.C., Pate, D. & Kalhan, S.C. (1991) Leucine kinetics and fuel utilisation during a brief fast in human pregnancy. *Metabolism* **40**, 1249–1256.

Dornhorst, A., Bailey, P.C., Anyaoku, V., Elkeles, R.S., Johnston, D.G. & Beard, R.W. (1990) Abnormalities of glucose tolerance following gestational diabetes. *Quarterly Journal of Medicine* **77**, 1219–1228.

Dornhorst, A., Nicholls, J.S., Probst, F. *et al.* (1991) Calorie restriction for treatment of gestational diabetes. *Diabetes* **40** (suppl. 2), 161–164.

Dunaif, A., Graf, M., Mandeli, J., Laumas, V. & Dobrjansky, A. (1987) Characterisation of groups of hyperandrogenic women with acanthosis nigricans, impaired glucose tolerance, and/or hyperinsulinaemia. *Journal of Clinical Endocrinology and Metabolism* **65**, 449–507.

Dunaif, A., Segal, K.R., Futterweit, W. & Dobrjansky, A. (1989) Profound peripheral insulin resistance, independent of obesity, in polycystic ovary syndrome. *Diabetes* **38**, 1165–1174.

Dunaif, A., Green, G., Futterweit, W. & Dobrjansky, A. (1990) Suppression of hyperandrogenism does not improve peripheral or hepatic insulin resistance in the polycystic ovary syndrome. *Journal of Clinical Endocrinology and Metabolism* **70**, 699–704.

Edwards, L.E., Dickes, W.F., Alton, I.R. & Hakanson, E.Y. (1978) Pregnancy in the massively obese: Course, outcome and obesity prognosis of the infant. *American Journal of Obstetrics and Gynecology* **131**, 479–483.

Felig, P., Marliss, E. & Cahill, G.F. (1969) Plasma amino acid levels and insulin secretion in obesity. *New England Journal of Medicine* **281**, 811–816.

Fitch, W. & King, J.C. (1987) Protein turnover and 3-methylhistidine excretion in non-pregnant, pregnant and gestational diabetic women. *Human Nutrition: Clinical Nutrition* **41C**, 327–339.

Franks, S. (1989) Polycystic ovary syndrome: a changing perspective. *Clinical Endocrinology* **31**, 87–120.

Freinkel, N. (1980) Of pregnancy and progeny. *Diabetes* **29**, 1023–1035.

Garbaciak, J.A., Richter, M., Miller, S. & Barton, J.J. (1985) Maternal weight and pregnancy complications. *American Journal of Obstetrics and Gynecology* **152**, 238–245.

Geffner, M.E., Kaplan, S.A., Bersch, N., Golde, D.W., Landaw, E.M. & Chang, R.J. (1986) Persistence of insulin resistance in polycystic ovary disease after inhibition of ovarian steroid secretion. *Fertility and Sterility* **45**, 327–333.

Gillmer, D.G., Beard, R.W., Brooke, F.M. & Oakley, N.W. (1975) Carbohydrate metabolism in pregnancy. Part 1—Diurnal plasma glucose profile in normal and diabetic women. *British Medical Journal* **3**, 399–404.

Ginsberg, J. & Cramp, D.G. (1977) Carbohydrate metabolism. In: Phillip, E.E., Barnes, J. & Newton, M. (eds) *Scientific Foundations of Obstetrics and Gynaecology*, pp. 467–479. London: Heinemann.

Goldzieher, J.W. & Green, J.A. (1962) The polycystic ovary. 1. Clinical and histological features. *Journal of Clinical Endocrinology and Metabolism* **22**, 325–338.

Grandjean, H., Sarramon, M.-F., de Mouzon, J., Reme, J.-M. & Pontonnier, G. (1980) Detection of gestational diabetes by means of ultrasonic diagnosis of excessive fetal growth. *American Journal of Obstetrics and Gynecology* **138**, 790–792.

Greene, G.W., Smiciklas-Wright, H., Scholl, T.O. & Karp, R.J. (1988) Postpartum weight change: How much of the weight gained in pregnancy will be lost after delivery? *Obstetrics and Gynecology* **71**, 701–707.

Gross, T., Sokol, R.J. & King, K.C. (1980) Obesity in pregnancy: Risks and outcome. *Obstetrics and Gynecology* **56**, 446–450.

Guillebaud, J. (1995). *Contraception*. Edinburgh: Churchill Livingstone.

Hales, C.N. & Barker, D.J.P. (1992) Type 2 (non-insulin dependent) diabetes mellitus: the thrifty phenotype. *Diabetologia* **35**, 595–601.

Herrera, E., Gomez-Coronado, D. & Lasuncion, M.A. (1987) Lipid metabolism in pregnancy. *Biology of the Neonate* **51**, 70–77.

Hoegsburg, B., Gruppuso, P.A. & Coustan, D.R. (1993) Hyperinsulinaemia in macrosomic infants of non-diabetic mothers. *Diabetes Care* **16**, 32–36.

Hytten, F.E. (1991). Weight gain in pregnancy. In: Hytten, F.E. & Chamberlain, G. (eds) *Clinical Physiology in Obstetrics*, pp. 173–203. Oxford: Blackwell Scientific Publications.

Hytten, F.E. & Leitch, I. (1971) *The Physiology of Human Pregnancy*. Oxford: Blackwell Scientific Publications.

Hytten, F.E. & Chamberlain, G. (1980) *Clinical Physiology in Obstetrics*. Oxford: Blackwell Scientific Publications.

Illingworth, P.J., Jung, R.T., Howie, P.W. & Isles, T.E. (1987) Reduction in postprandial energy expenditure during pregnancy. *British Medical Journal* **294**, 1573–1576.

Jialal, I., Naiker, P., Reddi, K., Moodley, J. & Joubert, S.M. (1987) Evidence for insulin resistance in nonobese patients with polycystic ovarian disease. *Journal of Clinical Endocrinology and Metabolism* **64**, 1066–1069.

Jovanovic-Peterson, L. & Peterson, C.M. (1991) Is exercise safe or useful for gestational diabetic women? *Diabetes* **20**, 179–181.

Kalhan, S.C., D'Angelo, L.J., Savin, S.M. & Adam, P.A.J. (1979) Glucose production in pregnant women at term gestation. *The Journal of Clinical Investigation* **63**, 388–394.

Kalkhoff, R.K., Kandaraki, E., Morrow, P.G., Mitchell, T.H., Kelber, S. & Borkowf, H.I. (1988) Relationship between neonatal birth weight and maternal plasma amino acid profiles in lean and obese nondiabetic women and in type 1 diabetic pregnant women. *Metabolism* **37**, 234–239.

Kannel, W.B., Brand, N., Skinner, J.J.J., Dawber, T.R. & McNamara, P.M. (1967) The relation of adiposity to blood pressure and development of hypertension. The Framingham Study. *Annals of Internal Medicine* **67**, 48–59.

Kiddy, D., Hamilton-Fairley, D., Bush, A. *et al.* (1990) Improvement in menstrual function and fertility in obese women with polycystic ovary syndrome treated with a 1000 calorie diet. *Clinical Endocrinology* **124** (suppl.), 253.

Kiddy, S.D., Sharp, P.S., White, D.M. *et al.* (1990) Differences in clinical and endocrine features between obese and non-obese subjects with polycystic ovary syndrome: an analysis of 263 consecutive cases. *Clinical Endocrinology* **32**, 213–220.

Kiddy, D.S., Hamilton-Fairley, D., Seppala, M., Koistinen, R., James, V.H.T. & Reed, M.J. (1989) Diet induced changes in sex hormone-binding globulin and free testosterone in women with normal or polycystic ovaries: correlation with insulin and insulin-like growth factor 1. *Clinical Endocrinology* **31**, 757–763.

Kissebah, A.H., Vydelingum, N., Murray, R. *et al.* (1982) Relation of body fat distribution to metabolic complications of obesity. *Journal of Clinical Endocrinology and Metabolism* **54**, 254–260.

Knopp, R.H., Magee, M.S., Raisys, V., Benedetti, T. & Bonet, B. (1991) Hypocaloric diets and ketogenesis in the management of obese gestational diabetic women. *Journal of American College of Nutrition* **10**, 649–667.

Knopp, R.H., Magee, M.S., Walden, C.E., Bonet, B. & Benedetti, T.J. (1992) Prediction of infant birth weight by GDM screening tests. *Diabetes Care* **15**, 1605–1613.

Kuhl, C. & Holst, J.J. (1976) Plasma glucoagon and the insulin: glucagon ratio in gestational diabetes. *Diabetes* **25**, 16–23.

Lind, T. (1975) Changes in carbohydrate metabolism during pregnancy. *Clinical Obstetrics and Gynecology* **395**, 1023–1028.

Lind, T., Billewicz, W.Z. & Brown, G. (1973) A serial study of changes occurring in the oral glucose tolerance test in pregnancy. *Journal of Obstetrics and Gynaecology of the British Commonwealth* **80**, 1033–1039.

Ludvik, B., Nolan, J.J., Baloga, J., Sacks, D. & Olefsky, J. (1995) Effect of obesity on insulin resistance in normal subjects and patients with NIDDM. *Diabetes* **44**, 1121–1125.

Magee, M.S., Knopp, R.H. & Benedetti, T.J. (1990) Metabolic effects of 1200-kcal diet in obese pregnant women with gestational diabetes. *Diabetes* **39**, 234–240.

Mahabeer, S., Jialal, I., Norman, R.J., Naidoo, C., Reddi, K. & Joubert, S.M. (1989) Insulin and C-peptide secretion in non-obese patients with polycystic ovarian disease. *Hormone and Metabolic Research* **21**, 502–506.

Maresh, M., Beard, R.W., Bray, C.S., Elkeles, R.S. & Wadsworth, J. (1989) Factors predisposing to and outcome of gestational diabetes. *Obstetrics and Gynaecology* **74**, 342–346.

Metzger, B.E., Bybee, D.E., Frienkel, N., Phelps, R.L., Radvany, R.M. & Vaisrub, N. (1985) Gestational diabetes mellitus; correlations between the phenotypic and genotypic characteristics of the mother and abnormal glucose tolerance during the first year postpartum. *Diabetes* **34** (suppl. 2), 111–115.

Metzger, B.E., Ravinikar, V., Vileisis, R.A. & Freinkel, N. (1982) 'Accelerated starvation' and the skipped breakfast in late normal pregnancy. *Lancet* **I**, 588–592.

Metzger, B.E. & Frienkel, N. (1987) Accelerated starvation in pregnancy: Implications for dietary treatment of obesity and gestational diabetes mellitus. *Biology of the Neonate* **51**, 78–85.

Millar, W.J. & Stephens, T. (1987) The prevalence of overweight and obesity in Britain, Canada, and United States. *American Journal of Public Health* **77**, 38–41.

Nagy, L.E. & King, J.C. (1984) Postprandial energy expenditure and respiratory quotient during early and late pregnancy. *American Journal of Clinical Nutrition* **40**, 1258–1263.

Nolan, C.J., Riley, S.F., Sheedy, M.T., Walstab, J.E. & Beischer, N.A. (1995) Maternal serum triglyceride, glucose tolerance, and neonatal birthweight ratio in pregnancy. *Diabetes Care* **18**, 1551–1556.

O'Sullivan, J.B. (1984) Subsequent morbidity among gestational diabetic women. In: Sutherland, H.W. & Stowers, J.M. (eds) *Carbohydrate Metabolism in Pregnancy and the Newborn*, pp. 174–180. Edingburgh: Churchill Livingstone.

Pasquali, R., Venturoli, S., Paradis, R., Capelli, M., Parenti, M. & Melchionda, N. (1982) Insulin and C-peptide levels in obese patients with polycystic ovaries. *Hormone and Metabolic Research* **154**, 284–287.

Pederson, J., Bojsen-Moller, B. & Poulsen, H. (1954) Blood sugar in newborn infants of diabetic infants of diabetic mothers. *Acta Endocrinologica* **15**, 33–52.

Pettitt, D.J., Baird, H.R., Aleck, K.A., Bennett, P.H. & Knowler, W.C. (1983) Excessive obesity in offspring of Pima Indian women with diabetes during pregnancy. *New England Journal of Medicine* **308**, 242–245.

Pettitt, D.J., Aleck, K.A., Baird, R., Carraher, M.J., Beneett, P.H. & Knowler, W.C. (1988) Congenital susceptibility to NIDDM. Role of intrauterine environment. *Diabetes* **37**, 622–628.

Pimblett, C. (1996) The dietary management of diabetes and pregnancy. In: Dornhorst, A. & Hadden, D.R. (eds) *Diabetes and Pregnancy. An International Approach to Diagnosis and Management*, pp. 139–153. Chichester: Wiley.

Prentice, A.M., Golberg, G.R., Davies, H.L., Murgatroyd, P.R. & Scott, W. (1989) Energy-sparing adaptations in human pregnancy assessed by whole body calorimetry. *British Journal of Nutrition* **62**, 5–22.

Prentice, A.M., Spaaij, C.J.K., Goldberg, G.R. *et al.* (1996) Energy requirements of pregnant and lactating women. *European Journal of Clinical Nutritional* **50** (suppl. 2), S82–S111.

Rimm, A.A., Werner, L.H., Yserloo, B.V. & Bernstein, R.A. (1975) Relationship of obesity and disease in 73,532 weight-conscious women. *Public Health of Reproduction* 90, 44–54.

Rizzo, T., Metzger, B.E., Burns, W.J. & Burns, K. (1991) Correlation between antepartum maternal metabolism and intelligence of offspring. *The New England Journal of Medicine* 325, 911–916.

Roberts, S.B., Savage, J., Coward, W.A., Chew, B. & Lucas, A. (1988) Energy expenditure and intake in infants born to lean and overweight mothers. *New England Journal of Medicine* 318, 461–466.

Robinson, S., Chan, S.-W., Spacey, S., Anyaoku, V., Johnston, D.G. & Franks, S. (1992a) Postprandial thermogenesis is reduced in polycystic ovary syndrome and is associated with increased insulin resistance. *Clinical Endocrinology* 36, 537–543.

Robinson, S., Coldham, N., Gelding, S.V. *et al.* (1992b) Leucine flux is increased whilst glucose turnover is normal in pregnancy complicated by gestational diabetes. *Diabetologia* 35 (suppl. 1), A683.

Robinson, S., Henderson, A., Beard, R.W., Johnston, D.G. & Elkeles, R.S. (1993a) Reduced insulin sensitivity and increased triglyceride in gestational diabetes. *Diabetes Medicine* 10 (suppl. 1), P8.

Robinson, S., Kiddy, D., Gelding, S.V. *et al.* (1993b) The relationship of insulin sensitivity to menstrual pattern in women with hyperandrogenism and polycystic ovaries. *Clinical Endocrinology* 39, 351–355.

Robinson, S., Viira, J., Learner, J. *et al.* (1993c) Insulin insensitivity is associated with a decrease in post prandial thermogenesis in normal pregnancy. *Diabetic Medicine* 10, 139–145.

Robinson, S., Andres, C., Gelding, S.V., Gray, I.P. & Franks, S. (1994) Specific two site radio-immunometric assay confirms hyperinsulinaemia in lean and obese PCOS subjects. *Journal of Endocrinology* 138 (suppl. 2), P228.

Robinson, S., Henderson, A.D., Gelding, S.V. *et al.* (1996) Dyslipidaemia is associated with insulin resistance in women with polycystic ovaries. *Clinical Endocrinology* 44, 277–284.

Ryan, E.A., O'Sullivan, M.J. & Skyler, J.S. (1985) Insulin action during pregnancy. Studies with the euglycemic clamp technique. *Diabetes* 34, 380–389.

Sanderson, D.A., Wilcox, M.A. & Johnson, I.R. (1994) Relative macrosomia identified by the individualised birthweight ratio (IBR). *Acta Obstetricia et Gynecologica Scandinavica* 73, 246–249.

Sebire, N. (1996) The influence of maternal obesity on pregnancy outcome. MA study of 174,048 pregnancies. London: Imperial College.

Segal, K.R. & Dunaif, A. (1990) Resting metabolic rate and postprandial thermogenesis in polycystic ovarian syndrome. *International Journal of Obesity* 14, 559–567.

Sheath, J., Grimwade, J., Waldron, K., Bickley, M., Taft, P. & Wood, C. (1972) Arteriovenous nonesterified fatty acids and glycerol difference in the umbilical cord at term and their relationship to fetal metabolism. *American Journal of Obstetrics and Gynecology* 113, 358–362.

Shoupe, D., Kumar, D.D. & Lobo, R.A. (1983) Insulin resistance in polycystic ovary syndrome. *American Journal of Obstetrics and Gynecology* 147, 588–592.

Spaaij, C.J.K., van Raaij, J.M.A., van der Heijden, L.J.M. *et al.* (1994) No substantial reduction of the thermic effect of a meal during pregnancy in well-nourished Dutch-women. *British Journal of Nutrition* 71, 335–344.

Spellacy, W.N., Miller, S., Winegar, A. & Peterson, P.Q. (1985) Macrosomia—maternal characteristics and infant complications. *Obstetrics and Gynecology* 66, 158–161.

Stowers, J.M., Sutherland, H.M. & Kerridge, D.J. (1985) Long-range implications for the mother; the Aberdeen experience. *Diabetes* 34 (suppl. 2), 106–110.

Thomas, C.R. (1987) Placental transfer of non-esterified fatty acids in normal and diabetic pregnancy. *Biology of the Neonate* 51, 94–101.

Thompson, G.N. & Halliday, D. (1992) Protein turnover in pregnancy. *European Journal of Clinical Nutrition* 46, 411–417.

van Raaij, J.M.A., Peek, M.E.M., Vermaat-Miedema, S.H., Schonk, C.M. & Hautvast, J.G.A.J. (1988) New equations for estimating body fat mass in pregnancy from body density or total body water. *American Journal of Clinical Nutrition* 48, 24–29.

Vessey, M.P., McPherson, K. & Johnson, B. (1977) Mortality in women participating in the Oxford/ Family Planning Association contraceptive study. *Lancet* **2**, 731–733.

Vessey, M., Lawless, M. & Yeates, D. (1982) Efficacy of different contraceptive methods. *Lancet* **1**, 841–842.

Warth, M.R., Arky, R.A. & Knopp, R.H. (1975) Lipid metabolism in pregnancy. III. Altered lipid composition in intermediate, very low, low and high-density lipoprotein fractions. *Journal of Clinical Endocrinology and Metabolism* **41**, 649–655.

Willis, D., Mason, H., Gilling-Smith, C. & Franks, S. (1996) Modulation by insulin of follicle stimulating hormone and luteinising hormone actions in human granulosa cells of normal and polycystic ovaries. *Journal of Clinical Endocrinology and Metabolism* **81**, 302–309.

....

CHAPTER 12

Pulmonary Function, Sleep Apnoea and Obesity

RONALD R. GRUNSTEIN

....

Introduction

Most physicians are aware of the links between obesity and a wide variety of common medical conditions including vascular disease, gallstones and diabetes. However, proper recognition of the powerful links between obesity and disordered pulmonary function and breathing, including obstructive sleep apnoea (OSA), has only occurred recently. This delayed awareness is due to several factors. There was a mistaken view that breathing disorders in obesity were rare or did not have serious consequences. Physicians tended to concentrate on awake abnormalities and unless the patient had obvious cardiorespiratory failure with severe obesity hypoventilation syndrome (OHS), little attention was paid to breathing in sleep. Snoring and daytime sleepiness, key features of these disorders, are often viewed with mirth detracting from their true importance as disease markers. In addition, the investigative techniques needed for the full assessment of such conditions have only recently been developed. The simultaneous measurement of the electroencephalographic and respiratory disturbances in OSA were first performed less than 30 years ago. Non-invasive measurement of arterial blood gases, especially oxygen saturation, is an even more recent technological advance. Finally, the advent of nasal continuous positive airway pressure (CPAP) (Sullivan et al., 1981), has not only provided a relatively simple method of treatment for most forms of sleep apnoea, including OHS, but has allowed a better understanding of the pathophysiology and consequences of these conditions.

Pulmonary function in obesity

Pulmonary function

Fat deposition in the neck, upper airway, chest wall and abdomen impairs the mechanical function of the respiratory system. While these changes may be obvious in the standing or sitting positions, the effect of obesity on pulmonary

Table 12.1 Pulmonary function changes with obesity.

Reduced:
  compliance (change of volume per unit of
    pressure)
  expiratory reserve volume (ERV)
  functional residual capacity
  vital capacity (VC)
  total lung capacity (TLC)
  forced expiratory volume (FEV)
Increased airway resistance
Restrictive pattern of spirometry
Ventilation-perfusion defect (reduced P_{O_2})
Increased P_{CO_2} (if hypoventilation in sleep is present)
'Shallower' breathing (smaller tidal volume for size)

function is pronounced in the supine position due to the effect of mass loading. The classic changes in pulmonary function with obesity are listed in Table 12.1, characterized by reduction in lung volumes and a restrictive lung abnormality on spirometry assessment.

Simple obesity, uncomplicated by sleep apnoea or lung disease, generally exerts only mild effects on pulmonary function (Ray *et al.*, 1983; Jenkins & Moxham, 1991). These reductions are typically in proportion to the degree of obesity. Although most studies of pulmonary function in obesity have used body mass index (BMI) or body-weight as indices of obesity, it would appear that measurements of central obesity correlate more closely with impaired lung function than BMI (Collins *et al.*, 1995). Patients with OHS tend to have more impaired lung function than patients without sleep-disordered breathing despite identical degrees of obesity (Rochester, 1995).

Gas exchange

Severely obese patients are often hypoxaemic, with a widened alveolar–arterial oxygen tension gradient (A-aP_{O_2}) (Rochester, 1995) but in some individuals hypoxaemia may be mild or absent. The Pa_{O_2} is most likely to be abnormal when obese subjects are supine, even if it is normal when they are sitting up. During voluntary breath holding, alveolar P_{O_2} falls much faster in obese subjects than in normal subjects, and the magnitude of the fall in 15 seconds is correlated with the severity of obesity, the reduction of functional residual capacity (FRC), and the oxygen consumption (Rochester, 1995).

Ventilation and perfusion are mismatched in obesity. The lung bases are well perfused, but they are underventilated owing to airway closure and alveolar

Table 12.2 Example arterial blood gases in obesity.

	Normal	Simple obesity	OHS
pH	7.4	7.4	7.4
Pa_{O_2}	90	72	57
Pa_{CO_2}	40	41	55
Base excess	0	0	+4

collapse. This effect is most pronounced in obese subjects with small lung volumes and in the supine position. The single-breath diffusing capacity (DLCO), a measure of alveolar wall function, is normal in simple obesity (Ray *et al.*, 1983), and slightly reduced in OHS (Sharp *et al.*, 1964). The physiological dead space (V_D), the ratio of dead space to tidal volume (V_D/V_T), and pulmonary mixing, as judged from nitrogen washout technique, are normal (Sharp *et al.*, 1964).

Typical blood gas composition is summarized in Table 12.2. Most patients with severe obesity are eucapnic, even though obesity produces a greater demand on the ventilatory system to maintain a normal P_{CO_2}. Patients with OHS are hypercapnic, and they have a lower P_{O_2} than patients with simple obesity (Leech *et al.*, 1987). The lower Pa_{O_2} in OHS results mainly from the increase in Pa_{CO_2}, but the A-aP_{O_2} is also somewhat larger in OHS. Patients with OHS uncomplicated obstructive airways disease can attain normal Pa_{CO_2} by voluntary hyperventilation (Leech *et al.*, 1991).

Respiratory mechanics

Compliance

Compliance of the respiratory system is low in obesity, mainly because of the effect of obesity on the chest wall. Part of the decrement in respiratory system compliance results from a fall in lung compliance. Compliance of the lung is decreased by approximately 25% in simple obesity, and by 40% in OHS (Sharp *et al.*, 1964). Some of the reduction is probably due to the increased pulmonary blood volume, and some to increased closure of dependent airways.

It is commonly believed that the increased weight pressing on the thorax and abdomen of markedly obese subjects makes the chest wall stiff and non-compliant. Although the excess weight presents an added load, it is of the threshold type, i.e., a weight that has to be lifted to inspire. This can be demonstrated by measuring chest wall or respiratory system compliance with the pulse airflow technique. The threshold load appears as if it were a resistance to flow, and the chest wall compliance *per se* is relatively normal in simple obesity.

Resistance

Subjects with simple obesity exhibit increased airway and respiratory system resistances, and the resistances are higher in patients with a higher BMI (Zerah *et al.*, 1993). The major reason for increased lung and respiratory system resistance in obesity is the reduction of lung volume. Specific airway conductance is approximately 50–70% of normal in eucapnic, obese subjects and OHS, and it is not correlated with BMI (Zerah *et al.*, 1993). In the supine position, there is a marked increase in resistance compared to controls (Yap *et al.*, 1995).

The ratio FEV_1/FVC (forced expiratory volume in 1 second/forced vital capacity) is normal in obese patients without underlying lung disease (Sharp *et al.*, 1964; Lopata & Onal, 1982; Ray *et al.*, 1983; Leech *et al.*, 1987; Zerah *et al.*, 1993). The same is true for OHS (Sharp *et al.*, 1964; Lopata & Onal, 1982; Leech *et al.*, 1987). This can be interpreted to mean that the source of the increased resistance lies in lung tissue and small airways, rather than in the large airways.

Work and energy cost of breathing

The work of breathing may be calculated as the work per litre of ventilation or the work per minute. The work of breathing is 60% higher than normal in obesity, and from the limited available data, 250% higher than normal in the OHS.

The energy cost of breathing can be estimated from the oxygen cost, which is the oxygen consumed by the respiratory muscles per litre of ventilation. The energy cost of breathing is four times higher than normal in obesity, and over seven times higher than normal in the OHS (Rochester, 1995).

Control and pattern of breathing

During quiet breathing at rest, the respiratory rate (RR) of eucapnic obese subjects is approximately 40% higher than in normal subjects. The duration of inspiration (T_i) as a fraction of total breath duration (T_{tot}) is normal. The tidal volume (V_T) is normal in simple obesity, both at rest and at maximal exercise (Rochester, 1995). Patients with OHS have a 25% higher RR and a 25% lower

V_T than subjects with simple obesity but T_i/T_{tot} remains normal. When V_T of the obese subject is normalized to body-weight, V_T/kg is approximately half normal at rest and only one-third normal at maximal exercise. The V_T/kg at maximal exercise is inversely correlated with the percentage of body fat.

Ventilatory drive

In most patients with simple obesity, ventilatory drive, measured by responses to chemical stimuli (hypercapnia, hypoxaemia), is normal. Patients with OHS typically have blunted ventilatory responses to hypoxia and hypercapnia, though typically there is a shift in carbon dioxide responsiveness. This is characterized by a normal slope of the ventilatory response to carbon dioxide albeit at a higher level of P_{CO_2} (Berthon-Jones & Sullivan, 1987).

Respiratory muscles and exercise capacity

Respiratory muscle function, measured by maximal inspiratory and expiratory pressures are normal in eucapnic obese subjects. In the severely obese, the diaphragm may be at mechanical disadvantage in the supine position. In OHS, inspiratory muscles are weaker. Maximal voluntary ventilation, an index of ventilatory endurance, is reduced in obesity, especially OHS (Sharp *et al.*, 1964; Ray *et al.*, 1983). There is little evidence of morphometric differences in respiratory muscles in obesity. Young adults with uncomplicated obesity have a near normal capacity for physical exercise. A similar situation to resting is seen in these subjects when exercising: they breathe faster with a smaller tidal volume.

Sleep-disordered breathing—background

Physiology

To the sleep researcher, humans exist in three states—wakefulness, non-rapid eye movement (NREM) sleep and rapid eye movement (REM or dreaming) sleep. NREM sleep is made up of four stages (1–4) and there are clear differences between NREM and REM sleep in many aspects of physiology. Sleep has profound effects on breathing and these effects vary in different sleep stages (usually most marked in REM sleep). Sleep may amplify the effect of various drugs (e.g., alcohol, opiates) on breathing. The influence of genetic variability in respiratory control, gender and age may also be altered by sleep. During sleep, the body is more reliant on automatic (metabolic) control mechanisms rather than behavioural control of breathing, which controls breathing, for example, during speech.

In normal individuals, there is a small reduction in ventilation, pharyngeal muscle tone and chemosensitivity to chemical stimuli (e.g., hypoxia or hypercapnia) during sleep. Short apnoeas may occur at sleep onset or in REM sleep. While breathing tends to be regular in NREM sleep, REM sleep is characterized by breathing irregularity. This breathing irregularity is most marked at times of eye movements (phasic REM). One important feature of REM is the loss of postural muscle tone which has the evolutionary advantage of preventing us from acting out our dreams and injuring our bed partners. This leaves humans heavily reliant on the diaphragm (a non-postural muscle) for breathing in REM sleep. However, individuals with defective respiratory muscle function (neuromuscular diseases) or muscles operating at a mechanical disadvantage (kyphoscoliosis, lung disease) will have impaired breathing in sleep, particularly REM sleep. In obesity, there are more complex mechanisms explaining the deterioration in breathing in REM sleep (see below). An obese individual, with additional problems such as lung or neuromuscular disease, will be at much greater risk of respiratory failure in sleep.

What is sleep apnoea?

Sleep-disordered breathing encompasses a spectrum of conditions linked by the loss of a normal pattern of breathing in sleep or in particular stages of sleep. At one end of the spectrum are individuals who snore (perhaps only intermittently) and have no disruption of sleep, so-called 'simple snorers'. As a majority of middle-aged adults are at least 'simple snorers', most clinicians dealing with sleep-disordered breathing consider that the spectrum of true sleep-breathing disorders begins with heavy snorers who may have markedly elevated upper airway resistance during sleep with accompanying arousals and sleep fragmentation (Guilleminault *et al.*, 1992; see below).

OSA is characterized by repetitive cessation of airflow during sleep (apnoea), secondary to collapse of the upper airway at the level of the pharynx (Remmers *et al.*, 1978) (Fig. 12.1). During apnoeas, futile respiratory efforts occur and hypoxaemia follows, which may be profound, until the apnoea is terminated by arousal and upper airway patency is re-established (Fig. 12.2). In the typical patient, after a few deep breaths (often loud snores), the cycle of events is repeated as often as 200–600 times per night (Fig. 12.3). As a result of recurrent arousals, sleep is dramatically fragmented with loss of normal sleep architecture. This, in turn, results in loss of vigilance or even severe sleepiness during the day (MacNamara *et al.*, 1993).

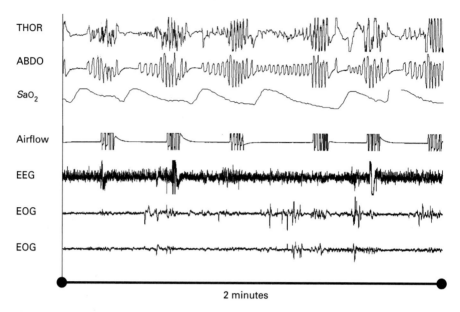

THOR

ABDO

SaO_2

Airflow

EEG

EOG

EOG

2 minutes

Fig. 12.1 Two-minute tracing of a patient with typical severe sleep apnoea. The apnoeas are obstructive as shown by continued respiratory effort during the apnoea (THOR, thoracic movement; ABDO, abdominal muscle respiratory effort.). The apnoeas are indicated by intermittent cessation of airflow and are occurring in REM sleep (shown by rapid eye movements on the EOG, electro-oculogram). There are falls in oxygen saturation (SaO_2) with each apnoea. On this 2-minute tracing, the electroencephalogram (EEG) is uninterpretable and needs to be analysed in 30-second periods to be visualized properly for arousals and other changes in EEG activity.

Some patients may not exhibit the classic pattern of OSA. Clinical significant upper airway obstruction may occur in the absence of complete collapse of the upper airway. Partial obstruction (hypopnoea) may produce similar pathophysiological events (i.e., hypoxaemia and arousal), yet there is evidence of persisting (albeit reduced) airflow. Even apparently normal oro-nasal airflow can be associated with persisting arousal and excessive daytime sleepiness, the so-called 'upper airway resistance' syndrome (Guilleminault *et al.*, 1992). In these patients, invasive measurements of intrathoracic pressure have shown huge swings in respiratory effort associated with arousal despite normal airflow. The resistance to breathing produced by a narrow upper airway leads to these increasing respiratory efforts. There appear to be neural inputs from respiratory effort sensors that will produce arousal and disturbed sleep. Obviously if patients can have sleep-disordered breathing in the presence of normal airflow this must lead to major problems defining disease. However, in many cases it is simply an issue of using the appropriate method of measurement. Simple measurement of flow using temperature sensitive devices such as thermistors or thermocouples

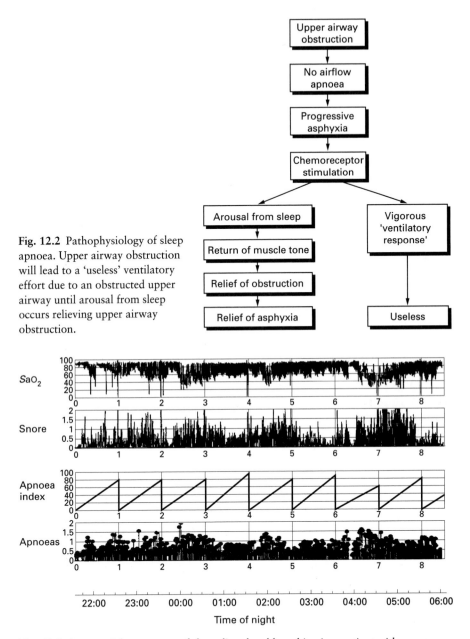

Fig. 12.2 Pathophysiology of sleep apnoea. Upper airway obstruction will lead to a 'useless' ventilatory effort due to an obstructed upper airway until arousal from sleep occurs relieving upper airway obstruction.

Fig. 12.3 An overnight summary of sleep-disordered breathing in a patient with severe OSA. The top panel shows repeated falls in oxygen saturation during sleep (Sao_2). At 05:00 there is a period of more prolonged falls in Sao_2 without return to baseline. There is likely to be associated hypoventilation in sleep. The patient continues to snore loudly in between apnoea with each line on the second panel indicating a loud snore. The lowermost panel shows individual apnoeas (approximately 500, indicated by 'lollipop' shapes) spread over the night. Above this is a summary of the apnoea index (number of apnoeas per hour). The apnoea index varies between 60–80 per hour.

may give potentially inaccurate information. In contrast, use of pressure transducers or respiratory effort detectors may give more exact information regarding flow limitation and provide a way of diagnosing patients with apparent normal airflow but high upper airway resistance.

At the other end of the spectrum, there are patients with severe respiratory failure in sleep and some respiratory failure awake. These patients may have prolonged periods of hypoxaemia usually due to reduced ventilation (lasting minutes) rather than apnoeas (which typically last for 10–60 seconds). There is progressive hypercapnia in sleep due to reduced gas exchange ('hypoventilation') and this leads to resetting of central chemoreceptors which allow tolerance of higher awake carbon dioxide tensions. Nevertheless, the prolonged exposure to hypoxaemia and hypercapnia will lead to pulmonary hypertension and often a degree of right-sided heart failure, 'cor pulmonale'. Patients with these severe forms of respiratory failure in sleep include patients with many types of chronic lung disease, respiratory muscle failure due to neuromuscular disorders and importantly for those with an interest in obesity, the OHS (see below).

Pathogenesis of sleep apnoea

Upper airway closure occurs when the pharyngeal intraluminal pressure (suction pressure applied to upper airway in inspiration) exceeds the forces that dilate the pharynx (Remmers et al., 1978; Sullivan et al., 1990). Most cases of OSA occur as a result of this phenomenon, though upper airway obstruction at the epiglottis or glottis may occur less frequently (Rubinstein et al., 1989a). Therefore in most cases of sleep apnoea, two sets of anatomical components and opposing forces determine the state of the upper airway in sleep (Fig. 12.4). The anatomical components are airway size and the physical properties of the pharyngeal walls; the forces include muscle tone/function, tissue weight and intraluminal (suction) pressure (Sullivan et al., 1990). In turn, muscle tone and suction pressure are influenced by sleep stage and relative respiratory drive to the diaphragm vs the upper airway dilator muscle (Fig. 12.4).

Most studies report that OSA patients have reduced upper airway dimensions (Fleetham, 1992). In a patient with reduced upper airway size, greater suction pressure is generated in inspiration. In the awake state, this is reflexly compensated for by increased upper airway dilator muscle activity, normalizing airflow resistance (Horner et al., 1991; Mezzanotte et al., 1992). However, during sleep, upper airway muscle activity falls, particularly in the genioglossus (Remmers et al., 1978) resulting in airway occlusion in OSA patients. Nevertheless, the specific or dominant mechanism for upper airway obstruction may vary between individuals. Also, although there is a compensatory mechanism of increased genioglossus activity operative in sleep apnoea (Mezzanotte et al., 1992), some

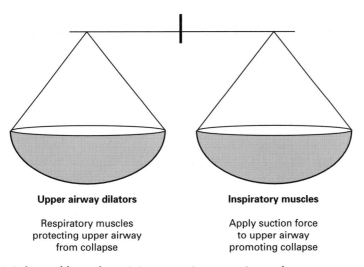

Upper airway dilators	Inspiratory muscles
Respiratory muscles protecting upper airway from collapse	Apply suction force to upper airway promoting collapse

Fig. 12.4 Balance of forces determining upper airway opening or closure.

patients have similar genioglossus muscle activity values to control subjects. Therefore, compensatory muscle activity may be increased in other muscle groups; alternatively, other mechanisms may be important in such patients.

Apart from upper airway motor defects, there may be defects in sensory mechanisms that normally protect the upper airway from closure (Larsson *et al.*, 1992). In sleep apnoea, clinical and histopathological changes have been identified that suggest chronic airway vibration and repeated occlusion may produce a defect in sensory control. In addition, recent studies in the English bulldog, an excellent animal model of sleep apnoea, suggest that modulation of serotinergic control of the upper airway may lead to upper airway closure (Veasey *et al.*, 1995).

Obesity and pathogenesis of obstructive sleep apnoea

There are a number of potential ways in which obesity may reduce upper airway size and therefore 'load' the balance of forces in favour of airway collapse. Studies employing different upper airway imaging modalities indicate that sleep apnoea patients have a decreased pharyngeal cross-sectional area during the awake state but this is not a universal finding (Fleetham, 1992). One problem is that measurement of cross-sectional area may be influenced by the level of neuromuscular tone at the time of the investigation. However, this will not affect volumetric measurements of upper airway structures. In general, obese sleep apnoea patients have larger tongues and smaller upper airway volumes (Fleetham, 1992). Magnetic resonance imaging (MRI) scans demonstrate altered upper airway shape in OSA patients, presumably due to small fat deposits. Excess fat deposition around the airway is not a universal finding in obese OSA patients (Schwab *et al.*, 1995) and well-matched controls are often difficult to obtain. Human upper airway pathological studies have rarely been described in sleep apnoea, though in one report more fat and muscle was observed in the uvula of sleep apnoea patients (Stauffer *et al.*, 1989). External neck circumference is increased in sleep apnoea and it has been suggested that this measurement explains most or all of the link between obesity and sleep apnoea (Katz *et al.*, 1990; Davies & Stradling, 1990). The hypothesis suggested by these studies is that neck circumference is an index of neck fat deposition and increased fatty tissue in the neck region which in turn promotes mass loading and obstruction of the upper airway in sleep leading to OSA (Koenig & Thach, 1988). However, in a wide weight range of sleep apnoea clinic patients, we observed that waist measurement provided similar or better statistical correlations with sleep apnoea (Grunstein *et al.*, 1993a). In contrast, in morbidly obese patients, neck size is a better predictor of sleep apnoea than other body anthropomorphic measures (Grunstein *et al.*, 1995a).

Abdominal obesity may reduce lung volumes particularly in the supine posture and reflexly influence upper airway dimensions. As lung volumes decrease from total lung capacity to residual volume, pharyngeal cross-sectional area decreases and pharyngeal resistance increases (Series *et al.*, 1990). Impaired respiratory muscle force has also been noted in obese patients (Lopata *et al.*, 1982). Cephalad movement of the trachea, as would occur with a decrease in lung volume, decreases upper airway size and increases pharyngeal resistance (Van de Graaf, 1988). Therefore, it is likely that obesity will promote sleep apnoea through a variety of mechanisms. In some patients, subcutaneous neck fat may be the critical 'load' that tips the balance in favour of upper airway closure in sleep. In other patients, abdominal fat loading may be important.

Finally and more speculatively, the central obesity–sleep apnoea link also may be related to abnormal upper airway muscle function. A reduction in type I and IIb muscle fibres in the middle pharyngeal constrictor muscle has been demonstrated in non-obese habitual snorers (Smirne *et al.*, 1991). Similar muscle fibre changes have been noted in other skeletal muscles in obesity (Wade *et al.*, 1990). Moreover, studies of sleep apnoea patients before and after weight loss have shown changes in upper airway function rather than structure (Rubinstein *et al.*, 1988) supporting a hypothesis of abnormal upper airway muscle function in obese patients with sleep apnoea.

Obesity hypoventilation syndrome

When awake, the majority of patients with sleep apnoea have normal arterial carbon dioxide tensions. In contrast, the original descriptions of the condition emphasized the minority of patients with OSA with awake respiratory failure who were labelled 'Pickwickian syndrome' (in honour of Joe, the fat boy, in Dicken's *Pickwick Papers*, see Kryger, 1985, for review). This terminology was used because a link with sleep apnoea was not recognized and many alternative theories were developed. One such theory was that obesity produced a load to breathing, which together with depressed chemosensitivity produced OHS (Rochester & Enson, 1974). The recognition that sleep apnoea was present in these patients and relief of upper airway obstruction by tracheostomy effectively treated the respiratory failure altered the understanding of the evolution of OHS. Upper airway obstruction is clearly a crucial factor in the pathogenesis of OHS (Sullivan *et al.*, 1990). However, since most OSA patients do not have hypercapnia when awake, upper airway obstruction alone is insufficient to cause OHS. Similarly, obesity is not a prerequisite to develop respiratory failure in OSA and obesity, *per se*, is associated with normal chemosensitivity. A number of recent studies have emphasized the multifactorial aetiology of awake respiratory failure in OSA. The key elements (Fig. 12.4) are a combination of obesity (increased upper airway loading and reduced lung volumes), airflow limitation, poor chemoreceptor function (particularly defective arousal responses to hypoxia) and possibly alcohol consumption (reducing upper airway tone and arousal responses to asphyxia) (Sullivan *et al.*, 1990).

Patients with chronic airflow limitation and sleep apnoea, labelled the 'overlap syndrome', also have awake hypercapnia. In fact, many 'blue bloaters' (chronic airflow limitation, hypercapnia, hypoxaemia with cyanosis, impaired chemosensitivity and cardiac failure) have sleep disordered breathing. However, it is important to stress that awake hypercapnia can occur in obese patients in the absence of any smoking history or lung disease (Leech *et al.*, 1987) (Fig. 12.5).

The term Pickwickian syndrome has historical interest, but can be replaced by OHS or OSA with awake respiratory failure which more accurately describes a syndrome within the spectrum of sleep-disordered breathing. Patients with OHS may have classical OSA in NREM sleep but will have prolonged hypoxaemia in REM sleep with hypercapnia (see Figs 12.3 and 12.6). Oxygen saturation rarely normalizes between dips in oxygen saturation in REM sleep. In more severe cases, oxygen saturation may be abnormal awake or prolonged falls in oxygen tension occurs even in NREM sleep with progressive hypercapnia. The pattern of breathing may look similar to patients with normal weight but OSA and lung disease.

Longitudinal studies demonstrating the development of OHS are lacking but almost certainly OHS is preceded by heavy snoring which is followed by the development of OSA. The severity of sleep-induced respiratory abnormalities

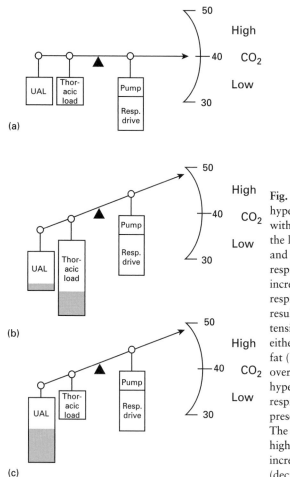

Fig. 12.5 Development of hypercapnia in OHS. In a patient with obesity without hypercapnia, the load of the upper airway (UAL) and thoracic cage on the respiratory system is balanced by increased respiratory drive and respiratory 'pump' activity (a). This results in normal carbon dioxide tension (Pco_2) wake. In OHS, either thoracic cage wall loading by fat (b) or upper airway loading (c) over time leads to progressive hypercapnia due to inadequate respiratory drive for the load presented to the respiratory system. The chemoreceptors tolerate a higher Pco_2 level without increasing ventilatory effort (decreased chemoreceptor activity).

is crucial in the development of OHS (Leech *et al.*, 1987). Patients with greater oxyhaemoglobin desaturation during sleep develop hypercapnic OSA compared to patients with eucapnic OSA. These results complement findings of other investigators who have found augmented ventilation in the postapnoeic period in patients who maintain awake eucapnia. During an apnoeic period, carbon dioxide will rise acutely. The longer the apnoea, the greater the rise in carbon dioxide will be. The apnoea will be terminated by arousal, which provides an opportunity to increase ventilation so that oxygen and carbon dioxide levels are returned to normal. If the ventilatory responses to either hypoxia or hypercapnia are depressed, the apnoeic periods will be extended and the degree of blood gas deterioration will be greater. In the postapnoeic recovery period, if the reflex responses are less sensitive or arousal depressed, normalization of

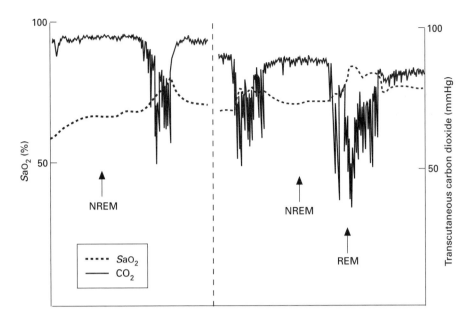

Fig. 12.6 Hypoxaemia and hypercapnia in a patient with OHS. Two panels, in early and later parts of the night, with oxygen saturation and carbon dioxide measured transcutaneously. In the left half of the panel, there is progressive hypercapnia indicated by increasing levels of transcutaneous carbon dioxide. The hypercapnia peaks during a period of hypoventilation in REM sleep (not marked as REM). In the right panel later in the night, there is more profound hypoxaemia with even higher levels of carbon dioxide. Such hypoxaemia and hypercapnia during sleep will almost always leads to hypercapnia awake due to resetting of chemoreceptor drive.

blood gases in this period will be compromised (Sullivan *et al.*, 1990). The length of apnoea and the degree of ventilation between apnoeas will determine the overall level of alveolar ventilation. In those patients able to compensate for the loss of ventilation during apnoeic periods by increased ventilation between events, overall eucapnia will be maintained. In contrast, if the compensatory mechanisms are poor, then minute ventilation will be reduced during sleep. This will eventually allow the resetting of the chemoreceptors (Berthon Jones & Sullivan, 1987) and progression to daytime carbon dioxide retention.

The progression of respiratory failure in sleep in OHS is shown schematically in Fig. 12.7. Sleep fragmentation as the result of repetitive arousals will in turn depress arousability leading to more prolonged impairment of gas exchange. The prolonged exposure to hypoxaemia and hypercapnia will over time lead to depression of chemosensitivity and further reduction in arousability to hypoxaemia and hypercapnia. Arousal responses may further be impaired in patients prescribed sedatives/hypnotics to improve 'insomnia', opiate analgesics to ease musculoskeletal pain or by consumption of alcohol. This 'vicious cycle'

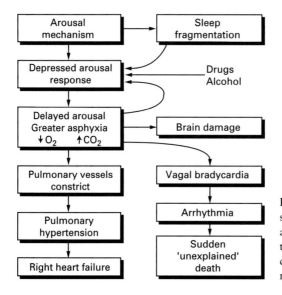

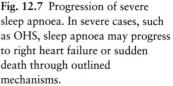

Fig. 12.7 Progression of severe sleep apnoea. In severe cases, such as OHS, sleep apnoea may progress to right heart failure or sudden death through outlined mechanisms.

will progress over time to cor pulmonale if left untreated. Alternatively, there is a risk of sudden death due to an arrhythmia in sleep (Rössner *et al.*, 1991).

Central apnoea

The term 'central apnoea' refers to a form of apnoea where breathing effort is not detected, in contrast to obstructive apnoea where breathing efforts are often vigorous (Bradley & Phillipson, 1992). However, the term central apnoea has been used in the past to describe patterns of breathing in OHS and other types of hypoventilation in sleep syndromes, e.g., neuromuscular disease. It is important to differentiate these 'central apnoeas' which tend to occur in patients with awake hypercapnia and reduced respiratory drive from central apnoeas classically occurring as part of the periodic breathing seen in patients with cardiac failure (Bradley & Phillipson, 1992), so called Cheyne–Stokes breathing. Other causes of central apnoea are periodic breathing due to strokes or rarely an idiopathic form. Sporadic central apnoeas may also occur in patients with severe OSA. The aetiology of central apnoea in the non-hypoventilating patient (i.e., normal carbon dioxide tension awake) is complex involving interplay between circulation time, brisk chemoreceptor drive and upper airway narrowing (Bradley & Phillipson, 1992).

Sleep-disordered breathing — clinical

Symptoms of sleep-disordered breathing

The dominant symptoms associated with OSA are heavy snoring and excessive daytime sleepiness (EDS). Witnessed apnoeas may be a reasonably specific symptom in patients but is relatively insensitive. Other symptoms are choking, palpitations, nocturia (due to excessive nocturnal urinary output) and gastro-oesophageal reflux (Table 12.3). Daytime symptoms include morning headaches, fatigue, poor memory and concentration, alteration in mood and impotence (McNamara et al., 1993). Sleepiness may be severe leading to sleep 'attacks' whilst driving ('active sleepiness') or may manifest itself as a constant struggle to stay awake during monotonous tasks with sleep occurring immediately on having a rest ('passive sleepiness').

The nature of these symptoms also emphasizes the importance of obtaining a history from the spouse, bed partner and other family members in the proper assessment of the OSA patient. Unless they are told, few if any patients are aware that they snore or stop breathing during sleep — yet this concerns many bed partners to the point where they initiate the medical consultation. Excessive sleepiness may be recognized by the patient, but often, for social or other reasons, this is either denied by the patient or considered to be 'normal' — again underlining the critical importance of confirmatory history from a family member, friend or workmate.

Examination of the upper airway may be important. Viewed from the mouth the uvula and soft palate are often swollen and oedematous in patients with sleep apnoea due to the vibration of soft tissues with snoring. The presence of

Table 12.3 Some symptoms of sleep-disordered breathing.

Snoring
Daytime sleepiness
Disrupted sleep at night
Choking in sleep
Dry throat
Palpitations in sleep
Nocturia
'Heartburn'
Headaches (day or night)
Fatigue
Poor memory and concentration
Alteration in mood, irritability
Impotence

such findings in an apparently asymptomatic patient should alert the physician to the presence of nocturnal upper airway obstruction. Considering the prevalence of sleep apnoea, pharyngeal examination as well as questions on snoring and sleepiness are mandatory in the clinical assessment of an obese patient.

Clinical sequelae

Psycho-social

EDS is characteristic but not pathognomonic of sleep apnoea. It is important to recognize that EDS may occur in a range of sleep disorders which may co-exist with OSA. Sleepiness in OSA is predominantly related to repetitive arousal and sleep fragmentation, but a direct effect of hypoxaemia is possible (Montplaisir *et al.*, 1992). OSA is also characterized by a range of EDS from simply increased sleep time in a previously short-sleeper to obtundation. Sleepiness may lead to both impaired work performance and driving (Findley *et al.*, 1989). Although poor performance in simulation tasks may be overcome by greater vigilance in the real-life situation, data from a number of centres demonstrate a higher actual accident rate for OSA patients compared to controls. Some studies have suggested sleep apnoea is a significant risk in commercial drivers. Treatment with nasal CPAP dramatically improves daytime sleepiness and even driving simulator performance. One problem is that patients may not be aware of their degree of sleepiness: information from partners and other family members is often helpful. There is also a relatively poor correlation between severity of OSA and daytime sleepiness and no simple test will accurately quantify daytime sleepiness. Such a test would be useful in prioritizing patients for treatment, assessing ability to work and drive, and evaluating response to therapy.

A number of studies have found OSA patients perform poorly on psychometric tests compared to controls and a variable degree of improvement occurs following nasal CPAP therapy (Bearpark *et al.*, 1987; Montplaisir *et al.*, 1992). Whether this is an effect of impaired concentration or actual deterioration in cognition and memory is a moot point. Follow-up tests may produce practice effects that need to be controlled for, as do other factors such as educational level and alcohol use. Few standard psychometric tests are designed to test for the subtle differences in cognition that are often reported by patients with OSA. Most studies have looked at small groups of patients with severe disease: it is not known whether cognitive impairment exists in milder forms of OSA.

Impaired psycho-social functioning has also been demonstrated in obesity (Sjöstrom *et al.*, 1992). Data from the Swedish Obese Subjects (SOS) study indicates that in equally obese men and women, a history of sleep apnoea is associated with impaired work performance, increased sick leave and a much higher divorce rate (Grunstein *et al.*, 1995b).

Cardiovascular sequelae of sleep apnoea

Patients with sleep apnoea clearly have acute cardiovascular changes as an immediate consequence of their breathing disturbance. However, it is more controversial whether these acute changes lead to chronic disturbances in cardio-vascular function or an increased incidence of vascular end-points (Working Group on OSA and Hypertension, 1993).

Acute effects. Obstructive apnoeas are accompanied by profound haemodynamic changes including increases in systemic and pulmonary arterial blood pressure. Individual apnoeas can be divided into three phases with regard to the observed effects on blood pressure, heart rate, sympathetic and parasympathetic nerve activity and cardiac output (Working Group on OSA and Hypertension, 1993). Phase 1 (recovery from the previous apnoea typically during the early part of the next apnoea) is typified by minor pleural pressure swings, minimal heart rate and muscle sympathetic nerve activity (SNA) change and modest changes in oxygen saturation. With progressive apnoea (phase 2), there is worsening hypoxaemia, increasing pleural pressure swings, bradycardia (and possibly bradyarrhythmias), heightened SNA and an overall rise in blood pressure. In phase 3, characterized by arousal and resumption of ventilation, oxygen saturation returns to normal. There are marked increases in heart rate, and blood pressure may rise to levels ranging from 200 to 300 mmHg. In phase 3, SNA increases, but this appears to be rapidly interrupted prior to the postapnoea peak in blood pressure (Fig. 12.8). There is a fall in stroke volume during apnoea, particularly at apnoea termination. Therefore, the combination of a fall in stroke volume and rise in blood pressure suggests a substantial increase in total peripheral resistance.

The potentiation of SNA activity during apnoea is likely to be due to a combination of apnoea and hypoxaemia. It has also been suggested that arousal is the primary stimulus for this blood pressure rise in phase 3 but other workers have provided evidence supporting a contributory role for hypoxaemia (Iwase *et al.*, 1992). Whatever the mechanism, the marked changes in cardiorespiratory behaviour, together with reported changes in cerebral blood flow, provide an environment for increasing the risk of various vascular disease end-points (Working Group on OSA and Hypertension, 1993).

Chronic effects. It is not known to what degree these acute cardiovascular changes produce chronic effects. Sleep apnoea patients are characterized by markedly

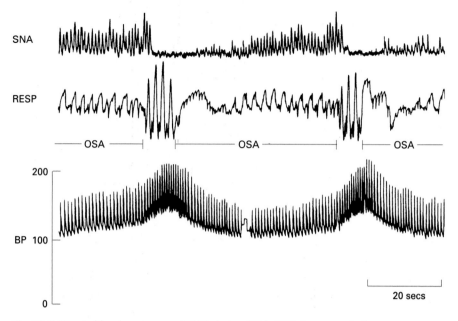

Fig. 12.8 Rise in blood pressure and SNA during OSA. SNA increases during apnoea abruptly terminating with resumption of breathing. Blood pressure peaks at this point also.

elevated sympathetic nerve traffic in the awake state and a potent pressor response to eucapnic hypoxia compared to controls (Hedner *et al.*, 1992). This pressor response is related to disease severity and is likely to be the result of exposure of the cardiovascular system to intermittent hypoxia during sleep. Patients with OSA have increased left ventricular mass (measured using echocardiography) compared to non-OSA patients with similar daytime blood pressure values (Hedner *et al.*, 1990). Left ventricular hypertrophy in OSA is partly due to increased afterload and also to afterload-independent effects such as increased SNA, causing a direct trophic effect on myocardium. In the rat, intermittent hypoxic exposure leads to persistent elevation of mean arterial pressure and both right and left ventricular hypertrophy (Fletcher *et al.*, 1992). Treatment of OSA can also improve left impaired left ventricular function in OSA. Malone and co-workers reported that nasal CPAP improved left ventricular function in men with OSA and idiopathic dilated cardiomyopathy, withdrawal of CPAP led to deterioration in myocardial function (Malone *et al.*, 1991). Irrespective of the effect on left heart function, pulmonary hypertension is not uncommon in OSA (Laks *et al.*, 1995). These observations in OSA have implications in analysis of data linking obesity and cardiac disease.

Is sleep apnoea a risk factor for hypertension? Despite a number of potential mechanisms for the development of sustained hypertension, there is no irrefutable evidence that OSA directly causes daytime hypertension (Working Group on OSA and Hypertension, 1993). Sleep apnoea is a common finding in hypertension clinic patients, but this may be due to shared confounding factors such as central obesity and increasing age (Stradling, 1991; Grunstein *et al.*, 1993a). Large-scale epidemiological studies often find an association between snoring (reported on questionnaire) and hypertension, but these studies are typically also confounded by co-existing obesity or interpretation is difficult as there are only a few cases of OSA or hypertension.

A number of more recent studies using large patient cohorts with or without detailed respiratory monitoring have strongly suggested that sleep apnoea is a risk factor for hypertension independent of obesity (Gislason *et al.*, 1993; Grunstein *et al.*, 1993a, 1995a; Carlson *et al.*, 1994; Hla *et al.*, 1994) (Fig. 12.9). It is important to recognize that hypertension may not correlate with the number of apnoeas per hour but other parameters such as frequency or intensity of arousal, the magnitude of the blood pressure response to individual apnoeas or extent of intra-thoracic pressure swings. The distribution of body fat needs to be assessed accurately in studies examining blood pressure in sleep apnoea patients. Abnormal circadian blood pressure patterns with an attenuated fall in blood pressure at night have been linked to relatively increased LV mass in hypertensive subjects. Some studies have suggested that OSA patients have a blood pressure rise or similar values in sleep to wakefulness.

Prospective studies examining the longitudinal development of hypertension in severe untreated OSA compared to matched controls are unlikely to be performed due to the ethical issues of not treating sleep apnoea. One potential method of avoiding the problems of confounding variables and interpretation of cross-sectional statistical data is to effectively treat OSA and examine the subsequent response of blood pressure. Factors such as weight loss and alcohol

Fig. 12.9 High prevalence of hypertension in OSA independent of obesity. Data adapted from Hla *et al.*, 1994 (Wisconsin Sleep Cohort) showing higher percentage of hypertensives in patients with OSA or subjective snorers relative to non-snorers. These findings were irrespective of whether the patients were overweight or obese (BMI > 27).

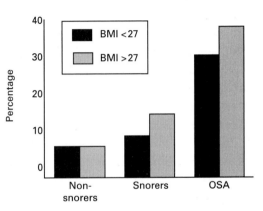

consumption need to be controlled. Recently, studies using either intra-arterial monitoring, automated daytime blood-pressure readings or 24-hour ambulatory blood-pressure monitoring have demonstrated a fall in blood pressure levels after CPAP treatment (Working Group on Sleep Apnoea and Hypertension, 1993).

OSA, stroke, myocardial infarction and death. The advent of nasal CPAP has prevented large studies investigating the natural history of untreated OSA. However, in certain sleep disorder centres established in the 1970s long-term data is available strongly suggesting that mortality risk is increased in untreated sleep apnoea. He *et al.* (1988) observed an increased cumulative mortality in untreated patients with an apnoea index (AI) >20 compared to AI <20. Tracheostomy or CPAP treatment but not uvulopalatopharyngoplasty (UPPP) reduced the mortality risk. These authors, however, did not provide information on cause of death but other studies suggest an excess of cardiovascular deaths in OSA. A number of groups have reported an increased risk of myocardial infarction and stroke in sleep apnoea (Hung *et al.*, 1990; Palomaki *et al.*, 1992). Snoring is a strong risk factor for sleep-related strokes while sleep apnoea symptoms (snoring plus reported apnoeas or EDS) increases cerebral infarction risk with an odds ratio of 8.0. Some emerging data directly links OSA with increased thrombotic tendency (Rångemark *et al.*, 1995). The ongoing multicentre Sleep Heart Health study in the U.S.A. may assist in the future for determining the influence of OSA on health outcome.

Endocrine and metabolic effects

Sleep apnoea patients are characterized by a neuroendocrine defect in growth hormone (GH) and testosterone secretion (Santamaria *et al.*, 1988; Grunstein *et al.*, 1989, 1993b; Grunstein, 1993). This is probably due to central effects of sleep fragmentation and hypoxaemia, as the hormonal changes are reversed by nasal CPAP treatment without associated weight change. It is likely that GH impairment in sleep apnoea is additive to the low GH levels seen in obesity. GH deficiency in OSA may explain impaired growth seen in children with upper airway obstruction which often improves following adenotonsillectomy (Stradling *et al.*, 1990). It is unknown whether these changes in GH and testosterone levels in adults with sleep apnoea are associated with measurable changes in body composition, body fat distribution, energy expenditure or bone density.

Recently two reports have suggested that insulin levels are increased in patients with sleep apnoea independent of obesity (Strohl *et al.*, 1995) or visceral fat mass (Grunstein *et al.*, 1995a). Other data strongly suggest reversal of sleep apnoea leads to increased insulin sensitivity in obese non-insulin-dependent

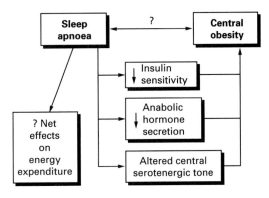

Fig. 12.10 Possible interaction between sleep apnoea and pathogenesis of central obesity (see text for discussion).

diabetes mellitus (NIDDM) patients (Brooks *et al.*, 1994). OSA may well be a confounder in some of the hormonal associations observed in central obesity. For example, low levels of testosterone have been reported in centrally obese individuals (Seidell *et al.*, 1990) but similarly low levels have been reported to be normalized by treatment of sleep apnoea without weight change (Grunstein *et al.*, 1989).

Does sleep apnoea promote weight gain? Anecdotally many patients report their snoring and apnoea to begin before significant weight gain. Perhaps the sleep fragmentation in heavy snoring or OSA promotes sleepiness and leads to reduced energy expenditure. Further falls in anabolic hormones (testosterone and GH) will lead to central fat accumulation. Reduction in insulin sensitivity seen in sleep apnoea may result from these and other changes in sympathetic activity (Grunstein *et al.*, 1995a). However, in severe sleep apnoea, energy expenditure is significantly increased in sleep (Stenlöf *et al.*, 1996). This would be expected to reduce weight over time assuming energy intake or other energy expenditure remains unaltered. However, daytime sleepiness will lead to a reduction in exercise and spontaneous physical activity. Reported eating increases in obese subjects with snoring and witnessed apnoeas (Grunstein *et al.*, 1995a). Finally, Hudgel and co-workers (1995) have reported that serotinergic tone in sleep apnoea may be altered. As summarized in Fig. 12.10, there is reason to speculate that sleep apnoea may promote central obesity but some pieces of the jigsaw remain undiscovered.

Clinical interaction of obesity and sleep-disordered breathing

The interaction between obesity and sleep apnoea is complex. Obesity is an important predisposing factor for the development of sleep apnoea but the exact mechanism of this link is unclear. As discussed, sleep apnoea is associated with increased rates of hypertension, stroke, ischaemic heart disease and mortality but obesity, in particular central obesity, is a major confounder of this association (Grunstein *et al.*, 1993a, 1995a). Whether sleep apnoea is a risk factor for these disorders or just a risk marker for central obesity is still somewhat controversial. However, evidence is accumulating regarding the importance of sleep apnoea to health in the obese patient.

Sleep-disordered breathing — epidemiology

Recognition of sleep-disordered breathing

Sleep-disordered breathing patients may present to a wide variety of medical practitioners. For example, a patient may complain of mood disturbance and tiredness and be seen by a psychiatrist. Others may present to a neurologist with a morning headache.

Clinical impression as a method of detection of sleep apnoea is associated with a surprisingly poor specificity and sensitivity (Strohl & Redline, 1996). However, symptoms such as sleepiness are common in the general community including obese patients (Vgontzas *et al.*, 1994) and may have more than sleep apnoea as an aetiology (Fig. 12.11). Sleepiness may be secondary to lack of sleep, medications or other sleep disorders. Snoring may also be under-estimated because the partner is not present at interview (Fig. 12.12) or the patient lives alone. Physical examination generally has poor predictive value though obvious pharyngeal crowding and tonsillar hypertrophy will be suggestive of upper airway obstruction (Hoffstein & Szalai, 1993).

A number of groups have proposed predictive equations for sleep apnoea detection in primary practice and most of these equations employ BMI as a variable in such calculations (Strohl & Redline, 1996). While some of these equations have reasonable specificity and sensitivity they do not apply to specific

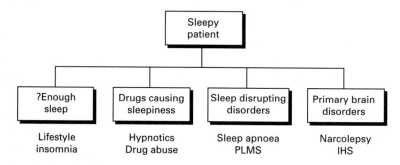

Fig. 12.11 Sleepiness in the obese patient. PLMS, periodic limb movement disorder; IHS, idiopathic hypersomnolence.

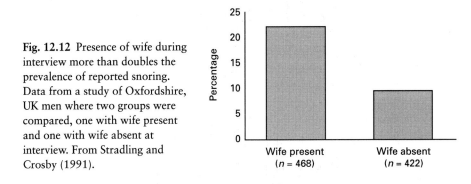

Fig. 12.12 Presence of wife during interview more than doubles the prevalence of reported snoring. Data from a study of Oxfordshire, UK men where two groups were compared, one with wife present and one with wife absent at interview. From Stradling and Crosby (1991).

groups such as women, children or the elderly. Overall such questionnaire methods of sleep apnoea detection have limited usefulness.

Breathing during sleep in obese children has attracted much less attention than in the adult population and no prevalence studies have been performed. It appears that obesity is not as dominant a factor in childhood apnoea as it is in adults (Mallory *et al.*, 1989; Leach *et al.*, 1992). However, it is important to recognize that OSA symptomatology and patterns of disordered breathing may be different to that seen in adults. Syndromes associated with obesity such as Prader–Willi or Down's syndromes frequently are associated with sleep apnoea.

Can we define what is sleep apnoea?

Unfortunately, there is no agreed definition of sleep apnoea. An apnoea is conventionally defined as a cessation of breathing for 10 or more seconds in adults but, as outlined above, there is a spectrum of disease and no particular cut-off point, where normality ends and disease begins. In some ways this is not unlike disease cut-offs for hypercholesterolaemia or diabetes where definitions change as research accumulates on the impact of having a fasting blood sugar level or cholesterol above or below a certain point. With respect to sleep apnoea, much of this type of longitudinal information is lacking due the expense of detailed sleep investigation of large community populations and the availability of effective treatment, such as nasal CPAP.

In the past, most researchers used a working definition of 5 apnoeas per hour of sleep (apnoea index > 5) to define sleep apnoea. However, this is an arbitrary cut-off which allowed researchers to communicate in a common 'language'. As sleep apnoea is increasingly recognized as a common disorder, such definitions are being reconsidered because airflow cessation may be incomplete, i.e., periods of hypoventilation and hypoxaemia with no audible upper airway obstruction, hypopnoea rather than apnoea (Gould *et al.*, 1988), or the breathing disturbance producing arousal may only be reflected by a change in upper airway resistance (Guilleminault *et al.*, 1992). Indeed it may be that, for different complications of sleep apnoea, different measurements may be important. For example, the important measurement index for daytime sleepiness may be some combination of arousals and sleep fragmentation while for hypertension the magnitude of the blood pressure changes during apnoea and arousal may be more important.

Most clinicians recognize OSA as a disorder characterized by repetitive apnoeas, loud snoring and excessive daytime sleepiness. However, in OSA the patient is often the last to realize the extent of the mental and physical effects of his or her disorder and a history obtained from a family member may be much more valuable. As discussed already, some forms of OSA may occur without the presence of snoring or apnoea but with obvious clinical effects (Guilleminault *et al.*, 1992). Similarly, EDS may not occur but instead the clinical picture may mimic an anxiety state, especially in females. Adult criteria for OSA may also not be appropriate in the paediatric age group (Rosen *et al.*, 1992).

Prevalence of sleep-disordered breathing

Most epidemiological studies to date have concentrated on self-reported snoring or some measure of OSA. Epidemiological studies fall into three categories: firstly, studies based solely on questionnaire data about habitual snoring and/or a history of witnessed apnoeas; secondly, studies in which questionnaires are validated by full polysomnographic sleep studies or nocturnal respiration monitoring in a random or selected subpopulation; and, finally, the most important are studies where all or most patients undergo full sleep studies or nocturnal respiratory monitoring.

Recent data from this last type of study has revealed that the prevalence of sleep apnoea in men is higher than previously estimated from questionnaire studies. Results from the Wisconsin Sleep Cohort Study (Young *et al.*, 1993), which measure OSA by full sleep studies, indicate that 9% of female and 24% of male middle-aged public servants have an apnoea index > 5 per hour (Fig. 12.13). Using a cut-off of 15 apnoeas per hour (a criterion which would satisfy most sleep researchers), 4% of women and 9% of men have sleep apnoea. Similar prevalence of OSA has been found by our group in an Australian rural community using home monitoring of breathing (Bearpark *et al.*, 1995). In this latter study, snoring, measured by a microphone, occurred in 80% of middle-aged males.

Sleep apnoea and obesity — epidemiology

All epidemiological investigations have consistently shown that obesity, especially

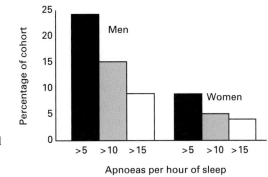

Fig. 12.13 Prevalence of sleep apnoea by sleep studies in the Wisconsin Sleep Cohort. Nine per cent of men and 4% of women had more than 15 apnoeas per hour of sleep.

central obesity, is strongly associated with adult sleep-disordered breathing (Grunstein *et al.*, 1993a; Young *et al.*, 1993; Bearpark *et al.*, 1995). Measurements of central obesity such as waist or neck measurements are tightly linked to OSA in sleep clinic populations (Grunstein *et al.*, 1993a). In the general population the association, although not as strong as in clinic cohorts, is still quite robust. For example in the Busselton Sleep Survey (Bearpark *et al.*, 1995), there is powerful effect of BMI in increasing the risk of SDB in the community (Fig. 12.14). There are no data on the prevalence of OHS in the population.

How many patients with OSA or OHS would be expected in an obesity clinic population? There is limited data on the prevalence of sleep apnoea in the obese population. Data from the SOS study, which examined 3034 subjects with BMI > 35, revealed a high rate of reported snoring and apnoea (Grunstein *et al.*, 1995a). Over 50% of obese men and one-third of obese women in this study reported habitual loud snoring. The same question administered to a random sample of Swedish males of similar age found that, in comparison, 15.5% of

Fig. 12.14 Obesity (measured by BMI, is an important predictor of sleep apnoea) in the Busselton Sleep Survey. With the odds ratio for BMI < 25 set at 1.0, a BMI of > 30 increased the odds ratio of either sleep apnoea (respiratory disturbance index > 10), desaturation during the night (min SaO_2 < 90) or heavy snoring (snoring for more than 50% of the night) by 5–18 times depending on the variable.

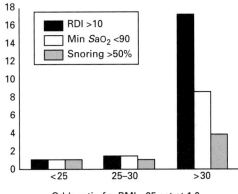

men were self-reported habitual snorers (Gislason *et al.*, 1988). Therefore, reported heavy snoring is 3 times more common in obese men compared to the general male population. As the prevalence of sleep apnoea is closely related to the prevalence of habitual snoring, it is clear that sleep apnoea is much more prevalent in the obese. In the SOS study, a history of frequent witnessed apnoeas (a sensitive marker of sleep apnoea in epidemiological studies), was reported by 33% of men and 12% of women. Studies based on questionnaires also *underestimate* the prevalence of sleep apnoea (Young *et al.*, 1993). Also the frequency of sleep-related hypoventilation in the obese is unknown. Therefore, although the exact prevalence of the spectrum of sleep-breathing disorders in the obese is unknown, it is clear that OSA and related conditions occur in a very high proportion of obese subjects.

Other risk factors for sleep apnoea

Age

OSA increases in prevalence with age and is commonly recognized in the 5th to 7th decades. High rates of OSA are recognized in the aged nursing home population. Some of the increase in prevalence with age is due to increased central fat deposition with age. There are very limited data on the prevalence of sleep apnoea in children.

Gender

In the past, it has been asserted that male/female ratio in sleep apnoea is 10:1 (Guilleminault *et al.*, 1988). More recent data demonstrate that this is incorrect and the ratio is closer to 2.5:1 (Young *et al.*, 1993; Bearpark *et al.*, 1995). Sleep apnoea is rare in premenopausal women and when it does occur it is frequently associated with morbid obesity (Guilleminault *et al.*, 1988) or maxillofacial abnormalities. The prevalence of OSA increases in women after the menopause leading to speculation that female sex hormones are protective or male hormones may promote OSA. These effects may be mediated by hormonal/gender influences on respiratory drive or upper airway function. The male upper airway has different mechanical properties compared to female airways (Brooks & Strohl, 1992). Alternatively, the increased prevalence in OSA after menopause may be secondary to changing body fat distribution in postmenopausal women.

A number of studies have suggested that androgen administration may promote, or hypogonadism may protect from, the development of sleep apnoea (for review see Grunstein, 1993). However, virtually all patients with androgen-induced apnoea already have some underlying disturbance of breathing in sleep. Moreover, androgen antagonists do not alter ventilatory control nor do they appear to have a therapeutic role in sleep apnoea (Stewart *et al.*, 1992).

The observation of a relatively low prevalence of sleep apnoea in pre-menopausal women compared to postmenopausal women has led to studies examining the therapeutic role of progestational hormones in sleep apnoea (for review see Grunstein, 1993). Progesterone levels fall after menopause and progestogens have been shown to stimulate ventilation during the luteal phase of the menstrual cycle, in pregnancy, in normal male subjects and in conditions of alveolar hypoventilation. In general the therapeutic results for progestogens in men with sleep apnoea have been discouraging.

Familial/genetic/maxillofacial

Sleep apnoea aggregates in families (Strohl & Redline, 1996). The risk of having OSA increases progressively with increasing numbers of affected relatives and this risk is independent of age, obesity and alcohol consumption (Strohl & Redline, 1996). Approximately 40–50% of variance in apnoeic activity can be attributed to familial factors. Such risk may be the result of similarities in facial structure affecting upper airway dynamics in sleep. Numerous studies employing orthodontic measurements such as cephalometry strongly suggest certain maxillofacial appearances, particularly Class II malocclusion, are linked with sleep apnoea. The Pierre–Robin syndrome is strongly associated with OSA because of mandibular shortening. Down's syndrome patients are predisposed to OSA due to oropharyngeal crowding, brachycephalic head shape and obesity. A recent report has identified a strong link between OSA and the connective tissue disorder, Marfan's syndrome (Cistulli & Sullivan, 1993). Nearly two-thirds of Marfan's syndrome sufferers have OSA and such patients, being tall and thin, do not have the typical body habitus of the sleep apnoea patient. The reason for the link between Marfan's syndrome and OSA is likely to be abnormal compliance of the upper airway due to abnormal connective tissue. One important consideration is that the intrathoracic pressure swings and blood pressure changes in OSA may provoke aortic dilatation and rupture, a common mode of death in Marfan's syndrome.

There are no data on the utility of screening family members of patients with OSA. However, it is clear that in obese patients familial maxillomandibular structure will interact to increase the likelihood of sleep apnoea (Ferguson *et al.*, 1995). This will explain why weight loss may not be enough to cure sleep apnoea in obese patients (Pillar *et al.*, 1994).

Race

There is some evidence that young African-Americans have a higher prevalence of OSA independent of obesity and lifestyle factors. There appears to be a high rate of sleep apnoea in Mexican-Americans possibly due to obesity. This is also the likely explanation for high rates of sleep apnoea in urbanized Polynesians, in Hawaii, Western Samoa and New Zealand.

Tobacco/alcohol use

Acute alcohol ingestion promotes apnoea development during later sleep. Some studies have suggested that lifetime alcohol consumption may be a risk factor for the development of OSA, particularly if accompanied by respiratory failure (Chan *et al.*, 1989). Other studies have failed to find a link between lifetime alcohol consumption and OSA (Jalleh *et al.*, 1992). Data from the Wisconsin Sleep Cohort suggests that smoking history may be a dose-dependent risk factor for OSA (Wetter *et al.*, 1994).

Vital capacity

A low vital capacity has been recognized as a risk factor for OSA and also for cardiovascular disease. This observation may be explained by low vital capacity being a marker for central obesity (Strohl & Redline, 1996).

Upper airway morphology

Apart from obesity, conditions causing narrowing of the upper airway will promote the development of sleep apnoea. These include fixed upper airway lesions (e.g., nasal obstruction, enlarged tonsils), macroglossia (acromegaly, amyloid, hypothyroidism) or neurological conditions impairing upper airway muscle tone (Grunstein *et al.*, 1993b).

Endocrine/metabolic disorders

A number of endocrine and metabolic disorders apart from obesity are associated with an increased prevalence of OSA. Hypothyroidism may lead to sleep apnoea by reducing chemosensitivity, myxoedematous infiltration of the upper airway and upper airway myopathy (Grunstein & Sullivan, 1988). Interestingly, hypothyroid rats have similar upper airway muscle fibre structure as reported in habitual snorers (Petroff *et al.*, 1992). It is controversial whether thyroxine treatment will cure sleep apnoea in hypothyroidism (Grunstein & Sullivan, 1988).

Obese hypothyroid patients have less improvement in sleep apnoea following thyroid hormone replacement. Sleep apnoea may also provoke cardiovascular complications when initiating thyroid hormone replacement (Grunstein & Sullivan, 1988).

Over 50% of patients with acromegaly have sleep apnoea and there is a higher than expected prevalence of central apnoea (Grunstein et al., 1991b). Increased biochemical activity GH and insulin-like growth-factor 1 levels are associated with the presence of central sleep apnoea. Treatment of acromegaly with the somatostatin analogue octreotide reduces sleep apnoea severity (Grunstein et al., 1994). Cushing's disease is also associated with sleep apnoea.

Investigation of OSA — is measuring sleep necessary?

Under ideal circumstances, a full sleep study is the most appropriate investigation for assessing OSA. It allows accurate quantification of breathing events and provides information on sleep fragmentation and arousals which may be just as important in producing clinical effects as the respiratory events. However, such studies are expensive, and, if current epidemiological surveys are accurate, full sleep studies for all cases of OSA may be beyond the reach of most health care systems.

However, it is important to differentiate 'screening' of asymptomatic individuals from patients who present with symptoms. Based on current knowledge, there is no justification to routinely screen for OSA as we do for high cholesterol or hypertension. However, patients presenting with sleepiness or other apparent complications of OSA may justify investigation.

There is no 'correct' approach — local resources and expertise will determine how sleep apnoea is investigated. Methods, using oximetry and/or more sophisticated respiratory monitoring (e.g., combinations of airway sound, airflow, chest wall movement, body position) are appropriate first-line investigations (Stradling, 1992). However, it is important to stress that negative respiratory monitoring tests for sleep apnoea, in the presence of positive symptoms from patient or bed partner, often warrants a close review and further investigation. In the obese patient, surface sensors may give misleading information or fall off more easily. Without measuring sleep one cannot be sure if investigation results are valid. It is important to understand the limitations of just measuring breathing and understanding the possibility of misdiagnosis despite full polysomnography. Large trials of the cost–benefit and reliability of home monitoring of sleep apnoea have not been performed.

It is important to confirm whether this high prevalence of OSA is paralleled by symptoms, impaired quality of life or other measurable adverse consequences. Epidemiological information will need to be more sophisticated to allow a better understanding of the relationship between sleep apnoea events and clinical effects. However, even a conservative view of the more recent epidemiological studies in OSA suggests a potentially huge investigative and therapeutic load for health care systems.

Treatment of sleep apnoea and snoring

The approach to treatment will vary according to severity of symptoms, severity of hypoxaemia in sleep and cost. As alluded to above, in the absence of significant data showing a deleterious effect of asymptomatic sleep apnoea, treatment for prognosis alone is probably inappropriate. Nevertheless, in a patient with 60 apnoeas per hour of sleep, hypoventilation in REM to an oxygen saturation of 50% and a history of cardiovascular disease, most clinicians would urge treatment regardless of symptoms. It is also important to realize that patient denial may produce an 'asymptomatic' patient—always check with relatives if there is a highly positive study in an asymptomatic patient. At the other end of the spectrum patients may want treatment for 'acoustic' reasons. Here it is important to verify that the snoring is really heavy and not just a surrogate marker for marital discord.

Weight loss

A number of studies have demonstrated a reduction in sleep apnoea severity after weight loss, either through caloric restriction or bariatric surgery. However, like other treatment modalities, it is important to fully re-assess patients after weight loss and ensure that there is no or little residual disordered breathing. Most published reports indicate that, although there is a reduction apnoea index, a significant degree of apnoea persists, which in most cases warrants further treatment (Table 12.4). Even weight loss associated with apparently successful

Table 12.4 Effect of weight loss on severity of OSA in patients who had sleep studies before and after weight loss.

Study	Apnoea index before	Apnoea index after	Comment
Smith *et al.* (1985)	55 ± 8	29 ± 7	Diet programme, 10% weight loss
Pasquali *et al.* (1990)	67 ± 23	33 ± 26	
Sugerman *et al.* (1992)	64 ± 39	26 ± 26	Gastric surgery
Suratt *et al.* (1992)	90 ± 32	62 ± 49	Very low calorie diet, 15% weight loss

bariatric surgery has limited efficacy in reducing sleep apnoea as many patients also have maxillofacial abnormalities predisposing them to OSA (Pillar *et al.*, 1994). Also it is unclear whether weight reduction leads to any clear changes in upper airway fat deposition.

Changing lifestyle factors

Some studies have suggested that reduction of smoking and alcohol consumption will lead to reduced self-reported snoring and reverse mild sleep apnoea (Braver *et al.*, 1995). Avoiding sleep deprivation is important as reduced sleep may influence upper airway tone and chemosensitivity. Drugs such as benzodiazepines or opiates should be avoided at bedtime, particularly in patients with severe OSA or OHS. Sleep fragmentation or deprivation may affect upper airway muscle tone so that good sleep habits and avoidance of sleep deprivation are important in the management of mild sleep apnoea.

Devices

Positive airway pressure

Until the early 1980s, tracheostomy was the main form of treatment available for sleep apnoea and was usually performed on patients with severe symptomatic disease. The advent of nasal CPAP revolutionized the management of OSA and allowed a wider range of patients to be treated (Sullivan *et al.*, 1981; Sullivan & Grunstein, 1993). However, although CPAP may be appropriate for upper airway resistance syndrome patients, it is rarely employed as a treatment for heavy snoring on its own.

CPAP is generated by an electro-mechanical blower which delivers airflow via wide-bore tubing to a nasal mask with a fixed expiratory resistance. Adjustment of flow allows a varying pressure to be generated at the nares. The pressure is determined by a sleep study when pressure is increased steadily during sleep until apnoea, snoring and hypoxaemia is eliminated. When the correct pressure is set, a rebound of slow-wave sleep and REM sleep occurs in many patients. CPAP treatment leads to normalization of sleep architecture, decreased upper airway oedema and a reduction in daytime sleepiness (Sullivan & Grunstein, 1994). It is important to stress that CPAP is not a cure for sleep apnoea. Cessation of treatment will lead to a recurrence of sleep-disordered breathing and accompanying symptoms though with regular CPAP use there is a decrease in the underlying level of sleep apnoea severity.

Nasal CPAP is an effective treatment, but compliance is variable (Grunstein, 1995). Recent studies using electronic monitors of compliance (effective machine run time) indicate that up to 50% of patients prescribed CPAP have difficulty with compliance. Different rates of compliance are reported by the same centres depending on the level of motivation provided to the patient. Problems affecting compliance with nasal CPAP include a sense of claustrophobia, mask air leaks, nasal congestion and dryness of the mouth and throat (usually associated with mask or mouth air leaks), and the inconvenience of using a machine. Patients with mild disease or those requiring high pressures are most likely to be non-compliant. Obese patients generally require higher CPAP pressures (Miljeteig & Hoffstein, 1993).

Over the past few years, there have been increasing technological advances in CPAP design with better fitting and sealing masks, built in humidification to reduce nasal side-effects and smaller, quieter motors. It would be expected that these changes will improve compliance to some extent. Recently, CPAP machines have been developed with special in-built sensors that automatically adjust to provide the lowest pressure needed to keep the upper airway patent (Berthon-Jones, 1993). These devices will allow a much lower mean pressure to be used across the night. With present CPAP machines, the pressure set is typically the pressure required to prevent disturbed breathing in REM sleep in the supine position. However, for most of the night (spent in NREM sleep and in various body positions) a lower pressure is adequate. Thus, an auto-adjusting CPAP may have several advantages in improving compliance but there is currently no evidence to support this hypothesis.

Devices that allow variation between the set inspiratory and expiratory pressures, known as bi-level positive airway pressure were originally introduced to improve compliance in CPAP users (Sanders & Kern, 1990). Although this compliance-improving role is unproven, this form of positive airway pressure therapy has been used increasingly in the management of severe respiratory failure in sleep, such as OHS (see below).

Mandibular advancement splints

The use of an orthodontic device designed to advance the mandible and thus increase the upper airway aperture, has produced a major reduction in sleep apnoea severity in several studies (Clark *et al.*, 1993) and is the subject of a large randomized clinical trial at present in Canada (A. Lowe, personal communication). Again the efficacy of these devices is likely to be reduced in the obese patient as skeletal factors are less important in the genesis of upper airway obstruction. Data on the prevalence of side-effects related to the temperomandibular joint is needed.

Other treatments

There is no drug that can be currently recommended as a definitive treatment for sleep apnoea (Grunstein *et al.*, 1991a). There is some promise in the use of serotonin agonists (Kopelman *et al.*, 1991; Veasey *et al.*, 1995) which may stimulate hypoglossal neurons to increase activity in sleep and avoid upper airway closure. However, currently available drugs have been disappointing (Hudgel *et al.*, 1995). Trials of upper airway electrical pacing to increase upper airway dilator tone are ongoing (Schwartz *et al.*, 1996).

Surgery

Tracheostomy

Prior to the introduction of nasal CPAP as a treatment for OSA, tracheostomy was the major therapeutic modality. Tracheostomy is only currently indicated in patients with severe OSA who have been unable to comply with CPAP or related therapies. Our clinical practice is to fully evaluate such patients as hospital admissions with repeat polysomnography, intensive support for nasal CPAP treatment including ear, nose and throat review, humidification of inspired air through the CPAP machine, and if necessary, customized CPAP masks (Sullivan & Grunstein, 1994). Tracheostomy can produce significant morbidity and may be a problem in the morbidly obese, fat-necked individual. However, skilful minimalist surgery and close follow up justifies tracheostomy as a therapeutic option in some patients.

Facial reconstructive surgery

Many patients with OSA have abnormalities in facial structure on cephalometry and correction of such factors by maxillofacial surgery (mandibular advancement, maxillomandibular surgery) will lead to cure in sleep apnoea (Riley *et al.*, 1989). However, the correlation of mechanical characteristics of the pharyngeal airway with cephalometry is only indirect and, moreover, such surgery is expensive, potentially requiring several operative procedures. Exact selection criteria are not available for this form of surgery, though it would appear to be inappropriate for obese patients (Hochban *et al.*, 1994).

Other groups have selected patients with maxillary constriction which frequently is part of the 'sleep apnoea facies' and expanded this region either surgically or with an orthodontic splint. Preliminary results appear promising (P. Cistulli, personal communication).

Uvulopalatopharyngoplasty (UPPP)

This operation was developed for the treatment of heavy snoring in Japan in the early 1950s involving a careful removal of uvula and part of the soft palate. A similar operation is used by veterinary surgeons to treat bothersome breathing in bulldogs, interestingly itself a breed of dog potentially useful as a large animal model of OSA (Hendriks *et al.*, 1987). The introduction of UPPP for the treatment of OSA into North America occurred in 1981 (Fujita *et al.*, 1981) but despite early enthusiasm the operation has never lived up to its promise as a 'cure' for sleep apnoea (Rodenstein, 1992). Accumulated data from many studies over the past decade suggests extreme caution in performing this form of surgery for OSA. There are no preoperative tests which satisfactorily predict the response to surgery. There is a significant morbidity and even mortality (Rodenstein, 1992). Excessive removal of palatal tissue will lead to velo-pharyngeal incompetence and nasal regurgitation and speech changes. Many studies report particularly poor results in obese patients. Current guidelines on sleep apnoea treatment indicate that UPPP may be appropriate for some heavy snorers but is inappropriate in most cases of sleep apnoea (Grunstein *et al.*, 1991a).

Recently, there has been great enthusiasm for UPPP performed with a surgical laser aiming at stiffening palatal tissue rather than complete removal. Again the early enthusiasm has led to widespread use of this form of surgery with heavy promotion in the media. However, meaningful outcome data are lacking. As in conventional UPPP, subjective reports of snoring improvement are not supported by objective benefit. There is clearly a 'placebo' effect in snoring surgery which has been demonstrated in other forms of surgical intervention, such as simple sternotomy for severe angina.

Management of sleep apnoea with awake respiratory failure including obese hypoventilation syndrome

Many centres prefer to manage these patients in hospital, even for brief periods. While most patients starting CPAP require only one night of sleep monitoring to adequately determine pressure, patients with sleep apnoea and awake respiratory failure require more detailed assessment. Patients are typically restless and may develop confusion during the night from severe hypoxaemia and hypercapnia making positive airway pressure initiation more difficult (Sullivan & Grunstein, 1994). In these decompensated patients, oxygen alone should be used with caution and with close monitoring of hypercapnia. This is one group in whom sedation or use of hypnotics is contraindicated. A frequently unfortunate scenario in our department is transfer of patients with progressive respiratory failure

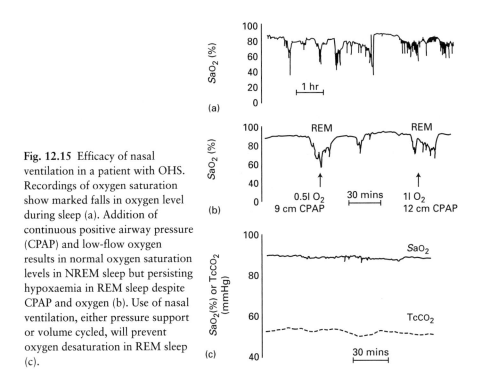

Fig. 12.15 Efficacy of nasal ventilation in a patient with OHS. Recordings of oxygen saturation show marked falls in oxygen level during sleep (a). Addition of continuous positive airway pressure (CPAP) and low-flow oxygen results in normal oxygen saturation levels in NREM sleep but persisting hypoxaemia in REM sleep despite CPAP and oxygen (b). Use of nasal ventilation, either pressure support or volume cycled, will prevent oxygen desaturation in REM sleep (c).

due to OHS who have been put into acute hypercapnic respiratory failure by a 'cocktail' of sedatives and high-flow oxygen requiring intubation and intensive care admission.

Until recently, high CPAP pressures or CPAP plus added oxygen were needed in the first weeks of treatment until blood gases improve (Piper & Sullivan, 1993; Sullivan & Grunstein, 1994) or respiratory failure was rapidly controlled by nasal ventilation or, in obtunded decompensated patients, by a short period of intubation (Piper & Sullivan, 1993; Sullivan & Grunstein, 1994). Currently, the advent of cheaper bi-level positive airway pressure systems have allowed better tolerated and effective treatment of hypercapnic respiratory failure in these patients (Fig. 12.15). Home use of these devices is then prescribed with or without oxygen, depending on the degree of intrinsic lung disease.

Summary

Obesity produces measurable reduction in pulmonary function and is strongly associated with breathing disorders in sleep, such as sleep apnoea and obesity hypoventilation.

Moderate to severe degrees of obesity lead to a restrictive abnormality in lung function due to the mechanical effects of central body fat. Similar fat deposition is linked to upper airway collapsibility in sleep and recent epidemiological data has identified obesity as a crucial risk factor in the development of OSA. Moreover, the combination of obesity-reduced pulmonary function and sleep apnoea leads to progressive respiratory failure in sleep finally resulting in awake respiratory failure (OHS).

Sleep-disordered breathing has a number of clinical consequences, including excess cardiovascular morbidity. Obesity is an important confounder of this association. Conservative measures such as weight reduction may reduce apnoea severity but long-term maintenance of weight reduction is a limiting factor. Treatment of sleep-breathing disorders has been advanced greatly by the use of positive airway pressure devices.

Acknowledgements

The author wishes to thank Dr A. Piper for assistance in preparation of figures for this chapter.

References

Bearpark, H., Elliott, L., Grunstein, R. *et al.* (1995) Snoring and sleep apnea. A population study in Australian men. *American Journal of Respiratory and Critical Care Medicine* 151, 1459–1459.

Bearpark, H., Grunstein, R., Touyz, S., Channon, L. & Sullivan, C.E. (1987) Cognitive and psychological dysfunction in sleep apnea before and after treatment with CPAP. *Sleep Research* 17, 303.

Berthon-Jones, M. (1993) Feasibility of a self-setting CPAP machine. *Sleep* 16, S120–S121.

Berthon-Jones, M. & Sullivan, C.E. (1987) Time course of change in ventilatory response to CO_2 with long-term CPAP therapy for obstructive sleep apnea. *American Review of Respiratory Disease* 135, 144–147.

Braver, H.M., Block, A.J., Perri, M.G. (1995) Treatment for snoring. Combined weight loss, sleeping on side, and nasal spray. *Chest* 107, 1283–1288.

Bradley, T.D. & Phillipson, E.A. (1992) Central sleep apnea. *Clinics in Chest Medicine* 13, 493–505.

Brooks, L.J. & Strohl, K.P. (1992) Size and mechanical properties of the pharynx in healthy men and women. *American Review of Respiratory Disease* 146, 1394–1397.

Carlson, J., Hedner, J., Ejnell, H. & Petterson, L.E. (1994) High prevalence of hypertension in sleep apnea patients independent of obesity. *American Journal of Respiratory and Critical Care Medicine* 150, 72–77.

Chan, C.S., Grunstein, R.R., Bye, P.T.B., Woolcock, A.J. & Sullivan, C.E. (1989) Obstructive sleep apnea with severe chronic airflow limitation—comparison of hypercapnic and eucapnic patients. *American Review of Respiratory Disease* 140, 1274–1278.

Cistulli, P. & Sullivan, C.E. (1993) Sleep apnea in Marfans syndrome. *American Review of Respiratory Disease* 147, 645–648.

Clark, G.T., Arand, D., Chung, E. & Tong, D. (1993) Effect of anterior mandibular positioning on obstructive sleep apnea. *American Review of Respiratory Disease* 147, 624–629.

Collins, L.C., Hoberty, P.D., Walker, J.F., Fletcher, E.C. & Peiris, A.N. (1995) The effect of body fat distribution on pulmonary function tests. *Chest* 107, 1298–1302.

Davies, R.J.O. & Stradling, J.R. (1990) The relationship between neck circumference, radiographic pharyngeal anatomy, and obstructive sleep apnoea. *European Respiratory Journal* 3, 509–514.

Ferguson, K.A., Ono, T., Lowe, A.A., Ryan, C.F. & Fleetham, J.A. (1995) The relationship between obesity and cranio-facial structure in obstructive sleep apnea. *Chest* 108, 375–381.

Findley, L., Fabrizio, M., Knight, H. *et al.* (1989) Driving simulator performance in patients with sleep apnea. *American Review of Respiratory Disease* 140, 529–530.

Fleetham, J.A. (1992) Upper airway imaging in relation to obstructive sleep apnoea. *Clinics in Chest Medicine* 13, 399–416.

Fletcher, E.C., Lesske, J., Behm, R. *et al.* (1992) Carotid chemoreceptors, systemic blood pressure and chronic episodic hypoxia mimicking sleep apnea. *Journal of Applied Physiology* 72, 1978–1984.

Fujita, S., Conway, W., Zorich, F. & Roth, T. (1981) Surgical correction of anatomic abnormalities in obstructive sleep apnea syndrome: uvulopalato-pharyngoplasty. *Otolaryngology—Head and Neck Surgery* 89, 923–934.

Gislason, T., Ahlmqvist, M., Ariksson, G., Taube, A. & Boman, G. (1988) Prevalence of sleep apnea syndrome amongst Swedish men. *Journal of Clinical Epidemiology* 41, 571–576.

Gislason, T., Benediktsdottir, B. & Bjornsson, J.K. *et al.* (1993) Snoring, hypertension and the sleep apnea syndrome. An epidemiologic survey of middle aged women. *Chest* 103, 1147–1151.

Gould, G.A., Whyte, K.F., Rhind, G.B. *et al.* (1988) The sleep hypopnea syndrome. *American Review of Respiratory Disease* 137, 895–898.

Grunstein, R.R. (1993) Endocrine and metabolic disturbances in obstructive sleep apnea. In: Saunders, N.A. & Sullivan, C.E. (eds) *Sleep and Breathing*, 2nd edn. New York: Marcel Dekker.

Grunstein, R.R. (1995) Sleep-related breathing disorders. 5. Nasal continuous positive airway pressure treatment for obstructive sleep apnoea. *Thorax* 50, 1106–1113.

Grunstein, R.R. & Sullivan, C.E. (1988) Hypothyroidism and sleep apnea. Mechanisms and management. *American Journal of Medicine* 85, 775–779.

Grunstein, R.R. & Sullivan, C.E. (1990) Neural control of respiration in sleep. In: Thorpy, M. (ed.) *Handbook of Sleep Disorders*, pp. 77–102. Basel: Marcel Dekker.

Grunstein, R.R., Handelsman, D.J., Lawrence, S.J. *et al.* (1989) Neurendocrine dysfunction in sleep apnea. Reversal by continuous nasal positive airway pressure. *Journal of Clinical Endocrinology and Metabolism* 68, 352–358.

Grunstein, R.R., Ellis, E.R., Hillman, D., McEvoy, R.D., Robertson, C.F. & Saunders, N.A. (1991a) Treatment of sleep disordered breathing. *Medical Journal of Australia* 154, 355–359.

Grunstein, R.R., Ho, K.Y. & Sullivan, C.E. (1991b) Sleep apnea and acromegaly. *Annals of Internal Medicine* 115, 527–532.

Grunstein, R.R., Wilcox, I., Yang, T.S., Gould, Y. & Hedner, J.A. (1993a) Snoring and sleep apnoea in men: association with central obesity and hypertension. *International Journal of Obesity* 17, 533–540.

Grunstein, R.R., Handelsman, D.J., Stewart, D.A. & Sullivan, C.E. (1993b) Growth hormone secretion is increased by nasal CPAP treatment of sleep apnea. *American Review of Respiratory Disease* 147, A686.

Grunstein, R.R., Ho, K.H., Sullivan, C.E. (1994) Effect of octreotide, a somatostatin analog, on sleep apnea in patients with acronegaly. *Annals of Internal Medicine* 121, 478–483.

Grunstein, R.R., Stenlöf, K., Hedner, J.A. & Sjostrom, L. (1995a) Impact of sleep apnea and sleepiness on metabolic and cardiovascular risk factors in the Swedish Obese Subjects (SOS) Study. *International Journal of Obesity* 19, 410–418.

Grunstein, R.R., Stenlöf, K., Hedner, J.A. & Sjostrom, L. (1995b) Impact of self reported sleep-breathing disturbances on psycho-social performance in the Swedish Obese Subjects (SOS) Study. *Sleep* 18, 635–643.

Guilleminault, C., Quera-Selva, M.A., Partinen, M. & Jamieson, A. (1988) Women and the obstructive sleep apnea syndrome. *Chest* 93, 104–109.

Guilleminault, C., Stoohs, R., Clerk, A., Simmons, J. & Labanowski, M. (1992) From obstructive sleep apnea syndrome to upper airway resistance syndrome: consistency of daytime sleepiness. *Sleep* 15, 513–516.

He, J., Kryger, M., Zorick, F., Conway, W. & Roth, T. (1988) Mortality and apnea index in obstructive sleep apnea. Experience in 385 patients. *Chest* 94, 9–14.

Hedner, J., Ejnell, H. & Caidahl, K. (1990) Left ventricular hypertrophy independent of hypertension in patients with obstructive sleep apnea. *Journal of Hypertension* 8, 941–946.

Hedner, J., Wilcox, I., Laks, L., Grunstein, R.R. & Sullivan, C.E. (1992) A specific and potent pressor effect of hypoxia in patients with sleep apnea. *American Review of Respiratory Disease* 146, 1240–1245.

Hendriks, J.C., Kline, L.R., Kovalski, R.J., O'Brien, J.A., Morrison, A.R. & Pack, A.I. (1987) The English Bull Dog: a natural model of sleep-disordered breathing. *Journal of Applied Physiology* 63, 1344–1350.

Hla, K.M., Young, T.B., Bidwell, T., Palta, M., Skatrud, J.B. & Dempsey, J. (1994) Sleep apnea and hypertension. *Annals of Internal Medicine* 120, 382–388.

Hochban, W., Brandenburg, U. & Peter, J.H. (1994) Surgical treatment of obstructive sleep apnea by maxillomandibular advancement. *Sleep* 17, 624–629.

Hoffstein, V., Zamel, N. & Phillipson, E.A. (1984) Lung Volume dependence of pharyngeal cross-sectional area in patients with obstructive sleep apnoea. *American Review of Respiratory Disease* 130, 175–178.

Hoffstein, V. & Szalai, J.P. (1993) Predictive value of clinical features in diagnosing obstructive sleep apnea. *Sleep* 16, 118–122.

Horner, R.L., Innes, J.A., Murphy, K. & Guz, A. (1991) Evidence for reflex upper airway dilator muscle activation by sudden negative airway pressure in man. *Journal of Physiology (Lond)* 436, 15–29.

Hudgel, D.W. (1995) Pharmacological treatment of obstructive sleep apnea. *Journal of Laboratory and Clinical Medicine* 126, 13–18.

Hudgel, D.W., Gordon, E.A. & Meltzer, H.Y. (1995) Abnormal serotonergic stimulation of cortisol production in obstructive sleep apnea. *American Journal of Respiratory and Critical Care Medicine* 152, 186–192.

Hung, J., Whitford, E.G., Parsons, R.W. & Hillman, D.R. (1990) Association of sleep apnoea and myocardial infarction in men. *Lancet* 336, 261–264.

Iwase, N., Kikuchi, Y. & Hida, W. (1992) Effects of repetitive airway obstruction in O_2 saturation and systemic and pulmonary arterial pressure in anesthetised dogs. *American Review of Respiratory Disease* 146, 1402–1410.

Jalleh, R., Fitzpatrick, M.F., Mathur, R. & Douglas, N.J. (1992) Do patients with the sleep apnea/hypopnea syndrome drink more alcohol? *Sleep* 15, 319–321.

Jenkins, S.C. & Moxham, J. (1991) The effects of mild obesity on lung function. *Respiratory Medicine* 85, 309–311.

Katz, I., Stradling, J., Slutsky, A.S. & Hoffstein, V. (1990) Do patients with obstructive sleep apnea have thick necks? *American Review of Respiratory Disease* 141, 1228–1231.

Koenig, J.S. & Thach, B.T. (1988) Effects of mass loading on the upper airway. *Journal of Applied Physiology* 64, 2294–2299.

Kopelman, P.G., Elliott, M.W., Simonds, A., Cramer, D., Ward, S. & Wedzicha, J.A. (1991) Short-term use of fluoxetine in asymptomatic obese subjects with sleep-related hypoventilation. *International Journal of Obesity* 16, 825–830.

Kryger, M.H. (1985) Fat, sleep, and Charles Dickens: literary and medical contributions to the understanding of sleep apnea. *Clinics in Chest Medicine* 6, 555–562.

Laks, L., Lehrhaft, B., Grunstein, R.R. & Sullivan, C.E. (1995) Pulmonary hypertension in obstructive sleep apnoea. *European Respiratory Journal* 8, 537–541.

Larsson, H., Carlsson-Nordlander, B., Lindblad, L.E., Norbeck, O. & Svanborg, E. (1992) Temperature thresholds in the oropharynx of patients with obstructive sleep apnea syndrome. *American Review of Respiratory Medicine* 146, 246–249.

Lavie, P., Berger, I., Yoffe, N. *et al.* (1992) Long-term morbidity and mortality of SAS patients. *Journal of Sleep Research* 1 (suppl. 1), 131.

Leach, J., Olson, J., Hermann, J. & Manning, S. (1992) Polysomnographic and clinical findings in children with obstructive sleep apnea. *Archives of Otolaryngology and Head and Neck Surgery* 118, 741–744.

Leech, J., Onal, E., Baer, P. & Lopata, M. (1987) Determinants of hypercapnia in occlusive sleep apnea syndrome. *Chest* 92, 807–813.

Leech, J., Onal, E., Aronson, R. & Lopata, M. (1991) Voluntary hyperventilation in obesity hypoventilation. *Chest* **100**, 1334–1338.

Lopata, M. & Onal, E. (1982) Mass loading, sleep apnea, and the pathogenesis of obesity hypoventilation. *American Review of Respiratory Disease* **126**, 640–645.

McNamara, S.G., Grunstein, R.R. & Sullivan, C.E. (1993) Obstructive sleep apnoea. *Thorax* **48**, 754–764.

Mallory, G.B. Jr, Fiser, D.H. & Jackson, R. (1989) Sleep-associated breathing disorders in morbidly obese children and adolescents. *Journal of Pediatriatrics* **115**, 892–897.

Malone, S., Liu, P.P., Holloway, R. *et al.* (1991) Obstructive sleep apnoea in patients with dilated cardiomyopathy. Effects of continuous airway pressure. *Lancet* **338**, 1480–1484.

Mezzanotte, W.S., Tagel, D.J. & White, D.P. (1992) Waking genioglossal electromyogram in sleep apnea patients versus normal controls (a neuromuscular compensatory mechanism). *Journal of Clinical Investigation* **89**, 1571–1579.

Miljeteig, H. & Hoffstein, V. (1993) Determinants of continuous positive airway pressure level for treatment of obstructive sleep apnea. *American Review of Respiratory Disease* **147**, 1526–1530.

Montplaisir, J., Bedard, M.A., Richer, F. & Rouleau, I. (1992) Neurobehavioural manifestations of obstructive sleep apnea syndrome before and after treatment with continuous positive airway pressure. *Sleep* **15**, S17–S19.

Palomaki, H., Partinen, M., Erkinjuntti, T. & Kaste, M. (1992) Snoring, sleep apnoea syndrome, and stroke. *Neurology* **42** (suppl. 6), 75–81.

Pasquali, R., Colella, P., Cirignotta, F. *et al.* (1990) Treatment of obese patients with obstructive sleep apnoea syndrome (OSAS): effect of weight loss and interference of otorhinolaryngoiatric pathology. *International Journal of Obesity* **14**, 207–217.

Petroff, B.J., Kelly, A.M., Rubinstein, N.A. & Pack, A.I. (1992) Effect of hypothyroidism on myosin heavy chain expression in rat pharyngeal dilator muscles. *Journal of Applied Physiology* **73**, 179–187.

Pillar, G., Peled, R. & Lavie, P. (1994) Recurrence of sleep apnea without concomitant weight increase 7.5 years after weight reduction surgery. *Chest* **106**, 1702–1704.

Piper, A.J. & Sullivan, C.E. (1993) Effects of short-term NIPPV in the management of patients with severe obstructive sleep apnea and hypercapnia. *Chest* **105**, 434–440.

Ray, C.S., Sue, D.Y., Bray, G., Hansen, J.E. & Wasserman, K. (1983) Effects of obesity on respiratory function. *American Review of Respiratory Disease* **128**, 501–506.

Rångemark, C., Hedner, J.A., Carlson, J.T., Gleerup, G. & Winther, K. (1995) Platelet function and fibrinolytic activity in hypertensive and normotensive sleep apnea patients. *Sleep* **18**, 188–194.

Remmers, J.E., De Groot, W.J., Sauerland, E.K. *et al.* (1978) Pathogenesis of upper airway occlusion during sleep. *Journal of Applied Physiology* **44**, 931–939.

Riley, R.W., Powell, N.B. & Guilleminault, C. (1989) Maxillofacial surgery and obstructive sleep apnea. A review of 80 patients. *Otolaryngology Head and Neck Surgery* **101**, 353–361.

Rodenstein, D.O. (1992) Assessment of uvulopalatopharyngoplasty for the treatment of sleep apnea syndrome. *Sleep* **15** (suppl.), S56–S62.

Rochester, D. (1995) *Obesity and abdominal distension.* In: Roussos, C. (ed.) *The Thorax*, pp. 1951–1973. New York: Marcel Dekker.

Rochester, D.F. & Enson, Y. (1974) Current concepts in the pathogenesis of the obesity-hypoventilation syndrome. *American Journal of Medicine* **57**, 402–420.

Rosen, C.L., D'Andrea, L. & Haddad, G.G. (1992) Adult criteria for obstructive sleep apnea do not identify children with serious obstruction. *American Review of Respiratory Disease* **146**, 1231–1234.

Rössner, S., Lagerstrand, L., Persson, H.E. & Sachs, C. (1991) The sleep apnea syndrome of obesity: risk of sudden death. *Journal of Internal Medicine* **230**, 135–142.

Rubinstein, I., Colaptino, N., Rotstein, L.E, Brown, I.G. & Hoffstein, V. (1988) Improvement in upper airway function after weight loss in patients with obstructive sleep apnoea. *American Review of Respiratory Disease* **138**, 1192–1195.

Rubinstein, I., Bradley, T.D., Zamel, N. & Hoffstein, V. (1989a) Glottic and cervical tracheal narrowing in patients with obstructive sleep apnea. *Journal of Applied Physiology* **67**, 2427–2431.

Rubinstein, I., Hoffstein, V. & Bradley, T.D. (1989b) Lung volume-related changes in the pharyngeal area of obese females with and without obstructive sleep apnea. *European Respiratory Journal* **2**, 344–351.

Sanders, M.H. & Kern, N. (1990) Obstructive sleep apnea treated by independently adjusted inspiratory and expiratory positive airway pressures via nasal mask: physiological and clinical implications. *Chest* **98**, 317–324.

Schwab, R.J., Gupta, K.B., Gefter, W.B., Metzger, L.J., Hoffman, E.A. & Pack, A.I. (1995) Upper airway and soft tissue anatomy in normal subjects and patients with sleep-disordered breathing. Significance of the lateral pharyngeal walls. *American Journal of Respiratory and Critical Care Medicine* **152**, 1673–1689.

Schwartz, A.R., Eisele, D.W., Hari, A., Testerman, R., Erickson, D. & Smith, P.L. (1996) Electrical stimulation of the lingual musculature in obstructive sleep apnea. *Journal of Applied Physiology* **81**, 643–652.

Seidell, J.C., Björntorp, P., Sjöström, L., Kvist, H. & Sannerstedt, R. (1990) Visceral fat accumulation in men is positively associated with insulin, glucose and C-peptide levels, but negatively with testosterone levels. *Metabolism* **39**, 897–901.

Series, F., Cormier, Y., Lampron, N. *et al.* (1990) Influence of passive changes of lung volume on upper airways. *Journal of Applied Physiology* **68**, 2159–2164.

Sharp, J.T., Henry, J.P., Sweaney, S.K., Meadows, W.R. & Pietras, R.J. (1964) The total work of breathing in normal and obese men. *Journal of Clinical Investigation* **43**, 728–739.

Sjöström, L., Larsson, B., Backman, L. *et al.* (1992) Swedish Obese Subjects (SOS). Recruitment for an intervention study and a selected description of the obese state. *International Journal of Obesity* **16**, 465–479.

Smirne, S., Iannaccone, S., Ferini-Strambi, L., Comola, M., Colombo, E. & Nemni, R. (1991) Muscle fibre type and habitual snoring. *Lancet* **337**, 597–599.

Smith, P.L., Gold, A.R., Meyers, D.A., Haponik, E.F. & Bleecker, E.R. (1985) Weight loss in mildly to moderately obese patients with obstructive sleep apnea. *Annals of Internal Medicine* **103**, 850–855.

Stauffer, J.L., Buick, M.K., Bixler, E.O. *et al.* (1989) Morphology of the uvula in obstructive sleep apnea. *American Review of Respiratory Disease* **140**, 724–728.

Stenlöf, K., Grunstein, R.R., Hedner, J.A. & Sjöstrom, L. (1996) Energy expenditure in sleep apnea. *American Journal of Physiology* **271**, E1036–E1043.

Stewart, D., Grunstein, R.R., Berthon-Jones, M., Handelsman, D.J. & Sullivan, C.E. (1992) Androgen blockade does not affect sleep disordered breathing or chemosensitivity in men with obstructive sleep apnea. *American Review of Respiratory Disease* **146**, 1389–1393.

Stradling, J.R., Thomas, G., Williams, P., Warley, A.H. & Freeland, A. (1990) Effect of adeno-tonsillectomy on nocturnal hypoxemia, sleep disturbance and symptoms in snoring children. *Lancet* **335**, 249–253.

Stradling, J.R. & Crosby, J.H. (1991) Predictors and prevalence of obstructive sleep apnoea and snoring in 1001 middle aged men. *Thorax* **46**, 85–90.

Stradling, J.R. (1992) Consensus report: sleep studies for sleep-related breathing disorders. *Journal of Sleep Research* **1**, 265–273.

Strohl, K.P., Novak, R.D., Singer, W. *et al.* (1994) Insulin levels, blood pressure and sleep apnea. *Sleep* **17**, 614–618.

Strohl, K.P. & Redline, S. (1996) Recognition of obstructive sleep apnea. *American Journal of Respiratory and Critical Care Medicine* **154**, 279–289.

Sugerman, H.J. (1992) Long-term effects of gastric surgery for treating respiratory insufficiency of obesity. *American Journal of Clinical Nutrition* **55** (suppl. 2), 597S–601S.

Sullivan, C.E., Issa, F.G., Berthon-Jones, M. & Eves, L. (1981) Reversal of obstructive sleep apnoea by continuous positive airway pressure applied through the nares. *Lancet* **1**; 862–865.

Sullivan, C.E., Grunstein, R.R., Marrone, O. & Berthon-Jones, M. (1990) Sleep apnea—pathophysiology: upper airway and control of breathing. In: Guilleminault, C. & Partinne, M. (eds) *Obstructive Sleep Apnea Syndrome: Clinical Research and Treatment*, pp. 49–69. New York: Raven Press.

Sullivan, C.E. & Grunstein, R.R. (1994) Continuous positive airway pressure in sleep disordered breathing. In: Kryger, M.H., Dement, W.C. & Roth, T.P. (eds) *Principles and Practice of Sleep Disorders Medicine*, pp. 559–570. Philadelphia: WB Saunders.

Suratt, P.M., McTier, R.F., Findley, L.J., Pohl, S.L. & Wilhoit, S.C. (1992) Effect of very low calorie diets with weight loss on obstructive sleep apnea. *American Journal of Clinical Nutrition* **56**, 182S–184S.

van de Graaff, W.B. (1988) Thoracic influence on upper airway patency. *Journal of Applied Physiology* **65**, 2124–2131.

Veasey, S.C., Panckeri, K.A., Hoffman, E.A., Pack, A.I. & Hendricks, J.C. (1995) The effects of serotonin antagonists in an animal model of sleep-disordered breathing. *American Journal of Respiratory and Critical Care Medicine* **153**, 776–786.

Vgontzas, A.N., Tan, T.L., Bixler, E.O., Martin, L.F., Shubert, D. & Kales, A. (1994) Sleep apnea and sleep disruption in obese women. *Archives of Internal Medicine* **154**, 1705–1715.

Wade, A.J., Marbut, M.M. & Round, J.M. (1990) Muscle fibre type and the aetiology of obesity. *Lancet* **335**, 805–808.

Wetter, D.W., Young, T.B., Bidwell, T.R., Badr, M.S. & Palta, M. (1994) Smoking as a risk factor for sleep-disordered breathing. *Archives of Internal Medicine* **154**, 2219–2224.

Working Group on OSA and Hypertension (1993) Obstructive sleep apnea and blood pressure — what is the relationship? *Blood Pressure* **2**, 166–682.

Yap, J.C., Watson, R.A., Gilbey, S. & Pride, N.B. (1995) Effects of posture on respiratory mechanics in obesity. *Journal of Applied Physiology* **79**, 1199–1205.

Young, T., Palta, M., Dempsey, J., Skatrud, J., Weber, S. & Badr, S. (1993) Occurrence of sleep disordered breathing among middle-aged adults. *New England Journal of Medicine* **328**, 1230–1235.

Zerah, F., Harf, A., Perlemuter, L., Lorino, H., Lorino, A.M. & Atlan, G. (1993) Effects of obesity on respiratory resistance. *Chest* **103**, 1470–1476.

CHAPTER 13

Obesity in Childhood

PETER S.W. DAVIES

Introduction

The physiological consequences and the subsequent increased morbidity and mortality associated with obesity have been documented elsewhere in this book. There are a number of reasons why obesity in childhood is of special concern, including the possibility of short- and long-term psychological and physiological damage. The psychological damage has been highlighted by abundant evidence produced over the years showing that obesity in childhood is associated with disturbed family interaction, poor peer interaction and poor self image (Lernar & Schroeder, 1971; Hammar et al., 1972; Sallade, 1973).

The short-term physiological impact of childhood obesity is less clear cut and the major physiological concerns relate to long-term obesity that begins in childhood and persists into adult life. Thus, the relationship between childhood obesity and later obesity is especially important.

One study that has investigated this relationship (Poskitt & Cole, 1977) suggested that only one in nine obese infants was still obese at the age of 5 years. Interpretation of such data can be difficult, and a similar study in adolescent girls (Durnin & McKillop, 1978) found that those who had a high percentage of body fat, i.e., greater than 30%, had also shown a high degree of obesity in infancy. The conclusion drawn from the study was that fat female infants did not necessarily become fat adolescents, but fat female adolescents tended to have been fat infants. Boys did not show the same trend with virtually zero correlation between infant and adolescent levels of body fat.

In another study (Roland-Cachera et al., 1987), the development of adiposity was followed in 164 subjects from the age of 1 month to adulthood using body mass index (BMI) as a measure of adiposity. Most fat infants did not remain fat, but twice as many fat as non-fat infants became fat adults. This study also showed the interesting relationship between 'adiposity rebound' and the development of obesity in later childhood. In normal development, BMI rises steeply in the first 12–18 months of life, followed by a gradual but sustained fall to a nadir at about 6 or 7 years of age. Following the nadir there is a gradual increase over time. Those individuals who showed a rise in BMI earlier than normal seem to be the children who became overweight and even obese during later childhood. While the relationship between childhood obesity and adult obesity is not absolute, the conclusion that might be drawn from the available literature is that while most fat children do not become fat adults, many fat adults were fat children.

Prevalence

In recent years a number of studies have indicated that the prevalence of obesity during childhood is increasing. There are, however, fewer data in this area than one might expect, primarily because of difficulty in the simple and accurate determination of body fat levels in children. Consequently there are little historical body composition data to which to compare more recent estimates.

One notable exception is the database collected within the U.S.A. National Health Examination Surveys (NHES) and National Health and Nutrition Examination Surveys (NHANES). A number of these surveys have been used to evaluate the changes in obesity in children since the early 1960s up to 1980 (Gortmaker et al., 1987). Using triceps skinfold measurements as an indication of body fat levels this group found that there was a 54% increase in the prevalence of obesity between 1963 and 1980 in children aged 6–11 years of age. Superobesity (defined as having a skinfold thickness greater than the 95th centile) increased by a staggering 98% over the same time period. Increases of a similar magnitude were seen in older children (12–17 years).

Similar data are provided by the National Studies of Health and Growth carried out in 1972, 1980 and 1990 on English and Scottish children. A review of growth data and body composition data in children aged between 4.5 and 12 years of age has recently been produced (Chinn & Rona, 1994). There were increases in weight for height in all groups between 1972 and 1990 except English boys. Triceps skinfold measurement, when expressed as a standard deviation score in order to adjust for age and sex simultaneously, also showed a significant increase in both sexes in both England and Scotland. Other, smaller studies (Guillaume et al., 1993; Maffeis et al., 1993; Al-Nuaim et al., 1996; Esposito-Del Puente et al., 1996) have indicated a high prevalence of obesity throughout Europe, North America and the Middle East.

A further finding which is particularly disturbing is that there has been significant increase in the magnitude of obesity in obese children and adolescents (Barth et al., 1997). Thus, there is evidence of increases in both the prevalence and degree of obesity at least in older children and adolescents. For younger children it is harder to find similar indications in the literature.

The National Diet and Nutrition Survey of children aged 1.5–4.5 years (Gregory *et al.*, 1995) carried out in the U.K. used BMI to assess body size and body composition. Interestingly, there was no significant difference in mean BMI in these children in comparison with a similar survey in 1968 (HMSO, 1975). Indeed, there was evidence that in some age groups mean weight was lower than the 1968 values, despite an estimated increase in mean stature of 3.5 cm over the same period.

Assessment of obesity in childhood

Method of assessment

There are numerous ways in which obesity *per se* and the relative degree of obesity might be assessed during childhood. These range from extremely expensive and probably unnecessarily complicated methods such as dual X-ray absorptiometry and total body electrical conductivity, to simple and probably less accurate anthropometric measurement of height and weight. These latter approaches, although relatively simple, can give meaningful information more specifically relating to the degree of obesity, rather than the absolute level of obesity in terms of percentage body fat. Probably the best way to combine simple measurements of height and weight is to use them in the form of weight/height^2, otherwise known as Quetelet's index or BMI.

BMI is a good index of body size and has been used for many years to assess nutritional status and body composition in adults (Khosla & Lowe, 1967; Garrow & Webster, 1985) and in children (Cole *et al.*, 1981; Maffeis *et al.*, 1993; Rolland-Cachera, 1993). In childhood, mean BMI changes markedly with age, therefore BMI needs to be assessed using age-related references. Such data have been published recently (Cole *et al.*, 1995).

Figure 13.1 shows the mean or 50th and 95th centile BMI for boys between the ages of 1 and 18 years and the 95th centile. The standard definition in adults of overweight and obesity is a BMI of between 25 and 30, and 30 plus, respectively. It is obvious from the illustration that these definitions could not be applied during childhood.

These new data (Cole *et al.*, 1995) also allow for any individual's BMI to be converted to a standard deviation score (SDS) thus adjusting for age and sex simultaneously.

Changes in BMI SDS over time can be used to monitor changes in body size in order to evaluate the success or otherwise of regimens designed to reduce body-weight or, more specifically, body fat.

Skinfold calipers have long been used to obtain measurements of skinfold thickness at different sites on the body. There are a number of advantages and

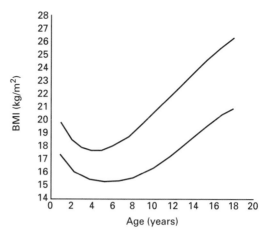

Fig. 13.1 The mean BMI and the 95th centile in boys from age 1 to 18 years. From Cole *et al.* (1995).

disadvantages to the use of skinfold calipers over just measurements of height and weight. Advantages include the fact that an actual measurement of fat thickness is obtained. Disadvantages include the fact that children, on the whole, do not find the measuring procedure enjoyable; and in some cases of obesity, measurements of skinfold thicknesses are not possible as the skinfold itself is greater than the caliper jaw aperture.

In recent years bioelectrical impedance has been used extensively in the assessment of body composition and obesity in childhood (Davies *et al.*, 1988; Gregory *et al.*, 1991; Danford *et al.*, 1992). It is a technique that is tolerated well by children, as it is painless and straightforward, and it gives an actual estimate of fatness, in terms of percentage body fat, via the electrical assessment of total body water and fat-free mass (FFM).

It has been proposed (Davies, 1994) that prediction equations developed from bioelectrical impedance equipment are less population specific than prediction equations based on skinfold thickness measurements. If this is proved to be correct then this would be an added advantage to using bioelectrical impedance in routine assessment of body composition in overweight children.

Aetiology of obesity in childhood

Genetics of obesity

The development of obesity certainly has a genetic component. It could be said that obesity will develop in childhood if the individual is genetically susceptible to the non-genetic influences on energy balance. The magnitude of the contribution of genetics to obesity is more contentious. Based upon a review of literature up

Table 13.1 The genetic and other contributors (in per cent) to BMI, subcutaneous fat mass, percentage body fat and fat mass. Bouchard *et al.* (1991).

	Genetics	Cultural transmission	Non-transmissible
BMI	5	30	65
Subcutaneous fat mass	5	30	65
Percentage body fat	25	30	45
Fat mass	25	30	45

to 1991, Bouchard and colleagues (Bouchard *et al.*, 1991) calculated the relative contribution of genetic, cultural transmission and non-transmissible influences on BMI, the amount of subcutaneous fat, percentage fat and fat mass. These data are shown in Table 13.1.

It is difficult to envisage, however, that genetics has influenced the aetiology of obesity in such a way as to be responsible for the increase in prevalence reported. As has been discussed elsewhere (Prentice & Jebb, 1995) the primary cause of the increasing prevalence of obesity must be environmental and/or behavioural influences on the population, as the gene pool has remained relatively constant over the period of time that has seen the rapid increase in levels of adult obesity in many countries of the world.

Energy intake

An energy intake greater, on average, than the energy expenditure of an individual will leave that individual with a positive energy balance. If that positive balance persists an increase in body-weight will occur. The difference between energy intake and energy expenditure in most people must be tightly controlled as the majority of people gain or lose little weight over time. As James (1985) describes, in the Framington Study, a long-term study of weight change over time, most subjects lost or gained no more than 5–10 kg over a 20-year period. Total energy turnover for an adult in this period would be close to 7000 MJ. If only a 1% imbalance occurred during this period, a 700 MJ positive energy balance would result in the deposition of 23 kg of body fat!

An excessive energy intake was for many years not thought to be a major contributing factor to the aetiology of obesity in childhood. Indeed in a recent study of energy metabolism in children (Fontvieille *et al.*, 1992) it was stated that 'most studies of energy balance do not indicate a greater calorie intake in obese children as compared with lean children'. The evidence to support that statement, however, is less than convincing.

Over 40 years ago a study on obese adolescent girls found that their energy intake was lower than found in controls (Johnson *et al.*, 1956). These data, however, were not adjusted for the differing body sizes of the obese and non-obese children, and therefore are difficult to interpret. Other studies (Hampton *et al.*, 1967; Baecke *et al.*, 1983) have also seemingly found the same phenomenon. All these studies attempted to assess energy intake using weighed dietary records. This approach places all the responsibility for an accurate measurement of food intake with the subject themselves. Recent work has shown that the technique is, not surprisingly perhaps, prone to bias, with under-recording found particularly in the obese (Southgate, 1986; Livingstone *et al.*, 1990). There are therefore few reliable data to suggest that obese children do in fact consume fewer calories than lean controls. Thus, overeating will, if continued over time, lead to an increase in body-weight and possibly to obesity. Having said that, there is now evidence that average energy intake in many populations is falling. For example, the British National Food Survey (HMSO, 1995) clearly indicates that the population is consuming less energy, on average, in the 1990s than in the 1970s. A number of recent studies have confirmed this trend in children of varying age groups.

The National Diet and Nutrition Survey of British Children aged 1.5–4.5 years (Gregory *et al.*, 1995) reported mean energy intake as being significantly lower at all ages than those reported by a similar survey in the late 1960s (HMSO, 1975). The average reduction was about 17%. A smaller study (Davies *et al.*, 1995) found similar results in the same age group, with estimations of energy intake calculated from measurements of energy expenditure being about 15% below previously reported values (FAO/WHO/UNU, 1985). Values of energy intake very similar to both these publications have been reported in a study based in Edinburgh (Payne & Belton, 1992).

Thus, at the population level it would seem that energy intake of children has declined over recent years and therefore, at population level, the influence of energy intake on the aetiology of obesity must be questionable based on current data. Nevertheless, it must be remembered that in any one individual an excess of energy intake over that expended will lead to weight gain.

Diet composition

As has been described, there are data that suggest, on average, that there has been a decline in energy intake in the paediatric population. The same data, however, also show that the composition of the diet has changed over the years, with fat contributing a larger proportion of energy intake and a concurrent fall in carbohydrate intake.

There is now mounting evidence that diet composition influences body size. Work with animal models (Herberg *et al.*, 1974; Hill *et al.*, 1983; Oscai *et al.*, 1984; Triscari *et al.*, 1985; Levin *et al.*, 1986; Oscai *et al.*, 1987; Jen, 1988; Hill *et al.*, 1989; Lucas *et al.*, 1989; Hill, 1990) has clearly shown that a high-fat diet induces obesity. Some such studies that used iso-calorific diets that differed in fat and carbohydrate content offer compelling evidence that diet composition is of importance in the aetiology of obesity, at least in animal models. Studies in adult humans (Dreon *et al.*, 1988; Kromhout *et al.*, 1988; Romieu *et al.*, 1988; Miller *et al.*, 1990; Tucker & Kano, 1992) have suggested that diets high in fat cause body fat levels to increase and diets high in carbohydrate are associated with lower levels of body fat. Carefully controlled studies that manipulate the diet also reinforce the argument that diet composition is important in weight maintenance and can influence body composition (Lissner *et al.*, 1987; Kendall *et al.*, 1991; Prewitt *et al.*, 1991).

One of the mechanisms proposed to explain this phenomenon is that a high-fat diet leads to the deposition of body fat due to the efficiency of the conversion of dietary fat into stored triglyceride. The metabolic cost of such a conversion is in the order of 3% of energy intake whereas the cost of storing dietary carbohydrate as body fat requires the expenditure of 23% of the ingested energy (Flatt, 1985). It has also been suggested that resting metabolic rate and the thermic effect of food differ according to diet composition, in that there is more potential for a thermogenesis effect following a high-carbohydrate, low-fat meal (Sims & Danforth, 1987).

Landsberg and Young (1983) have shown in animals that sympathetic nervous activity is increased following a high-fat meal which may influence energy balance via changes in adaptive thermogenesis. Differences in enzyme response to diet composition have been implicated in the relationship between diet composition and body composition. Specifically, high levels of dietary fat have been found to be directly related to levels and activity of lipoprotein lipase, the major rate-limiting enzyme for the conversion of dietary lipids into stored lipid.

Finally, there is evidence to suggest that in some individuals there is a blunted post-meal response to high-fat intakes, and that reduced post-meal fat oxidation leads to an increase in body size and potential obesity.

To date, there has been limited investigation into the effect of these possible phenomena in children (Gazzaniga & Burns, 1993; Oretega *et al.*, 1995; Rolland-Cachera *et al.*, 1995). In the first of these studies a significant positive correlation was found between percentage energy intake derived from fat and percentage body fat in a group of 48 children aged 9–11 years. However, in a subgroup of obese children (*n* = 18), the correlation was not significant. The second study found that the only nutrient intake in early childhood that was correlated with later BMI was percentage energy intake derived from protein. Again this study was of relatively few children ($n = 112$). In a cohort of 64 Spanish adolescents, divided into obese and non-obese groups based on their BMI, despite there being no differences in energy intake *per se*, the obese group derived a greater proportion of their energy from protein and fat (Oretega *et al.*, 1995). Finally, in a large cohort of pre-school children ($n = 1444$) no relationship was found between diet composition and body composition (Davies, 1997).

It is possible that if diet composition does influence body size there is a time course over which the influence takes place, and that pre-school children are too young for such a relationship to be revealed. If this was the case there may be a need to target education on good eating habits to parents and carers of pre-school children in order to prevent the potentially detrimental changes to body composition in later childhood.

Energy expenditure

Concurrent with a decline in total energy intake in children as described previously, there is now compelling evidence that total energy expenditure has also declined markedly over the last 30 years. One of the problems in attempting to measure total energy expenditure is that, until relatively recently, it was virtually impossible to measure energy output non-invasively and without impinging on the lifestyle of the individual. The development of the doubly labelled water technique in the 1980s (Schoeller & van Santen, 1982; Coward *et al.*, 1985) has now enabled a number of research centres to evaluate energy expenditure in various populations. It is the use of this technique that has shown a major reduction in energy expenditure at least in infants and young children. The reduction in total energy expenditure in young children is particularly disturbing as this most probably represents a major reduction in habitual levels of physical activity. Data that support that argument are strong.

Studies from three different centres, Phoenix (U.S.A.), Burlington (U.S.A.) and Cambridge (U.K.), all show remarkably similar results (Davies *et al.*, 1991, 1994; Fontvieille *et al.*, 1993a; Goran *et al.*, 1993). The Phoenix study involved 28 children, aged between 5 and 6 years of age. Mean total energy expenditure in these children was 24% below current recommendations of energy requirements (FAO/WHO/UNU, 1985). The Burlington study measured energy expenditure in a similar age group of children. In this case, mean energy expenditure was 23% below current recommendations. Finally, the Cambridge group have provided data from 167 children, aged 1 year old through to 6 years old, which show in most ages a reduction in total energy expenditure of between 15 and 25% in most cases. All these measurements of total energy expenditure, plotted in relation to current international guidelines for energy requirements are shown for boys and girls in Figs 13.2 and 13.3, respectively.

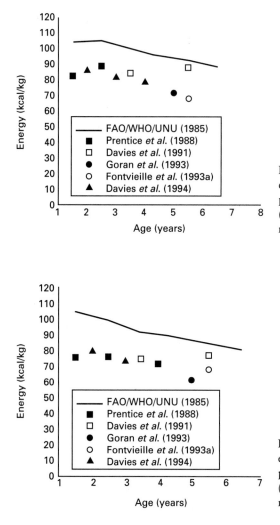

Fig. 13.2 Mean total energy expenditure for boys in 5 studies plotted against FAO/WHO/UNU (1985) recommendations of energy requirements.

Fig. 13.3 Mean total energy expenditure for girls in 5 studies plotted against FAO/WHO/UNU (1985) recommendations of energy requirements.

In an attempt to determine which components of total energy expenditure must have decreased in order to produce these changes, the relative magnitude of the components needs to be considered.

It is improbable that the energy cost of growth has been significantly reduced in recent years, even if average growth rates have changed. The energy cost of growth after the age of 1 year is an extremely small proportion of energy expenditure and only about 2% of energy intake. Therefore, even a major reduction in the energy cost of growth would not affect total energy expenditure greatly. Equally, it is difficult to conceive that the energy cost of thermoregulation has decreased dramatically in the last 30 years or so. There are few data to suggest that there has been a major reduction in recent years in resting metabolic rate per unit body-weight, which accounts for the majority of total energy expenditure.

The energy cost of activity is a much larger proportion of total energy expenditure than the energy cost of thermoregulation or the energy cost of growth. Consequently, there is considerable scope for a reduction of total energy expenditure to be associated with a reduction in the levels of physical activity. Indeed, it would be difficult to argue that changes in any or all of the other components could be responsible for a reduction in energy expenditure in the order of 20–25%. Physical activity levels are difficult to assess, which confounds objective assessment of changes that might have occurred in recent times.

Nevertheless, it is probable that a reduction in levels of physical activity is the major reason for the reduced measurements of total energy expenditure in young children. Indeed, Fontvieille et al. (1993a) showed a significant relationship between television viewing and body fatness, implicating reduced levels of activity in the aetiology of obesity. The same group also demonstrated a relationship between physical activity and body fatness in young male Pima Indians, a group prone to obesity (Fontvieille et al., 1993b). More recently, Davies et al. (1994) have shown a significant negative correlation between activity levels in pre-school children and body fatness. Thus, the reduction in total energy expenditure that seems to be occurring in young children may have important influences on body composition.

Treatment strategies

In adult obesity, three major types of treatment can be used: dietary intervention, a prescribed exercise programme and medication. The latter is not recommended for use in childhood (Dietz, 1993) and so the major focus of treatment in childhood obesity is the use of diet and exercise.

Dietary approaches

A reduction in daily energy intake is fundamental to initiate weight loss in any individual. The assessment of energy and nutrient intakes is not simple or straightforward. As has been previously discussed, methods which utilize weighed intakes often lead to under-reporting and it has been claimed that calorie intake determined from diet records have little clinical applicability (Dietz, 1993). Such records can seemingly be used to establish the pattern of food intake and to evaluate which food group is being over- or under-consumed (Dietz, 1993). In order to estimate the energy intake of any individual or their energy requirements, other approaches need to be utilized. It is now possible in many centres to measure resting metabolic rate with relative ease. Resting metabolic rate is by far the largest component of total energy expenditure in most individuals, and represents about 60% of total energy requirements. The major influence on the magnitude of resting metabolic rate is the amount of FFM. The remaining proportion of total energy expenditure comprises dietary-induced thermogenesis, non-dietary-induced thermogenesis, the energy cost of growth and physical activity. The thermogenic and other components are small in comparison with the energy cost of activity. Thus, if a resting metabolic rate can be measured and then increased by a factor to allow for the energy cost of activity, an estimate of energy requirement can be achieved. This has been the method adopted by the World Health Organization for many years (FAO/WHO/UNU, 1985). Some examples of allowance for activity are shown in Table 13.2.

If resting metabolic rate cannot be measured, it can be predicted using existing equations (Schofield, 1985). Once an estimated energy requirement for an individual is established, dietary guidelines can be produced that aim to provide fewer calories than required by the individual in order to promote weight loss. When weight loss occurs a re-evaluation of requirements should be carried out in due course as changes in body mass will influence the requirements, especially if FFM is lost during the weight loss. Such loss of lean tissue can be minimized by a more gradual weight loss.

Dietary intervention to reduce calorie intake needs to be tempered by the need to provide adequate micronutrients such as iron and calcium. Iron-deficient anaemia is one of the most common childhood nutritional disorders; any prescribed diet should maintain adequate intakes. Calcium, too, is especially important during childhood and any potential reduction in intake due to the reduction, of for example, intake of dairy products, should be carefully monitored.

A major advantage to those who aim to treat childhood obesity is that children are able, in some cases, to 'grow into their weight'. What is meant by this is that height may well increase for many years in an obese child and, even if weight simply remains stable, a more favourable body habitus will result. For example, a boy aged 8 years who is 1.3 m tall and weighs 30.5 kg would have a BMI close to the 90th centile (Cole *et al.*, 1995). Assuming that in 2 years time

Table 13.2 Some examples of the energy cost of activity as a multiple of basal metabolic rate in boys and girls.

	Boys	Girls
Light activity, i.e., sitting, standing, moving around, social activities, washing, play	1.6	1.5
Moderate activity, i.e., walking, household tasks, play	2.5	2.2
Heavy activity, i.e., work tasks	6.0	6.0

he is 1.4 m tall and that body-weight has increased by only 2 kg, his BMI would now be close to the 50th centile.

Many different dietary strategies can be employed. If traditional calorie counting is used, an often successful approach is the so-called traffic-light diet (Epstein *et al.*, 1990). In this diet, foods are colour coded, green, yellow or red depending upon the calorie density. Energy-dense foods are given a red coding and children are allowed only four red foods per week. This type of approach certainly simplifies the dietary intervention.

Another approach is to limit the intake of dietary fat. This strategy is based upon two facts. Firstly, the energy density of fat makes it easy to consume large numbers of calories quickly, and secondly, the evidence previously cited that suggests that a diet high in fat leads to obesity in animals and humans.

Role of exercise

In order to achieve a negative energy balance, and over time reduce body-weight, an exercise programme may be used in some cases of childhood obesity. A number of exercise regimens have been used, sometimes in conjunction with calorie restriction. Moreover, exercise is known to increase the FFM component of body-weight. This change in FFM has two different effects on weight loss. Firstly, the increase may mask or disguise the fact that the child is in fact losing body fat. This is because the density of the fat and FFM components of the body are not the same. If exercise does induce an increase in FFM, this might be interpreted as a reduced weight loss and the automatic assumption might be that fat loss has reduced. This may well not be the case. Secondly, as previously described, resting metabolic rate is dependent primarily upon the FFM of the individual, with the fat mass being much less metabolically active. The linear relationship between resting metabolic rate and FFM in a cohort of children and adolescents is shown in Fig. 13.4. An increase in FFM will therefore increase

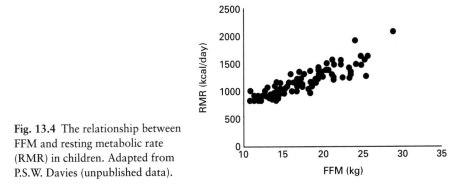

Fig. 13.4 The relationship between FFM and resting metabolic rate (RMR) in children. Adapted from P.S.W. Davies (unpublished data).

resting metabolic rate and hence total energy expenditure. This increase will contribute to a negative energy balance and the subsequent loss of body fat.

Any exercise programme for obese or overweight children and adolescents should be carefully designed and monitored. A number of key features should be addressed. These include the mode, frequency, duration and intensity of the programme designed. The mode of the exercise programme will vary depending on many factors. Swimming, walking or jogging, might be employed. Certainly, compliance with the exercise programme will increase if the child views the exercise programme as 'fun'. Team games might be considered so long as the overweight child is not self-conscious in taking part in the activity. Such decisions should always be made in consultation with the child.

While an increase in general levels of physical activity will be beneficial to weight loss, any formal exercise programme need to be designed in consultation with an exercise scientist or other specialist in the field. It should be remembered that motor ability mirrors closely the biological maturity of the child. For example, the time taken to complete a 2-mile walk decreases dramatically between the ages of 6 and 12 years and then plateaus at around the age of 13 in girls and 14 in boys. Thus, the biological maturity of the child should be taken into account if the exercise programme is to achieve goals.

The majority of studies of the effect of exercise on weight loss in children have combined an exercise programme with dietary intervention (Pena *et al.*, 1980; Epstein *et al.*, 1985; Hills & Parker, 1988; Pena *et al.*, 1989; Reybrouck, 1990). In most studies the subjects were at least 8 years of age. Two studies (Seltzer *et al.*, 1970; Blomquist *et al.*, 1985) that compared an exercise regimen alone with a control group failed to find a significant effect of the exercise programme on change in weight. It has been suggested that poor adherence to the exercise plan might have contributed to the poor results in these studies. Adherence to an exercise plan is an important issue and will be discussed in more detail later. In studies that have compared exercise and dietary intervention with dietary intervention alone, a number of different exercise modes, frequency, intensity and durations have been used. For example, one study (Reybrouck *et al.*, 1990) used a 2-hour walk every day plus daily aerobic exercise lasting 15–40 minutes, while another (Hills & Parker, 1988) used a weekly gymnastic session and three to four home-based aerobic session of about 20 minutes duration.

Children are more susceptible to heat-related injury than adults. They are much less able to dissipate heat through evaporation and rely more on radiation and convection. Much is still to be learnt about heat stress in children during exercise, but a conservative approach should be taken in hot climates. Injury, notably to bone and specifically to the epiphysial plates, should be a concern to any exercise prescriber.

Exercise adherence

The most professionally designed and appropriately structured exercise programme will be ineffective if the subject does not adhere to the regimen. Very little is known about adherence to prescribed exercise programmes in obese children, but some inference might be drawn from studies in other areas. A recent large-scale survey (Commonwealth of Australia, 1995) looked at so-called 'barriers' to taking part in regular physical activity. The major barriers and the percentage of individuals who cited each reason are shown in Table 13.3. While these data are based on adults, one might imagine similar responses in other groups. It is the role of the exercise scientist or prescriber to counteract these barriers and also to take the comments into account when attempting to prescribe a suitable programme for an overweight child. A recent review (Hillsdon *et al.*, 1995) attempted to find common features of successful intervention programme that aimed to increase levels of habitual physical activity in the population. The common features of successful programmes were that they were home-based programmes which used unsupervised informal exercise, with frequent professional contact, and used walking as the mode of exercise and a moderate level of intensity.

The future

There is abundant evidence that adult obesity has increased dramatically in recent years (Prentice & Jebb, 1995). Lifestyle factors must be predominantly the cause of this increase. The industrialized nations have an increasingly sedentary society with a relative abundance of food. Both of these conditions are extremely new in terms of human evolution. The response of the species to these changes has been to increase levels of adiposity. This increase is now being seen in younger and younger children in many societies.

Table 13.3 'Barriers' to taking part in regular physical activity.

	%
No time	34.6
Physically unable	24.3
Do not want to	13.4
Need encouragement	8.8
No chance to exercise	6.9
Exercise is too difficult	5.2
No facilities	2.5
No transport	2.3
Other	2.0

If the current trend is to be reversed, or at least stemmed, major changes are needed at all levels of society. The enhancement of public understanding of the health consequences of diet, nutrition and exercise requires the involvement of government in the determination and implementation of policies, educational programmes and resource allocation. The cost to society in terms of ill health is too large to ignore.

References

Al-Nuaim, A.R., Bamgboye, E.A. & Al-Herbish, A. (1996) The pattern of growth and obesity in Saudi Arabian male school children. *International Journal of Obesity* 20, 1000–1005.

Baecke, J.A.H., Van Staveren, W.A. & Burema, J. (1983) Food consumption, habitual physical activity, and body fatness in young Dutch adults. *American Journal of Clinical Nutrition* 37, 278–286.

Barth, N., Ziegler, A., Himmelmann, G.W. *et al.* (1997) Significant weight gains in a clinical sample of obese children and adolescents between 1985 and 1995. *International Journal of Obesity* 21, 122–126.

Blomquist, B.M., Borjeson, M., Larsson, Y., Persson, B. & Sterky, G. (1985) The effect of physical activity on the body measurements and work capacity of overweight boys. *Acta Paediatrica Scandanavia* 54, 566–572.

Bouchard, C., Després, J.P. & Tremblay, A. (1991) Genetics of obesity and human energy metabolism. *Proceedings of the Nutrition Society* 50, 139–147.

Chinn, S. & Rona, R.J. (1994) Trends in weight-for-height and triceps skinfold thickness for English and Scottish children, 1972–1982, and 1982–1990. *Paediatric and Perinatal Epidemiology* 8, 90–106.

Cole, T.J., Donnet, M.C. & Stanfield, J.P. (1981) Weight for height indices to assess nutritional status—a new index on a slide rule. *American Journal of Clinical Nutrition* 34, 1935–1943.

Cole, T.J., Freeman, J.V. & Preece, M.A. (1995) Body mass index reference curves for the UK, 1990. *Archives of Diseases in Childhood* 73, 25–29.

Commonwealth of Australia (1995) *Active and Inactive Australians.* Canberra: Office of Recreation Department.

Coward, W.A., Prentice, A.M., Murgatroyd, P.R. *et al.* (1985) Measurement of CO_2 and water production rates in man using $^2H_2^{18}O$ labelled H_2O: Comparison between calorimeter and isotope values. In: van Es, A.J.H. (ed.) *Human Energy Metabolism: physical activity and energy expenditure measurements in epidemiological research based upon direct and indirect calorimetry.* European Nutrition Report No. 5, pp. 126–128. Dean Haag: CIP-gegeres koninklijke.

Danford, L.C., Schoeller, D.A. & Kushner, R.F. (1992) Comparison of two bioelectrical impedance models for total body water measurements in children. *Annals of Human Biology* 19, 603–607.

Davies, P.S.W. (1994) Bioelectrical impedance measurement in children. *Age and Nutrition* 5, 102–106.

Davies, P.S.W., Hicks, C.J., Halliday, D. & Preece, M.A. (1988) The prediction of total body water using bioelectrical impedance in children and adolescents. *Annals of Human Biology* 15, 237–240.

Davies, P.S.W., Livingstone, M.B.E., Prentice, A.M. *et al.* (1991) Total energy expenditure during childhood and adolescence. *Proceedings of the Nutrition Society* 50, 14A.

Davies, P.S.W., Coward, W.A., Gregory, J., Tyler, H. & White, A. (1994) Total energy expenditure and energy intake in the pre-school child: A comparison. *British Journal of Nutrition* 72, 13–20.

Davies, P.S.W., Gregory, J., White, A. (1995) Energy expenditure in children aged 1.5 to 4.5

years: a comparison with current recommendations. *European Journal of Clinical Nutrition* **49**, 360–364.

Department of Health and Social Security (1975) *Report on Health and Social Subjects: 10. Nutrition Survey of Pre-School Children 1967–68.* London: HMSO.

Dietz, W.H. (1993) Therapeutic strategies in childhood obesity. *Hormone Research* **39**, 86–90.

Dreon, D.M., Frey-Hewitt, B., Ellsworth, N., WIlliams, P.T., Terry, R.B. & Wood, P.D. (1988) Dietary fat:carbohydrate ratio and obesity in middle-aged men. *American Journal of Clinical Nutrition* **47**, 995–1000.

Durnin, J.G.V.A., McKillop, M. (1978) The relationship between body build in infancy and percentage body fat in adolescence. A 14 year follow-up on 102 infants. *Proceedings of the Nutrition Society* **37**, 814.

Epstein, L.H., Wing, R.R., Penner, B.C. & Kress, M.J. (1985) The effect of diet and controlled exercise on weight loss in obese children. *Journal of Pediatrics* **107**, 358–361.

Epstein, L.H., Valoski, A., Wing, R.R. & McCurley, J. (1990) Ten year follow up of behavioural family based treatment for obese children. *Journal of the American Dietetics Association* **264**, 2519–2523.

Esposito-Del Puente, A., Contaldo, F., De Filippo, E. *et al.* (1996) High prevalence of overweight in a children population living in Naples (Italy). *International Journal of Obesity* **20**, 283–286.

FAO Nutrition Meeting Report Series, no. 52: WHO Technical Report Series no. 522 (1973) *Energy and Protein Requirements.* Geneva: Report of a joint FAO/WHO Ad Hoc Expert Committee.

FAO/WHO/UNU (1985) *Energy and Protein Requirements.* WHO Technical Report Series no. 724. Geneva: WHO.

Flatt, J.P. (1985) Energetics of intermediary metabolism. In: Garrow, J.S. & Halliday, D. (eds) *Substrate and Energy Metabolism in Man*, pp. 58–59. London: John Libbey.

Fontvieille, A.M., Dwyer, J. & Ravussin, E. (1992) Resting metabolic rate and body composition of Pima Indian and Caucasian children. *International Journal of Obesity*, **16**, 535–542.

Fontvieille, A.M., Harper, I.T., Ferraro, R.T., Sproul, M. & Ravussin, E. (1993a) Daily energy expenditure by five year old children, measured by doubly labelled water. *Journal of Pediatrics* **123**, 200–207.

Fontvieille, A.M., Krisha, A. & Ravussin, E. (1993b). Decreased physical activity in Pima Indians compared with Caucasian children. *International Journal of Obesity* **17**, 445–452.

Garrow, J.S. & Webster, J. (1985) Quetelet's Index (W/H^2) as a measure of fatness. *International Journal of Obesity* **9**, 147–153.

Gazzaniga, J.M. & Burns, T.L. (1993) Relationship between diet composition and body fatness, with adjustment for resting energy expenditure and physical activity, in pre-adolescent children. *American Journal of Clinical Nutrition* **58**, 21–28.

Goran, M.I., Carpenter, W.H. & Poehlman, E.T. (1993) Total energy expenditure in 4 to 6 year old children. *American Journal of Physiology* **264**, E706–E711.

Gortmaker, S.L., Doetz W.H., Sobel, A.M. & Wehter, C.A. (1987) Increasing pediatric obesity in the United States. *American Journal of Diseases in Childhood* **141**, 535–540.

Gregory, J.W., Greene, S.A., Scrimgeow, C.M. & Rennie, M.J. (1991) Body water measurements in growth disorders: a comparison of bioelectrical impedance and skinfold thickness techniques with isotope dilution. *Archives of Diseases in Childhood* **66**, 220–222.

Gregory, J.R., Collins, D.L., Davies, P.S.W., Hughes, J.M. & Clark, P.C. (1995) National diet and nutrition survey: children aged 1^1/$_2$ to 4^1/$_2$ years. London. HMSO.

Guillaume, M., Lapidus, L., Beckers, F., Drouget, B., Lambert, A.E. & Björntorp, P. (1993) Prevalence of obesity in Belgian Luxembourg. *International Journal of Obesity* **17** (suppl. 2), 36.

Hammar, S.L., Campbell, M.M. & Campbell, V.A. *et al.* (1972) An interdisciplinary study of adolescent obesity. *Journal of Pediatrics* **80**, 373–383.

Hampton, M.C., Hueneman, R.L., Shapiro, L.R. *et al.* (1967) Caloric and nutritional intake of teenagers. *Journal of the American Dietetics Association* **50**, 385–396.

Herberg, L., Doppen, W., Major, E. & Gries, F.A. (1974) Dietary-induced hypertrophic-hyperplastic obesity in mice. *Journal of Lipid Research* **15**, 580–585.

Hill, J.O. (1990) Body weight regulation in obese and obese-reduced rats. *International Journal of Obesity* **14** (suppl. 1), 31–45.

Hill, J.O., Fried, S.K. & DiGirolamo, M. (1983) Effects of a high fat diet on thermogenesis and brown adipose tissue in rats. *Life Sciences* **33**, 141–149.

Hill, J.O., Dorton, J., Sykes, M.N. & DiGirolamo, M. (1989) Duration of dietary obesity in rats influences resistance to obesity reversal. *International Journal of Obesity* **13**, 711–722.

Hills, A.P. & Parker, A.W. (1988) Obesity management via diet and exercise intervention. *Child: Care, Health and Development* **14**, 409–416.

Hillsdon, M., Thorogood, M., Anstiss, T. & Morris, J. (1995) Randomised controlled trials of physical activity promotion: a review. *Journal of Epidemiology and Community Health* **49**, 448–453.

James, L.P.T. (1985) Appetite control and other mechanisms of weight homeostasis. In: Blakres, K. & Waterloo, J.C. (eds) *Nutritional adaption in Man*, pp. 141–154. London: John Libbey.

Jen, K.L.C. (1988) Effects of diet composition on food intake and carcass composition in rats. *Physiology and Behavior* **42**, 551–556.

Johnson, M.L., Burke, B.S. & Mayer, J. (1956) Relative importance of inactivity and overeating in the energy balance of obese high school girls. *American Journal of Clinical Nutrition* **4**, 37–44.

Kendall, A., Levitsky, D.A., Strupp, B.J. & Lissner, L. (1991) Weight loss on a low fat diet: consequence of the imprecision of the control of food intake in humans. *American Journal of Clinical Nutrition* **53**, 1124–1129.

Khosla, T. & Lowe, C.R. (1967) Indices of obesity derived from body weight and height. *British Journal of Preventive and Social Medicine* **21**, 122–128.

Kromhout, D., Saris, W.H.M. & Horst, C.H. (1988) Energy intake, energy expenditure and smoking in relation to body fatness: The Zutphen Study. *American Journal of Clinical Nutrition* **47**, 668–674.

Landsberg, E. & Young, JB. (1983) The role of the sympathetic nervous system and catecholamines in the regulation of energy metabolism. *American Journal of Clinical Nutrition* **38**, 1018–1024.

Lernar, R.M. & Schroeder, C. (1971) Kindergarten children's active vocabulary about body build. *Developmental Psychology* **5**, 179.

Levin, B.E., Triscari, J. & Sullivan, A.C. (1986) Metabolic features of diet-induced obesity without hyperphagia in young rats. *American Journal of Physiology* **251**, R422–R440.

Lissner, L., Levitsky, D.A., Strupp B.J., Kalkwart, H.J. & Roe, D.A. (1987) Dietary fat and the regulation of energy intake in human subjects. *American Journal of Clinical Nutrition* **46**, 886–892.

Livingstone, M.B.E., Prentice, A.M., Strain, J.J. et al. (1990) Accuracy of weighed dietary records in studies of diet and health. *British Medical Journal* **300**, 708–712.

Lucas, F., Ackroff, K. & Sclafani, A. (1989) Dietary fat-induced hyperphagia in rats as a function of fat type and physical form. *Physiology and Behavior* **45**, 937–946.

Maffeis, C., Schutz, Y., Piccoli, R., Gonfiantini, E. & Pinelli, L. (1993) Prevalence of obesity in children in north-east Italy. *International Journal of Obesity* **17**, 287–294.

Miller, W.C., Lindeman, A.K., Wallace, J. & Niederpruem, N. (1990) Diet composition, energy intake and exercise in relation to body fat in men and women. *American Journal of Clinical Nutrition* **52**, 426–430.

Ministry of Agriculture Fisheries and Foods. (1995) *Household Food Consumption and Expenditure.* London: HMSO. 1940–94.

Oretega, R.M., Requejo, A.M., Andres, P., Lopez-Sobaler, A.M., Redondo, R. & Gonzalez-Fernandez, G. (1995) Relationship between diet composition and body mass index in a group of Spanish adolescents. *British Journal of Nutrition* **74**, 765–773.

Oscai, L.B., Brown, M.M. & Miller, W.C. (1984) Effect of dietary fat on food intake, growth and body composition in rats. *Growth* **48**, 415–424.

Oscai, L.B., Miller, W.C. & Arnall, D.A. (1987) Effect of dietary sugar and of dietary fat on food intake and body fat content in rats. *Growth* **51**, 64–73.

Payne, J.A. & Belton, N.R. (1992) Nutrient intake and growth in pre-school children. Comparison of energy intake and sources of energy with growth. *Journal of Human Nutrition and Dietetics* **5**, 287–298.

Pena, M., Bacallao, J., Barta, L., Regoly-Merel, A. & Tichy, M. (1980) The influence of physical exercise upon the body composition of obese children. *Acta Paediatrica Academiae Scientarum Hungaricae* **21**, 9–14.

Pena, M., Bacallao, J., Barta, L., Amader, M. & Johnson, F. (1989) Fiber and exercise in the treatment of obese adolescents. *Journal of Adolescent Health Care* **10**, 30–40.

Poskitt, E.M.E. & Cole, T.J. (1977) Do fat babies stay fat? *British Medical Journal* **1**, 7–9.

Prentice, A., Lucas, A., Vasquez-Velasquez, L., Davies, P.S.W & Whitehead, R.G. (1988) Are current dietary guidelines for young children a prescription for overfeeding. *Lancet* **ii**, 1066–1068.

Prentice, A.M. & Jebb, S.A. (1995) Obesity in Britain: gluttony or sloth? *British Medical Journal* **311**, 437–439.

Prewitt, T.E., Schmeisser, D., Bowen, P.E. *et al.* (1991) Changes in body weight, body composition and energy intake in women fed high and low fat diets. *American Journal of Clinical Nutrition* **54**, 304–310.

Reybrouck, T., Vinckx, J., Van Den Berghe, G. & Vanderschueren-Lodeweyckx, M. (1990) Exercise therapy and hypocaloric diet in the treatment of obese children and adolescents. *Acta Paediatrica Scandanavia* **79**, 84–89.

Rolland-Cachera, M.F. (1993) Assessment of obesity in children. *Nutrition Research* **13**, S95–S108.

Rolland-Cachera, M.F., Deheegar, M., Avorns, P. *et al.* (1987) Tracking the development of adiposity from one month of age to adulthood. *Annals of Human Biology* **14**, 219–229.

Rolland-Cachera, M.F., Deheeger, M., Ahrout, M. & Bellisle, F. (1995) Influence of macronutrients on adiposity development: a follow-up study of nutrition and growth from 10 months to 8 years of age. *International Journal of Obesity* **19**, 537–578.

Romieu, I., Willett, W.C., Stampfer, M.J. *et al.* (1988) Energy intake and determinants of relative weight. *American Journal of Clinical Nutrition* **47**, 406–412.

Sallade, J. (1973) A comparison of the psychological adjustment of obese and non-obese children. *Journal of Psychosomatic Research* **17**, 89–96.

Schoeller, D.A. & van Santen, E. (1982) Measurement of energy expenditure in humans by doubly labelled water. *Journal of Applied Physiology* **53**, 955–959.

Schofield, W.N. (1985) Predicting basal metabolic rate, new standards and review of previous work. *Human Nutrition: Clinical Nutrition* **39C** (suppl. 1), 5–41.

Seltzer, C.C. & Mayer, J. (1970) An effective weight control program in a public school system. *American Journal of Public Health* **60**, 679–689.

Sims, E.A.H. & Danforth, E. (1987) Expenditure and storage of energy in man. *Journal of Clinical Investigation* **76**, 1019–1024.

Southgate, D.A.T. (1986) Obese deceivers. *British Medical Journal* **292**, 1692–1693.

Triscari, J., Nauss-Karol, C., Levin, B.E. & Sullivan, A.C. (1985) Changes in lipid metabolism in diet-induced obesity. *Metabolism* **34**, 580–587.

Tucker, L.A. & Kano, M.J. (1992) Dietary fat and body fat: a multivariate study of 205 adult females. *American Journal of Clinical Nutrition* **56**, 616–622.

CHAPTER 14

....

Diabetes and Obesity

JOHN WILDING AND GARETH WILLIAMS

....

Introduction

Associations have been recognized for centuries between obesity and diabetes—indeed, Hindu physicians of 1500 years ago described a syndrome affecting older overweight patients who passed large volumes of sweet-tasting urine. Overall, non-insulin-dependent diabetes (NIDDM) is the most important medical consequence of obesity, because it is common, can inflict a wide range of damage on the individual, and is expensive to manage. NIDDM is rapidly becoming one of the major diseases in Western populations and will increasingly threaten developing countries. It accounts for 80–85% of the estimated 110 million diabetic patients world-wide, a number which is likely to reach 180 million by the year 2010 (WHO Study Group, 1997). In practical terms, obesity plays a major aetiological role in perhaps 80% of cases of NIDDM and remains a major obstacle to the successful long-term management of the disease. On this basis, obesity is arguably the most important problem in diabetes care world-wide.

Most of this chapter focuses on NIDDM. We shall first review the evidence that obesity predisposes to NIDDM and the ways in which increased fat mass might be diabetogenic; the interface between obesity and diabetes is of considerable scientific interest, and the mechanisms linking metabolism and the storage of energy are now being actively explored at the molecular level. The effects of overweight on insulin-dependent diabetes (IDDM) and chronic diabetic complications will also be considered. Finally, the impact of obesity on the practical management of NIDDM will be discussed, together with strategies to treat overweight in diabetes. We shall concentrate on human NIDDM, but where appropriate, will also consider relevant animal syndromes of obesity and NIDDM.

Obesity and NIDDM in humans

Many genetic and environmental factors interact to determine whether an individual will develop NIDDM. Obesity, especially in a truncal distribution, impairs insulin action and thus contributes to the insulin resistance which is a fundamental defect in the pathogenesis of NIDDM. The strong associations of obesity with NIDDM are highlighted by numerous cross-sectional surveys within and between populations, while longitudinal prospective studies indicate that obesity often precedes and predisposes to glucose intolerance.

Epidemiological associations of obesity with NIDDM

NIDDM becomes progressively commoner in populations with higher prevalences of obesity (Fig. 14.1). The diabetogenic effects of obesity have been graphically illustrated by certain 'experiments of acculturation', in which the sedentary overindulgence of the Western lifestyle has been rapidly inflicted on circumscribed populations that previously survived at subsistence level. The best-known examples include the Pima Indians of Arizona, the Micronesian Nauruan Islanders and Chinese immigrants to Mauritius (WHO Study Group, 1997). All these groups were previously lean and diabetes was a rarity, but the last few decades have witnessed the epidemic spread of obesity followed by a rising tide of NIDDM. At present, 80% of adult Pimas are obese and the prevalence of NIDDM (40% of adults, 70% of those over 60 years of age) is the highest in the world (Zimmet, 1982). These celebrated examples may over-estimate the diabetogenic impact of Westernization, because 'thrifty' genes

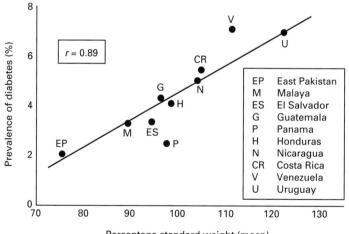

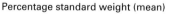

Fig. 14.1 Relationship between the prevalence of diabetes (predominantly NIDDM) and body-weight in 10 representative populations. Body-weight is expressed as the population mean, relative to a 'standard' weight which is given an arbitrary score of 100. From West (1978).

may have been selected during the previous struggle of these populations to survive under harsh conditions. Furthermore, weight gain in adult life may predispose particularly strongly to NIDDM in people who were malnourished *in utero* and in childhood (see later), and this was probably the case in many of these groups before the advent of Westernization.

Many studies have confirmed that NIDDM is commoner amongst overweight people and, more significantly, that the risk of developing the disease rises progressively with increasing fat mass, whether measured as body mass index (BMI) or percentage of 'ideal' body-weight. A massive study of over 50 000 North American men illustrates the diabetogenic hazards of obesity particularly clearly: the relative risk rises steadily once BMI exceeds the surprising low threshold of $24\,\text{kg/m}^2$, reaching 80 times that in lean subjects for individuals with a BMI of $> 35\,\text{kg/m}^2$ compared with those whose BMI was $< 23\,\text{kg/m}^2$ (Fig. 14.2a). The study also showed that weight gain after the age of 21 consistently increases the risks of developing diabetes and amplifies the effect of BMI at that age (Fig. 14.2b) (Chan *et al.*, 1994).

The anatomical distribution as well as the total bulk of adipose tissue is important in determining susceptibility to NIDDM. Vague first pointed out, over 40 years ago, the strong association with diabetes of 'android' (upper body, or truncal) obesity, characterized by an 'apple-shaped' deposition of subcutaneous and visceral fat affecting the abdomen (Vague, 1956). Truncal obesity is now recognized as an integral feature of the 'insulin-resistance' syndrome ('metabolic syndrome', or 'syndrome X'), together with dyslipidaemia, hypertension, hyper-insulinaemia and glucose intolerance (including NIDDM), a procoagulant tendency and accelerated atheroma formation (Fig. 14.3) (Reaven, 1988). Excess abdominal fat may itself contribute to the insulin resistance which has been suggested to underlie many if not all of the syndrome's abnormalities. By contrast, 'gynoid' obesity in a gluteo-femoral or 'pear-shaped' distribution is more weakly associated with syndrome X and with its ultimate end-point of premature death from atherosclerotic disease (Björntorp, 1994).

Abdominal fat deposition can be identified crudely by a high waist/hip ratio (WHR), and Fig. 14.4 shows the synergistic interaction of WHR with general adiposity (measured by BMI) on the 10-year risk of developing NIDDM in a Swedish population (Larsson *et al.*, 1994). Also illustrated in this figure is the over-riding importance of truncal rather than general obesity on ischaemic heart disease, which in this study was not influenced by BMI. The large study of American men suggests that waist circumference is also a strong predictor of diabetes (Chan *et al.*, 1994).

Non-invasive computed tomography and magnetic resonance imaging have made it possible to measure the individual components of abdominal fat, namely the subcutaneous and retroperitoneal depots (which both drain into the

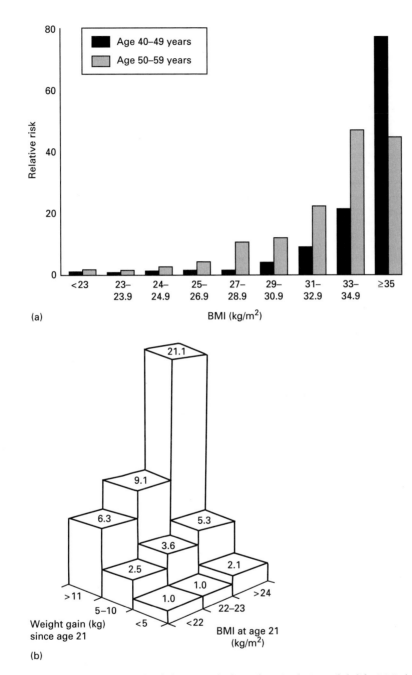

(a)

(b)

Fig. 14.2 Diabetogenic hazards of obesity and of weight gain during adult life. (a) Relative risks of developing diabetes in 5 years (risk defined as 1.0 for a BMI of < 23.0 kg/m²) as a function of BMI, in American men aged 40–49 and 50–59 years. (b) Relative risks of developing diabetes (defined as 1.0 for the lowest tertiles), as function of BMI at age 21 and of weight gained since that age. Data are from the Health Professionals' Follow-up Study of 51 529 American men. From Chan *et al.* (1994).

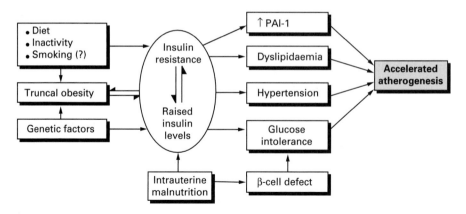

Fig. 14.3 Features of the 'insulin-resistance' syndrome (syndrome X). From Yki-Järvinen & Williams (1997).

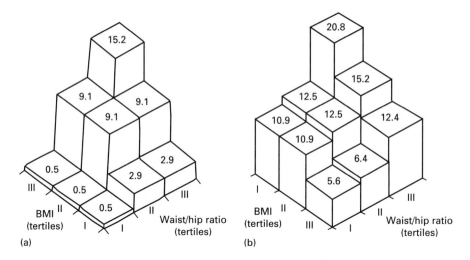

Fig. 14.4 Importance of truncal obesity (indicated by tertiles of WHR) in predicting the risk for developing (a) diabetes and (b) ischaemic heart disease (IHD). General obesity, measured as tertiles of BMI, synergizes with WHR in predicting NIDDM but has no predictive value for IHD (note reversed BMI tertiles). (a) From Larsson *et al.* (1985); (b) from Larsson *et al.* (1984).

systemic circulation), and the visceral fat in the mesentery and omentum which drains into the portal system and thus gains immediate access to the liver (Bergstrom *et al.*, 1990). Controversy persists as to which of these depots carries responsibility for the metabolic disturbances of syndrome X, particularly the insulin resistance and glucose intolerance. Several studies point to a dominant role of visceral fat, which would be consistent with the suggested metabolic effects of non-esterified fatty acids (NEFA) and other adipose tissue products on the liver, while others implicate the subcutaneous depot (Abate *et al.*, 1996; Lemieux *et al.*, 1996). The possible ways in which abdominal fat depots might specifically predispose to glucose intolerance are discussed below and in Chapter 8.

Overall, these data indicate that obesity (especially truncal) is strongly associated with glucose intolerance and NIDDM, but it must be remembered that correlation does not prove causation. At least 20% of NIDDM patients are not obese, and even in the highest-risk group with high BMI and WHR, over 80% of subjects will escape NIDDM (Colditz *et al.*, 1995). Obesity is therefore an important risk factor, but is neither sufficient nor obligatory for the development of NIDDM. As discussed below, obesity must interact to a variable degree with other inherited and/or acquired diabetogenic factors that determine insulin resistance and β-cell dysfunction, in order to lead to NIDDM in an individual.

Pathophysiological links between obesity and NIDDM

This section will focus on metabolic abnormalities of NIDDM and obesity and their possible genetic and environmental causes, and then will attempt to show how obesity might contribute to the causation of NIDDM. Firstly, relevant aspects of normal metabolism and the pathophysiology of NIDDM will be briefly reviewed (see Fig. 14.5).

NORMAL METABOLISM: THE KEY ROLE OF INSULIN

Insulin is synthesized and secreted by the β cells of the islets of Langerhans. It is cleaved from proinsulin under the action of specific proteolytic enzymes, liberating equimolar amounts of C-peptide. Normally, proinsulin is almost completely processed in this way and only small amounts of insulin precursors (proinsulin itself and its 'split products') enter the circulation. Insulin is coreleased with amylin (islet amyloid polypeptide, IAPP), which in humans and certain other species can polymerize to form insoluble amyloid fibrils that may accumulate within the islets, and that might contribute to β-cell failure in patients with NIDDM (Bennet *et al.*, 1994).

Under basal conditions, insulin is released in small regular pulses every 9–12 minutes (Matthews, 1991). Insulin secretion is rapidly stimulated by rises in the extracellular glucose concentration. The β cell senses ambient glucose levels through a tightly-yoked mechanism comprising the GLUT2 glucose transporter (which operates independently of insulin and therefore allows glucose to enter the β cell in proportion to its extracellular concentration) and glucokinase, the rate-limiting enzyme of the glycolytic pathway. Glycolysis metabolizes glucose to generate adenosine triphosphate (ATP), which closes ATP-sensitive K^+ channels in the β-cell membrane; this prevents K^+ ions from leaving the β cell and depolarizes the membrane, which in turn opens voltage-gated Ca^{2+} channels in the membrane and allows extracellular Ca^{2+} ions to enter the cell. The rise in cystosolic Ca^{2+} concentrations triggers exocytosis of the insulin-containing secretory granules (Howell, 1997).

Insulin action

Insulin begins the chain of events leading to its many biological actions by

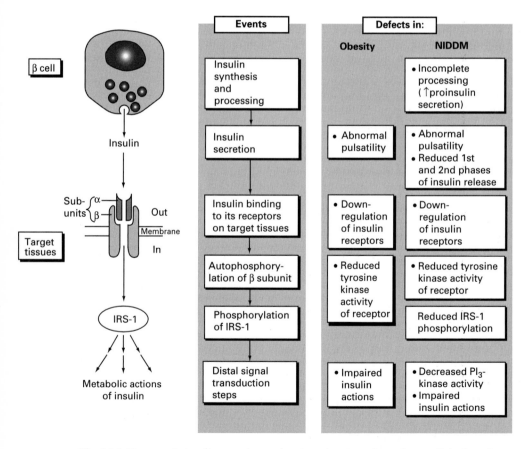

Fig. 14.5 Key steps in insulin secretion and action, showing where abnormalities have been identified in obesity and NIDDM. IRS-1, insulin receptor substrate-1.

binding to its receptors on the cell surface of its target tissues (Fig. 14.5). The insulin receptor comprises two entirely extracellular α subunits which include the insulin-binding site, each linked covalently to a β subunit that spans the cell membrane. The intracellular part of the β subunit includes a domain with tyrosine kinase activity that, following insulin binding, catalyses autophosphorylation, i.e., the transfer of phosphate groups from ATP to other tyrosine residues within the β subunit. The activated receptor then phosphorylates a 131-kDa protein, insulin receptor substrate-1 (IRS-1), which has multiple sites for binding and phosphorylating other intermediate proteins that transmit the signal of insulin binding to the cell's interior. Details of the subsequent events of signal transduction remain uncertain. After binding, the insulin–receptor complex is internalized, when the receptor may be either degraded or recycled back to the cell surface; high ambient insulin concentrations reduce ('down-regulate') the numbers of insulin receptors on target-cell surfaces (Maratos-Flier *et al.*, 1997).

Major metabolic actions of insulin

Insulin regulates all branches of metabolism; although diabetes is defined in terms of hyperglycaemia, disorders of insulin secretion or action also interfere with lipid and protein metabolism, and lipid disturbances may be particularly important in explaining the links between obesity and NIDDM.

Carbohydrate metabolism. Insulin lowers blood glucose concentrations through two distinct mechanisms (Fig. 14.6). Firstly, at the lower circulating levels found between meals, insulin suppresses the generation and secretion of glucose by the liver. Hepatic glucose output (HGO) is fuelled by both gluconeogenesis (the production of glucose from precursors such as lactate and alanine) and the breakdown of glycogen. Insulin inhibits gluconeogenesis, primarily at the level of phosphoenolpyruvate carboxykinase (PEPCK), its rate-limiting enzyme. It also promotes glycogen accumulation by stimulating glycogen synthetase while inhibiting glycogen phosphorylase. Insulin's actions on the liver are opposed by catecholamines in the circulation and released from hepatic sympathetic nerves, and by the other 'counter-regulatory' hormones, particularly glucagon, growth hormone and cortisol; these all therefore increase HGO and raise blood glucose.

The second glucose-lowering action of insulin is the stimulation of glucose uptake into peripheral tissues, particularly skeletal muscle (quantitatively the most important) and fat. Insulin enhances glucose uptake by stimulating the synthesis of the GLUT4 glucose transporter protein and, acutely, by inducing the translocation of GLUT4 units from the cell's interior to its surface (Fig.

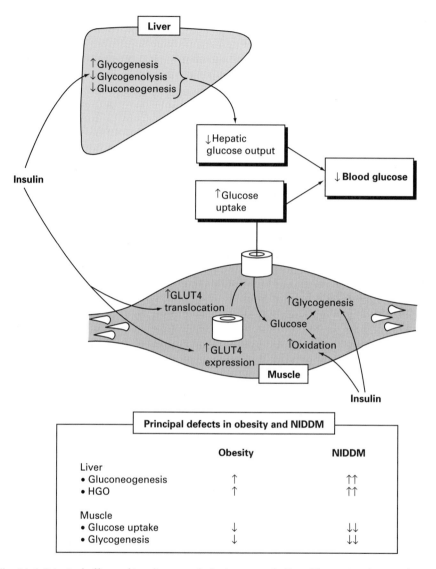

Fig. 14.6 Principal effects of insulin on carbohydrate metabolism. The major abnormalities in obesity and NIDDM are also shown. HGO, hepatic glucose output.

14.6). GLUT4 acts as a hydrophilic channel that allows the polar glucose molecule to follow its concentration gradient across the hydrophobic cell membrane. Relatively high insulin concentrations, as occur after eating, are required to increase glucose uptake. Insulin-stimulated glucose uptake is superimposed on basal levels of 'non-insulin-mediated glucose uptake' (NIMGU) which is facilitated by other glucose transporters, particularly GLUT1 and GLUT2.

The fate of glucose taken up by peripheral tissues is again governed by the balance between insulin and the counter-regulatory hormones. In muscle, glucose is either metabolized to produce ATP or is stored as glycogen; in fat, it is converted to glycerol-3-phosphate, which combines with NEFA to form triglyceride, and thus participates in lipogenesis.

Fat metabolism. One of insulin's main effects is to inhibit the breakdown of triglyceride (lipolysis) stored in adipose tissue, which liberates NEFA and glycerol. NEFA may be important in mediating insulin resistance by interfering with glucose metabolism in skeletal muscle and liver (Boden, 1997, and see below). Lipolysis is exquisitely sensitive to inhibition by insulin and is normally suppressed even by low basal insulin concentrations; it is therefore switched on substantially only when insulin levels fall further, e.g., during fasting. Lipolysis is strongly stimulated by catecholamines in the circulation or released from sympathetic nerve terminals in adipose tissue, and by other circulating counter-regulatory hormones. Total lipolysis is also enhanced when the fat mass is expanded, and there is some evidence that visceral adipose tissue may be more sensitive to catecholamine-induced lipolysis and more insensitive to the anti-lipolytic effects of insulin, as compared with other depots (Kruszynska, 1997).

PATHOGENESIS OF NIDDM

NIDDM is a heterogeneous collection of syndromes, due to variable interactions between numerous possible inherited and environmental factors that result in variable combinations of insulin resistance and insulin deficiency. The aetiology of NIDDM may therefore differ substantially between phenotypically similar individuals. The molecular basis of certain uncommon NIDDM syndromes (e.g., maturity-onset diabetes of the young, MODY) has now been elucidated, but the fundamental causes of the 'common' variant of NIDDM remain a mystery (Hattersley, 1997). Obesity is thought to predispose to NIDDM primarily by aggravating insulin insensitivity, through the postulated mechanisms described below.

Insulin resistance in NIDDM

Several aspects of insulin action are known to be impaired in NIDDM, notably in carbohydrate and lipid metabolism, and lead to hyperglycaemia and raised NEFA concentrations (Fig. 14.7). Blunting of insulin's normal ability to suppress gluconeogenesis and glycogenolysis in the liver leads to a sustained rise in HGO, which contributes to the generally increased basal blood glucose levels on which the exaggerated meal-time glycaemic peaks are superimposed. Recent

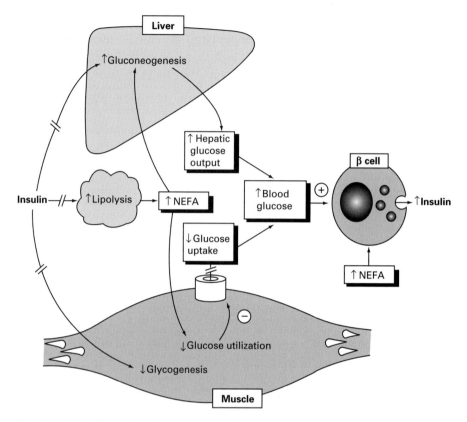

Fig. 14.7 Main effects of insulin resistance on lipid and carbohydrate metabolism. Interruption of insulin action, as in obesity and NIDDM, leads to increased HGO, decreased glucose uptake into muscle and thus to hyperglycaemia. Lipolysis is disinhibited, resulting in increased NEFA levels which may further exacerbate insulin resistance in liver and muscle. Hyperinsulinaemia is due mainly to increased insulin secretion, stimulated by raised glucose and NEFA levels: NEFA may also raise peripheral insulin levels by decreasing insulin clearance by the liver.

isotopic studies indicate that the main hepatic abnormality is the failure of insulin to inhibit gluconeogenesis (Consoli *et al.*, 1989; Jeng *et al.*, 1994). Insensitivity to insulin action in skeletal muscle, quantitatively the most important site of peripheral glucose disposal, results in hyperglycaemia after meals, when the rise in plasma insulin levels would normally stimulate GLUT4-mediated glucose uptake, thereby clearing glucose that enters the circulation from the gut. *In vivo* magnetic resonance spectroscopy and biopsy studies indicate that glycogen synthesis and glucose oxidation are both impaired, the former particularly so (Johnson *et al.*, 1991; Rothman *et al.*, 1991). Together, these defects in glucose handling are responsible for the basal and exaggerated postprandial hyperglycaemia of NIDDM.

The impact of insulin resistance on lipid metabolism has recently attracted much attention. Loss of insulin's anti-lipolytic action allows triglyceride in fat to break down, liberating glycerol (a substrate for gluconeogenesis) and NEFA (see Fig. 14.7). As discussed below, high NEFA levels may antagonize insulin

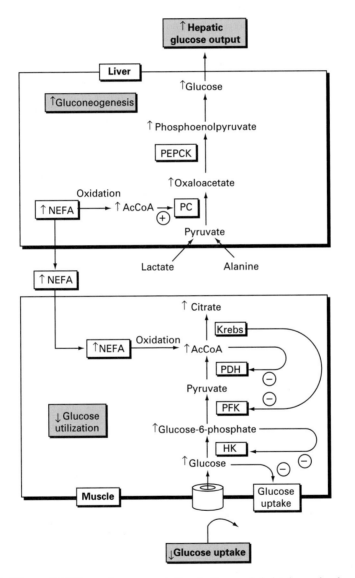

Fig. 14.8 Effects of NEFA on glucose metabolism in liver and skeletal muscle, showing the 'Randle' (glucose–fatty acid) cycle through which NEFA are postulated to impair glucose tolerance and induce insulin resistance. AcCoA, acetyl coenzyme; HK, hexokinase; Krebs, Krebs cycle; PC, pyruvate carboxylase; PDH, pyruvate dehydrogenase; PEPCK, phosphoenolpyruvate carboxykinase; PFK, phosphofructokinase. ⊖, inhibitor; ⊕ stimulation.

action, particularly when NEFA generated by visceral fat depots are delivered directly to the liver via the portal vein (Randle *et al.*, 1963; Boden, 1997; Fig. 14.8).

The raised glucose and NEFA concentrations initially stimulate insulin release (both are direct secretagogues), and the resulting hyperinsulinaemia is enough to overcome the effects of insulin resistance and tends to normalize blood glucose and NEFA (Kruszynska, 1997). Hyperinsulinaemia may be accentuated by high NEFA levels which may decrease the hepatic clearance of insulin (Peiris *et al.*, 1986). Chronically high glucose and NEFA levels may impair, rather than stimulate, β-cell function and may contribute to the decline in insulin secretion which leads to overt hyperglycaemia and NIDDM (Boden *et al.*, 1995; Fig. 14.9).

Mechanisms of insulin resistance in NIDDM. Insulin resistance is measured most commonly as the failure of high insulin concentrations to stimulate whole-body glucose disposal under hyperinsulinaemic, euglycaemic 'clamp' conditions. Insulin sensitivity spans a wide spectrum in all populations, and there is some overlap between apparently normal euglycaemic subjects and those with 'insulin-resistant' states such as NIDDM (Yki-Järvinen, 1995).

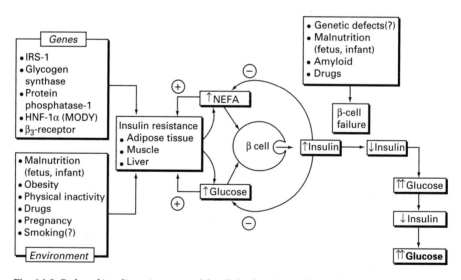

Fig. 14.9 Roles of insulin resistance and β-cell dysfunction in the pathogenesis of NIDDM. Initially, increased insulin secretion can compensate for insulin resistance, as hyperinsulinaemia can nearly normalize blood NEFA and glucose levels. Raised NEFA and glucose levels may exacerbate insulin resistance. Ultimately, insulin secretion fails, when the declining insulin levels allow blood glucose to rise rapidly into the diabetic range. HNF-1α, hepatic nuclear factor-1α.

Insulin resistance in NIDDM primarily affects postreceptor mechanisms rather than the insulin receptor itself (see Figs 14.5 and 14.6). Insulin receptor numbers may be reduced on target tissues, possibly through down-regulation in response to hyperinsulinaemia; perhaps because of the large number of 'spare' receptors, this does not appear to make an important contribution to insulin insensitivity (DeFronzo, 1988). Numerous mutations of the insulin receptor have been identified and some confer severe insulin resistance, but all are very rare and are not involved in common NIDDM (O'Rahilly & Moller, 1992). Various postreceptor defects have been identified in NIDDM (see Fig. 14.6). but most appear to be secondary to the metabolic disturbance of NIDDM rather than prime movers.

NIDDM has a strong genetic component, accounting for up to 80% of overall disease susceptibility (Fig. 14.9) (McCarthy et al., 1994). A single gene may be responsible in some families, but the combined effect of several diabetogenic genes seems more likely in most cases of 'common' NIDDM. The identity of these genes remains elusive, but many studies indicate that insulin resistance may be an inherited trait. Mutations in various candidate genes could confer insulin resistance, including those encoding metabolic enzymes or signal-transduction mediators (see Fig. 14.9). Some of these could plausibly explain certain metabolic abnormalities in NIDDM, as well as links between obesity, insulin resistance and glucose intolerance. For example, a point mutation (Trp64Arg) in the β_3-adrenoceptor which governs lipolysis in visceral adipose tissue is associated with various diabetogenic effects, including insulin insensitivity, obesity and an earlier onset of NIDDM; theoretically, the mutation could favour excessive lipolysis in visceral fat, leading to increased NEFA delivery to the liver and increased HGO (see below) (Kurabayashi et al., 1996). The possible role of 'thrifty' genes that favour energy storage as fat and that might therefore predispose to obesity is discussed below. At present, however, none of these genes has been assigned a dominant role in common NIDDM, and several have been positively excluded.

Various environmental factors may induce insulin resistance, perhaps beginning with malnutrition in utero and during early childhood. Several studies in different populations have now supported the original observations by Barker and Hales that glucose intolerance and other features of syndrome X were commoner in middle-aged people who were underweight at birth and at 1 year of age (Fall et al., 1995). This diabetogenic effect is more likely to be manifested if the subjects become overweight in later life, presumably because of the additional burden of obesity-related insulin resistance. Insulin resistance, especially in skeletal muscle, may be responsible and a recent study has demonstrated abnormalities in muscle metabolism in such subjects that may have been 'programmed' by poor nutrition in early life (Thompson *et al.*, 1997). The broad principles of this concept (rather cryptically named the 'thrifty phenotype') are now generally accepted, but its mechanisms and pathophysiological significance remain controversial.

Several other environmental or acquired factors are known to reduce insulin sensitivity, including obesity itself, reduced physical activity, pregnancy (due to the counter-regulatory effects of placental and ovarian hormones), glucocorticoids and other drugs, and perhaps smoking. Interestingly, raised blood glucose levels in established diabetes may further impair tissue insulin sensitivity, through ill-defined mechanisms ('glucotoxicity') (Yki-Järvinen, 1992).

β-cell dysfunction in NIDDM

This is the critical factor which determines whether or not an individual can maintain near-normoglycaemia by hypersecreting enough insulin to overcome the effects of insulin resistance, or will deteriorate into hyperglycaemia and NIDDM. Longitudinal studies have shown that insulin resistance precedes β-cell failure by several years, and that insulin levels fall at the transition from the prediabetic state of impaired glucose tolerance (IGT)—compensatory hyperinsulinaemia with only slightly elevated blood glucose levels—to overt NIDDM (DeFronzo, 1992). The bell-shaped profile that describes the natural history of β-cell function in NIDDM, rising to a plateau representing IGT before declining into β-cell failure and diabetes, has been termed the 'Starling curve' of the pancreas (Fig. 14.10) (DeFronzo *et al.*, 1992).

The causes of β-cell failure are not known. The normal pulsatile pattern of basal insulin secretion is disturbed in non-diabetic first-order relatives of some NIDDM patients with familial NIDDM and, at least in these pedigrees, β-cell dysfunction may be partly inherited (O'Rahilly *et al.*, 1986). Malnutrition in early life has also been suggested to impair insulin secretion as well as insulin action (Hales & Barker, 1992). In addition, acquired metabolic factors may contribute.

Hyperglycaemia *per se* may interfere with insulin secretion—another manifestation of glucotoxicity—as may raised NEFA levels (Yki-Jarvinen, 1992; Boden *et al.*, 1995). Amylin, the β-cell product cosecreted with insulin, acts on the β cell to inhibit insulin secretion, and it has been suggested but not proven that the accumulation within the islet of amyloid fibrils composed of polymerized amylin chains can damage the β cells. Proinsulin processing is defective in many patients with NIDDM, resulting in increased circulating levels of proinsulin and its split products, but it is not clear whether this represents a primary β-cell

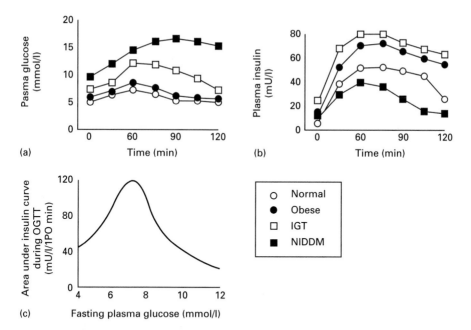

Fig. 14.10 Changes in (a) blood glucose and (b) insulin levels during the progression from normal glucose tolerance with compensatory hyperinsulinaemia in obese subjects to IGT with maximal hyperinsulinaemia, and finally to NIDDM with overt hyperglycaemia when β-cell failure leads to a fall in insulin levels. This sequence of events is described as the 'Starling curve' of the pancreas (c). From DeFronzo *et al.* (1992).

abnormality or results from the increased drive to produce and secrete insulin (Bennet *et al.*, 1994).

DIABETOGENIC EFFECTS OF OBESITY

The strong association of obesity with NIDDM could be explained in various ways. The generally accepted view is that obesity predisposes to NIDDM; it is assumed to do this by aggravating insulin resistance, and some proposed mechanisms are discussed below. An alternative model is that common factors — genetic and/or environmental — predispose to both obesity and NIDDM. An example of the latter may be 'thrifty' genes that favour storage of energy as fat, and that might therefore be selected through survival under conditions of recurrent famine. Thrifty genes might operate by impairing insulin action in skeletal muscle; this would have the dual effect of inducing insulin resistance in muscle and, under the influence of hyperinsulinaemia, of encouraging triglyceride deposition in fat. Both these effects would be enhanced under Westernized

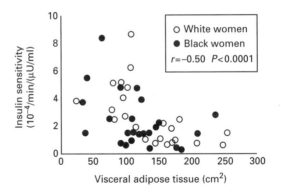

Fig. 14.11 Abdominal obesity is associated with insulin resistance. In this study of white and black American women, visceral fat mass was significantly inversely correlated with whole-body insulin sensitivity (S_I) under hyperinsulinaemic euglycaemic 'clamp' conditions, which largely reflects glucose uptake into skeletal muscle. Subcutaneous adipose tissue mass was not significantly correlated with S_I. Reproduced from Albu (1997).

conditions with readily available high-energy food, and could contribute to the rapid appearance of obesity and NIDDM in populations such as the Pima Indians and Nauruans (Neel, 1962).

In general, worsening obesity is accompanied by a decline in whole-body insulin sensitivity, and abdominal fat deposition is particularly strongly associated with glucose intolerance (Fig. 14.11). Obese patients who progress from normoglycaemia through IGT to overt NIDDM show the typical initial compensatory rise and subsequent decline in β-cell function (see Fig. 14.10). However, obesity is just one of several potential causes of insulin sensitivity, and even morbid obesity may not be enough to precipitate NIDDM in an individual (Bonadonna & DeFronzo, 1992). Nonetheless, in subjects with established NIDDM, the degree of obesity correlates closely with the severity of insulin resistance.

Numerous defects in insulin action and in intracellular signalling have been demonstrated in obese patients. These defects point to primarily postreceptor insulin resistance, and are broadly similar to but generally less severe than those in NIDDM (Figs 14.5 and 14.6). As with NIDDM, the primacy of these abnormalities is yet to be established.

Mediators of insulin resistance in obesity

The most likely explanation for insulin resistance worsening as fat mass increases is that specific adipocyte products can induce insulin insensitivity. Candidate diabetogenic factors include NEFA, tumour necrosis factor-α (TNF-α) and leptin (Fig. 14.12).

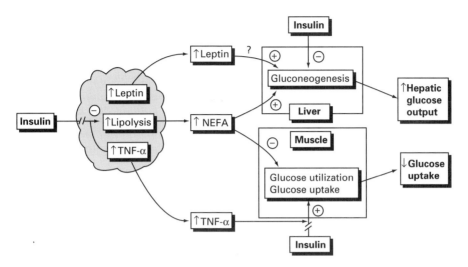

Fig. 14.12 Possible mediators of insulin resistance in obesity. Putative diabetogenic factors produced by fat include NEFA, TNF-α and possibly leptin.

Circulating levels of NEFA, liberated by lipolysis from adipocytes, are raised in obesity (Boden, 1997). The basal rate of lipolysis increases as fat mass rises, although the mechanism in unknown. High NEFA levels are thought to induce insulin insensitivity in liver and muscle, through the Randle (glucose–fatty acid) cycle (see Fig. 14.8) (Randle *et al.*, 1963). In muscle, acetyl CoA generated by the oxidation of NEFA inhibits pyruvate dehydrogenase, leading to reduced glucose utilization. The resulting increase in intracellular glucose flattens the transmembrane concentration gradient that drives glucose into the cell, leading to a secondary reduction in glucose uptake. In liver, the accumulation of acetyl CoA also interferes with glucose metabolism, by inhibiting pyruvate carboxylase and stimulating gluconeogenesis. Raised NEFA concentrations therefore lead to enhanced hepatic glucose production and decreased glucose uptake into muscle, thus tending to increase blood glucose concentrations and effectively opposing insulin action. Raised NEFA levels also inhibit the extraction of insulin by the liver, further increasing circulating insulin concentrations. NEFA secreted directly into the portal circulation could be particularly diabetogenic as they are delivered directly to the liver, and this could explain the reported association of visceral (mesenteric and omental) fat deposition with insulin resistance, hyperinsulinaemia and glucose intolerance (Abate *et al.*, 1996; Boden, 1997). However, as already mentioned, other studies have suggested that subcutaneous abdominal fat (which drains into the systemic circulation) has a greater metabolic impact.

TNF-α is a cytokine, first identified as a macrophage product and implicated in the metabolic disturbances of malignancy and chronic inflammation. The experimental actions of TNF-α include anorexia and weight loss (hence its alternative name, 'cachectin') and the induction of insulin resistance. TNF-α messenger RNA (mRNA) is present in adipose tissue and skeletal muscle, and its expression is increased in obese rodents and humans and correlates with BMI and plasma insulin levels. TNF-α may act in an endocrine and/or autocrine fashion upon fat and muscle to induce insulin resistance, and it has been shown to inhibit the tyrosine kinase activity of the insulin receptor, thus impairing insulin action (Hotamisligil & Spiegelman, 1994). Immunoneutralization of TNF-α in the *fa/fa* Zucker rat substantially improves insulin sensitivity, but initial trials of TNF-α antibodies in humans have proved disappointing; its role in the insulin resistance of human obesity therefore remains uncertain (Caro *et al.*, 1996). Recent studies have shown selectively increased expression of the TNFR2 (p80) TNF-α receptor in fat from obese humans and mice; this could modulate the biological activity of TNF-α and contribute to the metabolic disturbances of obesity, although the detailed mechanisms are yet to be clarified (Hotamisligil *et al.*, 1997).

Leptin, the product of the *ob* gene (see below and Chapter 3), may also contribute to the insulin resistance of obesity. In obese patients, plasma leptin levels rise broadly in parallel with body fat mass and with insulin resistance (Caro *et al.*, 1996). Most studies of leptin have focused on its anti-obesity actions and the secondary improvements in insulin resistance that follow weight loss. However, recent reports have shown that plasma leptin levels correlate with insulin resistance independently of obesity, and leptin has been shown to inhibit aspects of insulin action on hepatocytes *in vitro*, resulting in enhanced gluconeogenesis (Cohen *et al.*, 1996). The possible effects of leptin on insulin sensitivity are currently under investigation.

Links between obesity and NIDDM in animal syndromes

Many obese animals display insulin resistance and glucose intolerance, and some develop clinically obvious hyperglycaemia, generally without significant ketosis, analogous to human NIDDM. Although no single animal model perfectly matches the disease in humans, some have provided important insights into the pathophysiology of the condition and have been widely used to test both hypotheses and anti-diabetic drugs.

This section discusses the possible links between obesity and NIDDM in some of the classical single-gene rodent syndromes, namely the *ob/ob* and *db/db* mice and the *fa/fa* Zucker rat. Mutations in the genes encoding the adipocyte hormone leptin or its receptors are now known to be the fundamental lesions in these models. The *ob* (obese) mutation affects the leptin gene and prevents the production of biologically-active leptin (Zhang *et al.*, 1994), while the *db* (diabetes) and *fa* (fatty) mutations both affect the leptin receptor (OB-R), which exists in various isoforms (Tartaglia *et al.*, 1995; Chen *et al.*, 1996). The *db* mutation truncates the intracellular portion of the extended isoform (OB-Rb) that is expressed in the hypothalamus, removing the signal-transduction domain and thus conferring leptin insensitivity (Lee *et al.*, 1996). The *fa* mutation (Gln269Pro) lies in the extracellular portion of the receptor and may impair both leptin transport into the brain and neuronal sensitivity to leptin's appetite-suppressing action (Phillips *et al.*, 1996; Takaya *et al.*, 1996).

Leptin acts on the central nervous system (CNS), probably the hypothalamus, to inhibit feeding and stimulate thermogenesis, resulting in mobilization of fat and weight loss. *Ob/ob* mice are highly sensitive to the anti-obesity actions of leptin, which corrects obesity and insulin insensitivity and lowers blood glucose towards normal. Normal lean mice are less sensitive to leptin, while *fa/fa* rats are markedly leptin-insensitive and *db/db* mice are totally resistant (Campfield *et al.*, 1995; Cusin *et al.*, 1996). Leptin may act in part by inhibiting neurones in the hypothalamus which express neuropeptide Y (NPY) (Wang *et al.*, 1997) and it has been suggested that increased activity of these neurones may contribute to the obesity in these models (McKibbin *et al.*, 1991; Wilding *et al.*, 1993), and possibly also to the insulin resistance and other metabolic abnormalities (Zarjevski *et al.*, 1993) (Fig. 14.13). Other neural systems are evidently also

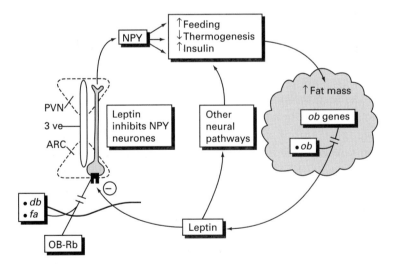

Fig. 14.13 Interactions between leptin and NPY-ergic neurones of the hypothalamic arcuate nucleus (ARC), in the control of energy homeostasis and body fat mass. The inhibitory effects of leptin on the NPY neurones are lost through the *ob* mutation (which prevents the production of biologically active leptin) and through the *db* and *fa* mutations in the OB-Rb leptin receptor isoform expressed by these (and other) neurones.

involved, as knockout of the NPY gene in *ob/ob* mice attenuates but does not totally correct obesity (Erickson *et al.*, 1996).

Mechanisms of insulin resistance and NIDDM

These models all develop morbid obesity, with visceral and subcutaneous fat deposition analogous to abdominal adiposity in humans. Whole-body insulin sensitivity falls progressively as fat mass increases, although tissues vary in their insulin insensitivity: the ability of insulin to stimulate glucose uptake into skeletal muscle and to lower blood glucose is eventually reduced by up to 80%, while white adipose tissue remains relatively insulin-sensitive so that the high prevailing insulin concentrations promote glucose uptake and its conversion into triglyceride (Zarjevski *et al.*, 1993).

The diabetogenic effects of obesity and insulin resistance depend on their severity and also on the age and the strain of the animal. As in humans, the critical factor is probably the animal's ability to produce enough insulin to overcome the effects of insulin resistance. In all these models, plasma insulin levels rise progressively to a plateau several-fold higher than in lean animals, and those models that progress to diabetes show a bell-shaped curve of β-cell function remarkably similar to that in human NIDDM (Fig. 14.10). *fa/fa* Zucker rats are only mildly glucose intolerant and remain near-normoglycaemic, although homozygosity for the *fa* gene in Wistar rats or in the ZDF (Zucker Diabetic Fatty) substrain leads to overt NIDDM. In *ob/ob* mice of the C57-BL and related strains, blood glucose remains normal until puberty and then rises steadily to overt NIDDM, with levels of 20–30 mmol/L. Spontaneous ketosis does not occur, and *ob/ob* mice can survive for many months without insulin. *db/db* homozygotes of the KSJ strain initially develop a non-ketotic, NIDDM-like syndrome, but plasma insulin levels fall in later life, leading to ketosis of variable severity and weight loss.

Insulin resistance in these syndromes is thought to be due to increased fat mass, possibly mediated by enhanced expression and circulating levels of TNF-α and raised NEFA concentrations as discussed above (Hotamisligil & Spiegelman, 1994; Boden, 1997). Clearly, although leptin may impair insulin action *in vitro* (Cohen *et al.*, 1996), it cannot explain insulin resistance in the *ob/ob* or *db/db* mice in which it is, respectively, absent and unable to act.

Other hazards of obesity in human diabetes

As well as predisposing to NIDDM, obesity has other adverse effects on diabetic patients (Table 14.1). As discussed below, it commonly impedes the successful management of NIDDM and of associated disease, notably hypertension and

Table 14.1 Impact of obesity in diabetes.

Exacerbates insulin resistance
- Predisposes to NIDDM
- Predisposes to gestational diabetes
- Increases requirements for antidiabetic drugs, including insulin

Increases other cardiovascular risk factors
- Raises blood pressure
- Induces dyslipidaemia (increased VLDL and triglycerides, reduced HDL)

May predispose to diabetic complications
- Macrovascular
- Microvascular

Fear of weight gain
- Unstable control in adolescents with IDDM
- Obstacle to stopping smoking

VLDL, very-low-density lipoproteins; HDL, high-density lipoproteins.

dyslipidaemia. Obesity is a major factor determining whether or not women who have had gestational diabetes will develop this again in subsequent pregnancies, and will ultimately fall prey to NIDDM (Moses, 1996).

Obesity in patients with IDDM has generally been neglected in comparison to NIDDM. By aggravating insulin resistance, which is present but less marked in IDDM than in NIDDM, obesity will increase insulin requirements. Conversely, excessive insulin dosages can lead to weight gain, presumably through the lipogenic effects of hyperinsulinaemia and possibly compounded by overeating during the hypoglycaemic episodes which become more frequent as insulin therapy is intensified (The Diabetes Control and Complications Trial Research Group, 1993). An extreme case, in children, is Mauriac's syndrome which comprises obesity, hepatomegaly (due to excessive glycogen deposition), growth failure and poor glycaemic control, often with both hyper- and hypoglycaemia. This is due to over-insulinization and can be reversed by reducing insulin dosages (Rosenbloom & Giordano, 1977).

Obesity, or the fear of it, can have devastating effects, especially in young patients with IDDM. These patients, almost exclusively female, reduce or omit insulin dosages, induce vomiting and/or abuse laxatives or diuretics in order to remain thin. This variant of 'eating disorder' behaviour is probably one of the commonest causes of 'brittle' or unstable diabetes, and often leads to recurrent episodes of diabetic ketoacidosis with an increased risk of developing chronic diabetic complications and of premature death (Kent *et al.*, 1994).

Obesity interacts with smoking in a particularly dangerous fashion in diabetic patients. Overall, smokers weigh less than non-smokers, primarily because of a reduced appetite, especially for sweet foods; conversely, those who stop smoking tend to gain weight, the average increases being about 5 kg or more. Smoking is undoubtedly used by some to prevent weight gain, and young women—the group in whom smoking is increasing most rapidly—are at particular risk. Smoking is especially hazardous for diabetic people, increasing the risks of arterial disease to about fourfold higher than in non-diabetic non-smokers (Dalloso & James, 1984; Hofstetter *et al.*, 1986; Stamford *et al.*, 1986; Stamler *et al.*, 1993). Despite widespread awareness of this problem, smoking is at least as common amongst diabetic patients as in the general population, and many diabetic people find it difficult to stop smoking. Fear of gaining weight is apparently a common motive, possibly reinforced by the diabetes care team's strong messages about the dangers of obesity. Logically, anti-smoking advice should have priority. Epidemiological data from non-diabetic populations suggest that the risks of continuing to smoke far outweigh those of any weight gain following smoking cessation (Stamler *et al.*, 1993). Fortunately, about 40% of diabetic people who stop smoking do not gain weight, and any increase can be limited by dietetic advice beforehand. Nicotine chewing gum or patches, and perhaps anti-obesity drugs, may be useful adjuncts in the weeks after stopping smoking.

In the long term, obesity may have adverse effects on chronic diabetic complications and survival in diabetic patients. There is some evidence that obesity is an independent risk factor for retinopathy and nephropathy (Ballard *et al.*, 1986; Barrett-Connor, 1989), although other studies have reported an apparently protective effect of overweight (Knowler, 1980). Given its associations with dyslipidaemia, hypertension and atherosclerosis, obesity would be predicted to enhance the risks of arterial disease in diabetic patients, and perhaps coronary heart disease and stroke which are the main causes of premature death in NIDDM. Surprisingly, this issue is unresolved, partly because of the paucity of long-term data in diabetic populations, and perhaps because of the confounding effects of diabetic patients who have lost weight through poor glycaemic control.

Management of obesity in diabetic patients

This section focuses on NIDDM, as weight loss has been traditionally regarded as the cornerstone (albeit structurally unsound) of therapy for the 80% of patients who are obese. The potential benefits of weight loss in NIDDM are undisputed, but the failure of most patients to reach even the most liberal of targets represents one of the thorniest problems in diabetes care. As with all obese people, the maintenance of weight loss—which is crucial to sustaining useful anti-diabetic effects—is particularly hard to achieve. Given the poor record of routine diabetic and lifestyle advice, other strategies including very-low-calorie diets (VLCD), anti-obesity drugs and surgery (gastric bypass or plication) are being explored.

Other problems in managing obese diabetic patients include the tendency of insulin and sulphonylureas to cause further weight gain.

Benefits of weight loss in NIDDM

Like all treatments, weight loss should ideally improve both the quality and the duration of life. Numerous short- and medium-term benefits of weight loss have been demonstrated in diabetic patients (Table 14.2), but the impact on the patient's quality of life and on the long-term outcomes of diabetic complications and survival have been little investigated.

In moderately or severely obese NIDDM patients, marked weight loss — which may not be sufficient to approach 'ideal' levels (corresponding to a BMI of $<25\,kg/m^2$) — can have spectacularly beneficial effects (Goldstein, 1992). In Wing's much-cited study of intensified dietetic and lifestyle measures, the mean fasting blood glucose and HbA_1 levels were nearly normalized in the group who lost over 14 kg, and all their subjects were able to reduce anti-diabetic treatment (including insulin), even though they remained on average 20–30% overweight (Wing et al., 1987). The glycaemic benefits of weight loss were striking when >10% of initial weight was lost, less marked with 5–10% loss, and non-existent below that threshold (Fig. 14.14). The most dramatic evidence comes from severely obese NIDDM patients, most of whom had an initial BMI of $>40\,kg/m^2$, who underwent gastric bypass surgery. Twelve months after surgery, the mean weight loss was 50 kg, corresponding to a 70% reduction in excess body-weight (Fig. 14.15). Before surgery, over 50% of patients had either NIDDM or IGT; postoperatively, 90% of these initially glucose-intolerant subjects (including 80% of those with NIDDM) became normoglycaemic and remained so for up to 14 years (Pories et al., 1995).

These encouraging data underline the importance of obesity in the pathogenesis of NIDDM and reinforce the rationale of developing effective anti-obesity measures as early, if not first-line, treatment of the disease. However, such results must be put into a realistic perspective. In practice, very few obese NIDDM patients lose enough weight to enjoy these benefits, and particularly, to be able to stop anti-diabetic drugs. In Wing's study, fewer than 5% of patients lost more than 14 kg; nonetheless, 25% lost between 5 and 10% of their initial weight, and this was enough to confer certain metabolic and other advantages (Fig.14.14). Weight loss is generally less useful for the 20% of NIDDM patients who are not obese and who may be relatively underweight because insulin deficiency rather than insulin insensitivity is their dominant metabolic problem; however, data from the U.K. Prospective Diabetes Study (UKPDS)

Table 14.2 Benefits of energy restriction and weight loss in NIDDM patients.

	Acute energy restriction	Long-term weight loss		
		3–10 kg	10–20 kg	>20 kg
Glycaemic control *†				
Fasting glucose	3 mmol/L fall	1–2 mmol/L fall	2–6 mmol/L fall	May be normalized
HbA$_{1c}$	NA	0–0.6% fall	1–3% fall	>2% fall
Lipid metabolism†				
LDL cholesterol		0.06–0.3 mmol/L fall	0.3–0.6 mmol/L fall	>0.6 mmol/L fall
Triglycerides		0.045–0.15 mmol/L fall	0.15–0.3 mmol/L fall	>0.3 mmol/L fall
HDL cholesterol	0.09 mmol/L fall	0.03–0.09 mmol increase	0.09–0.18 mmol increase	>0.18 mmol increase
Diastolic blood pressure‡		3–5 mmHg fall	5–10 mmHg	No data available

LDL, low-density lipoprotein; HDL, high-density lipoprotein.
* Wing et al. (1987).
† UKPDS, 1990.
‡ Treatment of Mild Hypertension Study, 1991.

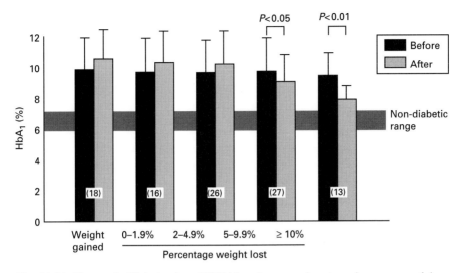

Fig. 14.14 Changes in HbA$_1$ in obese NIDDM patients as a function of percentage of the initial weight lost during the preceding 12 months. Subjects who gained weight are also shown. Numbers in parentheses are percentage of study population. Data from Wing *et al.* (1987).

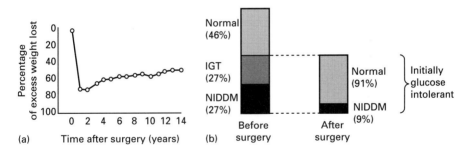

Fig. 14.15 Effects of gastric bypass surgery on (a) body-weight (expressed as per cent excess above 'ideal') and (b) on the glycaemic status of the patients who had either NIDDM or IGT before surgery. Pories *et al.* (1995).

suggest that fasting blood glucose may be lowered somewhat when non-obese patients lose weight (UKPDS Group, 1990).

Table 14.2 summarizes some metabolic and other changes that may result when moderately or severely obese (BMI > 30 kg/m^2) NIDDM patients lose 5–10% of their weight at diagnosis. These are representative data from the literature; different centres vary considerably in their ability to induce weight loss in their NIDDM patients, while individual patients differ in the extent to which blood glucose and other parameters will change in response to a given degree of weight loss.

Short-term (days to weeks) benefits of weight loss include increases in whole-body insulin sensitivity and falls in fasting and postprandial blood glucose and in glycated haemoglobin (HbA_{1c}) concentrations. Plasma triglycerides may also fall, while low-density lipoprotein (LDL) cholesterol falls and high-density lipo-protein (HDL) rises, with the HDL/LDL cholesterol ratio showing a favour-able rise (Dattilo & Kris Etherton, 1992). Blood pressure may decrease, even if dietary sodium intake is not restricted. In some studies, the fall in blood pressure in patients with moderate hypertension was as great as with routine anti-hypertensive drugs (Treatment of Mild Hypertension Research Group, 1991), although other reports (Wing *et al.*, 1987; Goldstein, 1992) show no such effect. The magnitude of all these changes varies considerably between studies.

Some acute changes are seen within a few days of dietary restriction, before appreciable losses of fat occur. Fasting and postprandial blood glucose levels can fall by as much as 5–10 mmol/L in patients treated with a VLCD (300 kcal/day), and can be virtually normalized even when the initial fasting value is up to 15 mmol/L (Gumbiner *et al.*, 1990); with less stringent energy restriction, falls of 2–3 mmol/L are more usual (Laakso *et al.*, 1988; Wing *et al.*, 1994). This fall in blood glucose may be enough to abolish glycosuria and alleviate osmotic diabetic symptoms of polyuria and thirst. HGO has been shown to decrease under these conditions, and the hepatic extraction of insulin may be enhanced, but the underlying mechanisms remain mysterious (Henry *et al.*, 1988).

Subsequent changes are mostly attributable to enhanced insulin sensitivity and/or the resulting fall in insulin levels. This in turn is presumably related to decreases in total body fat mass, and perhaps particularly in abdominal or visceral depots. Some therapies, e.g., increased physical exercise and perhaps D-fenfluramine, have been suggested to decrease visceral fat mass specifically (Marks *et al.*, 1996), but the relative effects of the various strategies have not been rigorously compared. Similar effects are seen whether weight is lost through dietary restriction, increased physical exercise, anti-obesity drugs or surgery; it is possible that measures which also improve insulin sensitivity independently of weight loss (e.g., D-fenfluramine) may have additional benefits, but this has not been systematically investigated. In addition to enhanced insulin sensitivity, some aspects of β-cell function may improve, including restoration of the normal pulsatile pattern of basal insulin secretion (Gumbiner *et al.*, 1990). This may simply reflect the general fall in blood glucose and alleviation of the 'glucotoxic' effects of hyperglycaemia on the β cell, although other factors (e.g., the fall in circulating leptin, which may inhibit insulin secretion) could also contribute.

In the longer term (months to years), blood glucose levels may fall further if weight loss continues, and a small proportion of newly diagnosed NIDDM patients (perhaps 5–10%) may remain normoglycaemic during the first year (UKPDS Group, 1995). Blood lipid levels and blood pressure can also be lowered (The Treatment of Mild Hypertension Research Group, 1991; Dattilo & Kris Etherton, 1992). The limiting factor is the maintenance of weight loss, and all these benefits will ultimately be negated by the typical pattern of weight loss for 3–6 months followed by a gradual return towards or even above the starting point. It is now clear that NIDDM is a disease of inexorable β-cell decline, irrespective of how it is treated (UKPDS Group, 1995). Accordingly, improvements in insulin sensitivity achieved by weight loss will have progressively less impact on blood glucose levels as insulin deficiency worsens (Fig. 14.16). Indeed, very few of those patients who initially respond to diet and lifestyle advice alone remain satisfactorily controlled after 1–2 years (Fig. 14.17).

The data in Table 14.2 show that relatively modest weight loss (5–10%) can have definite benefits in NIDDM patients. These levels of weight loss should provide rational and realistic treatment targets for the disease. The current European guidelines (Table 14.3; Alberti & Gries, 1988) suggest that BMI should be reduced to $<25\,kg/m^2$; clearly, this target will only be achieved by a few patients, and its stringency will demoralize many others.

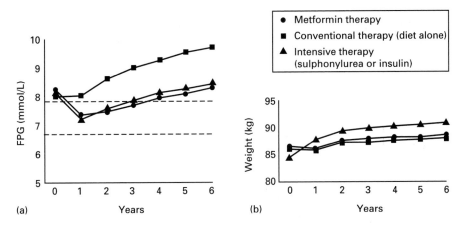

Fig. 14.16 (a) Changes in mean fasting plasma glucose (FPG) concentration and body in obese patients (>120% of ideal body-weight) with NIDDM, treated with diet alone, metformin or intensive therapy with a sulphonylurea or insulin. Diet alone generally fails to lower FPG to an 'acceptable' level (<7.8 mmol/L), even though diabetic symptoms improve when glucose falls below the renal threshold (usually ~10 mmol/L). Metformin, sulphonylureas or insulin initially lower FPG satisfactorily, but mean glucose tends to rise thereafter, at the same rate as in diet-treated patients, reflecting the inexorable decline in β-cell function. Dashed lines indicate thresholds for 'acceptable' and 'good' glycaemic control (see Table 14.3). (b) Effects on body-weight, showing the average 3–4 kg gain that tends to follow treatment with insulin or sulphonylureas.

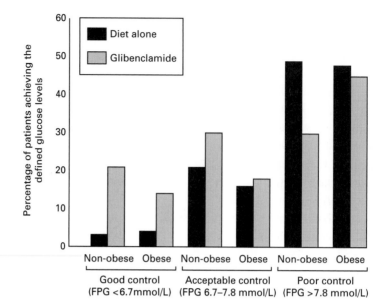

Fig. 14.17 Outcomes of diet alone and glibenclamide, in non-obese and obese NIDDM patients treated for 1 year after diagnosis, showing the percentages of patients that would achieve 'good', 'acceptable' and 'poor' levels of diabetic control as defined in Table 14.3. Data from UKPDS (1995).

Table 14.3 Suggested treatment targets for patients with NIDDM. From Alberti and Gries (1988).

	Good	Acceptable	Poor
Blood glucose (mmol/L)			
• Fasting	4.4–6.7	<7.8	>7.8
• Postprandial peak	4.4–8.9	<10.0	>10.0
HbA$_{1c}$(SD above non-diabetic mean)*	<2	<4	>4
Serum cholesterol (mmol/L)			
• Total	<5.2	<6.5	>6.5
• High-density lipoproteins	>1.1	>0.9	<0.9
Fasting serum triglycerides (mmol/L)	<1.7	<2.2	>2.2
BMI			
• Men	<25	<27	>27
• Women	<24	<26	>26
Blood pressure (mmHg)	<140/90	<160/95	>160/95

* Ranges for HbA$_{1c}$ concentrations vary considerably between centres and must be defined for each laboratory.
Note: Blood pressure and lipid targets are those defined for the general population and may not be appropriate for patients with diabetes.

Weight loss and long-term outcomes in NIDDM

At present, there are surprisingly few data about the effects of weight loss *per se* on diabetic complications or survival in NIDDM patients. This is mainly because of the practical impossibility of ensuring continued weight loss with standard dietetic strategies or the available anti-obesity drugs. One retrospective study has suggested that intentional weight loss during the first year after diagnosis of NIDDM was rewarded by proportional increases in survival, each 1 kg lost conferring an additional 3 months of life (Lean *et al.*, 1990). This potentially important finding needs to be confirmed in long-term prospective studies. The Swedish Obesity Study is now amassing long-term data following gastric plication surgery in morbidly obese subjects. Preliminary results suggest impressive benefits on the incidence of diabetes, with a reduction from 6.5% to less than 1% after 2 years, but it remains to be seen whether these benefits will influence survival (Sjöstrom, 1995).

Treatment of obesity in diabetic patients

In many cases, the management of the obese patient with NIDDM is a catalogue of defeatism and therapeutic despair. Very few patients benefit enough from standard dietetic and lifestyle advice to become non-diabetic, and most will follow a well-trodden route through a single oral hypoglycaemic agent (sulphonylurea or metformin) to a combination of oral agents. Ultimately, many are treated with insulin as the only available drug able to lower blood glucose towards normal. At present, anti-obesity drugs and VLCD are regarded as adjunctive measures, rather than first- or even second-line treatment (Fig. 14.18), even though the glucose-lowering effects of weight loss are potentially at least as powerful as those of the established oral hypoglycaemic drugs (Ha & Lean, 1997).

Routine dietary and lifestyle advice

Current dietary recommendations for people with diabetes (whether IDDM or NIDDM) differ very little from the guidelines for healthy eating advocated for the general population (Diabetes and Nutrition Study Group (DNSG) of the European Association for the study of Diabetes (EASD), 1995; Ha & Lean, 1997). The diet is designed both to limit hyperglycaemia and to reduce the risk of long-term macrovascular complications, and is low in fat (especially saturated) and relatively rich in complex carbohydrate and in dietary fibre (Fig. 14.19). This composition differs markedly from that of the low-sugar 'diabetic diet' which was promoted particularly during the 1960s and 1970s, and which by

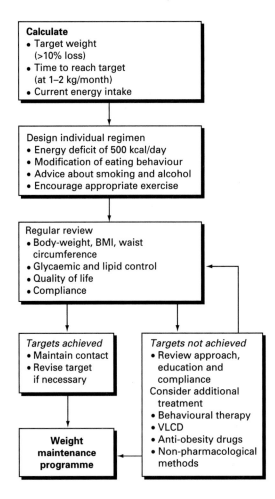

Calculate
- Target weight
  (>10% loss)
- Time to reach target
  (at 1–2 kg/month)
- Current energy intake

Design individual regimen
- Energy deficit of 500 kcal/day
- Modification of eating behaviour
- Advice about smoking and alcohol
- Encourage appropriate exercise

Regular review
- Body-weight, BMI, waist
  circumference
- Glycaemic and lipid control
- Quality of life
- Compliance

Targets achieved
- Maintain contact
- Revise target
  if necessary

Targets not achieved
- Review approach,
  education and
  compliance
Consider additional
treatment
- Behavioural therapy
- VLCD
- Anti-obesity drugs
- Non-pharmacological
  methods

**Weight
maintenance
programme**

Fig. 14.18 Algorithm for the practical management of NIDDM. Adapted from Williams (1994).

virtue of its higher fat content may actually have been atherogenic. In overweight patients, a weight-reducing diet should be prescribed, based on this general composition but allowing for the usual eating habits and preferences of the patient and his or her family. Total energy intake should be reduced by ~500 kcal/ day, based on calculated energy expenditure rather than the patient's dietary records (which are notoriously unreliable). The rationale of this general approach to all overweight patients, with or without diabetes, is discussed in Chapter 15.

Increased levels of physical activity will assist weight loss and will also improve insulin sensitivity, particularly enhancing glucose uptake into skeletal muscle. The current WHO guidelines for exercise in the general population (30 minutes exercise, sufficient to double the pulse rate, at least twice per week), are appropriate for many NIDDM patients, although a gentler graded exercise

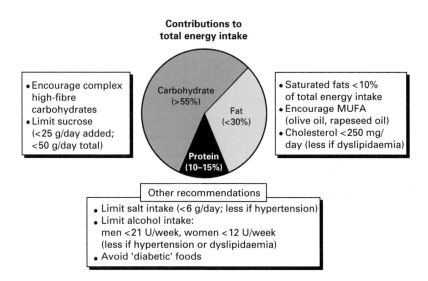

Contributions to total energy intake

- Encourage complex high-fibre carbohydrates
- Limit sucrose (<25 g/day added; <50 g/day total)

Carbohydrate (>55%)

Fat (<30%)

Protein (10–15%)

- Saturated fats <10% of total energy intake
- Encourage MUFA (olive oil, rapeseed oil)
- Cholesterol <250 mg/ day (less if dyslipidaemia)

Other recommendations
- Limit salt intake (<6 g/day; less if hypertension)
- Limit alcohol intake: men <21 U/week, women <12 U/week (less if hypertension or dyslipidaemia)
- Avoid 'diabetic' foods

Fig. 14.19 Recommended dietary composition for diabetic patients, and a strategy for prescribing a weight-reducing diet suitable for overweight subjects.

schedule may need to be built up for very obese subjects or those with coronary heart disease. NIDDM patients frequently have ischaemic heart disease (angina and myocardial dysfunction) which may be subclinical, and they should therefore have an electrocardiogram and perhaps echocardiography before undertaking an exercise programme.

Standard dietetic lifestyle advice often achieves weight loss of a few kilogrammes during the first few months, but most subjects who lose weight regain this within the first year after diagnosis. Up to 20% of patients show acceptable glycaemic control initially, with an improvement in or even loss of diabetic symptoms and most blood glucose measurements under 10 mmol/L; however, fewer than 5% of those in the UKPDS were able to maintain long-term near-normoglycaemia, with a fasting plasma glucose concentration of <6 mmol/L for 3 years (see Fig. 14.17). Dietary and lifestyle measures alone are unlikely to be effective if initial fasting plasma glucose exceeds 15 mmol/L (UKPDS Group, 1995).

Very-low-calorie diets

VLCDs, providing 300–400 kcal/day, are discussed in Chapter 16. Restricting energy intake to this degree can markedly decrease fasting and postprandial glucose levels within a few days and can abolish diabetic symptoms, even in patients with initially severe hyperglycaemia (fasting plasma glucose >15 mmol/L) (Hanefield & Weck, 1989; Uusitupa *et al.*, 1990). Insulin resistance

Table 14.4 Guidelines for the use of VLCDs in NIDDM. Reproduced from Ha and Lean (1997).

Indications	Contraindications
Rapid relief of hyperglycaemic symptoms	Cardiac disease
Rapid reductions in weight and blood glucose preoperatively	• Significant cardiac arrythmias
	• Recent myocardial infarction
Other obesity-related medical conditions, e.g., sleep apnoea	• Unstable angina
	• Decompensated cardiac failure
Severe obesity (BMI > 40), refractory to standard dietetic measures and with continuing poor diabetic control	Major organ failure
	Recent cerebrovascular accident
	Protein-wasting conditions
	Untreated hypothyroidism
	Drug abuse

is reduced acutely, with a decrease in HGO, even before appreciable body fat loss occurs, as discussed on p. 334.

VLCDs can be difficult to sustain for the many weeks or months which may be needed to lower body-weight towards the 'ideal' range, but in many cases can achieve the weight loss of > 10% which is known to improve blood glucose and lipid levels and blood pressure. In practical terms, VLCDs may be more acceptable if used to replace one or two meals each day rather than the entire energy intake. The strategy of using VLCDs periodically has been called into doubt because of evidence that weight 'cycling' may predispose to cardiovascular disease, which is particularly undesirable in NIDDM patients (see Chapter 10).

VLCDs currently have a minor role in the management of obese NIDDM patients, and are generally restricted to those with a BMI > 40 kg/m^2 who need to lose weight rapidly because of intercurrent medical problems or impending elective surgery. Guidelines for their use in NIDDM are shown in Table 14.4. As with all anti-obesity treatments, a major difficulty is the maintenance of weight loss when the VLCD is discontinued.

Anti-obesity drugs

Given that obesity is such a common and aetiologically important accompaniment of NIDDM, there are astonishingly few data on the potential anti-diabetic effects of weight-reducing drugs. In particular, there are no adequate studies on their long-term impact on diabetic control, complications or mortality.

The available anti-obesity drugs are limited by their efficacy and by the general reluctance of many physicians to prescribe them for extended periods; if used as anti-diabetic agents, they would need to be given indefinitely, as hyperglycaemia generally returns with the almost inevitable regain in weight when any weight-reducing measure is stopped. With continuing treatment, some subjects would undoubtedly lose enough weight (and maintain this) to remain near-normoglycaemic. An effective anti-obesity drug could therefore be used as monotherapy for NIDDM, but the long-term safety of the available drugs has not been ascertained, even in non-diabetic subjects. The average weight loss during the first few months of anti-obesity drug treatment (which appears to be a remarkably uniform 4–7 kg, irrespective of the agent used) should encompass a number of patients who lose the critical 10% of initial weight that confers beneficial effects on metabolism and blood pressure. Most of these patients would probably still require treatment with a sulphonylurea, metformin or even insulin; combinations of these drugs with the available anti-obesity agents have not yet been evaluated in the long term, and there are few short-term studies (Willey et al., 1994).

Individual anti-obesity drugs are described in detail in Chapter 19.

D-fenfluramine. This serotininergic agent reduces food intake and may also have a mild thermogenic action in humans. It was recently withdrawn following reports of vascular heart disease associated with its use, particularly in combination with phentermine. It has, however, provided some useful information about drug-induced weight loss in diabetic subjects. Its ability to induce and maintain weight loss has been confirmed in several reports, notably the large multi-national INDEX study (Guy-Grand et al., 1989), but as with all anti-obesity drugs, individual responses vary widely; during 3–12 months of treatment, about one-third of non-diabetic subjects may achieve weight loss that exceeds 10%, approximately twice as many as with placebo.

Its long-term effects in NIDDM subjects has not been investigated, but several short-term studies show that, in conjunction with diet and/or oral agents, D-fenfluramine has a relatively modest average glucose-lowering effect: fasting glucose may fall by 2 mmol/L and HbA_{1c} by up to 1% (Willey et al., 1994). In addition to its mobilization of body fat (which may preferentially involve visceral depots) (Marks et al., 1996), D-fenfluramine has an intrinsic insulin-sensitizing effect which can lower blood glucose before weight loss occurs. Glucose transport into muscle is apparently enhanced, but the mechanism of action is unknown (Davis & Faulds, 1996).

Phentermine. This agent is not recommended for use in the U.K. because of its potential for dependence, but is still used in some European countries and in the U.S.A., where (despite a worrying lack of basic safety information) its combination with D-fenfluramine was popular until the recent withdrawal of D-fenfluramine. Nonetheless, phentermine can decrease weight, and a few studies have demonstrated a significant glucose-lowering action, either alone or in combination with D-fenfluramine (Campbell *et al.*, 1977; Gershberg *et al.*, 1977).

Fluoxetine. This antidepressant, a selective serotonin reuptake inhibitor, is licensed in the U.K. to treat binge-eating but not for routine obesity. Its anti-obesity effects are variable and generally unimpressive, but some studies have shown a rather weak anti-diabetic effect in patients with NIDDM (Goldstein *et al.*, 1994).

New anti-obesity agents. These include sibutramine, an inhibitor of the reuptake of both serotonin and noradrenalin, and tetrahydrolipstatin (orlistat), an inhibitor of pancreatic and gastrointestinal lipases which inhibits fat absorption from the gut. Both drugs can induce weight loss comparable to that with D-fenfluramine (Bray *et al.*, 1995; Drent *et al.*, 1995), and are currently being investigated in the management of obese patients with NIDDM.

Effects of anti-diabetic drugs on body-weight

The choice of anti-diabetic drug may be influenced by the patient's weight and by the capacity of sulphonylureas and insulin to induce weight gain (see Fig. 14.16).

Sulphonylureas. These are widely used as first-line treatment for NIDDM patients, especially those who are not markedly obese. They lower blood glucose levels primarily by stimulating insulin secretion and, initially at least, raise plasma insulin concentrations. Insulin resistance may also improve somewhat, although this appears to be due to the general lowering of blood glucose levels and amelioration of 'glucotoxicity' in peripheral tissues, rather than a specific insulin-sensitizing action. Overall, fasting and postprandial glucose levels are lowered by up to 3 mmol/L, and HbA_{1c} by 0.5–1%; up to 20% of newly diagnosed patients achieve 'good', and up to 30% 'acceptable' control, those with obesity generally responding less impressively (Fig. 14.17).

Many NIDDM patients treated with sulphonylureas gain weight during the first 3–6 months; the average increase observed in the UKPDS was 3–4 kg (see Fig. 14.16). Weight gain tends to persist, and is largely attributable to increased fat mass. The degree of weight gain does not appear to depend on which sulphonylurea is used. Causative factors probably include the lipogenic effects of hyperinsulinaemia, and the tendency to overeat during hypoglycaemic episodes; some patients may also relax dietary restriction when they start specific anti-diabetic medication (UKPDS Group, 1995).

Metformin, a biguanide, has been widely used throughout Europe for over 30 years and has at last been acknowledged as a useful anti-diabetic drug in the U.S.A. (DeFronzo *et al.*, 1995). The closely related phenformin has been abandoned in most countries because it carries over 10 times the risk of lactic acidosis, a rare but frequently fatal complication of biguanides. Metformin does not stimulate insulin secretion, but instead enhances insulin action, notably decreasing gluconeogenesis in the liver and therefore HGO. It lowers blood glucose concentrations when these are raised (often by 2–3 mmol/L), but does not induce hypoglycaemia. Unlike the sulphonylureas, it usually does not cause weight gain, and some patients lose weight; there was no overall change in the obese NIDDM patients who received metformin in the UKPDS (UKPDS Group, 1995). Accordingly, it is often used as first-line drug treatment in obese NIDDM patients who have failed to respond to diet and lifestyle modification alone. The lack of weight gain is probably attributable to the fact that it induces neither hyperinsulinaemia nor hypoglycaemia. Metformin commonly causes mild and occasionally marked gastrointestinal symptoms including heartburn and dyspepsia and, although it has no specific anorectic action, these side-effects may help dietary compliance in some cases.

Combined oral treatment with a sulphonylurea and metformin. This is commonly used for patients who fail to respond adequately to either drug alone, irrespective of their weight. Addition of metformin may help to limit sulphonylurea-induced weight gain. Many patients remain poorly controlled on combined oral treatment for prolonged periods, while the patient and/or the doctor becomes persuaded of the need for insulin. Under these circumstances, body-weight may fall (usually with worsening diabetic symptoms) because of the catabolic effects of insulin deficiency.

Insulin is ultimately required by 30–50% of NIDDM patients, when β-cell function has declined to the point of absolute insulin deficiency, and because of the limited glucose-lowering efficacy of the oral agents, it is frequently used as the only means of controlling hyperglycaemia. One or two daily injections of long-acting insulin are often effective, but some patients with little endogenous insulin reserve also need short-acting insulin injections before the main meals to limit postprandial hyperglycaemia. Most patients starting insulin gain some weight, commonly 3–4 kg, as occurs with sulphonylureas.

Thiazolidinediones. This new group of 'insulin-sensitizing' drugs are currently being evaluated for the treatment and possibly prevention of NIDDM (Nolan *et al.*, 1994). Although they have been reported to cause weight gain at high doses in some animal models, they appear to have no significant effects on body-weight in clinical studies. Interestingly, some of these agents reduce circulating leptin concentrations, perhaps because of the decrease in insulin levels that accompanies the increase in whole-body insulin sensitivity (Nolan *et al.*, 1996).

Prevention of NIDDM

There is now evidence from many sources that treating obesity is an effective way of preventing NIDDM, even once IGT is present. The most dramatic benefits are seen following surgical intervention in morbid obesity (see p. 553); the ability of thiazolidinediones to prevent patients with IGT from progressing to NIDDM are promising, but require longer-term evaluation. Lifestyle modification is another approach, and is probably the most rational and desirable. The extent to which the grip of Westernization must be loosened is difficult, but not impossible to achieve in practice, as demonstrated by the Malmö study of Swedish men in their late forties, in which a moderate exercise and diet programme, which produced modest weight loss of 2–4%, was effective in preventing progression from IGT to diabetes (Eriksson & Lindgarde, 1991). Such interventions are likely to work predominantly by improving insulin sensitivity, and are likely to influence all aspects of the insulin-resistance syndrome (Torjesen *et al.*, 1997) (Fig. 14.20). On a world-wide scale, such programmes to reduce obesity may represent the best chance of reducing the incidence of diabetes in large populations.

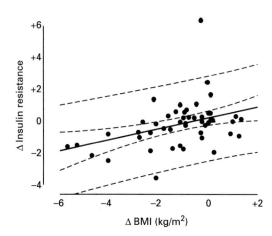

Fig. 14.20 Improvement in insulin resistance (calculated by mathematical modelling of fasting glucose and insulin levels) with weight loss during a programme of dietary modification and/or exercise, from the Oslo Diet and Exercise Study. From Torjesen *et al.* (1997).

References

Abate, N., Garg, A., Peshock, R.M., Straygundersen, J., Adamshuet, B. & Grundy, S.M. (1996) Relationship of generalized and regional adiposity to insulin sensitivity in men with NIDDM. *Diabetes* 45, 1684–1693.

Alberti, K.G.M.M. & Gries, F.A. (1988) Management of non-insulin-dependent diabetes-mellitus in Europe—a consensus view. *Diabetic Medicine* 5, 275–281.

Albu, J.B., Murphy, L., Frager, D.H. *et al.* (1997) Visceral fat and race-dependent health risks in obese non-diabetic premenopausal women. *Diabetes Care* 46, 456–462.

Ballard, D.J., Melton, L.J., Dwyer, M.S. *et al.* (1986) Risk-factors for diabetic-retinopathy—a population-based study in Rochester, Minnesota. *Diabetes Care* 9, 334–342.

Barrett-Connor, E. (1989) Epidemiology, obesity and non-insulin-dependent diabetes mellitus *Epidermiological Reviews* 11, 172.

Bennet, W.M., Smith, D.M. & Bloom, S.R. (1994) Islet amyloid polypeptide: does it play a pathophysiological role in the development of diabetes? *Diabetic Medicine* 11, 825–829.

Bergstrom, R.W., Newell-Morris, L., Leonetti, D.L., Shuman, W.P., Wahl, P.W. & Fujimoto, W.Y. (1990) Association of elevated fasting C-peptide concentration and increased abdominal fat distribution with development of NIDDM in Japanese-American men. *Diabetes* 39, 104–111.

Björntorp, P. (1994) Abdominal obesity and the metabolic syndrome. *Annals of Medicine* 24, 265–268.

Boden, G. (1997) Role of fatty acids in the pathogenesis of insulin resistance and NIDDM. *Diabetes* 46, 3–10.

Boden, G., Chen, X.H., Rosner, J. & Barton, M. (1995) Effects of a 48-h fat infusion on insulin-secretion and glucose-utilization. *Diabetes* 44, 1239–1242.

Bonadonna, R.C. & DeFronzo, R.A. (1992) Glucose metabolism in obesity. In: Björntorp, P. & Brodoff, B.N. (eds) *Obesity*, pp. 474–501. Philadelphia: J.B. Lippincott.

Bray, G.A., Ryan, D.H., Gordon, D., Heidingsfelder, S., Macchiavelli, R. & Wilson, K. (1995) Double-blind randomized trial of sibutramine in overweight subjects. *American Journal of Clinical Nutrition* 61, 912.

Campbell, C.J., Bhalla, I.P., Steele, J.M. & Duncan, L.J.P. (1977) Controlled trial of phentermine in obese diabetic patients. *The Practitioner* 218, 851–855.

Campfield, L.A., Smith, F.J., Guisez, Y., Devos, R. & Burn, P. (1995) Recombinant mouse *ob* protein—evidence for a peripheral signal linking adiposity and central neural networks. *Science* 269, 546–549.

Caro, J.F., Sinha, M.K., Kolaczynski, J.W., Zhang, P.L. & Considine, R.V. (1996) Leptin—the tale of an obesity gene. *Diabetes* 45, 1455–1462.

Chan, J.M., Stampfer, M.J., Ribb, E.B., Willett, W.C. & Colditz, G.A. (1994) Obesity, fat distribution and weight gain as risk factors for clinical diabetes in man. *Diabetes Care* 17, 961–969.

Chen, H., Charlat, O., Tartaglia, L.A. *et al.* (1996) Evidence that the diabetes gene encodes the leptin receptor—identification of a mutation in the leptin receptor gene in *db/db* mice. *Cell* 84, 491–495.

Cohen, B., Novick, D. & Rubinstein, M. (1996) Modulation of insulin activities by leptin. *Science* 274, 1185–1188.

Colditz, G.A., Willett, W.C., Rotnitzky, A. & Manson, J.E. (1995) Weight-gain as a risk factor for clinical diabetes-mellitus in women. *Annals of Internal Medicine* 122, 481–486.

Consoli, A., Nurjhan, N., Capani, F. & Gerich, J. (1989) Predominant role of gluconeogenesis in increased hepatic glucose-production in NIDDM. *Diabetes* 38, 550–557.

Cusin, I., Rohner Jeanrenaud, F., Stricker Krongrad, A. & Jeanrenaud, B. (1996) The weight-reducing effect of an intracerebroventricular bolus injection of leptin in genetically-obese fa/fa rats—reduced sensitivity compared with lean animals. *Diabetes* 45, 1446–1451.

Dalloso, H.M. & James, W.P.T. (1984) The role of smoking in the regulation of energy balance. *International Journal of Obesity* 8, 365–375.

Dattilo, A.M. & Kris Etherton, P.M. (1992) Effects of weight reduction on blood lipids and lipoproteins: a meta-analysis. *American Journal of Clinical Nutrition* 56, 320–328.

Davis, R. & Faulds, D. (1996) Dexfenfluramine—an updated review of its therapeutic use in the management of obesity. *Drugs* **52**, 696–724.

DeFronzo, R.A. (1988) The triumvirate—beta-cell, muscle, liver—a collusion responsible for NIDDM. *Diabetes* **37**, 667–687.

DeFronzo, R.A. (1992) Pathogenesis of type 2 (non-insulin dependent) diabetes mellitus: a balanced overview. *Diabetologia* **35**, 389–397.

DeFronzo, R.A., Bonadonna, R.C. & Ferrannini, E. (1992) Pathogenesis of NIDDM. A balanced overview. *Diabetes Care* **15**, 318–368.

DeFronzo, R.A., Goodman, A.M. & the Multicentre Metformin Study Group (1995) Efficacy of metformin in patients with non-insulin dependent diabetes mellitus. *New England Journal of Medicine* **333**, 541–549.

Diabetes and Nutrition Study Group (DNSG) of the European Association for the study of Diabetes (EASD) (1995) Recommendations for the nutritional management of patients with diabetes mellitus. *Diabetes Nutrition and Metabolism* **8**, 1–5.

Drent, M.J., Larsson, I. & William-Olsson, T. *et al.* (1995) Orlistat (RO 18-0647), a lipase inhibitor in the treatment of human obesity: a multiple dose study. *International Journal of Obesity* **19**, 221–226.

Erickson, J.C., Hollopeter, G. & Palmiter, R.D. (1996) Attenuation of the obesity syndrome of *ob/ob* mice by the loss of neuropeptide-y. *Science* **274**, 1704–1707.

Eriksson, K.F. & Lindgarde, F. (1991) Prevention of type-2 (non-insulin-dependent) diabetes-mellitus by diet and physical exercise—the 6-year Malmö Feasibility Study. *Diabetologia* **34**, 891–898.

Fall, C.H.D., Osmond, C., Barker, D.J.P. *et al.* (1995) Fetal and infant growth and cardiovascular risk-factors in women. *British Medical Journal* **310**, 428–432.

Gershberg, H., Kane, R., Hulse, M. & Pengsen, E. (1977) Effects of diet and an anorectic drug (phentermine resin) in obese diabetics. *Current Research Therapeutics* **22**, 814–820.

Goldstein, D.J. (1992) Beneficial health-effects of modest weight-loss. *International Journal of Obesity* **16**, 397–415.

Goldstein, D.J., Rampey, A.H., Enas, G.G., Potvin, J.H., Fludzinski, L.L.A. & Levine, L.R. (1994) Fluoxetine — a randomized clinical-trial in the treatment of obesity. *International Journal of Obesity* **18**, 129–135.

Gumbiner, B., Polonsky, K.S., Beltz, W.F. *et al.* (1990) Effects of weight loss and reduced hyperglycemia on the kinetics of insulin secretion in obese non-insulin dependent diabetes mellitus. *Journal of Clinical Endocrinology and Metabolism* **70**, 1594–1602.

Guy-Grand, B., Apfelbaum, M., Crepaldi, G., Gries, A., Lefèbvre, P. & Turner, P. (1989) International trial of long term dexfenfluramine in obesity. *Lancet* **2**, 1142–1145.

Ha, T. & Lean, M.E.J. (1997) Diet and lifestyle modification in the management of non-insulin-dependent diabetes mellitus. In: Pickup, J.C. & Williams, G. (eds) *Textbook of Diabetes*, 2nd edn, pp. 37.1–37.18. Oxford: Blackwell Science.

Hales, C.N. & Barker, D.J.P. (1992) Type 2 (non-insulin dependent) diabetes mellitus: the thrifty phenotype hypothesis. *Diabetologia* **35**, 595–601.

Hanefield, M. & Weck, M. (1989) Very low calorie diet therapy in obese non-insulin dependent diabetes patients. *International Journal of Obesity* **13**, 33–37.

Hattersley, A.T. (1997) Maturity-onset diabetes of the young. In: Pickup, J.C. & Williams, G. (eds) *Textbook of Diabetes*, 2nd edn, pp. 22.1–22.10. Oxford: Blackwell Science.

Henry, R.R., Brechtel, G. & Griver, K. (1988) Secretion and hepatic extraction of insulin after weight-loss in obese noninsulin-dependent diabetes mellitus. *Journal of Clinical Endocrinology and Metabolism* **66**, 979–986.

Hotamisligil, G.S. & Spiegelman, B.M. (1994) Tumor-necrosis-factor-alpha—a key component of the obesity-diabetes link. *Diabetes* **43**, 1271–1278.

Hotamisligil, G.S., Arner, P., Atkinson, R.L. & Spiegelman, B.M. (1997) Differential regulation of the p80 tumor necrosis factor receptor in human obesity and insulin resistance. *Diabetes* **46**, 451–455.

Hofstetter, A., Schutz, Y., Jéquier, E. & Wahren, J. (1986) Increased 24-hour energy expenditure in cigarette smokers. *New England Journal of Medicine* **314**, 79–82.

Howell, S.L. (1997) The biosynthesis and secretion of insulin. In: Pickup, J.C. & Williams, G. (eds) *Textbook of Diabetes*, 2nd edn, pp. 9.1–9.14. Oxford: Blackwell Science.

Jeng, C.Y., Sheu, W.H., Fuh, M.M., Chen, Y.D. & Reaven, G.M. (1994) Relationship between hepatic glucose production and fasting plasma glucose concentration in patients with non-insulin dependent diabetes mellitus. *Diabetes* 38, 744–751.

Johnson, A.B., Argyraki, M., Thow, J.C. *et al.* (1991) Impaired activation of skeletal muscle glycogen synthase in non-insulin-dependent diabetes mellitus is unrelated to the degree of obesity. *Metabolism* 40, 252–260.

Kent, L.A., Gill, G.V. & Williams, G. (1994) Mortality and outcome of patients with brittle diabetes and recurrent ketoacidosis (see comments). *Lancet* 344, 778–781.

Knowler, W.C. (1980) Increased incidence of retinopathy in diabetics with increased blood pressure. Asia year follow-up study in Pima Indians. *New England Journal of Medicine* 302, 645–650.

Kruszynska, Y.T. (1997) Normal metabolism: the physiology of fuel homeostasis. In: Pickup, J.C. & Williams, G. (eds) *Textbook of Diabetes*, 2nd edn, pp. 11.1–11.37. Oxford: Blackwell Science.

Kurabayashi, T., Carey, D.G.P. & Morrison, N.A. (1996) The beta-3-adrenergic receptor gene Trp64Arg mutation is overrepresented in obese women—effects on weight, BMI, abdominal fat, blood-pressure, and reproductive history in an elderly Australian population. *Diabetes* 45, 1358–1363.

Laakso, M., Uusitupa, M., Takala, J., Majander, H., Reijonen, T. & Penttila, I. (1988) Effects of hypocaloric diet and insulin therapy on metabolic control and mechanisms of hyperglycemia in obese non-insulin-dependent diabetic subjects. *Metabolism: Clinical and Experimental* 37, 109–1100.

Larsson, B., Svardsudd, K., Welin, L, Wihemsen, L, Björntorp, P. & Tibblin, G. (1994) Abdominal adipose tissue distribution, obesity and risk of cardiovascular disease and death: 13 year follow-up of participants in the study of men born in 1913. *British Medical Journal* 288, 1401–1404.

Lean, M.E., Powrie, J.K., Anderson, A.S. & Garthwaite, P.H. (1990) Obesity, weight loss and prognosis in type 2 diabetes. *Diabetic Medicine* 7, 228–233.

Lee, G.H., Proenca, R., Montez, J.M. *et al.* (1996) Abnormal splicing of the leptin receptor in diabetic mice. *Nature* 379, 632–635.

Lemieux, S., Prudhomme, D., Nadeau, A., Tremblay, A., Bouchard, C. & Després, J.P. (1996) 7-year changes in body-fat and visceral adipose-tissue in women—associations with indexes of plasma glucose-insulin homeostasis. *Diabetes Care* 19, 983–991.

Maratos-Flier, E., Goldstein, B.J. & Kahn, C.R. (1997) Insulin receptor and post-receptor mechanisms. In: Pickup, J.C. & Williams, G. (eds) *Textbook of Diabetes*, 2nd edn, pp. 10.1–10.22. Oxford: Blackwell Science.

Marks, S.J., Moore, N.R., Clark, M.L., Strauss, B.J.S., & Hockaday, R . (1996) Reduction of visceral adipose-tissue and improvement of metabolic indexes—effect of dexfenfluramine in NIDDM. *Obesity Research* 4, 1–7.

Matthews, D.R. (1991) Physiological implications of pulsatile hormone secretion. *Annals of the New York Academy of Sciences* 618, 28–37.

McCarthy, M.I., Froguel, P. & Hitman, G.A. (1994) The genetics of non-insulin-dependent diabetes mellitus: tools and aims. *Diabetologia* 37, 959–968.

McKibbin, P.E., Cotton, S.J., McMillan, S. *et al.* (1991) Altered neuropeptide Y concentrations in specific hypothalamic regions of obese (*fa/fa*) Zucker rats—possible relationship to obesity and neuroendocrine disturbances. *Diabetes* 40, 1423–1429.

Moses, R.G. (1996) The recurrence rate of gestational diabetes in subsequent pregnancies. *Diabetes Care* 19, 1348–1350.

Neel, J.V. (1962) Diabetes mellitus: a thrifty genotype rendered detrimental by 'progress'. *American Journal of Human Genetics* 14, 353–362.

Nolan, J.J., Ludvik, B., Beerdsen, P., Joyce, M. & Olefsky, J. (1994) Improvement in glucose-tolerance and insulin-resistance in obese subjects treated with troglitazone. *New England Journal of Medicine* 331, 1188–1193.

Nolan, J.J., Olefsky, J.M., Nyce, M.R., Considine, R.V. & Caro, J.F. (1996) Effect of troglitazone on leptin production—studies *in-vitro* and in human subjects. *Diabetes* 45, 1276–1278.

O'Rahilly, S. & Moller, D.E. (1992) Mutant insulin receptors in syndromes of insulin resistance. *Clinical Endocrinology* **36**, 121–132.

O'Rahilly, S.P., Nugent, Z., Rudenski, A.S. *et al* (1986) Beta-cell dysfunction, rather than insulin insensitivity, is the primary defect in familial type-2 diabetes. *Lancet* **2**, 360–364.

Peiris, A.N., Mueller, R.A., Smith, G.A., Struve, M.F. & Kissebah, A.H. (1986) Splanchnic insulin metabolism in obesity—influence of body-fat distribution. *Journal of Clinical Investigation* **78**, 1648–1657.

Phillips, M.S., Liu, W.Y., Hammond, H.A. *et al.* (1996) Leptin receptor missense mutation in the fatty Zucker rat. *Nature Genetics* **13**, 18–19.

Pories, W.J., Swanson, M.S., MacDonald, K.G. *et al.* (1995) Who would have thought it?—an operation proves to be the most effective therapy for adult-onset diabetes-mellitus. *Annals of Surgery* **222**, 339–352.

Randle, P.J., Garland, P.B., Hales, C.N. & Newsholme, C.A. (1963) The glucose fatty-acid cycle. Its role in insulin sensitivity and the metabolic disturbances of diabetes mellitus. *Lancet* **1**, 785–789.

Reaven, G.M. (1988) Role of insulin resistance in human disease. *Diabetes* **37**, 1595–1607.

Rosenbloom, A.L. & Giordano, B.P. (1977) Chronic overtreatment with insulin in children and adolescents. *American Journal of Diseases of Childhood* **131**, 881–885.

Rothman, D.L., Shulman, R.G. & Shulman, G.I. (1991) NMR studies of muscle glycogen synthesis in normal and non-insulin-dependent diabetic subjects. *Biochemical Society Transactions* **19**, 992–994.

Sjöstrom, L. (1995) The natural history of massive obesity. *Obesity Research* **3**, 317.

Stamford, B.A., Matter, S., Fell, R.D. & Papnek, P. (1986) Effects of smoking cessation on weight gain, metabolic rate, caloric consumption and blood lipids. *American Journal of Clinical Nutrition* **43**, 486–494.

Stamler, J., Vaccaro, O., Neaton, J.D., Wentworth, D. For the Multiple Risk Factor Intervention Trial Research Group (1993) Diabetes, and other risk factors and 12-year cardiovascular mortality for men screened in the Multiple Risk Factor Intervention Trial. *Diabetes Care* **16**, 434–444.

Takaya, K., Ogawa, Y., Isse, N. *et al.* (1996) Molecular-cloning of rat leptin receptor isoform complementary DNAS—identification of a missense mutation in Zucker fatty (*fa/fa*) rats. *Biochemical and Biophysical Research Communications* **225**, 75–83.

Tartaglia, L.A. Dembski, M., Weng, X. *et al.* (1995) Identification and expression cloning of a leptin receptor Ob-R. *Cell* **83**, 1263–1271.

The Diabetes Control and Complications Trial Research Group (1993) The effect of intensive treatment of diabetes on the development and progression long-term complications in insulin dependent diabetes mellitus. *New England Journal of Medicine* **329**, 977–986.

Thompson, C.H., Sanderson, A.L., Sandeman, D. *et al.* (1997) Fetal growth and insulin resistance in adult life: role of skeletal muscle morphology. *Clinical Science* **92**, 291–296.

Torjesen, P.A., Birkeland, K.I., Anderssen, S.A., Hjermann, I., Holme, I. & Urdal, P. (1997) Lifestyle changes may reverse development of the insulin resistance syndrome—the Oslo diet and exercise study: a randomized trial. *Diabetes Care* **20**, 26–31.

The Treatment of Mild Hypertension Research Group (1991) The treatment of mild hypertension study. A randomized, placebo-controlled trial of a nutritional-hygienic regimen along with various drug monotherapies. *Archives of Internal Medicine* **151**, 1413–1423.

UKPDS Group. (1990) UK Prospective Diabetes Study 7: response of fasting plasma glucose to diet therapy in newly presenting type II diabetic patients. *Metabolism* **39**, 905–912.

UKPDS Group. (1995) United Kingdom Prospective Diabetes Study (UKPDS). 13: Relative efficacy of randomly allocated diet, sulphonylurea, insulin, or metformin in patients with newly diagnosed non-insulin dependent diabetes followed for three years. *British Medical Journal* **310**, 83–88.

Uusitupa, M.I., Laakso, M., Sarlund H., Majander, H., Takala, J. & Penttila, I. (1990) Effects of a very-low-calorie diet on metabolic control and cardiovascular risk factors in the treatment of obese non-insulin-dependent diabetics. *American Journal of Clinical Nutrition* **51**, 768–773.

Vague, J. (1956) The degree of masculine differentiation of obesities, a factor determining predisposition to diabetes, atherosclerosis, gout and uric calculous disease. *American Journal of Clinical Nutrition* **4**, 20–34.

Wang, W., Bing, C., Al-Barazanji, K. *et al.* (1997) Interactions between leptin and hypothalamic neuropeptide Y neurones in the control of food intake and energy homeostasis in the rat. *Diabetes* **46**, 335–341.

West, K. (1978) *Epidemiology of Diabetes and its Vascular Lesions.* Amsterdam: Elsevier.

WHO Study Group. (1994) *Prevention of Diabetes Mellitus.* WHO techical report series; 844.

Wilding, J.P.H., Gilbey, S.G., Bailey, C.J. *et al.* (1993) Increased neuropeptide Y messenger RNA and decreased neurotensin messenger RNA in the hypothalamus of the obse (*ob/ob*) mouse. *Endocrinology* **132**, 1939–1944.

Willey, K.A., Molyneaux, L.M. & Yue, D.K. (1994) Obese patients with type 2 diabetes poorly controlled by insulin and metformin: effects of adjunctive dexfenfluramine therapy on glycaemic control. *Diabetic Medicine* **11**, 701–704.

Williams, G. (1994) Management of non-insulin dependent diabetes. *Lancet* **343**, 95–100.

Wing, R.R., Koeske,R., Epstein, L.H., Nowalk, M.P., Gooding, W. & Becker, D. (1987) Long-term effects of modest weight-loss in type-II diabetic patients. *Archives of Internal Medicine* **147**, 1749–1753.

Wing, R.R., Blair, E.H., Bononi, P., Marcus, M.D., Watanabe, R. & Bergman, R.N. (1994) Caloric restriction *per se* is a significant factor in improvements in glycemic control and insulin sensitivity during weight loss in obese NIDDM patients. *Diabetes Care* **17**, 30–36.

Yki-Järvinen, H. (1992) Glucose toxicity. *Endocrine Reviews* **13**, 415–431.

Yki-Järvinen, H. (1995) Role of insulin-resistance in the pathogenesis of NIDDM. *Diabetologia* **38**, 1378–1388.

Yki-Järvinen, H. & Williams, G. (1997) Insulin resistance in non-insulin-dependent diabetes mellitus. In: Pickup, J.C. & Williams, G. (eds) *Textbook of Diabetes*, 2nd edn, pp. 20.1–20.14. Oxford: Blackwell Science.

Zarjevski, N., Cusin, I., Rohner-Jeanrenaud, F. & Jeanrenaud, B. (1993) Chronic intracerebroventricular neuropeptide Y administration to normal rats mimics hormonal and metabolic changes of obesity. *Endocrinology* **133**, 1753–1758.

Zhang, Y., Proenca, R., Maffei, M., Barone, M., Leopold, L. & Friedman, J.M. (1994) Positional cloning of the mouse *obese* gene and its human homologue. *Nature* **372**, 425–432.

Zimmet, P. (1982) Type 2 (non-insulin dependent) diabetes mellitus—an epidemiological overview. *Diabetologia* **22**, 399–411.

......

CHAPTER 15

Clinical Assessment, Investigation and Principles of Management: Realistic Weight Goals

NICK FINER

......

Introduction

Despite the acceptance that obesity is a disease and also a risk for disease, governments, health care purchasers and providers are all extremely reluctant to direct medical resources to its prevention and treatment. In most countries, obesity is the Cinderella of medical specialties; its investigation and management often regarded as an unrewarding chore for endocrinologists and general physicians. These attitudes persist in medical schools, where the curricula devote little attention to teaching students how to evaluate or treat obesity. Most general practitioners in the U.K. accept the medical importance of obesity; in one survey (Cade & O'Connell, 1991) 98% of general practitioners questioned believed it part of their professional role to counsel the overweight or obese on the health risks of their excess weight. A study in the U.S. (Price, 1977) found a similar willingness of family physicians to counsel patients on the risks of obesity. However, both surveys showed a coexisting prejudice against obese patients, who were characterized as lazy and lacking in self-control. An analysis of 2333 respondents to a survey on slimming by the Consumer's Association of the U.K. found that half had been advised by their general practitioner to lose weight, and that 17% had been reassured about their weight, advised to join a slimming group or referred for specialist advice (1%). However, less than a third of the large majority, presumably being managed by the general practitioner, were asked to attend regularly for supervision (Ashwell, 1973). It is perhaps not surprising therefore that patients who present with obesity or its complications are treated differently to other patients. For example, an audit of referrals to one specialist obesity clinic found that 42% of patients had not been weighed, let alone had a body mass index (BMI) calculated; referral letters rarely gave information about medical history (only 25%), medication (40%) or physical examination findings (<10%) (Coomber et al., 1997).

It is hardly surprising that commercial organizations have moved into this comparative vacuum of mainstream medical treatment of obesity. In the U.S.A., the diet industry is worth more than $30 billion yearly (Ezzati et al., 1992).

Despite this, or perhaps as a result, the public is becoming sceptical about healthy lifestyle interventions (Rippe, 1996). Patients do, however, have the right to expect a level of professional competence from the doctors that is no less whether they consult for help with obesity, than for example, hypertension or asthma. The medical profession needs to know how to fit obesity management into the overall scheme of preventative medicine and health care. At the same time clinicians need to know why and how to incorporate treatment of obesity, regardless of its presentation, into everyday practice. This chapter considers the issues involved in managing obesity effectively, and how to approach the assessment, investigation and treatment of the obese individual.

Obesity management protocols

A number of professional, governmental and other bodies have drawn up guidelines for obesity management. These strategies for providing medical care to the obese provide useful and relatively consistent guidance for the clinician (Scottish Intercollegiate Guidelines Network, 1996; Price, 1997; Royal College of Physicians, 1997).

A National Institutes of Health Consensus Development Conference reported its conclusions in 1992 (NIH Technology Assessment Conference Panel, 1992). The report found that 33–40% of adult women and 20–24% of adult men were actively trying to lose weight, and that a further 28% of each group were trying to maintain weight. Strategies to restrict energy intake were more commonly used than exercise. The report suggested that the 'fundamental principle of weight loss and control is that for almost all people, a lifelong commitment to a change in lifestyle, behavioural responses and dietary practices is necessary' and that for the severely overweight, children, elderly, pregnant or lactating individual, a trained physician or other health professional should assess any contra-indications or underlying psychological problems. Furthermore, the NIH Technology Assessment Conference Panel advised that 'for persons of high medical risk, a properly trained physician should be involved in a multidisciplinary approach to care' (NIH Technology Assessment Conference Panel, 1992). Criteria for evaluating weight loss methods were also established (Table 15.1), and these are further amplified by recommendations of the Food and Nutrition Board of the Institute of Medicine, National Academy of Sciences (Committee to develop criteria for evaluating the outcomes of approaches to prevent and treat obesity, 1995) (Table 15.2) which detailed the selection of patients, the content of the treatment programme and the methods of assessing efficacy across the range of treatments.

In Scotland, a national strategy was developed under an initiative to produce 'evidence-based' guidelines (Scottish Intercollegiate Guidelines Network, 1996).

Table 15.1 Criteria for evaluating weight-loss methods or programmes suggested by NIH Technology Assessment Panel (NIH Technology Assessment Conference Panel, 1992).

- The percentage of all beginning participants who complete the programme
- The percentage of those completing who achieve various degrees of weight loss
- The proportion of weight loss maintained at 1, 3 and 5 years
- The percentage of participants who experience any adverse medical or psychological effects, and the kind and severity

Table 15.2 A comparison of the standards to which various treatment programmes (self-help, non-medically supervised commercial and medically supervised) should adhere, in terms of the selection of patients, supervision and assessment of outcome. Adapted from Committee to develop criteria for evaluating the outcomes of approaches to prevent and treat obesity (1995).

	Do-it-yourself programme	Non-clinical programme	Clinical programme
Who is appropriate?			
Decide on who is appropriate for the programme	Yes	Yes	Yes
Obtain information on health state and weight-loss goals of clients	Generally unable to do	Yes	Yes
Weight loss for those with obesity-related or other health problems	Encourage contact with health-care provider during programme		Yes
Weight loss for lactating women, children, significant renal or psychiatric disease, diabetes	Advise against without medical supervision	Medical supervision required for entry	May be appropriate
Weight loss for pregnant women, underweight or anorectic	Discourage	Discourage Entry	
Is the programme soundly based and safe?			
Encourage individuals with risk factors seek medical supervision	Yes	Yes	N/A
Assess clients for risk factors	N/A	N/A	Yes
Inform about potential risks of programme	Yes	Yes	Special responsibilities if special diets, drugs or surgery used

Continued

Table 15.2 (*Continued*).

	Do-it-yourself programme	Non-clinical programme	Clinical programme
Measure height, weight, BMI and waist/hip ratio	Encourage and instruct clients on how to measure and explain results	Measure and calculate; provide and interpret results to patient	
Physical assessment	Encourage clients to have assessment by health-care provider		Perform assessment
Psychological assessment	Provide test with guidance on use and scoring	Administer test(s)	
Diet and physical activity assessment	Inform clients of importance of these factors and give guidance on how to do so	Evaluate at beginning and end of treatment phase and 6 monthly during maintenance	
What is the evidence of success? Success judged by achievement of long-term weight loss	Yes	Yes	Yes
Judge ability to empower clients to eat more healthy diet, and improve health status, knowledge and quality of life	Yes	Yes	Yes
Contact with health care provider	Encourage clients, especially those with obesity-related co-morbidities		Yes

N/A, not applicable.

Published by the Scottish Intercollegiate Guidelines Network (SIGN) in line with the U.S. Institute of Medicine report (Committee to develop criteria for evaluating the outcomes of approaches to prevent and treat obesity, 1995), it focused on the integration of prevention and management; the SIGN guidelines also promulgated the concept that targets for management should be realistic and set according to current evidence of health benefits from modest degrees of weight loss. It also emphasized an integrated approach between primary and secondary care.

These expert reports were published at a time when evidence of the efficacy of anorectic medication was being re-evaluated and increasingly accepted, but before reports at the end of 1997 of potential serious side-effects from the fenfluramines alone or in combination with phentermine. Following the withdrawal of the fenfluramines, their recommendations on incorporating pharmacotherapy 'routinely' into their management schemes were withdrawn. The principles, however, of incorporating drugs into overall obesity treatment remain, and the imminent licensing of newer and hopefully safer drugs such as sibutramine and orlistat make it likely that further revisions of such integrated management strategies will shortly be needed.

Principles of management

Prevention

Preventing obesity must form part of obesity management. It is unrealistic to think that the health burden resulting from the rapid escalation of obesity world-wide can, or will, be met purely by a strategy of treatment, however effective (Garner & Wooley, 1991). Public health measures to limit weight gain should be accompanied by opportunistic intervention in the at-risk individual and the family. Although there are few directly applicable studies to support such a strategy, the SIGN guidelines reflect current opinion that prevention should be routinely incorporated into clinical management. This approach has been represented as a series of overlapping activities which together form an integrated management scheme (Fig. 15.1) (Gill, 1997).

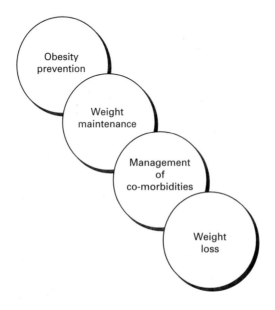

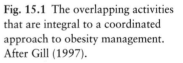

Fig. 15.1 The overlapping activities that are integral to a coordinated approach to obesity management. After Gill (1997).

Risk assessment

The medical risks of obesity have been addressed in earlier chapters, but it is these health risks that should form the core of the clinical assessment of the obese patient. The risks or existence of co-morbidities should strongly influence, but not necessarily determine, treatment. Clinicians should recognize, however, that the risks of obesity are greater than just those of the metabolic and organ-specific co-morbidities. Risk of impaired general health, mental health and well-being, and quality of life are likely to be of greater immediacy and importance to an obese individual than a future risk of developing diabetes, gallstones or colon cancer; such risks are often under-estimated not just by the patient but also by the doctor. Immediate symptoms are more likely to motivate lifestyle change and weight loss than future risk.

Conventionally the degree of obesity has been used as a surrogate for disease severity and to determine treatment. Garrow first used arbitrary cut-points of BMI to grade obesity (Garrow, 1981), and based treatment strategies according to these grades (Table 15.3). The underlying principles of this approach are sound and it is right that interventions which inherently carry greater risk (e.g., surgery) should be reserved for the more severe grades of obesity, while more modest interventions be used for lesser and more prevalent degrees of obesity. However, the focus on BMI, and the arbitrariness of the divisions (now modified by the World Health Organization from the original Garrow classification) serve to straight-jacket the clinician, and to ignore the need to fit treatment to the individual and vice versa. These BMI grades also under-estimate the risks

Table 15.3 Selection of treatment strategy appropriate to degree of obesity proposed originally by Garrow. Adapted from Garrow (1981).

BMI range	Grade 0 20–24.9	Grade 1 25–29.9	Grade 2 30–40	Grade 3 >40
Diet				
Very low calorie	No	No	No	Possibly
Conventional	No	Yes	Yes	Yes
Milk diet	No	Possibly	Yes	Yes
Drugs				
Anorectic	No	No	Possibly	Possibly
Physical training				
Exercise/activity	Yes	Yes	Possibly	No
Surgical				
Jaw wiring	No	No	Possibly	Yes
Gastroplasty	No	No	No	Possibly
Reassurance	Yes	Possibly	No	No

from what is often called 'moderate' obesity. The data from the Nurses Health Trial show clearly that risk of cardiovascular disease (Manson *et al.*, 1997) and non-insulin-dependent diabetes mellitus (NIDDM) (Carey *et al.*, 1997) increases in women from a BMI of around 23. More importantly BMI is an imperfect measure of risk. Fat distribution independently predicts risk and, particularly at modest degrees of obesity, is a better indicator of risk than BMI (Lundgren *et al.*, 1989; Han *et al.*, 1995; Carey *et al.*, 1997). While this and other schemes emphasize the role of conventional diets for all grades of obesity, they do not take into account individuals' previous experience or exposure to obesity treatment, nor the presence or absence of co-morbidities such as diabetes and hypertension that may justify more aggressive intervention at lower degrees of obesity. It is probably inappropriate to re-prescribe a 'conventional' reduced calorie diet as treatment to a 40-year-old man with diabetes and hypertension who has previously been unsuccessful with simple dietetic intervention.

Two schemes that amplified this approach have been published. Brownell and Wadden (1991) suggested a three-stage process in selecting treatment for an individual (Fig. 15.2); the first step was to classify the degree of obesity (again by somewhat arbitrary cut-points of overweight and obesity. The level of overweight dictated which of five steps of care would be reasonable to implement; the least costly and risky approaches being favoured for the lowest levels of obesity, while the most aggressive interventions (e.g., surgery) are reserved for the most severely obese. A third stage by which a number of patient and programme factors are considered can be used to ensure a proper match between programme, patient and disease severity.

Another model developed by Blackburn (Committee to develop criteria for evaluating the outcomes of approaches to prevent and treat obesity, 1995) (Fig. 15.3) is a dynamic stepped intervention that describes the steps to be taken according to outcome. It suggests that all patients enter the least intensive intervention first; progressive failure leads to increasing intensity of intervention. In the model, patients therefore may take 2 years or more to reach the criteria for treatment of eating disorders, or the use of drugs or very-low-calorie diets, and do so regardless of their degree of obesity. Both this and the Brownell and Wadden model seem unsuited to countries outside North America as provision of tertiary specialist centres or hospital nutrition clinics are scarce. As models they do, however, suggest a logical way to offer treatment, and importantly could be used to standardize the approach to treatment and so act as a basis for research and audit into outcome.

Figure 15.4 takes a different approach and suggests a way in which the various providers of treatments relevant to obesity can interact, and suggests that a suitable trained practice nurse could play a key role in treatment and support. Experience in the field of diabetes and asthma care, especially in the U.K., has

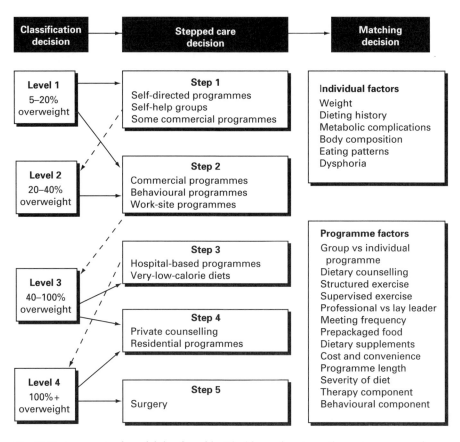

Fig. 15.2 A conceptual model developed by Blackburn showing a three-stage process for assigning treatment to an individual. The first step based on classification of the degree of obesity links with a limited choice of interventions that are themselves stepped in intensity, cost and risk. A third stage of matching is dictated by client and programme factors. The dashed lines show the lowest level of treatment likely to be effective. Redrawn from Brownell and Wadden (1991). Copyright (1991) by the Association for Advancement of Behavior Therapy. Reprinted by permission of the publisher.

shown how successful and cost effective specialist nurses can be. The scheme also suggests that there should be a two-way interplay between doctors, dietitians and nurses as opposed the existing top-down approach with doctors in the ascendancy. In addition the need to involve commercial slimming groups and sports clubs and to encourage patient support groups is recognized.

The SIGN guidelines (Fig. 15.5) draw together the principles of risk assessment from BMI, fat distribution and other factors into a didactic management strategy (Scottish Intercollegiate Guidelines Network, 1996). The guidelines are targeted at primary care physicians (general practitioners). This is a realistic approach since it is in this sector of health care that obesity, because of its

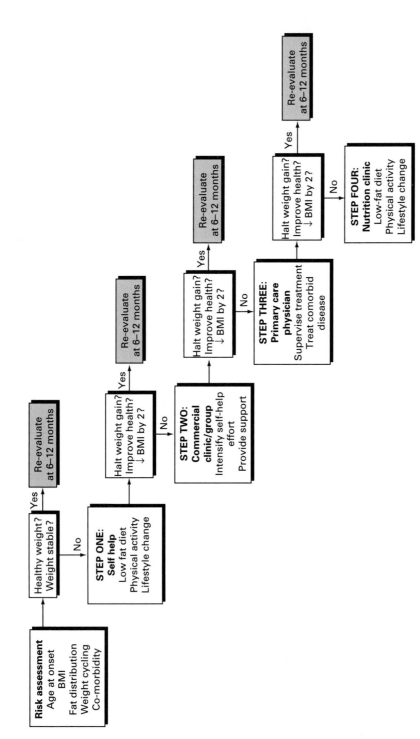

Fig. 15.3 A stepped care model of treatment developed by Blackburn. In this scheme all patients assessed to be at risk participate in step 1 over 3–6 months. Goals for treatment success and failure are set. If these are not met then increasingly aggressive interventions are applied. Redrawn from Committee to develop criteria for evaluating the outcomes of approaches to prevent and treat obesity (1995). Copyright (1995) by the National Academy Press, Washington, D.C.

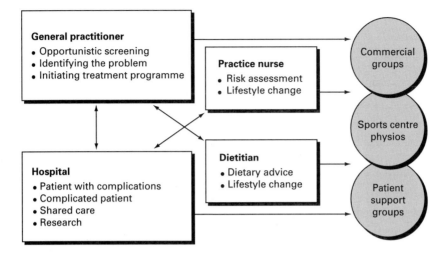

Fig. 15.4 A diagram to show how health-care services and professionals can interact to support each other and form a coordinated network of obesity treatment and supervision. At present the concept of an obesity-trained practice nurse is undeveloped, and dietitians are unable to refer patients for medical assessment. The involvement of commercial providers, especially slimming groups, is poorly integrated into more medical obesity management.

high prevalence, will necessarily have to be treated in the main. The SIGN guidelines direct the physician towards the more limited intervention of 'healthy eating' advice (and follow-up) to those of normal weight, or those with modest overweight (BMI 15–30 kg/m^2) but without significant risk factors. The guidelines emphasize that risk factors other than obesity be given priority. Thus, smoking cessation should be of a higher priority than weight loss (Wannamethee & Shaper, 1989), although weight management interventions are likely to be needed to limit weight gain on smoking cessation (Williamson et al., 1991).

Weight loss and weight-loss goals

Clinical assessment

The usual principles of medical consultation should apply to assessing the patient with obesity. Consultation can be facilitated by asking the patient to collect dietary or body-weight data prior to the first visit. In health systems, such as exist in the U.K. where medical care is free at the point of delivery, there is a high frequency of non-attendance at out-patient clinics. Obesity clinics seem particularly prone to attract a high rate of 'did not attend' patients, perhaps because patients have perceived the referral as inappropriate, unlikely to be

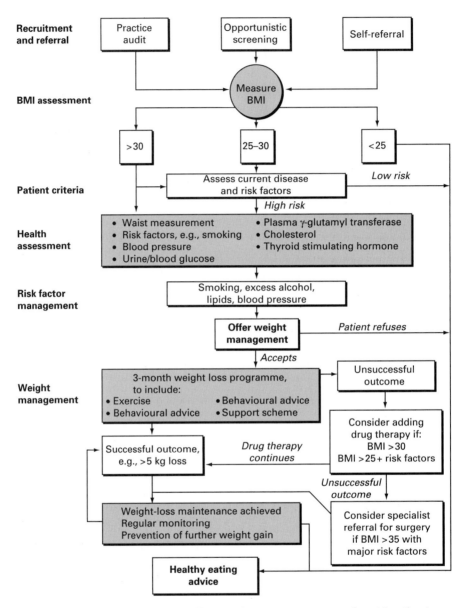

Fig. 15.5 The SIGN guidelines that offer a total management strategy from identification and recruitment of patients, to investigation and stepped treatment according to risk and outcome. The scheme allows for failure and incorporates pharmacological intervention in selected cases. The guidelines were drawn up prior to the withdrawal of the fenfluramines in 1997. Redrawn from Scottish Intercollegiate Guidelines Network (1996).

helpful, or are concerned that they will not be treated sympathetically. With this background it can be useful to have some form of (postal) pre-appointment screening to assess patients' motivation. The process can be combined with giving information and reassurance about the purpose of clinic attendance. At the same time, the patient will have time to put together details of their previous history, treatments and current dietary habits, removed form the stress of a one-to-one consultation.

The consultation room must be properly equipped for obese patients. This will necessitate larger-than-average chairs, access for wheelchairs or patients with mobility problems, couches that are large enough to accommodate a large patient safely, and that can be raised or lowered. Medical equipment of an appropriate size is essential. There is nothing more demeaning to the patient, and indicative of professional incompetence and thoughtlessness, than if the scales are inadequate for weighing, the blood pressure cuff too small, or the tape measure too short to surround the waist of the patient.

Obesity will usually have had a long previous history of development and treatment efforts. It involves multiple systems, often including psychiatric and social complications. The initial assessment is unlikely to take less than 45 minutes. It is particularly important for the doctor and patient to develop a good rapport, and this is unlikely if either are rushed. The consultation itself is likely to be an important part of treatment. For example, the information that the doctor elicits can raise patients' acceptance about the importance attached to exercise and activity. Table 15.4 outlines the areas to be covered at the initial visit.

Patients referred with obesity are particularly likely to bring a partner or friend to the first visit. Many clinics encourage this. There is, however, a difference of opinion amongst doctors as to whether the presence of a partner or friend is useful or antipathetic to the therapeutic environment. The presence of another person can act as a barrier to the patient being able to fully express his or her feelings and needs (Aitken, 1997), so that the patient feels pressurized to withhold or alter sensitive information, for example about sexual conflict, childhood or ongoing abuse, or about secret eating habits. It is best to try and get the best of both worlds. An initial interview with the patient alone will allow them to talk uninhibitedly; a joint interview with the accompanying person later (perhaps after the examination) allows an insight into how the patient interacts with others and vice versa. The presence of a spouse or partner is particularly useful in eliciting features of sleep quality, and whether there are features of sleep apnoea (snoring or apnoea attacks).

History

The history should start with the patient's presenting symptoms. Although obesity may be the obvious presenting complaint, and may have been stated as the purpose of the referral by the referring general practitioner, it is important to get the patient's perspective of his or her problem. This may differ considerably from the doctor's. The patient may believe he or she has been referred for treatment of a specific problem such as angina, depression, infertility, or arthritis. He or she may not yet have accepted that the overweight is the underlying cause of the symptoms, or be unready to enter obesity treatment. The concept of readiness to change was developed as a model to describe the wide range of attitudes, beliefs and cognition that surround health behaviours. Developed initially in relation to smoking cessation (DiClemente *et al.*, 1991), this model is increasingly being applied to obesity treatment (Rossi *et al.*, 1995). A number of measures have been developed (e.g., Dieting Readiness Test (Brownell, 1990), Weight Efficacy Life-Style Questionnaire (Prochaska *et al.*, 1992)) to try and predict outcome of treatment and may be usefully applied in a clinical setting.

Table 15.4 Checklist of the key points to be included in taking a history, examining and investigating a patient with obesity.

History	Presenting complaints
	History of weight gain
	History of weight losses and previous treatment
	Exercise and activity history
	Family history of obesity and co-morbidities
	Drug history and alcohol intake
	Social history
	(Dietary history)
	Past medical history (including psychiatric or eating disorders)
	Systems review
	Expectations from treatment
	Motivation/readiness
Examination	Height, weight, waist and hip circumference
	Skin changes
	Gonadal status
	Pulmonary hypertension, cor pulmonale
	Cardiac valvular disease
	Dyslipidaemia, xanthoma, xanthelasma, corneal arcus
	Diabetic retinopathy
	Hypothalamic–pituitary disease, visual fields, optic atrophy
	Goitre or signs of thyroid disease
Investigations	Free thyroxine and thyroid-stimulating hormone
	Fasting blood glucose
	Urine glucose
	Fasting cholesterol and triglycerides
	Electrocardiogram

More commonly, however, patients come with expectations for treatment; often, however, this is seen as something passive and it is hoped that 'the doctor will do something' for 'the weight problem'. Goal setting can usefully be integrated into the initial consultation by the appropriate emphasis on non-weight measures of health in the history taking.

The history of weight gain should be described in detail. The purpose of this is to elucidate a possible aetiology, but can also be used as a way of assessing the individual's insight and understanding of the factors causing weight gain. As with the history of complaints, such an approach can define at the outset the links between lifestyle, behaviour and body-weight control. It is also useful to distinguish a childhood onset from that occurring later in life either in relation to specific physiological 'critical periods' or illness. Although the strong genetic predisposition to obesity is well defined, single gene defects are extremely rare. Leptin deficiency due to gene mutation has been described in just one family (Montague et al., 1997) and obviously has potential therapeutic implications. It is likely that other gene predispositions will be identified by a bottom-up molecular biology approach, but also perhaps from careful definition of obesity phenotypes. A number of syndromes are associated with childhood-onset obesity, but the history in such cases is usually, but not always, obvious because of the associated clinical features (Table 15.5). Diseases, usually en-docrine or neuro-endocrine, involving the hypothalamus tend to have a much shorter history of weight gain compared to that seen in 'spontaneous' obesity; patients with these diseases usually present with symptoms specific to the disease rather than their obesity. An audit of more than 2 years' referrals to a hospital obesity clinic showed no new cases of endocrine disease (Finer & Zarb, 1984). A history of Cushing's disease (bruising, mood change, muscle weakness, hirsutism and buffalo hump fat) and hypothyroidism (cold intolerance, oedema and puffiness of the eyelids, dry skin and hair, and constipation) should be specifically sought. Later-onset obesity may relate to events such as pregnancy and the menopause in women, although it remains unclear as to how much the change in hormonal status directly accounts for the weight gain, compared to other changes in lifestyle that tend to accompany such events. Weight gain at the time of significant life events (e.g., marriage, job change, bereavement, smoking cessation) is important to identify in order to help the patient appreciate the importance of change in lifestyle to body-weight regulation.

Few patients will remember details of their weight throughout life, but there are often key landmarks at which weight may be recalled. These include marriage, childbirth or previous episodes of obesity treatment. An alternative to weight recall, especially if weights are not remembered, is to ask about clothing size, or use standard outline drawings of body size (Stunkard et al., 1983). The use of imprecise terms such as 'plump', 'chubby' and 'overweight' are often grossly inaccurate, with a general tendency to under-estimate the degree of overweight. Body size outlines are particularly useful for obtaining an idea of the degree of obesity of family members.

Table 15.5 Some of the commoner and more well defined genetic syndromes in which obesity is a prominent clinical manifestation.

Syndrome	Genetic association	Obesity features	Other features
Prader–Willi	15q11	Feeding difficulties at birth, overtaken by extreme hyperphagia and weight gain with generalized obesity from age 2–3. Short stature	Hypogonadism, hypotonia, small hands and feet, scoliosis, learning difficulties, behaviour problems
Bardet–Biedl	16q21, 11q13,15q22	Overlap with Lawrence–Moon–Bardet–Biedl syndrome (in which obesity is inconsistent); onset of generalized obesity in first 2 years. Short stature	Retinitis pigmentosa, hypogonadism, learning difficulties, polydactyly
Cohen	8q22–23	Truncal obesity from mid-childhood. Short stature	Hypotonia, delayed puberty with or without hypogonadism
Alström	Autosomal recessive	Normal height, truncal obesity from mid-childhood	Hypogonadism, blindness in infancy from retinal degeneration, deafness, insulin resistance
Albright hereditary osteodystrophy	Autosomal recessive	Childhood onset	Diabetes with severe insulin resistance, blindness due to retinal degeneration
Klinefelter's	XXY	Adult onset, with peripheral distribution. Tall with eunuchoid proportions	Hypogonadal, moderate learning difficulties, gynaecomastia

A history of previous obesity treatments and weight loss is likely to be revealing. Individuals who truly have had no previous advice or dietetic input can be identified and will probably need referral in due course for straightforward nutritional/dietetic counselling. On the other hand, the person who has already tried and failed on well-supervised diets and behavioural programmes may be a candidate for drug treatment, surgery, or even no treatment at all. It is unlikely to be productive to revisit previous battlegrounds of weight control, and doing so may only serve to accentuate failure and further diminish self-esteem. However, it often is possible to highlight what went wrong on previous attempts, and specifically address the issues raised in further treatment to forestall repetition of errors or omissions. Occasionally patients insist that they are unable to lose weight, whatever the intervention. They will often quote a history of hospital admission for starvation without weight loss. The doctor can be certain that such a history is incompatible with the known facts concerning human energy balance. Exploring or confronting such denial (or delusion) during the initial visit is unlikely to be helpful. It is better to reserve interpretations of these events to a later stage of the therapeutic relationship. Access to previous medical records, if available, rarely support such dramatic interpretations of past events, and are an important adjunct to a verbally obtained history.

Details of current levels of exercise and activity should be ascertained and at the same time motivation to increase activity, daily activities or exercise explored. A point-blank refusal to consider an increase in activity as a possibility (either from lack of fitness or time) suggests a poor prognosis for weight loss maintenance.

A family history of obesity may suggest a genetic predisposition. Asking about other members of the family can also be a way into considering family-based therapies or preventative action for children who appear to be at particular risk of obesity, either through their parental genes or eating habits. The risk of developing complications, particularly diabetes mellitus or coronary artery disease, can also be ascertained by a knowledge of the incidence of such diseases within the family. The weight of the spouse or partner, however, often reveals more about shared dietary habits and lifestyle, and the possibility of change.

Details of a drug history are important since a number of drugs are associated with weight gain. These include phenothiazines, tricyclic antidepressants, antihistamines, anti-convulsants, lithium, glucocorticoid steroids, anabolic and potent progestagenic steroids and, theoretically, beta-blockers. Chronic or recurrent hypoglycaemia from over-treated diabetes mellitus can stimulate appetite and food intake thereby leading to weight gain. Over-replacement with thyroid hormones, in patients with biochemically proven hypothyroidism, will also stimulate appetite (through decreasing satiety) (Sheikh & Finer, 1994) and this can outstrip the effect on raising metabolic rate. Although many women believe that the contraceptive pill and hormone replacement treatment lead to weight gain, the evidence is poor. Hormone replacement in postmenopausal women reverses the trend to visceral fat deposition (Haarbo et al., 1991), while conversely hypoandrogenaemia in men is associated with increased visceral fat and can be reversed with testosterone supplementation (Marin et al., 1992). Identifying patients on diuretics, especially if taken intermittently, may help to explain sudden shifts in body-weight that relate to fluid loss or gain rather than fat-mass changes. Smoking cessation may produce greater health gain than weight loss, but the effect on weight gain (and vice versa) is well described (Dallosso & James, 1984; Williamson et al., 1991).

The social history should include information about income, educational achievement and family dynamics. It is these aspects of life that often will determine not just motivation and understanding, but also the ability to change. 'Healthy eating' need not be more expensive than a poor quality diet, but sensitivity is needed in suggesting dietary changes which are not part of the patient's social milieu. Expense is not the only issue. A lack of storage or cooking facilities, a limited choice or difficulties in access to shops, or a partner on an overlapping work shift can all make change difficult. Relationships may be seriously undermined when one partner starts to lose weight. For example the often slim, inadequate husband may feel threatened if his obese wife loses weight, gains in assertiveness and starts socializing. The interview may highlight how easily changes in food-related habits can be altered.

Dietary habits can be usefully outlined in perhaps 5 minutes during the initial consultation, but a formal diet history will require a separate consultation with a trained dietitian. It is useful to ask the patient to keep a diet diary (and also to record any exercise or activity taken) for a week or so. This can be used as a basis for assessment. The patient can be asked to start recording before the first appointment and bring the diary on the first visit. This may lead to a more accurate record, since the patient will feel less pressured than when he or she knows the doctor's expectations communicated at the first consultation. The diaries provide qualitative data on meal and snack frequency, night-time or binge eating, and large variations in intake (for example at weekends). The records also provide limited nutritional information on, for example, sugar or fat-rich items in the diet, and alcohol intake. Alcohol is an important source of energy intake, especially for men. The distribution of energy from alcohol in men is markedly skewed: the mean percentage of energy from alcohol is 6.9% for men, but over a quarter of men (28%) receive more than 10% of their energy from alcohol, and 2.5% of those who drink obtain nearly 30% of their energy from alcohol (Gregory et al., 1990); the implication for reducing dietary energy intake is obvious. Self-monitoring and recording intake is a cornerstone of behavioural treatment and change (Dubbert & Wilson, 1984; Wadden &

Letizia, 1992), and may in itself improve the diet (Bellack *et al.*, 1974). This can be turned to clinical advantage: if weight is recorded and shown to fall during the period of self-monitoring there is a clear demonstration of what can be achieved by such a simple intervention. Detailed dietary assessments are of dubious value in the initial evaluation, since it is known that they are extremely inaccurate and patients can under-report energy intake by 30% (Prentice *et al.*, 1986; Lichtman *et al.*, 1993). Dietary energy prescription can be based on estimated energy expenditure (Lean & James, 1986) less a fixed deficit, typically of 200 kJ/500 kcal (2.09 MJ). This approach is not only more successful than fixed 500 kJ/1200 kcal (5.02 MJ) diets (Frost *et al.*, 1991), but also avoids the difficulty of knowing how to prescribe a diet to an obese patient reporting weight maintenance on 3000 kJ/750 kcal (3.14 MJ) daily.

To complete the full medical assessment, the history of previous illness and a check for symptoms from all body systems is needed. Weight loss is a symptom of many serious diseases; no physician wishes to congratulate a patient with undiagnosed colon cancer or thyrotoxicosis on their progressive weight loss. Knowing that a patient has a history of ischaemic heart disease may raise the priority for intervening, but will at the same time dictate extra caution at ensuring that weight loss is not overly rapid, and that exercise levels are not increased too rapidly. A history of gallstones or eating disorders would also mitigate against regimens producing prolonged rapid weight loss, especially very-low-calorie liquid diets since these are known to increase the risk of gallstone formation (Broomfield *et al.*, 1988). Previous gastro-intestinal disorders, e.g., lactose intolerance or severe constipation, should also influence the diet prescribed. A late menarche and the failure to establish a regular menstrual cycle may suggest the presence of polycystic ovary syndrome; such patients may need contraceptive advice since weight loss can restore fertility.

The end of the interview should also allow the patient to express a view about his or her expectations and hopes; these, both for weight loss and also for improved quality of life, are often unrealistic, and management will need to include re-focusing their goals. While health gain may be the stated aim of entering treatment, for most patients it is rate and absolute amounts of weight loss by which they judge their success. If this is their belief it is important that there is an opportunity to point out the medical aims of treatment.

Examination

Clinical examination must form part of any medical assessment, and this applies equally for the obese patient. An outline is shown in Table 15.4. Many obese patients fear having to undress and expose themselves, and sensitivity is needed to avoid embarrassment. Height should be measured (without socks and shoes) accurately with a stadiometer. Before weighing, the patient should be asked to remove shoes, outer clothing and empty his or her pockets of coins and other heavy items. Weight is most simply measured using electronic scales, although beam balances are satisfactory but more cumbersome and time consuming to use. It is essential that the scales are accurate and good practice dictates that they should regularly be calibrated against known weights. BMI can be calculated from height and weight, but does not always predict body fat accurately. Skinfold thickness measurements, while of use in epidemiological studies, are of little use in assessing total body fat in individual patients. If felt necessary, body fat can be assessed by investigative techniques discussed below. Fat distribution should be assessed clinically and used to refine an assessment of risk. Waist and hip circumference should be measured according to established methods (World Health Organization, 1989). Waist is taken as the midpoint between the lower rib margin and the iliac crest, and the hip defined as the widest point over the greater trochanters. In practice these landmarks may prove extremely difficult in the very obese (for whom a tape measure of 200 cm may be needed), particularly if there is a large abdominal 'apron' overhanging where the hip would be measured. Waist and hip circumferences probably add little to risk assessment in such patients with a BMI above 35. A number of other 'bedside' anthropometric measures have been developed to assess fat distribution (van der Kooy & Seidell, 1993) but are not used in routine clinical practice. The obese may understandably feel very sensitive about having these measurements made. It may be appropriate to leave them until the end of the examination, and for the doctor, rather than a nurse in a treatment room, to make the measurements. Visual inspection of the skin and fat distribution is important. Cold dry skin may raise the possibility of hypothyroidism (co-existing or causative of the obesity). Thin atrophic skin is a feature of corticosteroid excess which may results from Cushing's syndrome, although most commonly iatrogenic as a result of corticosteroid treatment. The presence of acanthosis nigricans (pigmented 'velvety' skin creases especially in the axillae) suggests insulin resistance; severe hirsutism in a woman may indicate polycystic ovary syndrome.

Blood pressure must be measured with an appropriately sized cuff; use of too small a cuff will falsely elevate the reading (Maxwell et al., 1982). Clinical examination of the heart may reveal left ventricular hypertrophy and/ or dilatation, or possibly valve lesions that might very rarely relate to previous exposure to certain anorectic drug regimens (Connolly et al., 1997). The presence of xanthelasma or xanthoma alerts to the presence of dyslipidaemias. Many severely obese people will have problems with lymphatic obstruction to the lower limbs, with swelling and lymphoedema sufficient to impair mobility. Venous insufficiency may also lead to ulceration of the legs. Retinopathies from associated diabetes or hypertension are important to diagnose so that they can be appropriately treated.

Respiratory problems are common in obesity, and a neck circumference of more than 43 cm (17 inches) suggests that obstructive sleep apnoea is likely (see Chapter 12). Cor pulmonale with pulmonary hypertension and oedema is a late complication. Abdominal and breast examination is significantly hindered by the presence of excessive body fat, but the clinician must be aware that breast and colon cancer incidences are increased in obesity. Abnormal gonadal status may suggest certain rare genetic syndromes, several of which include obesity (Table 15.5). Acquired hypothalamic–pituitary disease is often associated with obesity and if there is any suspicion of this it is worth checking visual fields, retinal and optic disk integrity.

Investigation

The diagnosis of obesity is self-evident being defined on anthropometric measurements; the role of investigation is to assess possible causes of obesity, and its complications (Kopelman, 1994). As discussed above, few diseases present as obesity, but it is wise to undertake a small number of routine tests (see Table 15.4).

Thyroid function tests (the most usual strategy is to measure free thyroxine and thyroid-stimulating hormone) are needed since thyroid disorders are common in the general population, and are often insidious in onset. Tri-iodothyronine is not useful in diagnosis, falling rapidly during under-feeding, and increasing in response to over-feeding (Danforth et al., 1979; Jung, 1984). While thyroid hormones have profound effects on energy metabolism (DuBois, 1927), disorders of thyroid function are a rare cause of obesity (Hoogwerf & Nuttall, 1984; Pears et al., 1990; Lessan & Finer, 1996).

Diabetes mellitus and dyslipidaemia are common complications of obesity, and screening for them with fasting blood glucose and lipid profile (after a 14-hour fast), as well as testing for urinary glucose, should be routine. The use of glycated haemoglobin for diagnosing diabetes mellitus has been suggested but is not yet established. A full blood count is useful both for screening purposes and as a crude nutritional measure; a raised mean corpuscular volume (MCV) raises the possibility of excessive alcohol intake or vitamin B_{12} or folic acid deficiency. Routine screening for Cushing's syndrome is unrewarding in the absence of specific clinical clues and interpretation of results from simple tests (such as plasma cortisol or urinary cortisol excretion) is not always straightforward in an obese patient. An electrocardiogram should be routinely recorded in view of the high prevalence of hypertension and cardiovascular disease in obesity.

Further investigation will be dictated by the clinical suspicion of coexisting pathology. Investigation of those with associated gonadal, menstrual or reproductive abnormalities will include measurement of testosterone, sex hormone binding globulin (SHBG), luteinizing hormone (LH) and follicle-stimulating hormone (FSH), and ovarian ultrasound. Obesity itself is associated with reduced SHBG concentrations, while in polycystic ovary syndrome a high LH and testosterone is to be expected. The finding of hypogonadism suggests further investigation for possible hypothalamic–pituitary disease (prolactin, dynamic pituitary function tests, magnetic resonance imaging (MRI) of the hypothalamus

Table 15.6 Further investigations that may form part of specialist investigation, research or audit activities.

Area of investigation	Possible indications	Tests or methodology
Metabolic rate	History of failure to lose weight on diet, proven hypothalamic disease	Resting metabolic rate by indirect calorimetry or 24-hour energy expenditure measurements by doubly-labelled water of whole-body calorimetry
Body composition	Risk assessment, treatment monitoring, dysmorphic features, borderline high BMI in fit individual	Bio-electrical impedance, whole-body plethysmography or underwater weighing, DEXA scanning (Jebb & Elia, 1993)
Insulin sensitivity	Acanthosis nigricans, other biochemical evidence for metabolic syndrome, dysmorphic fat deposition	Fasting insulin/C-peptide to glucose ratio, glucose:insulin minimal modelling techniques (Matsuda & DeFronzo, 1997)
Sleep study	History of sleep apnoea, daytime drowsiness	Overnight sleep monitoring with measurement of oxygen saturation, respiration, snoring (Grunstein & Wilcox, 1994)
Eating disorders	History of binge eating, previous anorexia nervosa	Questionnaire assessments such as Eating Disorder Inventory, BITE (Allison, 1995)
Genetics	Syndrome presentation, very early onset, strongly discordant family history	?Leptin measurement

and pituitary) or, in children, chromosomal or more detailed genetic analysis. If Cushing's disease is suspected, suppression of plasma cortisol at 9.00 AM after 1 mg of dexamethasone given at midnight the day before (the overnight dexamethasone suppression test) makes the diagnosis unlikely. Incomplete suppression, or a persisting strong clinical suspicion of adrenocortical excess, will require more detailed investigation with dynamic endocrine tests and radiological investigation of the pituitary and adrenals.

Further investigation may form part of research or clinic audit protocols and are listed in Table 15.6.

Treatment choices and goals

The possibilities for treatment are outlined in the various clinical guidelines referenced earlier in the chapter, and are considered in more detail elsewhere in this book. Treatment aims to improve health and well-being, and decrease the risks of ill health later in life; it does not aim to achieve cosmetic results (although this may form part of the patient's expectations). Central to the concept of health improvement is the realization that weight loss is only an initial phase of treatment, and that weight-loss maintenance is the principle goal. Judged by these criteria the literature makes it clear that treatment is still far from satisfactory, but the pessimism of some may be misplaced. It is true, however, that the longest-term studies show that long-term weight-loss maintenance is at present rarely achieved as a result of non-surgical treatment (NIH Technology Assessment Conference Panel, 1992, 1993), whether patients are attending hospital-based programmes (Kramer et al., 1989) or commercial slimming clubs (Volkamar et al., 1981). The situation as regards prevention in childhood obesity is more promising (Glenny et al., 1997).

Realistic goals and expectations

Ideas about success in obesity treatment have been profoundly influenced by the evidence that has increasingly accumulated, namely that modest degrees of weight loss produce significant health gain. Weight loss of 5–10% can be shown to improve blood pressure (Stamler et al., 1980; Tuck et al., 1981; Rissanen et al., 1985), dyslipidaemia (Kanaley et al., 1993) and diabetes mellitus (Hadden et al., 1975; Wing et al., 1987). These data have been further supported by results showing a decreased mortality with modest intentional weight loss (Williamson et al., 1995).

With this background it is legitimate to redefine successful treatment in terms of a decrease in the severity of obesity rather than a return to 'normal' weight. Figure 15.6 showing theoretical weight loss and regain curves in response to

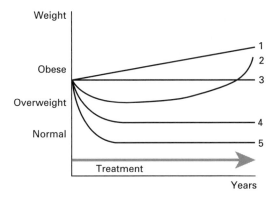

Fig. 15.6 Diagrammatic representation of the outcome of treatments for obesity. Line 1 represents the natural history of the disease with progressive weight gain. Line 3 represents weight stability. Partial success with weight falling to a level associated with decreased risk of ill health and potential partial amelioration of co-morbid disease is shown by line 4; line 5 would represent cure. Line 2 may be considered to be the only outcome to have totally failed, since weight loss is followed by regain above initial weight. After Rossner (1993).

treatment serves to reinforce the message that weight-loss maintenance is the desired goal of treatment. Thus, even weight stabilization without weight loss represents a modestly successful outcome compared to the natural history of progressive weight gain.

This background is needed in order to set goals for obesity treatment to the individual patient. Patients should be encouraged at the start of treatment to set their own goals. Classical learning theories dictate that unrealistic targets do not encourage or motivate. Unrealistic goals must be challenged, especially those which set up unrealistic expectations for rates or amounts of weight loss. Goals can be set, and tested for realism, in answer to questions such as 'How much weight each week do you expect to lose?' and 'How will your life be different when you lose weight?'. Encouraging achievable goals will lead to positive emotional responses, rather than ones that engender failure and negative thoughts (Brownell, 1997). It is not only the patients that need to have realistic expectations and goals. Commonly doctors, nurses and dietitians expect impossible and often undesirable rates of weight loss or target weights. Goal setting should not just apply to weight, but to other desirable behaviours such as increasing exercise and assertiveness, and can also relate to direct health benefits such as blood pressure reduction or improved diabetes control. Furthermore, this approach should be harnessed to encourage and teach the more difficult problem of weight-loss maintenance. However much the benefits of modest weight loss and weight loss maintenance are emphasized, patients are often reluctant to accept the messages and commonly have firmly held desires for ever-greater, and ever-faster weight loss. Dramatic weight loss can be achieved with surgical intervention, or potentially by pharmacotherapy, but there needs to be a valid risk:benefit expectation to justify such treatment. Goal setting in terms of compliance with other aspects of these treatments will still be relevant.

References

Aitken, H.A. (1997) A salutary lesson: family secrets. *British Medical Journal* **314**, 1718.

Allison, D.B. (1995) *Handbook of Assessment Methods for Eating Behaviors and Weight Related Problems. Measures, Theory and Research*. Thousand Oaks: Sage Publications Ltd.

Ashwell, M.A. (1973) A survey investigating patients' views on doctors' treatment of obesity. *Practitioner* **211**, 653–658.

Bellack, A.S., Rozensky, R. & Schwartz, J.S. (1974) A comparison of two forms of self-monitoring in a behavioral weight reduction program. *Behavior Therapy* **5**, 523–530.

Broomfield, P.H., Chopra, R., Bonorris B.G., Silverman, A.M., Schoenfield, L.J. & Marks, J.W. (1988) Effects of ursodeoxycholic acid and aspirin on the formation of lithogenic bile and gallstones during loss of weight. *New England Journal of Medicine* **319**, 1567–1572.

Brownell, K.D. (1990) Dieting readiness. *Weight Control Digest* **1**, 5–9.

Brownell, K.D. (1997) *The Learn Program for Weight Control*, 7th edn. Dallas: American Health Publishing Co.

Brownell, K.D. & Wadden, T.A. (1991) The heterogeneity of obesity: fitting treatment to individuals. *Behavior Therapy* **22**, 153–177.

Cade, J. & O'Connell, S. (1991) Management of weight problems and obesity: knowledge, attitudes and current practice of general practitioners. *British Journal of General Practice* **41**, 147–150.

Carey, V.J., Walters, E.E., Colditz, G.A. *et al.* (1997) Body fat distribution and risk of non-insulin-dependent diabetes mellitus in women: the nurses' health study. *American Journal of Epidemiology* **145**, 614–169.

Committee to develop criteria for evaluating the outcomes of approaches to prevent and treat obesity, F.a.N.B.I.o.M. (1995) *Weighing the Options. Criteria for Evaluating Weight-Management Programs*. Washington DC: National Academy Press.

Connolly, H.M., Crary, J.L., McGoon, M.D. *et al.* (1997) Valvular heart disease associated with fenfluramine-phentermine. *New England Journal of Medicine* **337**, 581–588.

Coomber, C., Finer, N. & Peterson, D.B. (1997) Quality of referrals to an obesity clinic. *International Journal of Obesity* **21**, S114 (abstract).

Dallosso, H.M. & James, W.P.T. (1984) The role of smoking in the regulation of energy balance. *International Journal of Obesity* **8**, 365–375.

Danforth Jr, E., Horton, E.S. & O'Connell, M. (1979) Dietary-induced alterations in thyroid hormone metabolism during overnutrition. *Journal of Clinical Investigation* **64**, 1336–1347.

DiClemente, C.C., Prochaska, J.O., Fairhurst, S.K., Velicer, W.F., Velasquez, M.M. & Rossi, J.S. (1991) The processes of smoking cessation: an analysis of precontemplation, contemplation and preparation stages of change. *Journal of Consulting and Clinical Psychology* **59**, 295–304.

Dubbert, P.M. & Wilson, G.T. (1984) Goal-setting and spouse involvement in the treatment of obesity. *Behavior Research and Therapy* **22**, 272–242.

DuBois, E.F. (1927) Diseases of the thyroid. In: DuBois, E.F. (ed.) *Basal Metabolism in Health and Disease*, pp. 287–342. Philadelphia: Lea & Febiger.

Ezzati, R.M., Massey, J.T., Waksburg, J., Chu, A. & Maurer, K.R. (1992) Sample design: third national health and nutrition examination survey. *Vital and Health Statistics* **2**, 113.

Finer, N. & Zarb, P. (1984) Clinical audit of an obesity clinic. *International Journal of Obesity* **8**, 474 (abstract).

Frost, G., Masters, K., King, C. et al. (1991) A new method of energy prescription to improve weight loss. *Journal of Human Nutrition and Dietetics* **4**, 269–373.

Garner, D.M. & Wooley, S.C. (1991) Confronting the failure of behavioural and dietary treatments for obesity. *Clinical Psychology Reviews* **11**, 573–578.

Garrow, J.S. (1981) *Treat Obesity Seriously: A Clinical Manual*. London: Churchill Livingstone.

Gill, T.G. (1997) Key issues in the prevention of obesity. *British Medical Bulletin* **53**, 229–237.

Glenny, A.-M., O'Meara, S., Melville, A., Sheldon, T.A. & Wilson, C. (1997) The treatment and prevention of obesity: a systematic review of the literature. *International Journal of Obesity* **21**, 715–737.

Gregory, J., Foster, K., Tyler, H. & Wiseman, M. Office of Population Census and Surveys, S.S.D., (eds) (1990) *The Dietary and Nutritional Survey of British Adults. A Survey of the Dietary Behaviour, Nutritional Status and Blood Pressure of Adults Aged 16 to 64 Living in Great Britain*, pp. 1–393. London: HMSO.

Grunstein, R.R. & Wilcox, I. (1994) Sleep-disordered breathing and obesity. In: Caterson, I.D., (ed.) *Obesity*, pp. 601–628. London: Baillière Tindall.

Haarbo, J., Marslew, U., Gotfredson, A. & Christiansen, C. (1991) Post-menopausal hormone replacement therapy prevents central distribution of body fat after the menopause. *Metabolism* **40**, 1323–1326.

Hadden, D.R., Montgomery, D.A., Skelly, R.J., Trimble, E.R., Weaver, J.A. & Wilson, E.A. (1975) Maturity onset diabetes mellitus—response to intensive dietary management. *British Medical Journal* **iii**, 276–278.

Han, T.S., van Leer, E.M., Seidell, J.C. & Lean, M.E.J. (1995) Waist circumference action levels in the identification of cardiovascular risk factors: prevalence study in a random sample. *British Medical Journal* **311**, 1041–1045.

Hoogwerf, B.J. & Nuttall, F.Q. (1984) Long term weight regulation in treated hyperthyroid and hypothyroid patients. *American Journal of Medicine* **30**, 681–686.

Jebb, S.A. & Elia, M. (1993) Techniques for the measurement of body composition: a practical guide. *International Journal of Obesity* **17**, 611–621.

Jung, R.T. (1984) Endocrinological aspects of obesity. *Clinics in Endocrinology and Metabolism* **13**, 597–612.

Kanaley, J.A., Andresen-Reid, M.L., Oenning, L., Kottke, B.A. & Jensen, M.D. (1993) Differential benefits of weight loss in upper-body and lower-body obese women. *American Journal of Clinical Nutrition* **57**, 20–26.

Kopelman, P.G. (1994) Investigation of obesity. *Clinical Endocrinology* **41**, 703–708.

Kramer, F.M., Jeffery, R.W., Forster, J.L. & Snell, M.K. (1980) Long-term follow-up of behavioural treatment for obesity: patterns of weight regain among men and women. *International Journal of Obesity* **13**, 123–136.

Lean, M.E.J. & James, W.P.T. (1986) Prescription of diabetic diets for the 1980s. *Lancet* **i**, 723–725.

Lessan, N.G. & Finer, N. (1996) Is hypothyroidism a cause of obesity? *Clinical Endocrinology* **151**, P106 (abstract).

Lichtman, S., Pisarka, K. & Berman, E. (1993) Discrepancy between self-reported and actual calorie intake and exercise in obese subjects. *New England Journal of Medicine* **327**, 1893–1898.

Lundgren, H., Bengtsson, C., Blohme, G., Lapidus, L. & Sjöstrom, L. (1989) Adiposity and adipose tissue distribution in relation to incidence of diabetes in women: results from a prospective population study in Gothenburg, Sweden. *International Journal of Obesity* **13**, 413–423.

Manson, J.E., Willet W.C. & Stampfer, M.J. (1997) The nurses' health study: body weight and mortality among women. *New England Journal of Medicine* **333**, 677–685.

Marin, P., Holmang, S., Jönsson, L. et al. (1992) The effects of testosterone treatment on body composition and metabolism in middle-aged obese men. *International Journal of Obesity* **16**, 991–997.

Matsuda, M. & DeFronzo, R.A. (1997) *In vivo* measurement of insulin sensitivity in humans. In: Draznin, B. & Rizza, R. (eds) *Clinical Research in Diabetes and Obesity*, Vol. I: *Methods, Assessment and Metabolic Regulation*, pp. 23–66. Totowa, NJ: Humana Press.

Maxwell, M.H., Waks, A.U., Schroth, P.C., Karam, M. & Dornfeld, L.P. (1982) Error in blood-pressure measurement due to incorrect cuff size in obese patients. *Lancet* **ii**, 33–36.

Montague, C.T., Farooqi, I.S., Whitehead, J.P. *et al.* (1997) Congenital leptin deficiency is associated with severe early-onset obesity in humans. *Nature* **387**, 903–908.

NIH Technology Assessment Conference Panel (1992) Methods for voluntary weight loss and control. *Annals of Internal Medicine* **116**, 942–949.

NIH Technology Assessment Conference Panel (1993) Methods for voluntary weight loss and control. *Annals of Internal Medicine*, **119**, 764–770.

Pears, J., Jung, R.T. & Gunn, A. (1990) Long term weight changes in treated hypothyroid and hyperthyroid patients. *Scottish Medical Journal* **35**, 180–182.

Prentice, A.M., Black, A.E., Coward, W.A. *et al.* (1986) High levels of energy expenditure in obese women. *British Medical Journal* **292**, 983–987.

Price, J.H., Desmond, S.M., Krol, R.A. (1997) Family practice physicians' beliefs, attitudes and practises regarding obesity. *American Journal of Preventative Medicine* **3**, 339–345.

Prochaska, J.O., Norcross, J.C., Fowler, J.L., Follick, M.J. & Abrams, D.B. (1992) Attendance and outcome in a work site weight control program: processes and stages of change as process and predictor variables. *Addictive Behaviors* **17**, 35–45.

Rippe, J.M. (1996) Overweight and health: communications challenges and opportunities. *American Journal of Clinical Nutrition* **63** (suppl.), 470S–473S.

Rissanen, A., Pieteinen, P., Siljamaki-Ojansuu, U., Pürainan, H. & Reissel, P. (1995) Treatment of hypertension in obese patients: efficacy and feasibility of weight and salt reduction programs. *Acta Medica Scandinavica* **218**, 149–156.

Rossi, J.S., Rossi, S.R., Velicer, W.F. & Prochaska, J.O. (1995) Motivational readiness to control weight. In: Allison, D.B. (ed.) *Handbook of Assessment Methods for Eating Behaviors and Weight-related Problems. Measures, Theories and Research*, pp. 387–430. Thousand Oaks: Sage Publications.

Rossner, S. (1993) Is obesity incurable? In: Ditschuneit, H., Gries, F.A., Hauner, H. *et al.* (eds) *Obesity in Europe 1993*, pp. 203–208. London: John Libbey & Co.

Royal College of Physicians (1997) *Overweight and Obese Patients. Principles of Management with Particular Reference to the Use of Drugs*, pp. 1–26. London: Royal College of Physicians.

Scottish Intercollegiate Guidelines Network (1996) *Obesity in Scotland. Integrating Prevention with Weight Management. A National Clinical Guideline Recommended for Use in Scotland.* Edinburgh: Royal College of Physicians, Scotland.

Sheikh, M. & Finer, N. (1994) Appetite and food consumption linkage in thyrotoxicosis: a model for states of increased energy expenditure. *International Journal of Obesity* **18** (suppl. 2), 115.

Stamler, J., Farinaro, E. & Mojonnier, L.M. (1980) Prevention and control of hypertension by nutritional-hygienic means. *Journal of the American Medical Association* **243**, 1819–1823.

Stunkard, A.J., Sorensen, T.I.A. & Schlusinger, F. (1983) Use of the Danish adopting register for the study of obesity and thinness. In: Kety, S., Rowland, L.P., Sidman, R.L. *et al.* (eds) *The Genetics of Neurological and Psychiatric Disorders*, pp. 115–129. New York: Raven.

Tuck, M.L., Sowers, J., Dornfeld, L.P., Kledzik, G. & Maxwell, M. (1981) The effect of weight reduction on blood pressure, plasma renin activity, and plasma aldosterone levels in obese patients. *New England Journal of Medicine* **304**, 930–933.

van der Kooy, K. & Seidell, J.C. (1993) Techniques for the measurement of visceral fat: a practical guide. *International Journal of Obesity* **17**, 187–196.

Volkmar, F.R., Stunkard, A.J., Woolston, J. & Bailey, J.F. (1981) High attrition rates in commercial weight loss programs. *Annals of Internal Medicine* **141**, 426–428.

Wadden, T.A. & Letizia, K.A. (1992) Predictors of attrition and weight loss in patients treated by moderate and severe caloric restriction. In: Wadden, T.A. & VanItallie, T.B. (eds) *Treatment of the Seriously Obese Patient*, pp. 383–410. New York: Guilford.

Wannamethee, G. & Shaper, A.G. (1989) Body weight and mortality in middle aged British men: impact of smoking. *British Medical Journal* **299**, 1497–1502.

Williamson, D.F., Madans, J., Anda, R.F., Kleinman, J.C., Giovino, G.A. & Byers, T. (1991) Smoking cessation and severity of weight gain in a national cohort. *The New England Journal of Medicine* **324**, 739–745.

Williamson, D.F., Pamuk, E.R., Thun, M., Flanders, D., Byers, T. & Heath, C. (1995) Prospective study of intentional weight loss and mortality in never-smoking overweight U.S. white women aged 40–64 years. *American Journal of Epidemiology* **141**, 1128–1141.

Wing, R.R., Koeske, R. & Epstein, L.H. (1987) Long-term effects of modest weight loss in Type 2 diabetic patients. *Annals of Internal Medicine* **147**, 1749–1753.

World Health Organization. (1989) *Measuring Obesity: Classification and Distribution of Anthropometric Data*. Nutr UD, EUR/ICP/NUT 125, Copenhagen: WHO.

CHAPTER 16

Dietary Treatment of Obesity

CAROLYN D. SUMMERBELL

Introduction

The aim of treating the obese patient is to produce long-term behaviour changes in lifestyle, particularly towards healthy eating and appropriate physical activity levels, in order to reduce body-weight, and the responsibility for these changes should lie with patient rather than the health professional. This chapter outlines the range of dietary treatments which are offered by health professionals for the treatment of the obese patient. Particular attention is given to the description and efficacy of low-fat diets, which are the 'slimming diets of today'. Weight-loss programmes, special diets and foods that are purported to aid weight loss will be reviewed in brief.

Most dietary treatments of obesity involve a reduction in energy intake and, in theory, most are simple to adhere to. However, in practice most obese patients find compliance to low-energy diets extremely difficult, particularly in the long term. Therefore, this chapter also reviews the long-term effectiveness of dietary treatments of obesity.

Since the effectiveness of dietary treatments of obesity appears to be poor, particularly in the long term, this chapter also focuses on the way in which health professionals currently deliver advice on weight reduction and how this may be improved. Factors relating to service delivery (rather than patient characteristics) which appear to predict success will be highlighted. Finally, the process of helping obese patients to change their eating habits will be discussed since it appears that this process may be more important than the type of dietary treatment advocated in terms of successful weight loss.

This chapter does not deal with the important dietary issues involved in the prevention of obesity nor the maintenance of ideal weight in the ex-obese, even though these issues may be even more important (and difficult) than those involved in the treatment of obesity. However, factors involved in the prevention of relapse which improve the long-term efficacy of dietary treatments for obesity should be built into the design of weight-loss programmes (HEA, 1995).

Dietary treatments for obesity

There is a variety of dietary treatments and adjuncts to treatment which may be used in the management of obesity and they should be used in a combination which suits the individual (Garrow, 1988; Brownell & Wadden, 1991). This section reviews the range of dietary treatments and adjuncts to treatment which are available and provides some guidance on matching treatments to patients.

Basic principles

Assessment of dietary intake

A first step in making changes is a shared awareness and understanding of the patient's present position. In order to begin education on new eating habits, one must be aware of old habits, regardless of the type of dietary treatment used. Although there are a number of tools which will assess dietary intake (Bingham, 1987), the most common methods used in this setting are the diet history and the 7-day unweighed diet diary methods. The 7-day unweighed diet diary is deemed to be the most useful method in this context (BDA, 1996), and is best obtained by asking the obese patient to keep a food diary for 1 week before the first visit to the clinic (although an audit by Macqueen and Frost (1995) suggested that the practice of sending diaries, as part of a 'weight-reduction pack', in advance of the first visit does not improve treatment outcome at 3 months). The diary may be provided by the health professional or simply recorded in a notebook bought by the patient. The patient must be given clear instructions on how to complete the diary, either verbally or, preferably, in written format in the diary provided. Although foods do not need to be weighed, a reasonable description of the types of foods and quantities consumed, in household measures, needs to be given. Also, a written example of how the patient may complete a day's food intake in the diary is also useful.

How the formation collected in diet diaries may be used in the dietary treatment of obesity

The completed diary then becomes the basis for discussion of eating habits so that decisions about changes can be made with the patient. Any changes must be (as far as possible) acceptable to the patient in terms of palatability and practicality, otherwise the patient will not comply with the dietary advice. An understanding of the patient's lifestyle, including financial and time constraints, and cultural issues if appropriate, is also important. The health professional should ensure that any advice will not compromise other aspects of healthy eating (Gibney, 1992), such as micronutrient intake, and will maintain a high protein/energy ratio to achieve better nitrogen retention and thus minimize loss of fat-free mass (Garrow, 1991).

Dietitians have the skills required to give such advice, but other health professionals normally do not, unless they are given additional training (BDA, 1996). Unfortunately, it is not practically possible for dietitians to advise most obese patients seeking treatment, and the issues around other health professionals giving dietary advice to obese patients is discussed later.

The diary may indicate an erratic eating pattern, with problems such as irregular meals, periods of fasting, excessively restrained eating, frequent snacking, grazing or binge eating. Stabilizing eating behaviour may therefore be necessary prior to any attempt to reduce weight (Haus et al., 1994), and referral to a clinical psychologist may be appropriate if the eating pattern is deemed to be abnormal (although many patients refuse to see a clinical psychologist and many centres do not have a clinical psychologist to refer patients to).

It may be useful to ask for additional information in the diet diary, such as relating mood or circumstances to eating, or monitoring physical activity, to help identify behaviour changes which may be needed.

As well as providing a record of reported food intake and eating behaviour at baseline, the diet diary can be used throughout treatment to review and plan for future treatment. A diet diary encourages the patient to be actively involved in treatment, and to take responsibility for making dietary and other behaviour changes. It may also provide an indication of the patient's motivation, and ways of improving motivation, and implementing change.

The problems associated with under-reporting of energy intake by obese patients

A common problem in developing dietary advice for the obese patient on the basis of the reported food and drink consumed in a food diary is that the energy intake of the reported diet is significantly less than that estimated from predictive equations for that obese person in energy balance. (Predictive equations for obese individuals have been reviewed by Heshka et al. (1993) who recommends using those formulated by Fleisch (1951) or Robertson and Reid (1952).) Indeed, there is a wealth of evidence which shows that energy intakes reported by the obese are significantly lower than would be feasible if they were to maintain their level of obesity (Black et al., 1991). Many authors have concluded from this evidence that the obese under-report their habitual energy intake during the study period. This may well be the case, but there is also the possibility that obese patients actively diet when asked to record their food intake and indeed report a true intake of their dieting behaviour. Support for this explanation is provided by the frequent (but not published) observation that people often lose weight when they are asked to record their food intake, even when these people are students studying for a nutrition degree. If the low energy intakes reported by obese patients are a result of true dieting behaviour, one might predict that if obese patients were asked to record their food intake for long enough they would either lose weight (and on this basis one may use continuous recording of food intake in a diary as an adjunct to therapy — see below), or report food intake associated with relapse. Unfortunately, little work around the use of long-term continuous food records in obese patients has been carried out.

Regardless of the explanation for the low energy intakes reported by obese patients, the health professional must accept that it may not be possible to obtain a comprehensive record of their food intake from a 7-day diary. If the obese patient is reporting true dieting behaviour then the diet which they consume during relapse will remain a mystery, and may be completely different in terms of foods eaten, quantities consumed, and eating behaviour compared to the diet they consume while losing weight. If the low energy intakes reported by the obese patient are a result of under-reporting then it may be possible to predict true dietary intake if the patient is under-reporting the quantity of all foods and drinks consumed by the same degree (since one could simply multiply the amount of food eaten by the same factor required to obtain the estimated energy intake from the reported energy intake), i.e., non-specific under-reporting. However, the limited evidence on under-reporting suggests that the obese tend to under-record food from snacks compared with meals (Heitmann & Lissner, 1995; Summerbell et al., 1996), and particularly from snacks consumed during the evening (Beaudoin & Mayer, 1953), compared with individuals of ideal weight, i.e., specific under-reporting. Therefore, since snacks tend to be made up of different foods and drinks and have a different macronutrient composition compared with meals (Summerbell et al., 1995), specific under-reporting means that it is impossible to predict true dietary intake from a 7-day diet diary.

Is it worth assessing food intake in obese patients?

With these caveats, is it still useful to use a 7-day diary to assess food intake in obese patients? The British Dietetic Association believes that, in clinical practice, it is (BDA, 1996). Apart from gleaning an insight into any possible behavioural

problems (as discussed in How the information collected in diet diaries ...,
above), it is also useful to have written information on which to base the
consultation.

However, the health professional should also calculate the patient's energy
intake from predictive equations since having an estimate of energy intake is
useful in calculating the true energy intake which will be required to lose weight;
1000 kcal/day below the estimated requirement will normally produce a weight
loss of 0.5–1.0 kg/week (Garrow, 1988). A possible scenario (and one which is
not uncommon in obesity clinics) may arise whereby the health professional
advises the obese patient to consume a diet which contains more energy than
that which the obese person reports to consume. Although some patients may
be alarmed at such advice, Frost et al. (1991) have shown that this approach to
formulating dietary advice works well.

In an attempt to improve (i.e., get nearer to the truth) the diet reported in a
7-day diary by obese patients, the health professional could ask additional
questions about food intake. This may be seen as validating their reported food
intake, but equally it may be viewed at attempting to 'trick' the patient into
revealing the truth. Although there are no standard questions or questionnaires
which are designed for this specific purpose, one could ask about the frequency
(say, per week) of consumption of certain types of foods, e.g., energy-dense
foods and take-aways, and cross reference this information with that in the diet
diary. Questions around eating behaviour may also be useful, and a question
which has been found to be particularly useful is 'Do you normally lose weight
or gain weight when on holiday' since many obese patients report losing weight
on holiday. This response implies that the obese patient does not overeat when
with other people. Indeed, there is evidence to show that many obese individuals
do not overeat in public places (Coll et al., 1979), but do so in private, particularly
at home during the evening (Brandon, 1987). This information can then be
used in helping the obese patient to identify triggers for overeating and alter
behaviour to reduce food intake (although I am not suggesting the prescription
of extended holidays for obese patients paid for by the health service!).

Hope for a useable tool to assess true dietary intake comes from two recently
published studies which have developed food frequency questionnaires that
appear to capture realistic energy intakes (Fricker et al., 1989; Lindroos et al.,
1993). Further research is needed to assess the reliability and validity of these
questionnaires.

Setting goals and rate of weight loss

Setting goals is also an important part of the weight-loss process but, as highlighted in Chapter 15, these goals must be realistic. Goals should be in terms of changes in eating habits and other behavioural changes as well as weight loss. For patients with 20 kg or more to lose, intermediate targets should be set. If this is not done the desired goal is often too far away from the starting point, and patients may well give up as they realize the long and difficult task they have set themselves.

The obese person should also be clear about the expected rate of weight loss. As stated above, if a person consumes 1000 kcal/day less than they would normally, then they should lose between 0.5–1.0 kg/week. But on no scientific basis, some people will be disappointed with a weight loss of less than 3 kg a week, and the obese person may give up on a diet because in their view it is not working, whereas in fact it is. Indeed, it has been shown that patients who have unrealistically high initial expected weight loss did not lose weight and consequently drop out of the programme (Bennet, 1986). It is important to help patients accept moderate, achievable expectations of weight loss, and to discourage unrealistic goals for the rate of loss and target weight.

The impact of information from other sources

It is easy to forget that the dietary advice given by the health professional is only part of the information required by the patient to change eating behaviour. Two salient points regarding information from other sources need to be kept in mind when treating the obese patient. Firstly, patients present with a wide variation in their baseline knowledge of the energy value of foods; some are real experts and know much more than most health professionals. The advice given by the health professional will be combined with the knowledge which the patient already has, rather than over-ride the patient's baseline knowledge, and it is this combined knowledge which will form the basis of changes which the patient makes to his or her diet. Explicit in this first point is the value of asking the patient appropriate questions and listening to the answers, and adapting the advice given using this information. Secondly, the constant and often more compelling background information on dieting from other sources, particularly from media and friends and family, will influence the changes to eating behaviour made by the patient as time goes by. Indeed, the patient may request advice from the health professional regarding a specific diet or food which they have heard will enhance their weight loss (or even cause weight loss without the tedium of dieting). Regardless of the credibility of reported claims for such diets or foods, it is important that the health professional addresses them seriously and does not dismiss them as simply ridiculous; if the patient thought that these claims were ridiculous they would not have asked for advice on them in the first place.

The range of dietary treatments used by health professionals

Conventional reducing diets

The key to conventional reducing diets is to advocate a diet lower in energy than the patient's estimated energy expenditure. In the past (and unfortunately still today by some), doctors routinely prescribed a 1000 kcal/day diet to all obese patients seeking to lose weight. Often the usefulness of this advice was (is) made even worse by giving the patient a standard diet sheet in the form of a prescription, regardless of the patients preferences, needs and limitations. In light of the basic principles of dietary treatments for obesity listed above it is not surprising that the efficacy of such dietary advice was (is) poor. Indeed, Frost *et al.* (1991) have demonstrated that prescription of very severe reductions of food intake may be less effective in the achievement of sustained weight loss than more moderate changes. They showed that a deficit of 500 kcal/day (from estimated) is sufficient for most obese people to achieve continuing weight loss of an average of 0.5 kg/week.

Regardless of the energy content of the reducing diet, it requires skill to be able to manipulate the patient's existing diet to one which contains fewer calories but takes into account the patient's needs, preferences and limitations. It would be easy to suggest that the patient simply eats less of everything, but it would be prudent to try and advise changes which make the diet as satiating as the existing diet in the hope that these changes are maintained in the long term. An example of how this may be achieved for a 60-year-old man who was rather 'set in his ways' is given in Tables 16.1 and 16.2. The diet suggested not only contains less energy than his existing diet while taking into account the patient's needs, preferences and limitations, but also contains about the same volume of food as the existing diet. It has been shown that diets high in dietary fibre are more satiating that low-fibre diets (see below), although a recent study has shown that fibre content does not explain all of the variability in the satiating capacity of foods (Holt *et al.*, 1995). In clinical practice the health professional needs to recommend a number of options for all meals and snacks consumed by the patient which contain a similar energy value but add variety (both in terms of nutritional value and palatability) to the diet.

Calorie counting. A conventional reducing diet may be formulated by counting the energy content of foods and drinks consumed each day to ensure that no more energy is consumed than desired. Labelling regulations now make calorie counting an easy task since all foods (except small sweets) must reveal their energy content. Calorie counting is not normally recommended by health professionals because it is thought to cause obsessional behaviour (although

Table 16.1 Existing diet consumed by a 60-year-old obese man who was 'rather set in his ways' and recommended reducing diet.

(a) Existing diet	Grams	(b) Recommended diet	Grams
Breakfast		*Breakfast*	
2 slices of white toast	54	porridge	180
butter	14	honey	15
marmalade	30	1 mug of tea (with skimmed milk)	30
1 mug of tea (with whole milk)	30		
Lunch		*Lunch*	
sandwich made with:		sandwiches made with:	
2 slices of white bread	60	4 slices of wholemeal bread	140
butter	20	low-fat spread	28
boiled egg	40	boiled egg	40
mayonnaise	20	tomato	40
1 packet of crisps	30	cucumber	20
1 apple	112	tuna	40
1 Mars bar	68	mayonnaise	10
1 mug of tea (with whole milk)	30	1 banana	200
Afternoon		*Afternoon*	
1 mug of tea (with whole milk)	30	1 mug of tea (with skimmed milk)	30
Dinner		*Dinner*	
Cornish pastie	260	beef stew	200
chips	180	baked potato	180
ketchup	40	baked beans	135
1 slice of white bread	30	rice pudding	200
butter	10	1 mug of tea (with skimmed milk)	30
1 mug of tea (with whole milk)	30		
Evening		*Evening*	
2 pints of beer	1136	1 pint of beer	568
		1 mug of tea (with skimmed milk)	30
		2 slices wholemeal bread (toasted)	70
		low-fat spread	14
		jam	10

there is little evidence to support this fear). However, it is important to understand that, regardless of the advice given by health professionals, a large majority of patients will still use calorie counting as a method of controlling their food intake, particularly those patients who have used some private slimming clubs in the past. Indeed, a form of calorie counting is implicit in the advice given by some slimming clubs (see below) and, in its favour, has the advantage of helping people understand the composition of foods and to control their own intake.

Table 16.2 Energy and macronutrient intake of the existing diet (described in Table 16.1a) compared with the recommended diet (described in Table 16.1b) of a 60-year-old man, who was 'rather set in his ways'.

Nutritional composition	Existing diet	Recommended diet
Total calories	3415	2414
Percentage of energy from:		
Protein	7	15
Carbohydrate	37	50
Fat	49	30
Alcohol	7	5
Sugars (g/day)	110	98
Fibre (g/day)	18	43

'Low-calorie' products. A common advertising slogan is that a product can be 'part of a low-calorie diet'. But *any food can be part of a low-calorie diet.* One could incorporate a chocolate bar or a packet of crisps into a low-calorie diet, as long as the other foods and drinks consumed were adjusted accordingly. A classic example of this type of advertising is that for Special K breakfast cereal which, per 100 g, contains more calories compared with most other breakfast cereals including All-Bran, Cornflakes, Grapenuts, muesli, Puffed Wheat, Rice Crispies, Shredded Wheat, Sugar Puffs and Weetabix.

The range of 'low-calorie' foods and ready-made meals is increasing all the time which suggests that they are a popular choice for some people. Although some 'low-calorie' products are highly palatable, they tend to be more expensive compared with direct alternatives which are not advertised as 'low calorie'. The health professional may need to give advice on the value of such products to patients.

Abuse of nutritional terminology. Some manufacturers abuse the public's confusion around nutritional terminology in their advertising of certain products so that these products appear relatively 'low calorie'. For example, all types of sugar contain the same amount of calories per weight even though some sugars, for some reason, sound lower in calories than others. Some names of different types of sugars include sucrose, glucose, galactose, maltose, lactose, fructose, brown sugar, beet sugar, corn syrup and partially inverted sugar syrup. A classic example of how a food manufacturer can use the public's misconception that some forms of sugar are lower in calories than others is an advert for Mars bars which appeared a few years ago. The advert informed the consumer that Mars bars are 'full of glucose which gives you energy'. The advert could equally well have read 'full of sugar which gives you calories'. **Energy = Calories**. This type of advertising highlights the point that the advice given by health professionals on weight-reducing diets may involve a degree of education around the true calorie content of foods.

Use of 'special foods' which are designed to aid weight loss. Like 'low-calorie' foods, the availability and use of sugar and fat substitutes have increased dramatically. The names of substitutes which are available, their chemical formula and long-term safety and their characteristics are detailed elsewhere (Gries, 1994). Research suggests that both sugar and fat substitutes may be useful in helping obese people lose weight (Kanders *et al.*, 1994; Cotton *et al.*, 1996, respectively).

In addition to sugar substitutes, a number of 'bulk' sweeteners are approved for use in the U.K. in foods often formulated for diabetics. These are modified sugars or alternative sugars, e.g., sorbitol, isomalt, mannitol, xylitol, hydrogenated glucose syrups. All have about the same energy value as sucrose, but are not absorbed as quickly as natural sugars and are not cariogenic. However, they are highlighted here since they are sold as 'sugar-free' and many people may believe this means that they are also calorie-free. Similar confusion occurs regarding beers and lagers which claim that 'all the sugar has been turned to alcohol' and some people believe this means that they are free from calories. Unfortunately, these 'strong' beers and lagers contain more calories than their weaker alternatives.

Healthy eating

The type of weight-reducing diet advised by health professionals has moved from one which is simply low in energy to one which is low energy but also in line with the healthy eating guidelines of today (COMA, 1994). These guidelines have been translated by the Health Education Authority into a useable teaching tool called the Balance of Good Health (HEA, 1996, Fig. 16.1). The healthy eating low-energy diet is simply one which conforms with this balance, but is also lower in energy than the energy requirements of the obese patient. The rationale for this move towards healthy eating is twofold. Firstly, healthy eating reducing diets can also promote health in terms of reducing avoidable mortality from diseases other than obesity which are thought to be exacerbated by an excess of saturated fat and sugar, and a deficiency of dietary fibre and antioxidant vitamins and minerals. Secondly, they are thought to promote

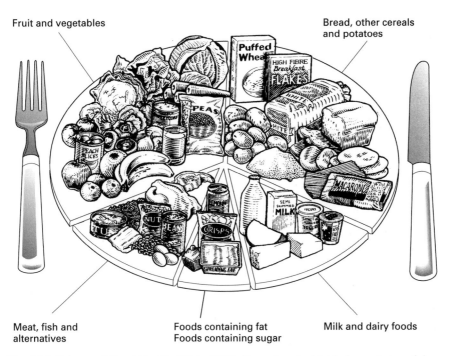

Fruit and vegetables

Bread, other cereals and potatoes

Meat, fish and alternatives

Foods containing fat
Foods containing sugar

Milk and dairy foods

Fig. 16.1 Balance of Good Health (HEA, 1996). Reproduced with kind permission of the Health Education Authority.

long-term compliance (although there is little evidence to support this claim) since they are not specially designed for obese people (and therefore inappropriate for people who have lost weight), i.e., if the ex-obese continue to eat a healthy diet then they should not regain the weight lost. Healthy eating reducing diets also have the advantage that the obese member(s) of a family does not need to prepare different foods compared with the non-obese member(s) of a family, they simply need to eat smaller quantities.

Nutritional and calorie value of 'healthy foods'

The nutritional and calorie value of 'healthy foods' is as variable as all other foods, and the important message is that *'healthy foods' do not necessarily contain more nutritional value or fewer calories compared with foods which are not labelled as 'healthy foods'*. The only way of assessing the calorie content of these foods is by reading the food labels, and the health professional should help the patient understand the importance of this in the education process.

Low-fat diets

As stated above, healthy eating diets are normally low in fat, but low-fat diets have become the 'slimming' diets of choice today. The specific rationale for this popularity is unclear, but there is evidence that energy from fat is more liable to be deposited as fat compared with carbohydrate and protein (see Chapter 6), and that high-fat foods promote over-consumption of food (Blundell *et al.*, 1995). It appears that this information has trickled down to the media and in the process been interpreted as 'low-fat diets are the most effective weight-loss diets'. As will be shown later, the efficacy of low-fat diets in terms of weight loss is not 100%, and part of the current popularity towards low-fat diets may simply be that a diet (whatever it may be) will always be number one in the popularity stakes at any one time, but that with time the number one position will be replaced by a different dietary regimen.

Low-fat foods. The range of reduced and low-fat foods now on the market has increased dramatically in the past 10 years in response to changing consumer demands. Reduced fat varieties of most dairy foods are now available and popular with people who want to lose weight. If a product is labelled as low fat a patient trying to lose weight may be tempted to buy it, but what does low fat mean? Firstly, if a food is labelled as low fat, this says very little about the fat content of the product and nothing about it's energy content. Certainly, low fat does not necessarily imply low energy. For example, yogurt is a naturally low fat food, and different types of yogurts contain similar amounts of fat — 'natural yogurt', 'flavoured yogurt' and 'fruit yogurt' all contain about 1 g of fat per 100 g. However, 'natural yogurt', contains 52 kcal/100 g whereas 'flavoured yogurt' contains 81 kcal/100 g and 'fruit yogurt' contains 95 kcal/100 g. The difference is in the sugar content — 'natural yogurt' does not have any sugar added to it whereas 'flavoured yogurt' and 'fruit yogurt' have appreciable quantities of sugar added to them.

Many foods are labelled as reduced fat, low fat, lower fat, very low fat, light or lite. However, these labels mean very little, certainly there is no legislation which governs the labelling of foods with these descriptors. Many products are naturally low in fat — yogurt, breakfast cereals, jams and honey, all fruits and vegetables, etc. To inform the consumer that these foods are low in fat is not very helpful. What the consumers wants to know is whether a product is lower in fat compared with a direct alternative. For example, whether products labelled as low-fat crisps, milk, biscuits, cheese are indeed significantly lower in fat than the equivalent products which are not labelled as low fat. Again, there is no legislation which governs how much lower in fat a product must be, compared with it's alternative, to be called low fat. The difference may be significant or negligible. To find out what the difference is the consumer must look at the labels, and assess whether the difference means that it is worthwhile buying the low-fat product (often products labelled as low fat are much more expensive than their alternative).

Low-cholesterol foods. Foods which are labelled as low cholesterol are not necessarily low in fat. A good example of this is polyunsaturated margarine which is low in cholesterol but very high in fat (as are all margarines and butters). Indeed, polyunsaturated margarine contains the same number of calories as any other margarine or butter, and if a patient wants to lose weight it does not really matter which spreading fat they choose — the important point is that the patient eats less of the spreading fat they choose to use, or chooses a low-fat spread.

Fat substitutes. These are discussed above.

Efficacy of low-fat diets on weight loss

Information on the efficacy of low-fat diets in terms of weight loss comes from a number of studies which vary in their aims and design.

Observational

Low fat vs control, isoenergetic to maintain weight. Despite attempts to hold energy intake constant, Prewitt *et al.* (1991) observed that weight loss was greater at 20 weeks when subjects followed a low-fat diet compared with a control diet during the 4-week run-in period. Similar changes were observed in obese and non-obese women.

Cross-over design

Low fat vs medium/high fat, isoenergetic to maintain weight. A retrospective study of liquid diets of precisely known composition with widely varied fat content showed that there was no detectable evidence of significant variation in body-weight over 15–56 days (Leibel *et al.*, 1992). Similar results were reported from a randomized study which assessed adherence to one of four fat-modified diets (goal: % fat: 38%, 30%, 38%, 28%) in 118 mildly hypercholesterolaemic subjects (Sarkkinen *et al.*, 1994).

Low fat vs control, both ad libitum. When ideal-weight females were randomly assigned to a low-fat diet followed (with a wash-out period in between) by a control diet, or vice versa, weight loss was greater during the low-fat phase

(Kendall *et al.*, 1991). In a non-randomized study using a latin square design, Lissner (1987) showed that the cause of greater losses in weight on low-fat diets is due to the fact that people spontaneously consume less energy on low-fat diets. The study by Lissner is particularly important because the low-, medium- and high-fat diets consisted of foods which were similar in appearance and palatability, i.e., the greater degree of weight loss (and therefore energy intake) associated with low-fat diets is not a result of low-fat diets being less palatable, but a result of the fact that low-fat diets are less energy dense and more satiating.

Low fat, low energy vs low energy. Racette *et al.* (1995) also found that a greater weight loss was observed in obese women randomly assigned to a low-energy diet compared with a low-fat diet, even though both diets were prescribed to approximately 75% of each subject's basal metabolic rate.

Low fat ad libitum vs low energy. Hammer *et al.* (1989) observed greater losses of weight in obese women randomly assigned to a low-energy diet compared with a low-fat diet, although it was extremely restrictive (800 kcal/day).

Controlled trials

Low fat ad libitum vs control. In a non-randomized controlled trial aimed at investigating the effect of diet on blood lipids, spontaneous loss of weight was observed in the intervention group who received advice on a low-fat/high-fibre diet (Raben *et al.*,1995).

It has also been noted in studies which have evaluated the efficacy of low-fat diets for postmenopausal women receiving therapy for early breast cancer that individuals randomized to low-fat diets experience modest reductions in body-weight over time, even though weight loss was not an intervention objective (Buzzard *et al.*, 1990; Sheppard *et al.*, 1991; White *et al.*, 1992; Chlebowski *et al.*, 1993).

However, a randomized controlled trial (RCT) (Mattes, 1993) of two low-fat diets (one which omitted all discretionary fat sources and one which included fat-modified discretionary foods) and a control diet, found no significant changes in body-weight over a 12-week period, although the low-fat groups tended to lose more weight.

Low fat vs control, isoenergetic to maintain weight. An RCT which evaluated the efficacy of low-fat diets for the prevention of non-melanoma skin cancer (Black *et al.*, 1995) observed that patients on the low-fat diet lost more weight than those who continued to consume their usual diet.

Low fat, low energy vs low energy. In trials where weight loss was the intervention objective, low-fat diets (at the same energy level) did not induce a greater weight loss than a control diet in both a non-randomized (Alford *et al.*, 1990) and a randomized study (Golay *et al.*, 1996). However, Baron *et al.* (1986) found that dieters randomized to a low-carbohydrate/low-fibre diet tended to lose more weight than those randomized to a higher-carbohydrate/higher-fibre diet, although those subjects in the low-carbohydrate/low-fibre diet group complained of more problems in dieting.

Low fat ad libitum vs low energy. Schlundt *et al.* (1993) found that over 20 weeks patients randomized to be counselled to restrict energy lost more weight than those in the *ad libitum* low-fat group. However, incomplete follow-ups 9–12 months later suggested that the two approaches were equivalent at this time point. Shah *et al.* (1994) found that over 6 months there was no difference in weight lost between dietary groups, but patients randomized to the low-fat group reported an improvement in palatability, satiety and quality of life, whereas scores for these factors diminished in the low-energy group. Another RCT of similar design (Jeffery *et al.*, 1995), but lasting 18 months, again found no difference in weight loss between patients on the low-fat *ad libitum* diet and the low-energy diet. However, Jeffery noted that women in the low-fat group rated the diet as being more palatable, and experienced greater reduction in binge eating scores, suggesting that this approach warrants further study.

Other data from randomized controlled trials

Singh *et al.* (1992) assessed the efficacy of a cardioprotective diet in patients with acute myocardial infarction. Five hundred and five patients were assigned to diet A (low-fat diet) or diet B (low-fat diet plus advised to eat more fruit, vegetables, nuts and grain products). After 1 year, body-weight fell significantly in patients in group A compared with those in group B. Hjermann *et al.* (1981) assessed the effect of a low-fat diet and smoking on the incidence of heart disease and found that, after 4 years, the intervention group had a significantly lower body mass index compared with baseline, but the control group did not. However, the results from this study are confusing since, although all patients in the intervention group received advice on low-fat diets, only those who were also overweight received advice on reducing energy intake.

Other RCTs have assessed the efficacy of multiple risk factor reduction on coronary atherosclerosis and clinical cardiac events (Ornish *et al.*, 1990; Schuler *et al.*, 1992; Haskell *et al.*, 1994), and have offered advice on low-fat diets, but also weight reduction and exercise. It is difficult to assess from these studies what proportion of weight loss was ascribed to the low-fat, and what proportion to the other intervention strategies.

In conclusion, summarizing the data is difficult since there are a number of confounding variables: baseline weight, sex, number of subjects, length of study period, level of percentage energy from fat, total energy intake, specific advice given on weight loss, etc. However, from the information available, low-fat diets appear to cause weight loss compared with habitual diets since they are less energy dense, and not because they are less palatable. Low-fat diets do not appear to be more effective compared with low-energy diets in terms of weight loss in the obese (Summerbell *et al.*, 1998). However, low-fat diets do appear to be more palatable, improve quality of life, and reduce binge eating scores compared with low-energy diets.

High-fibre diets. High-fibre diets rose to popularity in the 1980s with the publication of the *F-Plan diet* written by Audrey Eyton, but are currently not very popular. The rationale behind their effectiveness is that if one consumes enough fruit and vegetables, wholemeal bread, pasta, rice and beans (foods which are not energy dense) one will have little appetite remaining for other foods which are energy dense, and so the patient will consume a diet low in energy. Certainly the evidence suggests that high-fibre diets can be effective in the short term (Rabast, 1994) but, as they are seen as specific for weight loss rather than overall health, compliance to them in the long-term is likely to be poor.

Very-low-calorie diets. Very-low-calorie liquid diets (VLCDs) are nutritionally complete and provide about 600 kcal/day in the form of drinks. A modification of this approach is to substitute two to three meals each day with a liquid formula diet. VLCDs are produced by a number of manufacturers and tend to be expensive compared with other dietary treatments for obesity listed above. The use of such diets should not be recommended by health professionals for the majority of obese patients since these diets do not help the patient make permanent eating and other behavioural changes to their diet which are necessary if weight loss is to be maintained. However, the efficacy of VLCDs in terms of weight loss is good in the short term (Jebb & Goldberg, 1998) and therefore there may be instances when the health professional deems their use to be appropriate. For example the severely obese patient who needs to lose weight quickly because of an urgent obesity-related medical problem but claims not to be able to lose weight on other dietary treatments for obesity such as those listed above (although a milk-only diet may be as useful as a VLCD under these circumstances—see below). If VLCDs are used, care needs to be taken to ensure that the diet is used as part of a treatment package to prevent weight gain in the long term. Some patients may use VLCDs from time to time regardless of the fact that they are not the diet of choice recommended by the health professional. However, rather than dismiss the patient's use of VLCDs out of hand, the health professional should work with and educate the patient to ensure that the use of this type of diet is minimized and when it is used it is done so as safely as possible. The range of VLCDs, and a number of concerns associated with their use, has been reviewed by an expert committee in detail elsewhere (DoH, 1987).

The milk diet. The milk-only diet is a simple, cheap and readily available version of VLCDs. Its use as a dietary treatment for obesity was pioneered by Professor John Garrow in his obesity clinic (Garrow *et al.*, 1989), and an RCT which assessed the short-term (over 16 weeks) efficacy of the milk diet vs a conventional weight-reducing diet has recently been published (Summerbell *et al.* in preparation). Patients on the milk diet lost significantly more weight than those on the conventional weight-reducing diet, although part of the reason for this success may be that the milk diet was novel to the patients, and that this novelty may have worn off with time. A milk diet may be advocated to certain patients, for the same reasons as one would advocate a VLCD (see above). However, considering the advantages of the milk diet over a VLCD, one can see little reason for ever advising a patient to use a VLCD.

Nibbling vs gorging. There are occasionally reports in the media which purport that the frequency of eating may effect the rate of weight loss, particularly that nibbling promotes weight loss as compared with gorging. Indeed, a special diet called 'The Body Clock Diet' has been proposed on this basis (Gatty, 1978). However, recent evidence suggests that feeding frequency has little impact on energy balance (Summerbell *et al.*, 1996), although being 'allowed' to eat more often may confer some psychological benefit to the patient.

The range of dietary treatments used by the private sector

Slimming clubs

The dietary treatments offered by slimming clubs are conventional reducing diets with a 'twist'. Some clubs, such as Weight Watchers U.K., use a form of calorie counting to help the patient control their energy intake. Foods are given 'points' on the basis of their energy value and their saturated fat content, and there are no 'forbidden' foods. The client is allowed to eat foods up to the value of a given number of 'points' which is calculated on the basis of their body-weight (heavier clients being allowed more points). Clients following a

Weight Watchers diet are advised to eat a healthy diet, are allowed 5 'free' foods per day, and get 'bonus' points for exercise. Other slimming clubs, such as Slimming World, do not use calorie counting. Clients are advised to follow one of two diet plans; original and green. Both contain a list of 'free' foods, healthy extras (which are allowed in moderation), and 'sins'. Clients are allowed between 5 and 15 'sins' a day, and a chocolate bar such as a Mars bar is 15 'sins' whereas a glass of wine is 5 'sins'.

The main concern from health professionals about slimming clubs is that they are profit-making, but this may act in their favour since one could argue that if patients were unconvinced that they were worthwhile they would not enrol. Believing a dietary treatment will work may be an important factor in the efficacy of that dietary treatment (Chapter 17).

It is difficult to assess the efficacy of the advice offered by slimming clubs since this would require an RCT which has never been (and is never likely to be) conducted. However, there is no reason to believe that the dietary treatments advocated by slimming clubs are less effective than those advocated by health professionals. When Biesalski (1994) compared the results from a Weight Watchers study with a clinical study (both performed in Sweden) he found that the Weight Watchers group had lost significantly more weight than the clinical group at 24 months. This does not show that obese people who attend slimming clubs fare better than those who attend hospital obesity clinics (since different 'types' of people attend different 'types' of treatment), but it does show that slimming clubs are effective for a certain 'type' of person.

In what circumstances can the health professional recommend patients to use slimming clubs? It would seem sensible to recommend the use of slimming clubs to patients who believe that they are the best option for them and can afford them, although it may be prudent to ask the patient to make a follow-up appointment in, say, 3 months. The health professional should also suggest the patient comes back to clinic if weight loss stops or they have any medical problems.

Special diets

There is a myriad of special diets which are purported to aid weight loss (Liebermeister, 1994). They all work on the principle that consuming a low-calorie diet will stimulate weight loss, but few admit to such a simple claim. The diets are usually explained in paperbacks, and are widely available in bookshops. They claim to be offering something 'different', perhaps even an as yet unknown metabolic pathway which the diet can disturb in the favour of weight loss. Whatever the claim, it is always compelling (which one would expect as otherwise the author would not make any profit from writing the

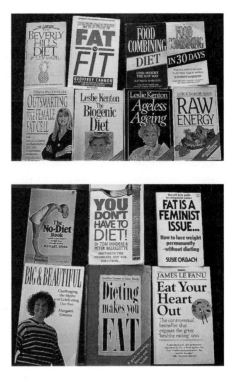

Fig. 16.2 Examples of best-selling slimming books.

book). Perhaps what is most distressing is that some of these books claim that weight loss, using their diets, will not be difficult. All patients find losing weight by dieting difficult, and sometimes impossible, but never easy.

Some of the diet books which have attracted popularity in the U.K. over recent years are shown in Fig. 16.2. Perhaps the most popular diet over recent years has been The Food Combining Diet (Marsden, 1993). The book helpfully provides a no-hassle 28-day menu plan, which does not involve calorie counting and encourages the consumption of fruit and vegetables. Marsden claims that the diet will not only enable the reader to achieve pain-free weight loss, but also improve health and spirits to a remarkable degree (she claims that the diet has a built-in cleansing programme which helps to improve elimination of toxins).

The diet is based on the principles of the Hay diet, a diet which separates foods that 'do not digest well together so that the body can use the food we eat more efficiently and without clogging up the system'. Essentially, the reader should not eat foods rich in protein at the same time as foods rich in starch or sugar (no more fish and chips!). Marsden explain why — 'Given that proteins take longer to digest than starches and that starches take longer than vegetables and fruit, mixing them together on the same plate or in the same mouthful can cause some people's digestive system a great deal of grief. Have sympathy for those poor old enzymes and acids down there in the dark, trying to sort out the muddle of which stays in the stomach for several hours and which moves on more quickly to the next department …. Mix starches with protein at the same meal and the digestive system won't know if it is functioning on acid foot or alkaline horseback'.

This basic premise of the diet is confusing. Surely, if the foods which Marsden suggests do not digest well together are eaten separately, then the foods eaten will be absorbed more efficiently and thus provide more calories. However, it is clear why the diet can cause weight loss. Diets which restrict food choice are liable also to result in a decrease in energy intake (Rolls, 1986). Restriction of food choice combined with the consumption of lots of fruits and vegetables is why the Hay diet promotes weight loss.

Quackery and 'health foods' which claim to aid weight loss

'Health foods' constitute a group of products which, as far as the consumer is concerned, fall on the boundary between foods and medicines. In many cases their advertising usually includes the implication, which may be explicit, that the consumption of the product will confer health benefits on the consumer. Of particular relevance to this chapter is the health claims made about products which are purported to aid weight loss.

A case in point which was reported in the *Healthwatch Newsletter* (Garrow, 1995) related to a slimming product named 'Autoslim' which was advertised in 1993 in a U.K. national newspaper. The advert claimed that the product would 'cause steady weight loss day after day'. As a result of taking this preparation 'your body's metabolism will activate and actually start to burn off excess calories and fat'. The metabolic situation created was described as a 'fat furnace'. The product was supplied by order only but with a money-back guarantee. The product came with a sheet describing 'Newton's special diet plan' on which the customer was allowed to eat unlimited amounts of fresh fruit and vegetables, lean meat and fish, but no white bread, cakes, nuts, sugar, sweets, milk, cheese or fat in any form.

After the trading standards officer was alerted to the existence of 'Autoslim' the product was analysed and was found to contain trivial amounts of some amino acids, but these were in any case supplied in far greater amounts by the normal diet, and would cause no significant change in metabolic rate. The company was prosecuted for supplying goods to which a false description was applied because 'Autoslim' had no effect on body-weight or weight reduction. The defence was that the diet advice supplied with the product would cause weight reduction if followed, and the product might motivate customers to keep to the diet. The defendants were found guilty on all charges, fined a total of £6000, and ordered to pay the costs of prosecution, estimated at about £5000.

There are many products on the market like 'Autoslim', and the health professional who treats obese patients needs to keep abreast of such products so that they can give sound advice on them if needed. As highlighted above, information from other sources may be more compelling than the advice offered by the health professional but, regardless of its credibility, it should be treated seriously. If you have any concerns about slimming products which you believe are untrue you should notify the relevant authorities.

Adjuncts to dietary advice

A number of adjuncts to dietary advice are dealt with in other chapters in this book, but briefly:

Behaviour modification. Some simple behaviour modification techniques of some description should always be used as an adjunct (Chapter 17).

Exercise. The addition of exercise to a dietary treatment programme for weight loss may improve weight loss (Garrow & Summerbell, 1995). As discussed by Saris (Chapter 18), it is important to suggest an increase in energy output in a way which is appropriate for the obese patient, and which they will continue.

Drugs and surgery. The use of drugs (Chapters 19 and 20) and surgery (Chapter 21) as adjuncts to dietary treatments should only be recommended when dietary treatments alone are deemed ineffective for an obese patient. The main problem of using drugs or surgery for the treatment of obesity is that the patient does not learn to alter their behaviour or take responsibility for their weight loss, unless the treatments are used as part of a treatment package.

Long-term effectiveness of dietary treatments for obesity

The efficacy of dietary treatments for obesity, using weight loss as the outcome, is good in the short term (Bennett, 1987) but poor in the long term (Garner & Wooley, 1991). However, the results of long-term studies are difficult to interpret for five reasons.

1   There is usually a large drop-out rate from long-term treatment and it is not known whether drop out is a result of the patient not losing weight and believing that the advice offered by the health professional is useless, or whether it is a result of the patient losing weight and believing that they do not require any advice from the health professional.

2   When one looks at the data from long-term studies in more detail there are clearly some patients who do well while others do badly. An audit by Pearson *et al.* (1989) illustrates the problem. Their audit of hospital-based dietetic treatment of obesity involved 100 overweight patients seen individually and followed up for 24 weeks. At 24 weeks only 50% were still attending. Of these, 28% were successful (defined as weight loss of 50% or more of that desired), 24% partially successful (weight loss of 33–50% of that desired) and 48% unsuccessful (weight loss of less than 33% of that desired). In the knowledge that some dietary treatments will suit some patients better than others, and some methods of service delivery of these treatments will suit some patients better than others, one could argue that those patients who appear to fail in long-term studies are not suited to either the dietary treatment (see above) or the method of service delivery (see below), or both (rather than the failure being attributed to patient characteristics). This argument also suggests that those patients who appear to fail in long-term studies would succeed under different circumstances.

3   While the results of long-term studies are disappointing, generalizing to the whole overweight and obese population is not justified. Most people attempt to lose weight on their own, with books or in commercial programmes (Brownell, 1993). Brownell surveyed more than 20 000 readers of *Consumer Reports* magazine, and of those who reported losing a significant amount of weight (mean = 15 kg) and maintaining the loss, 72% had done so on their own, compared with 20% in commercial programmes, 3% with diet pills, and only 5% in a health care setting. Therefore, it could be argued that obese people who enrol in hospital-based trials are resistant to dietary treatment. Furthermore, obese patients who actively seek treatment are more likely to suffer from binge-eating problems and have more psychopathology than is true of obese people who do not seek treatment or ideal weight controls (Fitzgibbon *et al.*, 1993), and obese patients who actively seek treatment and remain in weight loss programmes because they do not lose weight are more likely to suffer from binge-eating problems and have more psychopathology than ex-obese patients who once actively sought treatment but left the weight-loss programme because they had achieved weight loss (Vigus *et al.*, 1995). Therefore, the poor results from long-term studies must, at least in part, be biased since the patients who are recruited to these studies are more obviously the most difficult treat.

4   The quality of dietary treatment for obese patients for weight loss by health professionals in long-term studies may be poor. When one examines data from audits which have been carried out in a specialist obesity clinic where patients receive high quality advice there is evidence that those who stay in such a programme do continue to lose weight over time when treated by diet alone (Pacy *et al.*, 1987). For men at 1–3 months, 4–6 months, 7–12 months and > 13 months attendance mean weight loss was 5.0 kg ($n = 9$), 12.4 kg ($n = 4$), 12.4 kg ($n = 5$) and 13.0 kg ($n = 7$), respectively. For women at the same time intervals

mean weight loss was 4.0 kg (n = 42), 6.5 kg (n = 23), 10.0 kg (n = 21) and 17.0 kg (n = 41). However, drop-out rate was high (25 men and 127 women were initially selected for audit). Similar results have been observed in other specialist obesity clinics (Grace et al., 1998).

5   Given that the rest of the population is gaining weight at the rate of 0.45–0.91 kg (1–2 lb) a year, weight maintenance over the long term could be classified as success (Rossner, 1995).

Evidence for long-term effectiveness of dietary treatments for obesity from randomized controlled trials

For obvious reasons there are no data from RCTs on the efficacy of long-term dietary treatment vs no dietary treatment for obese patients using weight loss as the outcome since such a study would not be ethical.

There are, however, many RCTs on the efficacy of long-term dietary treatments vs dietary treatments in conjunction with behaviour modification, exercise, drugs or surgery. As shown in the relevant chapters of this book, these studies show that, in general, using an adjunct to dietary treatment is more effective than simply using diet alone. Furthermore, most of these studies show that dietary treatments alone are not efficacious in the long term. These studies need to be viewed with caution since the aim of them was to assess the efficacy of the adjunct, and the quality of dietary advice may have been poor.

There are only three long-term (at least 1 year) RCTs which have assessed the efficacy of one type of dietary treatment vs another, and these (Baron et al., 1986; Ryttig et al., 1989; Jeffery et al., 1995) have recently been systematically reviewed (Glenny et al., 1997). The authors concluded that, unfortunately, these studies were ambiguous about the advantages of increased dietary fibre and restricted fat.

Is it worth dieting?

Based on the evidence, there are some who argue that it is not worth dieting in the first instance if weight is to be regained because there is evidence that weight cycling is worse than staying obese (discussed in detail in Chapter 22). Dieting is a worthwhile activity (Garrow, 1994) *but it must be undertaken seriously.* Obese patients who have succeeded in losing weight are faced with the challenge of maintaining the lifestyle changes they have made for the rest of their lives. Treatments must help patients to recognize the possibility of relapse, and develop strategies to manage it (Biesalski, 1995). Maintenance of lost weight requires continued monitoring and support and acquisition of a different set of skills and behaviour modifications compared with those required for weight loss (Fairburn & Cooper, 1996). Specific relapse recognition and prevention techniques developed for use in addictive behaviour (Perri *et al.*, 1993) should be considered. Furthermore, providers of treatment must recognize that long-term monitoring and support of post-obese patients may be necessary.

Certainly, from my own clinical experience, changing the type of dietary treatment (see above) or service delivery (see below) when the patient stops losing weight (and before they 'give up' altogether), on the principle that 'a change is as good as a rest', can help. Diets and dieting are seen by most patients as boring after the initial weight loss phase, and changing from, say, a low-fat diet to a milk-only diet for a short period of time may relieve this boredom, reinstate compliance and thus stimulate further weight loss.

The way in which dietary treatments are delivered and how this may be improved

The efficacy of dietary treatments for weight loss may be improved if the way in which this advice is delivered is changed. A number of issues around service delivery are outlined below.

Who should deliver dietary advice to obese patients?

Clearly, dietitians have the knowledge and skills to give dietary advice, but other health professionals usually do not since they had little and often poor training in nutrition as students, particularly medical doctors (Summerbell, 1996). Murray *et al.* (1993) found that while primary care workers had a broad understanding of health eating recommendations, they had difficulty in translating knowledge into practical dietetic advice tailored to the individual. However, since it is impossible in general practice to refer all obese patients to dietitians for dietary advice, other health professionals should ensure that their knowledge and skills in this area are adequate. Effective strategies to improve health professionals' management of obesity are currently being reviewed (Harvey *et al.*, 1998).

It appears that knowledge and skills around treating obesity are not the only barriers health professionals face in terms of being effective. Health professionals (including some dietitians) have negative beliefs about overweight and obese patients and, while viewing their treatment as important, see it as both difficult and professionally unrewarding (Cade & O'Connell, 1990). Health professionals who treat obese patients need to acquire and maintain a positive attitude towards the efficacy of treatment (while appreciating that it is a difficult task). Health professionals who have a negative attitude towards the efficacy of obesity treatment should not treat obese patients.

Furthermore, weight-loss programmes which use a multidisciplinary approach using dietitians, medical doctors and psychologists, such as that reported by Fitzwater *et al.* (1991), may be more effective than programmes which use only one member of the primary health care team.

Those patients who do not do well in general practice, primarily because they claim that they do not lose weight on 1000 kcal (or less)/day, should be referred to specialist obesity clinics which are set up to treat the more challenging patient (Kopelman, 1993). Sadly, such clinics are few and far between.

For those patients who prefer to use private slimming clubs, the dietitian has a responsibility to offer training on issues around weight loss to the people who run them. For those patients who prefer to try 'special diets and foods' (see above), little can be done to improve the advice which is given in conjunction with the sale of these products. However, dietitians (and other interested health professionals) can help by reporting any unfounded claims made for these products to the relevant authorities, and also by giving sound advice through the media (e.g., local radio, women's magazines, newspaper articles, television).

Individual or group therapy

Group therapy may be preferred by some patients compared to individual therapy, and although Adams *et al.* (1983) found no difference in outcome between individual vs group weight-loss programmes in general, they found that men participating in group sessions and women seen in individual sessions were the most successful in maintaining weight loss over time. Furthermore, Bush *et al.* (1988) found that men who attended men-only group programmes attended more frequently and lost more weight than men on mixed programmes. Certainly, the men-only slimming club, GutBusters, reports success (Egger *et al.*, 1996). In contrast to these results, Hakala *et al.* (1993) showed that group counselling starting with an in-patient period led to rapid weight reduction, but a better and more sustained effect (over 5 years) was achieved by individual counselling, especially in men. In conclusion, Hayaki and Brownell (1996) suggest that group interventions may be at least as effective as individual interventions, presumably due to the social support created among individuals in the group. For the health professional, the problem of identifying at the outset of treatment those patients who would fare better in group compared with individual therapy, and vice versa, will hopefully become clearer in the light of further research.

Aside from the issue of efficacy, group therapy has the advantage that it is more cost-effective compared with individual therapy, and in general practice should be considered as a useful option even though most dietetic departments in the U.K. only offer treatment on an individual basis (Cowburn & Summerbell, 1998). Good models of practice include a non-profit making slimming club which uses dietitians as group leaders (Bush *et al.*, 1988), and a weight-reduction programme led by a public health nurse (Karvetti & Hakala, 1992) which has now been adopted nation-wide in the Finnish primary health-care system.

Frequency of visits

It appears that weight loss is largely predicted by the number of clinic visits rather than treatment duration (Fitzwater *et al.*, 1991), suggesting that appointments every 4 weeks, say, result in greater losses in weight compared with appointments every 8 weeks. (Unfortunately, no study has assessed the ideal time interval between visits in terms of weight loss.)

However, this evidence needs to be used with caution in the light of the knowledge that weighing patients may contribute to the negative psychological state of the individual (Ogden & Evans, 1996), although Lavery and Loewy (1993) found that the more frequently subjects weighed themselves, the more successful they were at weight loss during a 2-year period. Perhaps regular clinic visits with weighing may be the best combination in terms of weight loss for some obese patients, but not for others. Further research which identifies those patients who benefit from regular weighing needs to be conducted.

Place and time of consultation, transportation and child-care issues

Community-based weight-loss programmes have the advantage over health service-based programmes since they are able to treat large numbers of obese people, many of whom probably would not spontaneously seek professional help (but with time may well gain more weight and need professional advice). Part of the reason why these programmes are so popular is that they are convenient, i.e., they take place at work or home and do not impinge on the individuals 'leisure' time. Community approaches to weight control encompass worksite interventions (including weight-loss competitions at the worksite), intervention by home correspondence and multi-modal community strategies and, although they result in modest weight losses, they do so at lower costs than clinical interventions (Brownell, 1986; Jeffery, 1993).

On a less formal basis slimming clubs at work may prove useful, but at this level of intervention the quality of the advice given may be poor. The health professional should offer advice and support to individuals who run such weight-loss programmes since the effectiveness of these clubs will determine the number of obese patients seeking professional help in the future.

Murphree (1994) concluded that if patients in a primary health-care setting should have any success at all it was important to develop programmes which included new approaches to transportation and child-care issues. Rossner (1995) supports her findings, commenting that 'Elegant and theoretically adequate hypocaloric exercises will never result in weight loss if the obese patient cannot find transportation or a baby-sitter while she attends the weight loss session!'

Use of a continuous diet diary

As stated earlier, the use of continuous recording of food intake in a diet diary may improve compliance to dietary treatment and therefore efficacy. However, a study which is designed to address this issue has yet to be reported.

Spouse involvement

The involvement of a spouse or partner in the patient' weight-control programme is an important adjunct to weight loss (Black & Threlfall, 1989). Examples of the ways partners may augment treatment efficacy include reinforcing skills acquired during treatment and extending therapy time throughout the week. Further supporting the positive impact of spouse involvement, Pratt (1989) found that inclusion of the client's spouse in weight-reduction programmes was associated with low attrition rates.

   Another advantage of involving of a spouse or partner in the patient's weight-control programme was reported recently (Franson & Rossner, 1994). It appears that if the spouse or partner is overweight and is involved in the programme, then they are also likely to loose weight. This has implications for the use of family-based interventions.

Understanding how people make behaviour changes

The efficacy of dietary treatments for weight loss may be further improved if the health professional understands how people make behaviour changes, and apply these principles in practice. Successful weight loss depends on doing the right things (type of dietary treatment combined with type of service delivery) at the right time (stages) (HEA, 1995). Five stages of change are proposed: precontemplation, contemplation, preparation, action and maintenance. If the patient is not in the action phase then the advice will be wasted. The health professional therefore needs to steer the patient into the action phase before giving dietary advice.

References

Adams, S.O., Grady, K.E., Lund, A.K., Mulkaida, C. & Wolf, C.H. (1983) Weight loss: long term results in an ambulatory setting. *Journal of the American Dietetic Association* **83**, 306–310.

Alford, B.B., Blankenship, A.C. & Hagen, R.D. (1990) The effects of variations in carbohydrate, protein, and fat content of the diet upon weight loss, blood values, and nutrient intake of adult obese women. *Journal of the American Dietetic Association* **90**, 534–540.

Baron, J.A., Schori, A., Crow, B., Carter, R. & Mann, J.I. (1986) A randomized controlled trial of low carbohydrate and low fat/high fibre diets for weight loss. *American Journal of Public Health* **76**, 1293–1298.

BDA (1996) Position paper on the treatment of obesity. London: British Dietetic Association.

Beaudoin, R. & Mayer, J. (1953) Food intake of obese and non-obese women. *Journal of the American Dietetic Association* **29**, 29–34.

Bennett, G.A. (1986) Expectations in the treatment of obesity. *British Journal of Clinical Psychology* **25**, 311–312.

Bennett, W. (1987) Dietary treatments of obesity. *Annals of the New York Academy of Sciences* **499**, 250–263.

Biesalski, H.K. (1994) Essential requirements of long-term treatment of obesity. In: Ditschuneit, H., Gries, H., Hauner, H. *et al.* (eds) *Obesity in Europe 1993*, pp. 219–226. London: John Libbey & Co.

Bingham, S. (1987) The dietary assessment of individuals; methods, accuracy, new techniques and recommendations. *Nutrition Abstracts and Reviews* **57**, 705–742.

Black, D.R. & Threlfall, W.E. (1989) Partner weight status and subject weight loss: implications for cost-effective programs and public health. *Addictive Behaviours* **14**, 279–289.

Black, A.E., Goldberg, G.R., Jebb, S.A., Livingstone, M.B.E., Cole, T.L. & Prince, A.M. (1991) Critical evaluation of energy intake using fundamental principles of energy physiology: 2. Evaluating the results of published surveys. *European Journal of Clinical Nutrition* **45**, 583–599.

Black, H.S., Thornby, J.I., Wolf, J.E. *et al.* (1995) Evidence that a low-fat diet reduced the occurrence of non-melanoma skin cancer. *International Journal of Cancer* **62**, 165–169.

Blundell, J.E., Cotton., J.R., Delargy, H. *et al.* (1995) The fat paradox: fat-induced satiety signals versus high fat consumption. *International Journal of Obesity* **19**, 832–835.

Brandon, J.E. (1987) Differences in self-reported eating and exercise behaviours and actual self-concept congruence between obese and non-obese individuals. *Health Values* **11**, 22–33.

Brownell, K. (1986) Public Health approaches to obesity and it's management. *Annual Review of Public Health* **7**, 521–533.

Brownell, K.D. (1993) Whether obesity should be treated. *Health Psychology* **12**, 339–341.

Brownell, K.D. & Wadden, T.A. (1991) The heterogeneity of obesity: fitting treatments to individuals. *Behaviour Therapy* **22**, 153–177.

Bush, A., Webster, J., Chalmers, G. *et al.* (1988) The Harrow Slimming Club: report on 1090 enrolments in 50 courses, 1977–1986. *Journal of Human Nutrition and Dietetics* **1**, 429–436.

Buzzard, I.M., Asp, E.H., Chlebowski, R.T. *et al.* (1990) Diet intervention methods to reduce fat intake: nutrient and food group composition of self-selected low-fat diets. *Journal of the American Dietetic Association* **90**, 42–50.

Cade, J. & O'Connell, S. (1990) Management of weight problems and obesity: knowledge, attitudes and current practice of general practitioners. *British Journal of General Practice* **41**, 147–150.

Chlebowski, R.T., Blackburn, G.L., Buzzard, I.M. *et al.* for the Women's Intervention Nutrition Study (1993) Adherence to a dietary fat intake reduction program in postmenopausal women receiving therapy for early breast cancer. *Journal of Clinical Oncology* **11**, 2072–2080.

Coll, M., Meyer, A. & Stunkard, A.J. (1979) Obesity and food choices in public places. *Archives of General Psychiatry* **36**, 795–797.

COMA (1994) Nutritional aspects of cardiovascular disease. *Report of the Cardiovascular Review Group Committee on Medical Aspects of Food Policy*. Report on Health and Social Services no. 46. London: Department of Health.

Cotton, J.R., Weststrate, J.A. & Blundell, J.E. (1996) Replacement of dietary fat with sucrose polyester: effects on energy intake and appetite control in nonobese males. *American Journal of Clinical Nutrition* **63**, 891–896.

Cowburn, G. & Summerbell, C. (1998) A survey of dietetic practice in obesity management. *Journal of Human Nutrition and Dietetics* **11** (in press).

DoH (1987) The use of very low calorie diets in obesity. *Report of the Working Group on very low calorie diets. Committee on Medical Aspects of Food Policy.* Report on Health and Social Services no. 31. London: Department of Health.

Egger, G., Bolton, A., O'Neill, M. & Freeman, D. (1996) Effectiveness of an abdominal obesity reduction programme in men: the GutBuster 'waist loss' programme. *International Journal of Obesity* 20, 227–231.

Fairburn, C.G. & Cooper, Z. (1996) New perspectives on dietary and behavioural treatments for obesity. *International Journal of Obesity* 20 (suppl. 1), S11–S12.

Fitzgibbon, M.L., Stolley, M.R. & Kirschenbaum, D.S. (1993) Obese people who seek treatment have different characteristics than those who do not seek treatment. *Health Psychology* 12, 342–345.

Fitzwater, S.L., Weinsier, R.L., Wooldridge, N.H., Birch, R., Liu, C. & Bartolucci, A.A. (1991) Evaluation of long-term weight changes after a multidisciplinary weight control program. *Journal of the American Dietetic Association* 91, 421–429.

Fleisch, A. (1951) Le metabolisme basal standard et sa determination au moyen du 'Metabocalculator'. *Helvitica Medica Acta* 1, 23–44.

Franson, K. & Rossner, S. (1994) Effects of weight reduction programs on close family members. *International Journal of Obesity* 18, 648–649.

Fricker, J., Fumeron, F., Clair, D. & Apfelbaum, M. (1989) A positive correlation between energy intake and BMI in a population of 1312 overweight subjects. *International Journal of Obesity* 13, 673–681.

Frost, G., Masters, K., King, C. et al. (1991) A new method of energy prescription to improve weight loss. *Journal of Human Nutrition and Dietetics* 4, 369–373.

Garner, D.M. & Wooley, S.C. (1991) Confronting the failure of behavioural and dietary treatments for obesity. *Clinical Psychology Reviews* 11, 729–780.

Garrow, J.S. (1988) *Obesity and Related Disease.* Edinburgh: Churchill Livingstone.

Garrow, J.S., Webster, J.D., Pearson, M., Pacy, P.J. & Harpin, G. (1989) Inpatient–outpatient randomised comparison of Cambridge diet versus milk diet in 17 obese women over 24 weeks. *International Journal of Obesity* 13, 521–529.

Garrow, J.S. (1991) The safety of dieting. *Proceedings of the Nutrition Society* 50, 493–499.

Garrow, J.S. (1994) Should obesity be treated? *British Medical Journal* 309, 654–655.

Garrow, J.S. (1995) Slimming products: a success in court. *Healthwatch Newsletter* 18, 8.

Garrow, J.S. & Summerbell, C.D. (1995) Meta-analysis: effect of exercise, with or without dieting, on the body composition of overweight subjects. *European Journal of Clinical Nutrition* 49, 1–10.

Gatty R. (1978) *The Body Clock Diet.* London: Victor Gollance.

Gibney, M.J. (1992) Are there conflicts in dietary advice for the prevention of different diseases? *Proceedings of the Nutrition Society* 51, 35–45.

Gilbert, S. & Garrow, J.S. (1983) A prospective controlled trial of outpatient treatment for obesity. *Human Nutrition: Clinical Nutrition* 37C, 21–29.

Glenny, A.-M., O'Meara, S., Melville, A., Sheldon, T.A. & Wilson, C. (1997) The treatment and prevention of obesity: a systematic review of the literature. *International Journal of Obesity* 21, 715–737.

Golay, A., Allaz, A.F., Morel, Y., de Tonnac, N., Tankova, S. & Reaven, G. (1996) Similar weight loss with low- or high-carbohydrate diets. *American Journal of Clinical Nutrition* 63, 174–178.

Grace, C., Summerbell, C. & Kopelman, P. (1998) An audit of dietary treatment modalities and weight loss outcomes in a specialist obesity clinic. *Journal of Human Nutritiun and Dietetics* 11 (in press).

Gries, F.A. (1994) Artificial aids in stabilising weight loss. In: Ditschuneit, H., Gries, F.A., Hauner, H. et al. (eds) *Obesity in Europe 1993,* pp. 209–217. London: John Libbey & Co.

Hakala, P., Ritva-Liisa, K. & Ronnemaa, T. (1993) Group vs individual weight reduction programmes in the treatment of severe obesity — a five year follow-up study. *International Journal of Obesity* 17, 97–102.

Hammer, R.L., Barrier, C.A., Roundy, E.S., Bradford, J.M. & Fisher, A.G. (1989) Calorie-restricted low-fat diet and exercise in obese women. *American Journal of Clinical Nutrition* 49, 77–85.

Harvey, E.L., Glenny, A.-M., Kirk, S.F.L. & Summerbell, C.D. (1998) Protocol for a systematic review of health professionals' Management of obesity. *Journal of Human Nutrition and Dietetics* **11** (in press).

Haskell, W.L., Alderman, E.L., Fair, J.M. *et al.* (1994) Effects of intensive multiple risk factor reduction on coronary atherosclerosis and clinical events in men and women with coronary artery disease. *Circulation* **89**, 975–990.

Haus, G., Hoerr, S.L., Mavis, B. & Robinson, J. (1994) Key modifiable factors in weight maintenance: fat intake, exercise and weight cycling. *Journal of the American Dietetic Association* **94**, 409–413.

Hayaki, J. & Brownell, K.D. (1996) Behaviour change in practice: group approaches. *International Journal of Obesity* **20** (suppl. 1), S27–S30.

Heitmann, B.L. & Lissner, L. (1995) Dietary under-reporting by obese individuals. Is it specific or non-specific? *British Medical Journal* **311**, 986–989.

Heshka, S., Feld, K., Yang, M.-U., Allison, D.B. & Heymsfield, S.B. (1993) Resting energy expenditure in the obese: A cross-validation and comparison of predictive equations. *Journal of the American Dietetic Association* **93**, 1031–1036.

Hjermann, I., Velve Byre, K., Holme, I. & Leren, P. (1981) Effect of diet and smoking intervention on the incidence of coronary heart disease. *Lancet* **2 (8259)**, 1303–1310.

Holt, S.H.A., Brand Miller, J.C., Petocz, P. & Farmakalidis, E. (1995) A satiety index of common foods. *European Journal of Clinical Nutrition* **49**, 675–690.

HEA (1995) *Obesity in Primary Care*. London: Health Education Authority.

HEA (1996) *Balance of Good Health*. London: Health Education Authority.

Jeffery, R.W. (1993) Minnesota studies on community-based approaches to weight loss and control. *Annals of Internal Medicine* **119**, 719–721.

Jebb, S.A. & Goldberg, G.R. (1998) Efficacy of very low energy diets and meal replacements in the treatment of obesity. *Journal of Human Nutrition and Dietetics* **11** (in press).

Jeffery, R.W., Hellerstedt, W.L., French, S. & Baxter, J.E. (1995) A randomized trial of counselling for fat restriction versus calorie restriction in the treatment of obesity. *International Journal of Obesity* **19**, 132–137.

Kanders, B.S., George, L., Blackburn, L. & Lavin, P.T. (1994) The long-term effect of aspartame on body weight among obese women. In: Ditschuneit, F.A., Gries, H., Hauner, V. *et al.* (eds) *Obesity in Europe 1993*, pp. 247–252. London: John Libbey & Co.

Karvetti, R.-L. & Hakala, P. (1992) A seven year follow-up of a weight reduction programme in Finnish primary health care. *European Journal of Clinical Nutrition* **46**, 743–752.

Kendall, A., Levitsky, D.A., Strupp, B.J., & Lissner, L. (1991) Weight loss on a low-fat diet: consequences of the imprecision of the control of food intake in humans. *American Journal of Clinical Nutrition* **53**, 1124–1129.

Kopelman, P. (1993) Place of obesity clinics in the NHS. *British Journal of Hospital Medicine* **49**, 533–535.

Lavery, M.A. & Loewy, J.W. (1993) Identifying predictive variables for long-term weight change after participation in weight loss program. *Journal of the American Dietetic Association* **93**, 1017–1024.

Leibel, R.L., Hirsch, J., Appel, B.E. & Checani, G.C. (1992) Energy intake required to maintain body weight is not affected by wide variation in diet composition. *American Journal of Clinical Nutrition* **55**, 350–355.

Liebermeister, H. (1994) Novelties and curiosities: miracle diets in the treatment of obesity. In: Ditschuneit, H., Gries, F.A., Hauner, H. *et al.* (eds) *Obesity in Europe 1993*, pp. 263–267. London: John Libbey & Co.

Lissner, L., Levitsky, D.A., Strupp, B.J., Kalkwarf, H.J. & Roe, D.A. (1987) Dietary fat and the regulation of energy intake in human subjects. *American Journal of Clinical Nutrition* **46**, 886–892.

Lindroos, A.-K., Sjöström, L. & Lissner, L. (1993) Validity and reproducibility of a self-administered dietary questionnaire in obese and non-obese subjects. *European Journal of Clinical Nutrition* **47**, 461–481.

Macqueen, C. & Frost, G. (1995) Does higher quality information improve the attendance rate or treatment outcome of obese patients? *Journal of Human Nutrition and Dietetics* 8, 137–139.

Marsden, K. (1993) *The Food Combining Diet*. London: Thorsons.

Mattes, R.D. (1993) Fat preference and adherence to a reduced-fat diet. *American Journal of Clinical Nutrition* 57, 373–381.

Murphree, D. (1994) Patient attitude toward physician treatment for obesity. *Journal of Family Practice* 38, 45–48.

Murray, S., Narayan, V., Mitchell, M. & Witte, H. (1993) Study of dietetic knowledge among members of the primary health care team. *British Journal of General Practice* 43, 229–231.

Ogden, J. & Evans, C. (1996) The problem with weighing: effects on mood, self-esteem and body image. *International Journal of Obesity* 20, 272–277.

Ornish, D., Brown, S.E., Scherwitz, L.W. *et al.* (1990) Can lifestyle changes reverse coronary heart disease? *Lancet* 336, 129–133.

Pacy, P.J., Webster, J.D., Pearson, M. & Garrow, J.S. (1987) A cross-sectional cost/benefit audit in a hospital obesity clinic. *Human Nutrition: Applied Nutrition* 41A, 38–46.

Pearson, G.C., de Looy, A.E. & Webster, J. (1989) Analysis of the dietetic treatment of obesity. *Journal of Human Nutrition and Dietetics* 2, 371–377.

Perri, M.G., Sears, S.F. & Clarke, J.E. (1993) Towards a continuous care model of obesity management. *Diabetes Care* 16, 200–209.

Pratt, C.A. (1989) Development of a screening questionnaire to study attrition in weight-control programs. *Psychological Reports* 64, 1007–1016.

Prewitt, T.E., Schmeisser, D., Bowen, P.E. *et al.* (1991) Changes in body weight, body composition, and energy intake in women fed high- and low-fat diets. *American Journal of Clinical Nutrition* 54, 304–310.

Rabast, U. (1994) Dietary fibre in the treatment of obesity. In: Ditschuneit, H., Gries, F.A., Hauner, H. *et al.* (eds) *Obesity in Europe 1993*, pp. 279–283. London: John Libbey & Co.

Raben, A., Due Jensen, N., Marckmann, P., Sandstrom, B. & Astrup, A. (1995) Spontaneous weight loss during 11 weeks' *ad libitum* intake of a low fat/high fibre diet in young, normal weight subjects. *International Journal of Obesity* 19, 916–923.

Racette, S.B., Schoeller, D.A., Kushner, R.F., Neil, K.M. & Herling-Iaffaldano, K. (1995) Effects of aerobic exercise and dietary carbohydrate on energy expenditure and body composition during weight reduction in obese women. *American Journal of Clinical Nutrition* 61, 486–494.

Robertson, J.D. & Reid, D.D. (1952) Standards for the basal metabolism of normal people in Britain. *Lancet* i, 940–943.

Rolls, B.J. (1986) Sensory-specific satiety. *Nutrition Reviews* 44, 93–101.

Rossner S. (1995) Long-term intervention strategies in obesity treatment. *International Journal of Obesity* 19 (suppl. 7), S29–S33.

Ryttig, K.R., Tellnes, G., Haegh, L., Boe, E. & Fagerthun, H. (1989) A dietary fibre supplement and weight maintenance after weight reduction: a randomised double blind placebo controlled long-term trial. *American Journal of Clinical Nutrition* 13, 165–171.

Sarkkinen, E.S., Agren, J.J., Ahola, I., Ovaskainen, M.-L. & Uusitupa, M.I.J. (1994) Fatty acid composition of serum cholesterol esters, and erythrocyte and platelet membranes as indicators of long-term adherence to fat-modified diets. *American Journal of Clinical Nutrition* 59, 364–370.

Schlundt, D.G., Hill, J.O., Pope-Cordle, J., Arnold, D., Virts, K.L. & Katahn, M. (1993) Randomised evaluation of a low fat *ad libitum* carbohydrate diet for weight reduction. *International Journal of Obesity* 17, 623–629.

Schuler, G., Hambrecht, R., Schlierf, G. *et al.* (1992) Regular physical exercise and low-fat diet: effects on progression of coronary artery disease. *Circulation* 86, 1–11.

Shah, M., McGovern, P., French, S. & Baxter, J. (1994) Comparison of a low-fat, *ad libitum* complex carbohydrate diet with a low-energy diet in moderately obese women. *American Journal of Clinical Nutrition* 59, 980–984.

Sheppard, L., Kristal, A.R. & Kushi, L.H. (1991) Weight loss in women participating in a randomized trial of low-fat diets. *American Journal of Clinical Nutrition* 54, 821–828.

Singh, R.B., Rastogi, S.S., Verma, R. *et al.* (1992) Randomised controlled trial of cardioprotective diet in patients with recent acute myocardial infarction: results of one year follow-up. *British Medical Journal* **304**, 1015–1019.

Summerbell, C.D. (1996) Teaching nutrition to medical doctors: the potential role of the State Registered Dietitian. *Journal of Human Nutrition and Dietetics* **9**, 349–356.

Summerbell, C.D., Moody, R.C., Shanks, J., Stock, M.J. & Geissler, C. (1995) Sources of energy from meals vs snacks in 220 people in four age groups. *European Journal of Clinical Nutrition* **49**, 33–41.

Summerbell, C.D., Moody, R.C., Shanks, J., Stock, M.J. & Geissler, C. (1996) Relationship between feeding pattern and body mass index in 220 free-living people in four age groups. *European Journal of Clinical Nutrition* **50**, 513–519.

Summerbell, C.D., Jones, L.V. & Glasziou, P. (1998) The long-term effect of advice on low-fat diets in terms of weight loss: an interim meta-analysis. *Journal of Human Nutrition and Dietetics* **11** (in press).

White, E., Shattuck, A.L., Kristal, A.R. *et al.* (1992) Maintenance of a low-fat diet: follow-up of the women's health trial. *Cancer Epidemiology, Biomarkers and Prevention* **1**, 315–323.

Vigus, J., Tata, P., Judd, P., Bowyer, C. & Evans, E. (1995) Which way to treat obesity? Emotional, eating and behavioural issues in dieting. *Journal of Human Nutrition and Dietetics* **8**, 105–118.

CHAPTER 17

Cognitive–Behavioural Treatment of Obesity

JANE WARDLE AND LORNA RAPOPORT

The problem of obesity

Obesity is a problem both because of the significant health risks associated with it and because of its effect on psychological well being. These two facets of obesity are mirrored in motives for treatment, with some patients being motivated by their wish to improve their health and others by their wish to improve their appearance, although in both cases the immediate goal is weight loss. Obesity is also increasing rapidly in Western industrialized countries, and now affects more than 15% of adults in the U.K. (Bennett, 1995). Consequently it is a problem in terms of public health as well as at the level of the individual (Seidell, 1995).

The rapidly rising prevalence of obesity has not only stimulated medical attention, but has also contributed to the theories of the aetiology of obesity. In the past obesity has been conceptualized largely in the terms of the inadequacies of the individual—either psychological or biological. However, the realization that obesity prevalence can double (Prentice & Jebb, 1995) or even treble, as has happened in some of the recently industrialized Pacific islands (Hodge et al., 1996), over a relatively short time period, strongly implicates the changing physical and social structure of the modern industrial environment as a major cause. This leads to a quite different model of obesity, in which individuals may vary in susceptibility, but the proximal cause is the obesity-promoting environment.

Psychologists' involvement in obesity treatment has also reflected a range of different ways of conceptualizing obesity (Rodin et al., 1989). The psycho-dynamic perspective proposes that obesity has a psychogenic cause, i.e., that the individual's psychological state, combined with the unconscious meaning of food and eating, leads to overeating (Kaplan & Kaplan, 1957). According to this model, treating the underlying psychological difficulties, usually with some form of psychotherapy, should cure the weight problem. However, there has not been any convincing evidence for an underlying psychopathology in obesity, nor any particular personality type associated with obesity. Furthermore, no controlled trials of psychotherapy have yet been carried out to support the therapeutic claims. Finally, it seems implausible that population levels of psychopathology have been rising enough to explain the increase in obesity.

The behavioural model of obesity also stemmed from theories about an underlying abnormality, but of eating behaviour rather than psychopathology. It was originally proposed that an 'obese eating style' (either innate or acquired) was the cause of obesity, and therefore that learning new patterns of eating would reduce overeating and thereby control body-weight (Ferster *et al.*, 1962). However, the obese eating style proved hard to demonstrate outside the laboratory, and later research suggested than eating abnormalities were more likely to be a function of the obese person's prolonged dieting than to be the underlying cause of the disorder (Nisbett, 1968). Behavioural treatment programmes were then re-conceptualized in terms of strategies for developing control over food choices and eating behaviour, as means of maintaining a negative energy balance. This involved helping obese individuals to work out how to modify both their environments and their reactions to environmental stimuli. Behavioural methods were therefore applied to changing eating habits for the better, regardless of their origins (Brownell & Kramer, 1989). The model underlying behavioural treatment is consistent with the idea that environmental change is decreasing energy expenditure, while the increasing convenience and availability of highly palatable foods promotes energy intake — hence a positive energy balance is becoming more common.

The development of cognitive–behavioural treatments

Animal learning research had demonstrated that effective control over behaviour could be exerted through manipulating reinforcement contingencies (Skinner, 1953). In the application of these ideas to the human field the concept of reinforcement was extended to include self-administered rewards, the so-called 'self-control' model (Mahoney & Arnkoff, 1978). Among the earliest reports of behavioural treatment of obesity were the case series based on the self-control model of behaviour change, which demonstrated an impressive degree of weight loss (Stuart, 1967). The essential elements of the behaviourally based, self-control approach were a phase of recording of the target behaviour (self-monitoring) which was designed to identify situational consistencies in the problem behaviour (functional analysis), followed by negotiation of behaviour change goals and sub-goals designed to modify eating in key situations. Intervention strategies included 'stimulus control', i.e., regulating exposure to cues which might trigger excessive eating, and the use of self-administered rewards in relation to compliance with the sub-goals. With the development of cognitive approaches to behaviour change, the behavioural programmes were modified to include identifying and modifying 'self-defeating' cognitions (Meichenbaum, 1977). Treatment approaches of this kind have now been used widely for over 30 years under the general heading of cognitive-behaviour therapy (CBT).

A great many outcome studies have been published which consistently support the efficacy of CBT (in all its manifestations) over no treatment, or simple dietary treatment. However, the enthusiasm of the early days has been followed with a more sober evaluation in the light of longer-term follow-up studies (Foreyt *et al.*, 1982; Brownell & Wadden, 1992; Wilson & Fairburn, 1993). Initial weight losses are usually modest, averaging little more than 5–10% of initial weight, and it is unusual for there to be further weight loss once the active treatment phase is ended. There is also a tendency for a gradual return to the original weight. Most authorities would agree that the CBT approach has offered the most consistently effective results apart from surgical treatments, and probably represent the gold-standard of current treatment. Nevertheless, there is still room for considerable improvement, both in terms of treatment outcome and in the dissemination of the CBT methods to a wider audience.

In this chapter we shall describe the principal components of CBT for obesity, discuss the newer developments in psychological treatment of obesity, and consider the implications of developments in the genetics of obesity and the pharmacological management of obesity, for behavioural treatment programmes.

Assessment for cognitive–behavioural treatment

Behavioural treatments of all kinds have in common an initial phase in which motivation for treatment is evaluated, the history and current state of the presenting condition is assessed, a formulation of the problem is prepared, and a treatment programme is planned in consultation with the patient. Unlike some other treatment approaches, elements of the assessment process, such as keeping records of cognitions or behaviour, continue throughout the programme and may contribute to redefining the goals as treatment progresses.

Assessment of motivation

Patients present for obesity treatment through various routes and with a range of expectations of the treatment process. They also vary in the key features of their weight problem which concern them — with health and appearance being the most common issues. Some patients hope to solve life problems other than weight through psychological treatment, and it may be necessary to deal with significant emotional or social problems before initiating weight-control treatment. Patients also vary in the commitment which they bring to treatment and the extent to which they are ready to tolerate the discomforts associated with effective treatment. Psychological models of 'readiness to change' have been attracting increasing interest recently as a way of explaining variation in compliance with treatment advice. The 'stages of change' model is the most widely used and it identifies a sequence of stages from precontemplation (not even considering change) through contemplation, preparation, action and maintenance (Prochaska et al., 1992). It can safely be assumed that any patient who is attending a clinic appointment is beyond the precontemplation stage so far as *wanting* to lose weight is concerned. Indeed most obese patients have tried to lose weight before — the majority, many times. However, it cannot be assumed that all patients are equally ready to make significant and sustained alterations in behaviour. It is not uncommon for a patient to say that he or she is 'desperate to lose weight', 'will do anything', or 'must change now or never', but to prove unwilling to keep food records, walk a few extra miles a week or modify family meals to any significant degree. The motivational assessment should therefore focus not only on the hoped-for outcome (weight loss), but also on the behavioural changes which will be required to achieve that outcome.

One form of motivational assessment which has been used both to measure and modify motivation for behaviour change, is the decisional balance assessment (Prochaska et al., 1994). A substantial body of research shows that while expressed motivation to change is a predictor of outcome in treatment, the individual's evaluation of the balance of perceived costs and benefits of change may be a more significant factor. In the smoking field, successful quitters rate benefits higher, and costs lower, at the start of a treatment programme, than those who *seem* equally committed, but in fact fail to quit (Prochaska et al., 1994). The same approach could be applied in relation to changing diet or activity levels by getting the patients to list and evaluate the barriers and benefits to changing both diet and exercise. Although this approach is used primarily for assessment, it has also been argued that a non-directive, patient-centred approach of this kind not only allows patients to express their ambivalence about change, but may even help them to change. This process is known as motivational interviewing (Miller, 1996) and has been found to be an effective method of increasing patients' adherence to treatment.

Assessment of weight and body image

Although the focus of behavioural treatment is towards the future, it is essential to establish the pattern of weight and weight change over the lifetime, the family history of weight, and the history of previous attempts at weight control — and this can be done by interview. This information provides some indication of the weight trajectory, the likely familial (genetic) loading of obesity and the prospects for success of the present attempt.

The initial assessment should be followed with some system of monitoring weight change throughout treatment and follow-up. During the active treatment phase, regular weighing can reinforce positive behavioural changes and highlight problems. However, most authorities recommend only relatively infrequent weighing, both because fat loss is likely to be very gradual and therefore there is no point in frequent assessment, and because weight loss is not a perfect indicator of fat loss, e.g., variation in water retention causes weight to vary, so short-term changes may be a poor indication of the underlying trend. In the maintenance phase, weight monitoring could be an important element of long-term weight control. A monthly weight record, combined with an action plan to be initiated when weight goes beyond a predetermined threshold, could be a useful strategy.

Assessment of body image

Body image is not evaluated routinely in relation to obesity treatment, but there is increasing interest in including it as a significant target of treatment, both in its own right and as a means of improving adherence to treatment advice. A negative body image is likely to be associated with avoidance of exposure — which could include avoidance of social occasions, sexual behaviour or of active pursuits. The level of body image distress can be gauged from interview, and supplemented with one of the instruments designed to assess body shape dissatisfaction in eating disorders such as the Body Shape Questionnaire (Cooper et al., 1987) or the Body Image Avoidance Questionnaire (Rosen et al., 1991).

Assessment of eating behaviour

A history of the patient's eating and dieting behaviour along with their current eating patterns provides some of the basic information for developing a treatment programme. It also provides the opportunity to explore eating pathology such as binge eating (see below), night eating and emotional eating. In addition, extreme dietary restraint (usually achieved only episodically by obese people) is also a potential problem. Assessment for eating disorders, including binge eating, can be carried out through a standardized interview with the Eating Disorder Examination (Fairburn & Cooper, 1993).

Records of food intake are used by dietitians to get a snapshot of the quality and quantity of the patient's diet. In CBT programmes, the eating diary is also a key feature not only of the assessment, but also of the treatment itself. During the assessment phase, records of food intake are kept along with information on the setting of consumption (e.g., mood, speed of eating, the situation), and the events subsequent to the meal, to identify the stimuli which predict overeating, and the succeeding factors which might be reinforcing overeating (a so-called *functional analysis*). During the treatment phase, the diary can be used to record progress towards particular behavioural goals, and highlight new problems. There may also be other benefits of a food record. If the recorded energy intake is substantially below the estimated energy needs, and yet weight is not being lost, then the patient must be under-reporting their food intake (Prentice *et al.*, 1989). Tackling the patient's inability to be honest (to others or themselves) about what they eat—or possibly their inability to be aware of what they eat, can be an important step in helping them to acknowledge their problem. Adherence to self-monitoring can also serve as a simple compliance indicator—if the patient who alleges his or her commitment to lose weight cannot even complete a food record, then it is clear that there are serious motivational conflicts to be tackled. The final advantage is that the self-monitoring process in itself has been found to be beneficial in reducing food intake—albeit in the short term. Few people, normal weight or obese, keep a good mental account of what or when they eat, and so a written record provides a much better basis for planning and monitoring change.

Formal assessment of eating behaviour using psychometric measures can also be useful to characterize the individual patient and help to guide treatment goals, although there are few instruments designed specifically for obese patients. Assessment of restrained and disinhibited eating can be done with either the Dutch Eating Behaviour Questionnaire (Van Strien *et al.*, 1986a) or the Three Factor Eating Questionnaire (Stunkard & Messick, 1985). The patient's confidence in controlling their eating can be assessed with the Eating Self Efficacy Scale (Glynn & Ruderman, 1986), and social–environmental support for change, with Sallis' measure of 'social support for dietary change' (Sallis *et al.*, 1987).

A significant minority of obese patients will have more serious problems of control and patterning of eating, describing episodes of excessive eating similar to those reported by patients with bulimia nervosa. In the draft criteria for the DSMIV, a 'new' disorder, binge-eating disorder (BED) has been defined, characterized by episodes of binge eating at least twice a week for 6 months, with the episodes involving eating to uncomfortable excess and being distressed (Spitzer *et al.*, 1993). Elements of the binge-eating problem can be assessed at interview focussing primarily on the presence and frequency of binge eating (Marcus & Wing, 1987), or a formal measure, such as the Eating Disorder Examination (Fairburn & Cooper, 1993) can be used.

Assessment of physical activity

Physical activity assessment plays a relatively minor role in many treatment programmes, but there is increasing interest in the longer-term efficacy of activity changes and it may be appropriate to give physical activity equal status to controlling food intake (Foreyt & Goodrick, 1995). An activity record of some sort is therefore important, both to monitor activity levels and to highlight to the patient the importance attached to activity. The recording can be linked to any special activities which the obese individual may be taking up to improve fitness, e.g., the frequency and duration of swimming or walking. Alternatively, it is possible to get a crude measure of overall activity with a pedometer. Some patients enjoy using such a simple method of activity recording and they can find it reinforcing to chart the daily pedometer totals and to try to keep them above a target level. Finally, there is increasing evidence that sedentariness, in contrast to activity, may be a key factor in weight control (Epstein et al., 1995). This subtle distinction means that one focus of treatment could be to reduce 'sitting time' without necessarily specifying particular activities, and therefore that sitting time could be a feature of the daily diary.

Assessment of health risk

Conventionally, obesity treatments focus on weight loss. However, there is a growing realization that the principal reason for concern about obesity is the morbidity and mortality risk (Van Itallie & Lew, 1992). Consequently, if possible, it is useful to assess cardiovascular disease (CVD) risk factors such as fat distribution (based on waist/hip ratio or waist circumference), serum lipid levels, and blood pressure. Smoking is also a significant risk factor, and advice on quitting smoking needs to be included as part of any lifestyle interventions which are intended to reduce CVD risk.

Assessment of general psychological well being

Although the main focus of obesity treatment has to be weight and weight-related risk factors, a thorough psychological assessment should take account of associated psychological factors which are likely to affect any programme. The importance of this is emphasized by the results of the Swedish Obesity Study, which found poor psychosocial functioning in obese adults (Sullivan, 1993). These could include low self-esteem, depression, difficulties in assertiveness, and interpersonal or sexual difficulties. Problems of this kind might influence the treatment approach or might be severe enough to compromise the efficacy of treatment and therefore need to be dealt with before the CBT programme begins.

The elements of cognitive–behavioural treatment

Stimulus control

Stimulus control is one of the central elements of behavioural treatment. It derives from the idea that eating is triggered by a range of external or internal cues, such as being in an environment where eating usually occurs. The triggering process could be part of an innate repertoire of responses to the sight, smell or taste of food, it could be learned as a result of repeated associations between particular stimuli and eating, or it could be part of a coping repertoire — for example to ameliorate negative moods. Controlling eating at the final stage of this chain is known to be difficult, but controlling exposure to cues earlier in the chain should be easier. In other words, stimulus control is substituted, in part, for self-control.

The basic approach consists of identifying the chain of events leading up to problem eating, and developing strategies to intervene early on in the chain, e.g., not simply trying to resist eating when tempting foods are present, but reducing the chance that tempting foods would be present. One of the simplest examples would be to avoid buying highly palatable foods, or if there must be such foods, to store them so that they are not easily on view. Some stimulus control strategies such as avoiding shopping when hungry are applicable over the long term. Others, such as avoiding buffet-style meals, are valuable in the acute phase, but in the longer term the individual will need to learn other self-control strategies (see Exposure treatment, below).

Stimulus control methods can also be adapted to increase activity and decrease sedentary behaviour. Simple re-organizations of homes and workplaces (e.g., moving commonly used equipment further away) can induce more walking. Arrangements to carry out activities with friends can increase the chance of adherence to exercise plans.

Modifying self-defeating cognitions

Many obese people report a variety of negative thoughts or ways of thinking about weight and weight control. With the development of cognitive approaches to therapy, the investigation and modification of negative thoughts came to be an accepted part of behavioural programmes. In the case of obesity, Mahoney & Mahoney (1976) were among the first to describe the kind of ways of thinking which compromise treatment compliance in obesity. Examples include 'all or nothing' thinking (e.g., either 'I am strictly dieting' or 'I might as well give up entirely', as moderate control is useless) and 'catastrophizing' ('my failure to lose weight over 1 week means that the programme is useless'). The usual technique is to ask patients to recall or record their thoughts about their eating (and activity) behaviour. This record is then discussed in the treatment sessions to give the patient the chance to consider the evidence for and against the ideas that they have recorded. They can also develop arguments against some of the negative thoughts and then practise challenging them at the times that they occur in everyday life. There have not been any systematic comparisons of behaviour therapy with and without the cognitive approach, but clinical experience suggests that for some patients it is very helpful, and for many it has the advantage of a novel addition to the methods of self-control which they usually use.

Learned self-control

Obese patients will often say that they cannot exert self-control over their eating in certain provoking situations. Emotional states such as anger or anxiety are among the cues which many obese people associate with greater difficulty in controlling eating, while cueing from external factors (e.g., attractive foods) has been discussed above. It is important to remember that external and emotional eating are *not* unique to obesity and may not play a causal role, but they will certainly compromise adherence to treatment (Rodin, 1980). The stimulus-control approach discussed above is based on reducing exposure to the stimuli which precipitate eating, but in the longer term the obese person may wish to eliminate the association between such stimuli and the urge to eat.

Exposure with response prevention is a well-recognized behavioural technique for modifying responses. Assuming that the externally cued eating is a learned response, prolonged exposure to the eliciting cues without performance of the behaviour should extinguish the conditioned responses. This method has been used with bulimic patients to help them learn to look at, or taste, binge food without having a binge (Fairburn & Wilson, 1993). It can be adapted to help the obese person develop control over situations which normally trigger abandonment of the diet. Exposure first induces a dramatic increase in the urge to eat, but this reduces over 5–30 minutes providing a vivid demonstration of the development of control. In 'homework' assignments the patient can follow a self-exposure programme with problem foods or situations, progressing through a hierarchy of situations varying in difficulty level.

In emotional eating, emotional arousal is the conditioned stimulus for eating, probably having developed as a result of repeated associations between emotion and eating. This association can develop in dieters because lapses of control are more likely in a negative emotional state, when people feel less motivated by long-term goals. Repetitions of feeling upset and eating may eventually condition the individual to develop the physiological responses which precede eating (increased salivation, increased insulin secretion, decreased blood sugar), whenever they become emotionally aroused. Thus, what begins as a dietary lapse can become a conditioned urge to eat. One way of achieving the necessary unreinforced exposure (extinction) is to use imagined mood stimuli, combined with real food exposure. Alternatively music or films can be used to arouse emotions, combined with exposure to increasingly difficult foods. Again, it may be possible to 'prescribe' self-control practice as part of the homework.

In some cases, eating may be serving as a form of self-medication for negative emotional states, designed to modify the mood disturbance. In those cases, self-control treatment may need to be supplemented with training in strategies for managing emotional distress (see below).

Stress management

The place of stress in the control of diet or weight is ill-understood. Stressful life events have sometimes been linked to weight gain (Van Strien *et al.*, 1986b), dieters themselves often attribute their problems of dietary control to stress, and stress is widely believed to induce a preference for high-fat or 'comfort' foods. However, the experimental literature on the effects of stress on diet suggest more complex effects (Greeno & Wing, 1994). Animal studies indicate that *anorexia* is a more common reaction to stress than *hyperphagia* (Robbins & Fray, 1980). Human studies also identify extreme stress (and distress) with loss of appetite and weight, but lesser degrees of stress have variable effects. Variation in the response may depend on the individual, the type and amount of stress, and the availability of other coping resources such as social support. Clinically, it is possible to establish whether or not stress is associated with poorer dietary control by keeping a stress record in parallel with the dietary record. If stress appears to be a factor in loss of dietary control, then training in stress management could be useful. This chapter is not the place for a detailed description of stress management, but the principal features are early identification of sources of stress, the use of relaxation and positive self-talk to mitigate the acute stress responses, and development of appropriate resources to manage both the source of stress and the persistence of the stress response (problem-focused and emotion-focused coping) (Friedman *et al.*, 1994).

The other reason for considering stress management is that recent research developments have suggested that stress could play a part in promoting abdominal fat storage (Björntorp, 1996). At present, this is largely limited to observations that abdominal obesity is linked with life stress in epidemiological studies (which do not necessarily indicate causal effects) and to some suggestions that there are biochemical pathways which could account for the effect (Rebuffe-Scrive *et al.*, 1992). Nevertheless, these observations strengthen the case for either including an element of stress management in obesity treatment programmes, or recommending stress management to obese patients with demonstrable problems in stress-induced eating.

Setting behavioural goals

Behavioural treatment programmes commonly identify a number of goals and sub-goals which will define a successful treatment outcome, and in traditional obesity treatment these are defined in terms of weight loss. The ultimate goal would be the achievement of a weight (or body mass index (BMI)) within the normal range, and most obese patients, whatever their previous experience with treatment, seem to have extremely optimistic expectations when they join a new programme.

The plethora of sobering reviews of the outcome of treatment of obesity have led many authorities to question the practice of setting the goal of 'normal weight' if it is manifestly unachievable. An unrealistic goal sets the patient up for failure and may lead him or her to attribute failure to personal shortcomings rather than the real shortcomings of obesity treatment. Unrealistic goals can also lead patients (and health professionals) to undervalue modest weight losses, and thus to eschew treatment approaches which claim only modest outcomes. It is also clear that even very modest weight losses can have beneficial health effects (Goldstein, 1992).

However, there are likely to be problems associated with setting weight goals which reflect the reality that weight losses at best are unlikely to exceed 5–10% of initial body-weight. Firstly, this might deter many patients from even joining the programme, since there are many commercial alternatives which promise extraordinary and rapid weight losses. There is also the possibility that the unrealistic expectations are a source of positive (if illusory) motivation. However, observations from other areas of behaviour change suggest that the process of accepting a realistic goal could itself be therapeutic. For example, the most effective treatments for chronic pain encourage the patient to resume normal activities *despite* pain rather than seek 'a cure'. By analogy, acknowledging the chronicity and challenge of weight control might result in a better outcome than the continuing search for a magical solution. In some cases, where the weight history reveals persistent weight gain, even stabilization of weight would be a beneficial long-term outcome.

The second issue for setting treatment goals is the time perspective. Most treatment goals relate to weight loss during the active treatment period, but the real challenge is not short-term loss, but long-term maintenance. The popular image of weight control suggests that a person 'goes on a diet', loses weight, and then resumes normal eating. However, this pattern will result in almost certain regain to, or even above, the initial weight. The only realistic perspective is one in which the individual recognizes that eating and activity patterns will have to change permanently, and that weight control is a long-term, not a short-term, goal.

The third issue is the nature of the goals. In practice the goal of obesity treatment is weight loss, but it is important to remember that the reasons for weight loss are to improve cardiovascular and metabolic risk (or other secondary complications of obesity) and to improve body image. Weight loss offers the ideal solution, but it is not the only solution. Cardiovascular and metabolic risks are susceptible to changes in dietary quality and physical fitness, even if weight change is minimal (Law, 1994). In cases where patients have shown a consistently poor treatment response (e.g., little or no weight loss) and especially where their weight has been steadily rising, weight stability combined with lower CVD risk could provide an acceptable goal for that individual.

Changes in weight and health risk of course represent the overall treatment goals, but behavioural programmes usually include specified sub-goals. In the case of obesity treatment these are likely to include specific behaviour changes (e.g., in eating or activity) which are targeted over the treatment period. One of the key characteristics of behavioural treatments is the inclusion of short-term goals, achievement of which can sustain motivation. The process of negotiating and agreeing these short-term goals can serve as a form of behavioural rehearsal, which, if used effectively, should contribute directly to a positive treatment outcome.

Contemporary obesity treatment might therefore look for modest and sustained changes in weight or risk factors, representing a shift in expectations both for patients and health professionals. This also implies a shift in resources since if obesity is acknowledged to be a chronic problem, it may need to be managed through long-term care.

Improving body image

Body dissatisfaction is almost synonymous with obesity among women in Western cultures. In the past this has been seen as understandable, not least because many health professionals share the view that obesity is unattractive and connotes a lack of self-control. Indeed self-disgust is sometimes seen as 'healthy', since it should motivate the individual to change. However, there is increasing recognition that a poor body image could contribute to low self-esteem and thereby have an adverse influence on self-efficacy. Furthermore a realistic appraisal of the likely outcome of treatment suggests that most obese adults will still be well above a 'normal weight' after the treatment programme has ended. Consequently, it could be important to focus on improving body image regardless of the level of weight loss. A poor body image is also likely to be associated with avoidance of physical display—including physical activities requiring self-exposure—and so modifying body image could improve adherence to treatment advice.

Little is known about the cause of variation of body image, either among the obese or the normal weight. Anthropological research indicates enormous cultural differences, with obesity being most stigmatized in Western cultures. There is also a consistent gender difference with women of all weights reporting more body dissatisfaction than men. What is not clear is why some overweight women have such a negative body image, while others—equally fat—accept their shapes. However, evidence is emerging which implicates both social factors (e.g., teasing) and attributional factors (e.g., negative attitudes towards obesity) in the development of a negative body image (Grilo et al., 1994).

There are few reports of methods of improving body image among the obese (Rosen, 1996), the literature from body image disturbance among patients with bulimia nervosa or normal weight women provides some guidance (Butters & Cash, 1987). However, in these conditions there is an implication that the negative body image is 'abnormal', i.e., others would not rate that individual as being too fat. In other words body shape dissatisfaction is analysed as a form of dysmorphophobia. This is not necessarily the case among the obese, who really are fatter than is generally thought to be attractive. Significant prejudice is well established, and fat people will experience teasing, insults, embarrassment and outright discrimination (Allon, 1982). Achieving a better body image necessitates learning self-acceptance *despite* an appearance which falls short of cultural ideals of beauty, and learning to cope with the stigma of overweight (Sobal, 1991). In this respect, the literature on helping people accept disfigurement or disability may also provide some helpful guidance. The key changes towards a better body image are both cognitive and behavioural and include not equating a non-ideal appearance with personal unacceptibility (a cognitive change), and not allowing body appraisal to influence choices of activity (a behavioural change). Clinical experience suggests that a group-based treatment programme has many advantages in helping obese adults to develop more 'weight-blindness' in their evaluation of themselves and their future plans.

Disordered eating patterns and binge eating

Patterning of eating has attracted only limited attention in obesity management, although the 'night eating syndrome' was described by Stunkard many years ago (Stunkard, 1959). However, many obese patients report some degree of disturbance of eating patterns. Most commonly this involves an eating pattern which varies considerably from day to day, it may also involve long periods of restriction and other phases of frequent excessive consumption.

One problem with irregular eating patterns is that they can prevent the development of conditioned hunger and satiety. Evidence from animal eating suggests that eating (and the anticipatory physiological changes) can be conditioned to environmental cues — thus, hunger develops when mealtime cues are present. Likewise meal size is controlled by the (learned) interval between eating and the next meal — so the animal tends to eat larger meals in anticipation of a longer meal-to-meal interval. It is possible that normal human eating operates on similar lines, so with a regular meal pattern the activation of hunger is conditioned to mealtime cues, and meal size is related to the expected inter-meal interval. This provides a strong rationale for establishing a regular meal pattern early on in treatment, perhaps before implementing caloric restriction.

If obese patients report any binge eating, then it is important to carry out a thorough investigation of their eating behaviour, and establish the history and current state of binge eating (Marcus, 1993). In the past, patients with binge eating have been treated identically with obese non-binge eaters. However, most authorities now recommend that if binge eating is a significant problem, then help in developing normal eating patterns and regaining control over eating should be considered, as well as the weight-control element of treatment. Modifications of the treatment programmes used for bulimia nervosa provide a model for treatment (Porzelius et al., 1995), but there is no agreement yet over whether these should be introduced before, after, or in parallel with weight control. A conservative approach would suggest starting therapy with an emphasis on a regular meal patterns, reduction of restraint, and strategies to reduce binge frequency (stimulus control, stress management and exposure as appropriate). This could be followed with advice on healthy eating and increased physical activity.

The crucial question is whether a weight-control regimen can be safely instituted among individuals with BED. Clinicians working on the treatment of bulimia have often suggested that re-instatement of dietary restraint can precipitate a recurrence of binge eating. By analogy, dieting may be contra-indicated in obese patients who binge eat. However, it is possible that more conservative dietary regimens, with a stronger focus on physical activity, can be used safely as long as there is careful supervision and binge frequency is closely monitored.

Long-term maintenance

It is often observed that short-term weight loss is considerably easier than long-term maintenance of loss. Several different procedures have been tried as a means of reducing relapse, including booster sessions and relapse training (Perri, 1992). In both cases the patient is encouraged to acknowledge the likelihood of relapse, and either return to treatment, or be prepared to deal with dietary lapses to avoid them becoming relapses. This latter approach calls on the model developed in the management of alcoholism, where the 'abstinence violation effect' has been identified as a factor in relapse (Marlatt, 1990). The therapeutic strategy is principally cognitive—challenging the thought processes which otherwise lead from 'I've failed' through 'I'm a failure' to 'I might as well give up trying'. Unfortunately there is no clear evidence that either relapse training, or booster sessions make a substantial difference in the long term. However, there is a new emphasis in obesity treatments on the need for permanent lifestyle changes. This is not yet reflected in most commercial programmes—which still promise rapid weight loss and fail even to mention the longer term. Patients themselves also prefer the short-term perspective and find it hard to face up to the inevitable conclusions which must be drawn from looking back over their personal histories of weight loss and regain.

A shift of perspective is required to acknowledge that the tendency to gain weight will not just go away. In this context the idea of a genetic predisposition to weight gain may be helpful to the individual. Acceptance of the chronicity of the condition may assist patients in taking a lifelong perspective on diet and activity. Patients need to develop a lifestyle in which activity is made as easy as possible, and a low-fat, prudent diet becomes their normal eating pattern. This might require some longer-term adjustments to identify alternative sources of pleasure and social activity, if eating had hitherto played a significant role. At this point the individual needs to weigh up the advantages and disadvantages of such significant long-term changes, and they should feel free to reach their own decision, albeit informed by an understanding of the medical perspective.

The treatment context

The techniques of CBT have been described largely within the context of an individually-based treatment model, with treatment provided by a psychologist within a health-care setting. However, all of these factors could vary, and some variation might produce a better outcome, or at least prove to be more cost-effective. Systematic comparison of individual vs group treatment has not produced any clear answer in terms of weight loss. But, many behavioural programmes are routinely offered on a group basis, and many cognitive–behavioural therapists perceive the group environment as favourable. Comparison of group-based vs individual treatments has received little attention for measures other than weight loss (Hakala et al., 1993), but clinical experience suggests that the sense of solidarity which stems from a successful group can boost self-esteem, improve social support and enhance exercise compliance. Given the longer-term perspective which is required, a group may also provide for continuation on a self-help basis, or a mixture of self-help and intermittent therapist contact, thereby cutting down on treatment costs.

The professional expertise required is another area of uncertainty. Many commercial weight-loss programmes are run by leaders with little experience other than having been through the treatment themselves. If the key element in change is the group process, combined with a modicum of dietary advice and general support, then specific psychological expertise is a luxury. If the specific skills of psychologists contribute significantly to outcome, then a psychologist-led programme will provide the most effective model.

To develop better treatments for the future, advances in the understanding of the psychology and biology of obesity, and advances in behaviour change techniques, need to be translated into new treatments. This requires a specialist resource to develop and evaluate new treatments. It is possible that a limited number of specialist centres can do the development work, while trained, non-specialists can deliver treatments on a wide scale. The sheer scale of the obesity problem is a potent argument against an exclusively specialist service. There could never be enough psychologists or dietitians to treat the entire obese population, so if CBT programmes are to be accessible to many overweight people, they must be deliverable by non-specialists, or even by lay group leaders, preferably within the context of a properly quality-controlled and supervised training programme. Research into the specific competencies required by non-specialist providers of CBT for obesity is therefore essential.

The other consideration is that obesity treatment should *not* be given by psychologists without adjunctive dietary advice, since psychologists do not, without special training, have adequate knowledge of nutrition. It is not sufficient to rely on patients' *apparent* dietetic knowledge, since the psychologist is in no position to evaluate its accuracy. Psychological and dietetic expertise in combination may offer the most effective alliance for obesity treatment, and there is a strong tradition of programmes which start with a very restrictive dietetic regimen (e.g., very-low-calorie diets), followed by a 'maintenance' dietetic regimen, both in parallel with CBT.

The newer perspective

There have been some radical changes in thinking about obesity over the past few decades. The assumption of an underlying psychopathology has not stood the test of time. The 'cure', which was always thought to be just over the horizon, has not materialized, and health professionals no longer expect to find a simple solution. We now realize that the goal for obesity treatment must be long-term behaviour change, designed to reduce the health risks and psychosocial costs associated with obesity. More realistic treatment expectations, which recognize that a modest weight loss is the most likely outcome, could help patients and health professionals find more acceptable treatments.

New drug treatments for obesity are being developed at a spectacular pace (see Chapter 19). Some promise a hope of weight loss for people who have failed with dietary or behavioural treatments, others focus on producing modest, long-term changes. However, it is unlikely that any drug will be found which can entirely cure obesity, and unlikely that any drug could be prescribed on the scale that would be required if all overweight people were to be treated. The best outcome is likely to be achieved if drug treatment and behavioural treatments can be delivered synergistically, and this will require medical and behavioural scientists to work closely together to develop treatment strategies that allow the different elements of treatment to complement and enhance each other, rather than to compete.

The steady rise in obesity prevalence over the past few decades in almost all of the developed world has emphasized the influence of environmental factors and highlighted the need to seek preventive approaches. At the same time, the role of inherited genetic factors in obesity has become well established, with a growing knowledge of the way genes influence the process of fat storage. Contemporary views hold that genes contribute strongly to individual variation in weight (Sorensen, 1995), while environmental factors, which vary over time and place, determine the level of phenotypic expression of genetic susceptibility. We also understand that a genetic aetiology is no bar to control of weight through modulation of energy balance, but control may be more difficult for those who have such susceptibility, and that their efforts at control have to be lifelong. The implication of current trends in weight, which have led to more than half the U.K. population being defined as fatter than is optimal for health, have emphasized the need for community efforts at prevention at the level of the public health as well as the individual.

Research developments have also highlighted the ignorance and cruelty of social attitudes to obesity, and the need to promote, among obese people themselves, the general public and health professionals, a better understanding of obesity. We should aim to reduce prejudice and discrimination against obese people, as against any other group who are disadvantaged relative to their fellow human beings.

Apart from prejudice and discrimination, obese people are also susceptible to exploitation of their desperation to lose weight. An enormous commercial weight-loss sector exists in most developed countries, which has developed with little or no regulation or evaluation. Obese people have a right to appropriate information and guidance to help them to avoid harmful and uneffective treatments (Institute of Medicine, 1995).

References

Allon, N. (1982) The stigma of overweight in everyday life. In: Wolman, B.B. (ed.) *Psychological Aspects of Obesity*, pp. 130–174. New York: Van Nostrand Reinhold Co.

Bennett, N. (1995) *Health Survey for England 1993*. London: HMSO.

Björntorp, P. (1996) The regulation of adipose tissue distribution in humans. *International Journal of Obesity* **20**, 291–302.

Brownell, K.D. & Kramer, F.M. (1989) Behavioral management of obesity. *Medical Clinics of North America* **73**, 185–201.

Brownell, K.D. & Wadden, D.A. (1992) Etiology and treatment of obesity. *Journal of Consulting and Clinical Psychology* **60**, 505–517.

Butters, J.W. & Cash, T.F. (1987) Cognitive-behavioral treatment of women's body-image dissatisfaction. *Journal of Consulting and Clinical Psychology* **55**, 889–897.

Cooper, P., Taylor, M., Cooper, Z. & Fairburn, C. (1987) Development of the Body Shape Questionnaire. *International Journal of Eating Disorders* **6**, 485–490.

Epstein, L.H., Valoski, A.M., Vara, L.S. *et al.* (1995) Effects of decreasing sedentary behaviour and increasing activity on weight change in obese children. *Health Psychology* **14**, 109–115.

Fairburn, C.G. & Cooper, Z. (1993) The eating disorder examination. In: Fairburn, C.G. & Wilson, G.T. (eds) *Binge Eating: Nature, Assessment and Treatment*. New York: The Guilford Press.

Fairburn, C.G. & Wilson, G.T. (1993) Binge eating: definition and classification. In: Fairburn, C.G. & Wilson, G.T. (eds) *Binge Eating: Nature, Assessment and Treatment* pp. 3–14. New York: The Guilford Press.

Ferster, C.B., Nurnberger, J.I. & Levitt, E.B. (1962) The control of eating. *Journal of Mathetics* **1**, 87–109.

Foreyt, J. & Goodrick, K. (1995) The ultimate triumph of obesity. *Lancet* **346**, 134–135.

Foreyt, J.P., Mitchell, R.E., Garner, D.T., Gee, M., Scott, L.W. & Gotto, A.M. (1982) Behavioural treatment of obesity: results and limitations. *Behavior Therapy* **13**, 153–161.

Friedman, R., Shackelford, A., Reiff, S. & Benson, H. (1994) Stress and weight maintenance: the disinhibition effect and the micromanagement of stress. In: Blackburn, G.L. & Kanders, B.S. (eds) *Obesity—Pathophysiology, Psychology and Treatment*, pp. 253–263. New York: Chapman & Hall.

Glynn, S.M. & Ruderman, A.J. (1986) The development and validation of an Eating Self-Efficacy Scale. *Cognitive Therapy and Research* **10**, 403–420.

Goldstein, D.J. (1992) Beneficial health effects of modest weight loss. *International Journal of Obesity* **16**, 397–415.

Greeno, C.G. & Wing, R.R. (1994) Stress induced eating. *Psychological Bulletin* **115**, 444–464.

Grilo, C.M., Wilfley, D.E., Brownell, K.D. & Rodin, J. (1994) Teasing, body image, and self-esteem in a clinical sample of obese women. *Addictive Behaviors* **19**, 443–450.

Hakala, P., Karvetti, R.-L. & Rönnemaa, T. (1993) Group vs individual weigh reduction programmes in the treatment of severe obesity—a five year follow-up study. *International Journal of Obesity* **17**, 97–102.

Hodge, A.M., Dowse, G.K., Gareeboo, H., Tuomilehto, J., Alberti, K.G.M.M. & Zimmet, P.Z. (1996) Incidence, increasing prevalence, and predictors of change in obesity and fat distribution over 5 years in the rapidly developing population of Mauritius. *International Journal of Obesity* **20**, 137–146.

Institute of Medicine. (1995).

Kaplan, H.I. & Kaplan, H.S. (1957) The psychosomatic concept of obesity. *Journal of Nervous Mental Diseases* **125**, 181–201.

Law, M.R., Wald, N.J. & Thompson, S.G. (1994) By how much and how quickly does reduction in serum cholesterol concentration lower risk of ischaemic heart disease? *British Medical Journal* **308**, 367–373.

Mahoney, M.J. & Arnkoff, D. (1978) Cognitive and self-control therapies. In: Garfield, S.L. & Bergin, A.E. (eds) *Handbook of Psychotherapy and Behavior Change*, pp. 689–723. New York: Wiley.

Mahoney, M.J. & Mahoney, K. (1976) Cognitive ecology: cleaning up what you say to yourself. In: *Permanent Weight Control*, pp. 46–68. New York: W.W. Norton & Co Ltd.

Marcus, M.D. (1993) Binge eating in obesity. In: Fairburn, C.G. & Wilson, G.T. (eds) *Binge Eating: Nature, Assessment and Treatment* pp. 77–96. New York: The Guilford Press.

Marcus, M.D. & Wing, R.R. (1987) Binge eating among the obese. *Annals of Behavioral Medicine* **9**, 23–27.

Marlatt, G.A. (1990) Cue exposure and relapse prevention in the treatment of addictive behaviours. *Addictive Behaviour* **15**, 395–399.

Meichenbaum, D. (1977) *Cognitive-Behavior Modification*. New York: Plenum Press.

Miller, W.R. (1996) Motivational interviewing: Research, practice and puzzles. *Addictive Behaviors* **21**, 835–842.

Nisbett, R.E. (1968) Taste, deprivation, and weight determinants of eating behavior. *Journal of Personality and Social Psychology* **10**, 107–116.

Perri, M.G. (1992) Improving maintenance of weight loss following treatment by diet and lifestyle modification. In: Wadden, T.A. & Van Itallie, T.B. (eds) *Treatment of the Seriously Obese Patient*, pp. 456–477. London: The Guilford Press.

Porzelius, L.K., Houston, C., Smith, M., Arfken, C. & Fisher, E. Jr. (1995) Comparison of a standard behavioral weight loss treatment and a binge eating weight loss treatment. *Behavior Therapy* **26**, 119–134.

Prentice, A.M., Black, A.E., Murgatroyd, P.R., Goldberg, G.R. & Coward, W.A. (1989) Metabolism or appetite: questions of energy balance with particular reference to obesity. *Journal of Human Nutrition and Dietetics* **2**, 95–104.

Prentice, A.M. & Jebb, S.A. (1995) Obesity in Britain: gluttony or sloth. *British Journal of Medicine* **311**, 437–439.

Prochaska, J.O., DiClemente, C.C. & Norcross, J.C. (1992) In search of how people change. *American Psychologist* **47**, 1102–1114.

Prochaska, J.O., Velicer, W.F., Rossi, J.S. *et al.* (1994) Stages of change and decisional balance for 12 problem behaviors. *Health Psychology* **13**, 39–46.

Rebuffe-Scrive, M., Walsh, U.A., McEwen, B. & Rodin, J. (1992) Effect of chronic stress and exogenous glucocorticoids on regional fat distribution and metabolism. *Physiological Behavior* **52**, 583–590.

Robbins, T.W. & Fray, P.J. (1980) Stress-induced eating: fact, fiction or misunderstanding. *Appetite* **1**, 103–133.

Rodin, J. (1980) The externality theory today. In: Stunkard, A.J. (ed.) *Obesity*, pp. 226–239. Philadelphia: W.B. Saunders.

Rodin, J., Schank, D. & Striegel-Moore, R. (1989) Psychological features of obesity. *Medical Clinics of North America* **73**, 47–66.

Rosen, J.C., (1996) Improving body image in obesity. In: Thompson, J.K. (ed.) *Body Image, Eating Disorders and Obesity*, pp. 425–440. Washington, D.C.: American Psychological Association.

Rosen, J.C., Srebnik, D., Saltzberg, E. & Wendt, S. (1991) Development of a Body Image Avoidance Questionnaire. *Psychological Assessment* **3**, 1–6.

Sallis, J.F., Grossman, C.M., Pinski, R.B., Patterson, T.L. & Nadev, P.R. (1987) The development of scales to measure social support for diet and exercise behaviours. *Preventive Medicine* **16**, 825–836.

Seidell, J.C. (1995) Obesity in Europe: scaling an epidemic. *International Journal of Obesity* **19**, S1–S4.

Skinner, B.F. (1953) *Science and Human Behavior*. New York: Macmillan.

Sobal, J. (1991) Obesity and nutritional sociology: a model for coping with the stigma of obesity. *Clinical Sociology Review* **9**, 125–141.

Sorensen, T.I. (1995) The genetics of obesity. *Metabolism* **44** (suppl. 3), 4–6.

Spitzer, R.L., Yanovski, S., Wadden, T. *et al.* (1993) Binge eating disorder: its further validation in a multisite study. *International Journal of Eating Disorders* **13**, 137–153.

Stuart, R.B. (1967) Behavioural control over eating. *Behaviour Research and Therapy* **5**, 357–365.

Stunkard, A.J. (1959) Eating patterns and obesity. *Psychiatric Quarterly* **33**, 284–294.

Stunkard, A.J. & Messick, S. (1985) The Three-Factor Eating Questionnaire to measure dietary restraint, disinhibition and hunger. *Journal of Psychosomatic Research* **29**, 71–83.

Sullivan, M., Karlsson, J., Sjöstrom, L. *et al.* (1993) Swedish Obese Subjects (SOS) — an intervention study of obesity. Baseline evaluation of health and psychosocial functioning in the first 1743 subjects examined. *International Journal of Obesity* **17**, 503–512.

Thomas, P.R. (ed.) *Weighing the options: Criteria for Evaluating Weight Management Programs.* Washington, D.C.: National Academy Press.

Van Itallie, T.B. & Lew, E.A. (1992) Assessment of morbidity and mortality risk in the overweight patient. In: Wadden, T.A. & Van Itallie, T.B. (eds) *Treatment of the Seriously Obese Patient*, pp. 3–32. New York: The Guilford Press.

Van Strien, T., Frijters, J.E.R., Bergers, G.P.A. & Defares, P.B. (1986a) Dutch Eating Behaviour Questionnaire for assessment of restrained, emotional and external eating behaviour. *International Journal of Eating Disorders* **5**, 295–315.

Van Strien, T., Rookus, M.A., Bergers, G.P., Frijters, J.E. & Defares, P.B. (1986b) Life events, emotional eating and change in body mass index. *International Journal of Obesity* **10**, 29–35.

Wilson, G.T. & Fairburn, C.G. (1993) Cognitive treatments for eating disorders. *Journal of Consulting and Clinical Psychology* **61**, 261–269.

CHAPTER 18

Exercise and Obesity

MARLEEN A. VAN BAAK AND WIM H.M. SARIS

Introduction

Traditionally, exercise has been recommended as an important strategy for prevention of obesity and as an effective adjunct to its treatment. It has become evident that not only the increase in energy expenditure during exercise is important in this respect. Much information has accumulated regarding additional beneficial effects of exercise in obesity. This chapter will focus on the effects of acute and regular exercise (training) in obesity and will address recommendations for exercise programmes in obese patients.

Physical activity and prevention of obesity

Many cross-sectional studies (e.g., Tremblay *et al.*, 1990b; Rissanen *et al.*, 1991; Williamson *et al.*, 1993) show a negative correlation between level of physical activity and body mass. However, it may be argued that a low level of physical activity is a consequence rather than a cause of obesity. The question of cause or consequence is best answered by prospective studies. Several large observational studies in Europe and the U.S.A. have investigated the relationship between level of physical activity and body-weight changes prospectively. A study by Rissanen *et al.* (1991) in over 12 000 adult Finns with a median follow-up of 5.7 years showed that the risk of substantial weight gain (≥ 5 kg/5 years) was increased in persons with low levels of leisure physical activity at baseline. Their risk of substantial weight gain was almost twice that in physically active subjects. The National Health and Nutrition Examination Survey (NHANES-1) in the U.S.A. (in over 9000 adults with a follow-up of around 10 years) found no association between recreational physical activity at baseline and subsequent weight gain (Williamson *et al.*, 1993). However, low physical activity at follow-up was strongly related to major weight gain (> 13 kg) over the preceding 10 years. In addition the relative risk for major weight gain was increased in persons with low physical activity both at baseline and at follow-up. The authors suggest that low physical activity may be both a cause

Table 18.1 Odds ratios (OR) and 95% confidence intervals (95%CI) of body-mass gain ≥5 kg and BMI ≥26 at the end of 10-year follow-up according to self-assessed leisure time physical activity (LTPA) in Finnish men and women. Adapted from Haapanen *et al.* (1997).

Change in LTPA during follow-up	Men OR (95%CI)	Women OR (95%CI)
Physically active all the time	1.00	1.00
Become physically active	1.15 (0.76–1.73)	1.07 (0.72–1.59)
Become physically inactive	1.96 (1.39–2.75)	2.49 (1.72–3.60)
Physically inactive all the time	1.62 (1.18–2.20)	1.61 (1.17–2.21)

and a consequence of weight gain. Blair (1993) evaluated possible determinants of weight gain in over 10 000 American men at high risk for coronary heart disease who were participants in the Multiple Risk Factor Intervention Trial (MRFIT). Weight gain was defined as an increase in body-weight of >5% of baseline weight over the course of the study, 6 or 7 years. Baseline physical activity and an increase in activity level during the trial were inversely related to weight gain. Similar results were obtained in another Finnish study (Haapanen *et al.*, 1997). In a group of over 5000 working-aged men and women the risk of clinically significant body mass gain (>5 kg during the 10-year follow-up) was higher in men and women who decreased their physical activity during the 10-year follow-up or were inactive all the time than in subjects who were active all the time (Table 18.1).

Although it should be kept in mind that reliable measurements of physical activity levels in this type of studies are difficult to obtain, these large epidemiological studies support the notion that a high level of physical activity protects against increases in weight and obesity. A high level of physical activity can be attained by regular exercise, which can be defined as planned, structured, repetitive and purposeful physical activity (McArdle *et al.*, 1996).

Exercise and weight reduction

Numerous experimental studies have shown that, in the short term, adults lose weight when they increase their physical activity by exercise. Wilmore (1995) reviewed a total of 53 studies in the literature on weight changes with exercise training without changes in diet. Although the variation between individual studies was large, on average a 6-month period of training would result in a loss of 1.6 kg of body mass, a loss of 2.6 kg of fat mass and a gain of 1.0 kg of fat-free mass (FFM). Garrow and Summerbell (1995) did a meta-analysis of the effect of exercise on weight changes in overweight subjects. The average body mass index (BMI) of subjects in the eight studies that were included in the analysis varied between 25 and 30 kg/m² indicating that the results concern

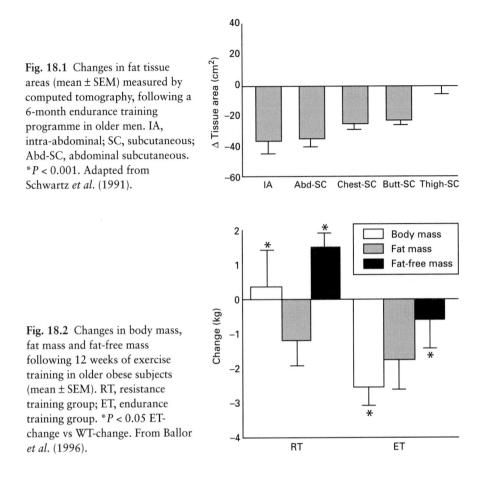

Fig. 18.1 Changes in fat tissue areas (mean ± SEM) measured by computed tomography, following a 6-month endurance training programme in older men. IA, intra-abdominal; SC, subcutaneous; Abd-SC, abdominal subcutaneous. *$P < 0.001$. Adapted from Schwartz *et al.* (1991).

Fig. 18.2 Changes in body mass, fat mass and fat-free mass following 12 weeks of exercise training in older obese subjects (mean ± SEM). RT, resistance training group; ET, endurance training group. *$P < 0.05$ ET-change vs WT-change. From Ballor *et al.* (1996).

mildly obese persons. Endurance exercise training without dietary restriction caused an average weight loss of 3 kg over 30 weeks in men and of 1.4 kg over 12 weeks in women, with little effect on FFM. Resistance exercise training (one study in men, one in women) had little effect on weight, but increased FFM about 2 kg in men and 1 kg in women. A meta-analysis of 11 studies by Ballor and Keesey (1991), in which less stringent inclusion criteria were used, confirms that resistance training preserves or increases FFM.

Although there are some indications that weight loss due to exercise training is less in lean women than in lean men (Andersson *et al.*, 1991; Ballor & Keesey, 1991; Meijer *et al.*, 1991b), the meta-analysis by Garrow and Summerbell (1995) does not confirm this difference in overweight men and women.

There is evidence that, with exercise training, fat is preferentially lost from the central regions of the body in men and women with large abdominal fat depots (Després *et al.*, 1985; Schwartz *et al.*, 1991; Kohrt *et al.*, 1992) (Fig. 18.1). Schwartz *et al.* (1991) concluded that the reduction of abdominal fat was directly related to the initial size of the depot.

These experimental results indicate that exercise training induces moderate subsequent weight and fat loss, which may be slightly more pronounced in overweight than in lean subjects. Resistance exercise training may preserve or increase FFM (Fig. 18.2).

Combined effects of exercise and dietary restriction on body-weight

The combined effects of dietary restriction and exercise training on body-weight have been reviewed extensively (Donnelly *et al.*, 1991; Saris, 1993; Saris, 1995; Garrow & Summerbell, 1995). Donnelly *et al.* (1991) showed that the average weight loss over seven studies with a duration varying between 21 and 112 (mean 62) days was approximately 1 kg higher when exercise training was added to a very-low-calorie diet (500–800 kcal/day) than with the diet alone (9.7 vs 8.6 kg). Garrow and Summerbell (1995) found a 1.5-kg difference in weight loss between low-calorie diets (< 1000 kcal/day; duration 8–16 weeks) and the same diet plus exercise (12.7 vs 11.2 kg; mean of 11 studies). In less severe energy restriction diets (> 1000 kcal/day; duration 5–26 weeks) the difference was 0.8 kg (7.6 vs 6.8 kg; mean of 10 studies). From these studies it is clear that adding exercise training to an energy-restricted diet results in a moderate extra weight loss that is small compared to the weight loss attained by the dietary treatment alone.

Most reviews also addressed the question whether adding exercise to an energy-restricted diet reduces or prevents the reduction of FFM accompanying such diets. Although the results are not fully conclusive, the majority of studies indeed suggests that this is the case (Donnelly *et al.*, 1991, Prentice *et al.*, 1991; Saris, 1993; Ballor & Poehlman, 1994; Saris, 1995; Garrow & Summerbell, 1995). The meta-analysis by Garrow and Summerbell (1995) indicates that for every 10-kg weight loss by diet alone, the expected loss of FFM is 2.9 kg in men and 2.2 kg in women. When the same weight loss is achieved by exercise combined with dietary restriction, the expected loss of FFM is reduced to 1.7 kg in men and women. Resistance exercise may result in a more effective preservation of FFM during a period of energy restriction than endurance training (Ballor *et al.*, 1996).

Exercise and weight maintenance

Although exercise training results in only modest (extra) reductions of body-weight when prescribed alone or in combination with dietary restriction, there is increasing evidence that regular exercise is of crucial importance for successful weight maintenance after a period of weight loss.

Subjects who perform regular exercise after a period of weight loss maintain their weight loss better than inactive subjects (Fig. 18.3) (Kayman *et al.*, 1990;

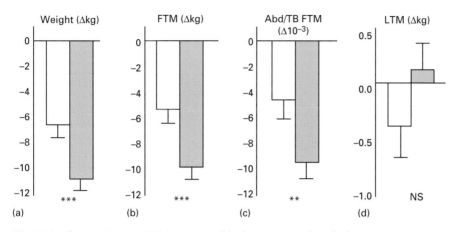

Fig. 18.3 Changes (mean ± SEM) in (a) total body mass (Weight), (b) fat mass (FTM), (c) abdominal-to-total body fat mass (Abd/TB FTM) and (d) lean body mass (LTM) from baseline to follow-up (9 months) in a group of overweight postmenopausal women enrolled in a 3-month diet-plus-exercise intervention, that either continued to exercise after the intervention (filled bars) or discontinued to exercise (open bars) after the intervention. **P < 0.01, ***P < 0.001, NS not significant. From Svendsen *et al.* (1994).

Van Dale *et al.*, 1990; Holden *et al.*, 1992; Svendsen *et al.*, 1994; DePue *et al.*, 1995; Hensrud *et al.*, 1995). A 4-year follow-up study by Hensrud *et al.* (1995) showed that in a group of 24 obese women who had lost at least 10 kg (mean 13 kg) under tightly controlled conditions, those women who reported self-selected regular exercise at follow-up had gained less weight than non-exercisers (6 vs 13 kg). The results of these studies may, however, be biased by the fact that exercise was self-selected. Two other studies, in which subjects were initially randomized into a diet-only group and a diet-plus-exercise group, however, show similar results. Pavlou *et al.* (1989) studied the long-term effects of several weight-reduction programmes with or without exercise in members of the Boston Police Department and the Metropolitan District Commission. He reported that the mean weight of the diet-only group had almost returned to pretreatment levels by 18–36 months, whilst weight loss was largely maintained in the diet-plus-exercise group. In the diet-plus-exercise group 72% of the men were still exercising at follow-up, in the diet-only group 84% had remained inactive. When only those who continued to exercise in the original diet-plus-exercise group were included, maintenance of weight loss was nearly 100%. When only the subjects who remained inactive in the original diet-only group were included weight regain was almost 100%. Kempen (1996) randomly assigned 24 obese women to a diet-only and a diet-plus-exercise group. After the diet period of 8 weeks, the women in the diet-plus-exercise group continued to exercise two times per week for 90 minutes for 1 year. Adherence to the exercise sessions was 85% (range 77–98%). Women in the diet-plus-exercise group lost more

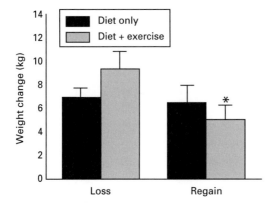

Fig. 18.4 Weight loss during an 8-week very-low-calorie diet and weight regain over 1 year (mean ± SEM) in obese women randomly divided over two groups: D, diet only; DE, diet plus exercise (during the dietary intervention and the 1-year follow-up). *$P < 0.05$ vs loss. Adapted from Kempen (1996).

weight during the diet period and regained less weight after 1 year than women in the non-exercise group (Fig. 18.4). Thus, these randomized studies support the evidence obtained in studies where exercise was self-selected, that exercise contributes significantly to the long-term success of weight-loss programmes.

These data clearly show that exercise is effective in preventing weight gain and is also an important adjunct during dietary treatment of obesity, not only because of increased weight loss, but also because of a more favourable ratio between the loss of fat and FFM. However, the most promising action of exercise may lie in its contribution to weight maintenance after weight loss. Which characteristics of exercise explain its effects on body-weight regulation? Looking at the energy balance equation, exercise may hypothetically interfere with the energy expenditure as well as the energy intake side of the equation.

Exercise and energy expenditure

Total daily energy expenditure (24-hour EE) can be divided into several components: resting metabolic rate (RMR), which accounts for approximately 60–70% of 24-hour EE; the energy cost of feeding (TEF, thermic effect of feeding), approximately 10% of 24-hour EE; and the thermic effect of physical activity or exercise (TEE), which is the most variable component and may vary from 15% of 24-hour EE in sedentary people, 30–40% in active people, to even 400% in professional cyclists under extreme circumstances (Saris *et al.*, 1989). Acute exercise may affect all three components of 24-hour EE. Apart from the acute effects, regular exercise or training may have additional effects.

Energy expenditure during exercise in lean and obese individuals

Energy expenditure increases during exercise. Figure 18.5 shows total energy expenditure during recreational activities such as walking, running and cycling in normal-weight subjects, per minute or per distance covered. Since energy

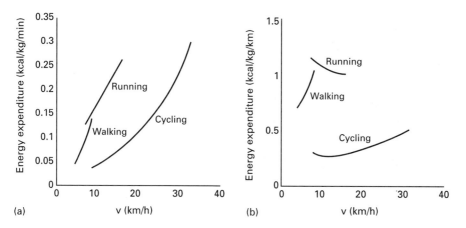

Fig. 18.5 Energy expenditure during walking, cycling and running at different speeds (v) (in kcal/kg/min (a) and kcal/kg/km (b)) in healthy, untrained adults. From Van Baak (1979).

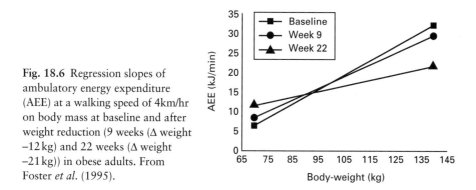

Fig. 18.6 Regression slopes of ambulatory energy expenditure (AEE) at a walking speed of 4km/hr on body mass at baseline and after weight reduction (9 weeks (Δ weight −12 kg) and 22 weeks (Δ weight −21 kg)) in obese adults. From Foster et al. (1995).

expenditure is expressed per kilogram body mass, energy expenditure at a certain speed or distance increases with body mass. Obese subjects were not included in these studies. A study by Skinner et al. (1973) showed no differences in mass-specific aerobic demand for lean, obese and weighted-lean individuals. On the other hand, Weigle et al. (1988) and Foster et al. (1995) both showed that weight loss caused a larger reduction in the non-resting energy cost of walking than predicted from the reduction of body-weight (Fig. 18.6). This rather indicates an inefficient locomotor pattern in obesity. Foster et al. (1995) suggested that in the obese more mechanical work has to be done during walking to overcome friction between thighs and between the arms and torso, and the arms and legs have to swing more widely to move around thighs and torso. Similarly, the net efficiency during cycle ergometry is negatively correlated with body mass (Berry et al., 1993).

Table 18.2 gives a selection of total energy expenditure (resting energy expenditure plus the additional energy cost of exercise) during a number of other

Table 18.2 Energy cost of various physical activities expressed as METs (ratio of work metabolic rate to resting metabolic rate). Adapted from Ainsworth *et al.* (1993).

Activity	METs
Aerobics	6.0
Bicycling, 12–13.9 mph, leisure, moderate effort	8.0
Bicycling, 100 W stationary bicycle ergometer	5.5
Rowing ergometer, 100 W	7.0
Running, jogging	7.0
Running, 6 mph	10.0
Soccer, casual	7.0
Stair-treadmill ergometer	6.0
Tennis, singles	8.0
Tennis, doubles	6.0
Walking, 3 mph, level, firm surface	3.5
Walking, brisk, 3.5 mph, level, firm surface	4.0

recreational physical activities. A more detailed list of activities can be found in McArdle *et al.* (1996) or Ainsworth *et al.* (1993). It should be realized that these are average values applicable under average conditions, and to the average person. To obtain the extra energy expended during the activity, resting energy expenditure (1 MET, approximately 1 kcal/kg/hr) has to be subtracted from the values in the table. The net energy cost of exercise (total – resting energy expenditure) varies roughly between 2 (leisure walking) and 20 kcal/kg/hr (cross-country skiing).

Training and energy expenditure during exercise

Regular exercise or training may lead to more efficient movement patterns, independent of weight loss: the energy cost of running at a certain speed is approximately 15% lower in trained than in untrained runners (Costill, 1986); in swimming, differences between elite and untrained swimmers may be even larger, up to 50% (Holmér, 1974); the energy cost of cycling is approximately 25% lower in trained cyclists riding racing bicycles compared to untrained subjects riding a touring bicycle (Van Baak, 1979).

Postexercise energy expenditure

Energy expenditure may remain elevated for some time during recovery from acute exercise. A number of different processes appear to be responsible for the excess postexercise oxygen consumption (EPOC) (Table 18.3). The total magnitude of EPOC depends on intensity and duration (Fig. 18.7) of the exercise performed. The highest value has been reported by Bahr *et al.* (1987):

Table 18.3 Causes of excess postexercise oxygen consumption (EPOC).

- Resynthesis of ATP and CP
- Resynthesis of glycogen from lactate
- Oxidation of lactate
- Replenishment of oxygen stores (haemoglobin and myoglobin)
- Thermogenic effects of elevated body temperature
- Thermogenic effects of noradrenalin and adrenalin
- Elevated heart rate, respiration and other physiological functions
- Increased triglyceride fatty acid cycling

ATP, adenosine triphosphate, CP, creatine phosphokinase

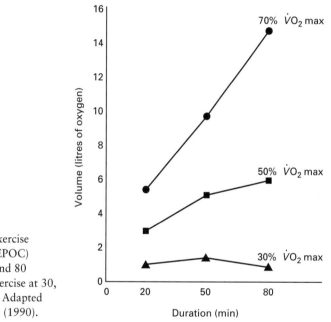

Fig. 18.7 Excess postexercise oxygen consumption (EPOC) resulting from 20, 50 and 80 minutes of treadmill exercise at 30, 50 and 70% $\dot{V}O_2$ max. Adapted from Gore and Withers (1990).

EPOC amounted to 32 (or approximately 150 kcal) over 720 minutes after 80 minutes of cycling exercise at 70% $\dot{V}O_2$ max, which would make a considerable contribution to 24-hour EE (Saris & Van Baak, 1994). Poehlman *et al.* (1991), however, indicated that an exercise prescription of low to moderate exercise, aimed at the general public, would result in an EPOC of maximally 30 kcal per exercise bout.

From the available literature on EPOC, it can be concluded that in lean subjects energy expenditure remains increased for a longer period of time than the duration of the exercise bout itself, but that the total magnitude of EPOC is small in comparison with the energy expended during exercise. EPOC has not been studied in obese individuals.

Training and resting metabolic rate

Several studies have addressed the question whether regular exercise affects RMR, independent of the acute effects of exercise described above. The results of cross-sectional studies, comparing untrained and trained individuals, are inconclusive. Some authors found no significant correlation between $\dot{V}O_2$ max, as an index of training status, and RMR (Davis *et al.*, 1983; Ravussin & Bogardus, 1989; Schulz *et al.*, 1991), others did (Poehlman *et al.*, 1989). Tremblay *et al.* (1986) reported a higher RMR in trained than in untrained men. In a later study these investigators showed that β-adrenergic stimulation was involved in the increased RMR in a highly trained group of men (Tremblay *et al.*, 1992). Longitudinal training studies in lean as well as obese men and women, on the other hand, in majority showed no effect on RMR measured between 12 and 96 hours after the last training session (Davis *et al.*, 1983; Poehlman *et al.*, 1986; Tremblay *et al.*, 1986; Bingham *et al.*, 1989; Frey-Hewitt *et al.*, 1990; Meijer *et al.*, 1991b; Buemann *et al.*, 1992; Segal *et al.*, 1992).

Another issue is whether exercise training reduces or even prevents the fall in RMR that is associated with energy-restricted diets. Although the majority of studies suggests a positive effect (Prentice *et al.*, 1991; Saris & Van Baak, 1994), the evidence is not very strong. Those studies which do find less reduction of RMR usually conclude that the mechanism is partly a reduced loss of FFM and partly an elevation of metabolic activity per unit of FFM (Prentice *et al.*, 1991).

In conclusion, although cross-sectional studies indicate that RMR may be increased in highly trained subjects compared to untrained subjects, exercise training programmes generally do not lead to an increase in RMR in lean or obese individuals. The addition of a training programme during a period of dietary restriction in obese individuals, on the other hand, may reduce the decrease in RMR accompanying a negative energy balance.

Thermic effect of feeding

Considerable inconsistency exists regarding the acute effects of exercise on the thermic effect of a meal ingested after an exercise bout (Saris & Van Baak, 1994; Segal, 1995). Several studies suggest that exercise may increase TEF in lean (Zahorska-Markiewicz, 1980; Young *et al.*, 1986) or obese subjects (Segal *et al.*, 1987, 1992); other studies failed to find an effect of exercise in lean (Segal *et al.*, 1987, 1992; Bahr & Sejersted, 1991) or obese (Zahorska-Markiewicz, 1980) individuals. Apart from the difficulty of measuring TEF, inconsistencies may be related to meal size and composition, the timing of the

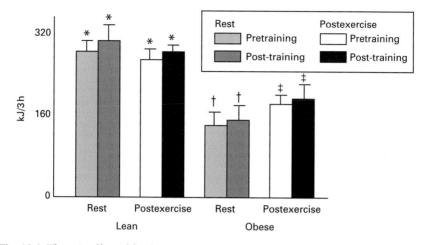

Fig. 18.8 Thermic effect of food (means ± SEM) at rest and after 1-hour exercise, before and after training, in lean and obese subjects. *$P < 0.01$ lean vs obese; †$P < 0.05$ rest vs postexercise; ‡$P < 0.05$ pretraining vs post-training. Adapted from Segal (1995).

meal and exercise, the intensity and duration of the exercise, and differences in the characteristics of the subjects (Segal, 1995).

Cross-sectional studies which compared TEF in trained and untrained subjects have yielded conflicting results (Saris & Van Baak, 1994). Some studies found a positive relationship between $\dot{V}O_2$ max and TEF (Davis *et al.*, 1983; Hill *et al.*, 1984; Poehlman *et al.*, 1989), others could not detect a difference between trained and untrained men (Thörne & Wahren, 1989; Schulz *et al.*, 1991).

Longitudinal training studies showed no effect of training on TEF in lean men and women (Davis *et al.*, 1983; Poehlman *et al.*, 1986) or moderately overweight men (Tremblay *et al.*, 1990a). Well-controlled studies by Segal and colleagues (Segal, 1995), in which the effect of exercise training was studied independent of changes in body mass and body fat in lean and obese subjects matched for FFM, suggest that TEF is not affected by training in lean subjects, neither at rest nor after an acute bout of exercise. In obese subjects, in which TEF was found to be blunted, TEF was increased roughly 40% by acute exercise after training, although under resting conditions TEF was not affected by training (Fig. 18.8). However, the absolute increment of total energy expenditure due to this effect is small.

24-hour energy expenditure

As discussed in the preceding paragraphs exercise increases energy expenditure during the exercise bout itself and may elevate postexercise energy expenditure.

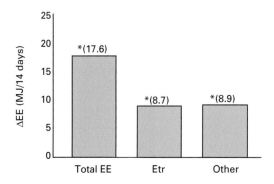

Fig. 18.9 Increase in (components of) energy expenditure (ΔEE) as a result of training in obese boys. Numbers in parentheses indicate SEM. *$P < 0.01$. Total EE, total energy expenditure over 14 days; Etr, energy expenditure during training hours (total of 10 training hours); Other, energy expenditure during non-training hours of the day (total of 14 days). From Blaak *et al.* (1992).

Effects on RMR and TEF, if any, are probably small. From this it cannot be concluded automatically that exercise also elevates 24-hour EE, since it is possible that non-exercise physical activity changes due to an exercise bout or training, either in a positive or in a negative direction.

Toth and Poehlman (1996) have reviewed the available literature on the effects of training on 24-hour EE. In all studies that measured 24-hour EE with the doubly labelled water technique (Bingham *et al.*, 1989; Meijer *et al.*, 1991a; Goran & Poehlman, 1992; Blaak *et al.*, 1992; Racette *et al.*, 1995) an increase in 24-hour EE after training was found, varying between 17 and 956 kcal/day. The increase was not always statistically significant. Only one study (Blaak *et al.*, 1992) included obese subjects (Fig. 18.9). Since in these studies the doubly labelled water technique was used to assess 24-hour EE under free-living conditions, this increased 24-hour EE is an average over a longer period (7–14 days), thus including days with and without exercise-training bouts. Preliminary evidence suggests that men may increase their non-exercise-training physical activity to a greater extent than women in response to exercise training. (Meijer *et al.*, 1991a; Blaak *et al.*, 1992).

Exercise and energy intake

In the preceding section the effects of acute and regular exercise on the energy expenditure side of the energy balance equation has been described. In this section interaction of exercise with energy intake will be discussed. This aspect has been less extensively studied, probably because of the difficulties associated with the accurate measurement of energy intake.

The classical study by Mayer *et al.* (1956) in 213 male employees of a jute mill in West Bengal, India, with a wide range of physical activity during work, showed that energy intake was tightly coupled to the energy demand of the job above the level described as 'light work' (Fig. 18.10). In sedentary employees

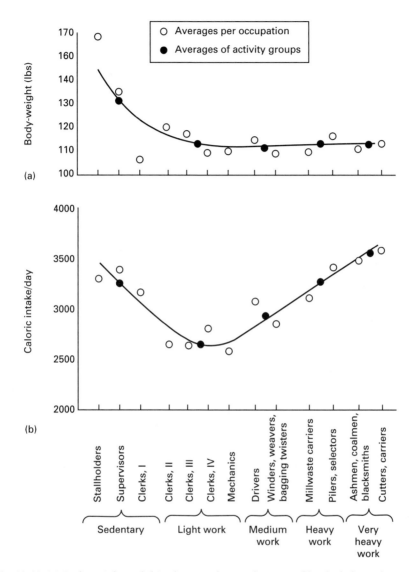

Fig. 18.10 (a) Body-weight and (b) caloric intake as a function of level of physical activity at work, in an industrial male population in West Bengal. From Mayer *et al.* (1956).

food intake was increased inappropriately, resulting in increased body mass. Although this study has major shortcomings in design and analysis, the general conclusion is supported by animal research (Oscai, 1973). Studies that have actually measured the effect of increasing physical activity on energy intake experimentally will be discussed in the next paragraphs.

Postexercise energy intake

Studies on the effects of exercise on energy intake during a postexercise meal are scarce. King *et al.* (1994, 1995) studied energy intake during a test meal provided 15 minutes after an exercise session (50 minutes at 70% $\dot{V}O_2$ max) in lean men and women. In men hunger ratings were reduced immediately after exercise. The duration of this exercise-induced anorexia had disappeared within 15 minutes and food intake during the test meal was unaffected by the previous exercise (King *et al.*, 1994). Thompson *et al.* (1988) reported similar results in lean males. In lean women the transient anorectic effect was absent; as in men, food intake was unaffected by a preceding exercise bout (King & Blundell, 1995). These data suggest that, although hunger may be transiently suppressed by intense exercise in males, energy intake between 15 and 60 minutes postexercise is not affected in lean males and females. Data on obese individuals are not available.

24-hour energy intake

Although the results presented above do not indicate a compensatory increase in food intake shortly after exercise, it is possible that compensation occurs later. Several studies have addressed this question in lean and obese men and women. Studies by Woo and colleagues (1982, 1985) showed that 19 days of mild or moderate treadmill walking, increasing total daily energy expenditure to 114% and 129% of sedentary energy expenditure, respectively, induced a significantly negative energy balance in obese women, but no significant change in lean women. Nevertheless, energy balance with moderate activity in lean women (–116 kcal/day) was similar to that with mild activity in obese women (–114 kcal/day) (Fig. 18.11). Durrant *et al.* (1982) reported similar results in obese and lean men and women. Staten (1991) found that 1 hour of exercise at 68% $\dot{V}O_2$ max during 5 days increased energy intake in lean men, but did not change energy intake in lean women. Men did not fully compensate for the energy expended during exercise and thus both men and women were in negative energy balance during the training period.

   Overall these studies seem to suggest that lean subjects compensate the energy expended during exercise to a larger extent by increasing the energy intake than obese subjects. This difference is in agreement with the general finding that the body-weight reduction with exercise training is more pronounced in obese than in lean persons. However, the variability appears to be large. One of the factors responsible for this variability may be the degree of dietary restraint or disinhibition (Keim *et al.*, 1990). Another factor that appears to have significant influence is the composition of the diet. Several studies show

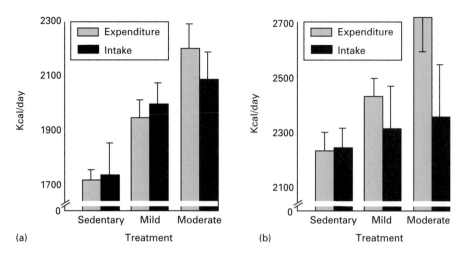

Fig. 18.11 Energy expenditure and energy intake (mean ± SEM) in (a) normal-weight ($n = 5$) and (b) overweight women ($n = 6$) who were sedentary, mildly physically active or moderately active for 19 days. Adapted from Woo *et al.* (1985).

that larger compensation and even overcompensation of the exercise-induced increase in energy expenditure takes place on a high-fat diet (Food Quotient (FQ) < 0.85) compared to a high-carbohydrate diet (FQ > 0.85) (Tremblay *et al.*, 1994b; King & Blundell, 1995; King *et al.*, 1996) (Fig. 18.12). These observations are in agreement with the notion that carbohydrate balance is regulated and that replenishment of the carbohydrate stores after exercise requires a larger energy intake on a high-fat diet than on a high-carbohydrate

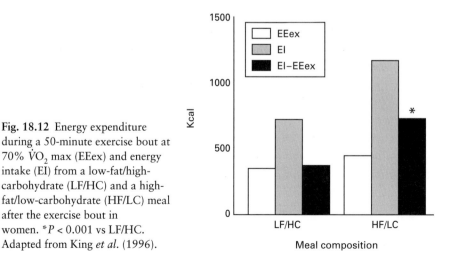

Fig. 18.12 Energy expenditure during a 50-minute exercise bout at 70% $\dot{V}O_2$ max (EEex) and energy intake (EI) from a low-fat/high-carbohydrate (LF/HC) and a high-fat/low-carbohydrate (HF/LC) meal after the exercise bout in women. *$P < 0.001$ vs LF/HC. Adapted from King *et al.* (1996).

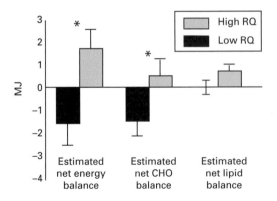

Fig. 18.13 Estimated net postexercise energy, carbohydrate (CHO) and lipid balance over 48 hours (mean ± SEM) in subgroups with a high RQ or with a low RQ during a 90-minute exercise bout at 60% $\dot{V}O_2$ max. Net energy balance was estimated from the difference between postexercise energy intake and control (rest) energy intake minus the energy cost of exercise above resting level. Net carbohydrate and lipid balance were calculated accordingly. Alméras *et al.* (1995), with permission from Elsevier Science.

diet (Flatt, 1987). This finding underlines the importance of a low-fat diet during weight loss and weight maintenance. In addition, Alméras *et al.* (1995) showed that energy intake after 90 minutes of exercise at 60% $\dot{V}O_2$ max was higher in men with a high respiratory quotient (RQ), indicating relatively low fat oxidation, during exercise than in men with a low RQ, indicating high fat oxidation. Thus, subjects with a low exercise RQ were more predisposed to a negative energy balance than subjects with a high RQ during exercise (Fig. 18.13).

Macronutrient preference

Cross-sectional studies indicate that trained individuals consume a larger proportion of carbohydrates in their diet than untrained people (Saris 1989; Horber *et al.*, 1996). Physical activity and fat content of the diet are strongly and inversely related in American adults (Simoes *et al.*, 1995). Whether these differences are guided by a higher carbohydrate oxidation during exercise in the more active individuals remains to be clarified. However, a predilection towards carbohydrates as a means to maintain energy balance may account in part for the relative ease with which active people seem to balance calories (Wood, 1996).

Exercise and the balance between energy expenditure and energy intake

The regulatory system that controls body(fat) mass and links energy intake to energy expenditure is not fully known. However, hormones such as insulin, produced by the pancreas, leptin, produced in adipose tissue, neuropeptide Y (NPY) and corticotropin-releasing hormone (CRH), both produced in the hypothalamus, are likely to play an important role. Acute exercise and exercise training lower plasma insulin levels. Preliminary data suggest that exercise has no acute effect on plasma leptin concentration in humans (Leijssen *et al.*, 1997). Training also does not affect basal leptin concentration, independent of changes in fat mass in older women (Kohrt *et al.*, 1996). Reductions in insulin and leptin may stimulate NPY production in the hypothalamus, which in turn will increase energy intake. In rats it has been shown that exercise increases NPY (Richard, 1995). Exercise also elevates CRH- and CRH receptor-mRNA in the hypothalamus (Richard, 1995). Richard hypothesizes that the stimulation of the CRH system by exercise may, by inhibition of the NPY system, explain the potential of exercise to create a negative energy balance.

Exercise and substrate utilization

Any intervention aimed at inducing weight loss in overweight persons should promote a negative fat balance. Exercise increases energy expenditure and substrate oxidation in skeletal muscles. Fatty acids are an important energy source for the exercising muscles. Moreover, due to the depletion of glycogen stores during exercise, fat oxidation is favoured following exercise. These combined effects result in increased fat oxidation. Exercise therefore allows fat oxidation to be in balance with fat intake at a lower body fat content (Flatt, 1995).

Substrate utilization during exercise

During exercise oxygen consumption rises and increased amounts of substrates have to be made available to be used as fuels in the exercising muscles. Increased activity of the sympathetic nervous system plays an important role in the mobilization of substrates from their stores in the body (Fig. 18.14). Hormonal changes (insulin, glucagon, growth hormone, adrenalin) support the actions of the sympathetic nervous system. In addition, the sympathetic nervous system regulates the cardiovascular adaptations necessary for the transport of oxygen and substrates to and waste products from the exercising muscles.

During the first minutes of submaximal aerobic exercise muscle glycogen breakdown is the main source of energy. As exercise continues, blood-borne substrates (glucose and non-esterified fatty acids (NEFAs)) become more important (Fig. 18.15). Although blood glucose concentration usually does not change during non-exhaustive exercise, the turnover of blood glucose is

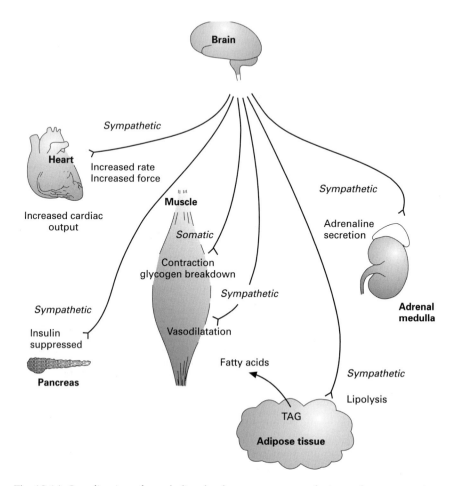

Fig. 18.14 Coordination of metabolism by the nervous system during endurance exercise. From Frayn (1996).

increased. The liver provides extra glucose by increased hepatic glycogenolysis and gluconeogenesis. The blood concentration of NEFAs initially falls, but gradually increases during prolonged exercise above resting levels, indicating that adipose tissue lipolysis is not strictly matched to muscle NEFA utilization. Another source of fatty acids during exercise are the triglyceride stores present within the skeletal muscles. At moderate exercise intensity (65% $\dot{V}O_2$ max) utilization of fatty acids increases and that of carbohydrates decreases with time (Romijn *et al.*, 1993) (Fig. 18.15), which is reflected by a gradual decrease of the RQ during prolonged exercise at this intensity.

The composition of the substrate mix utilized during exercise depends not only on duration but also on the intensity of exercise and the training status

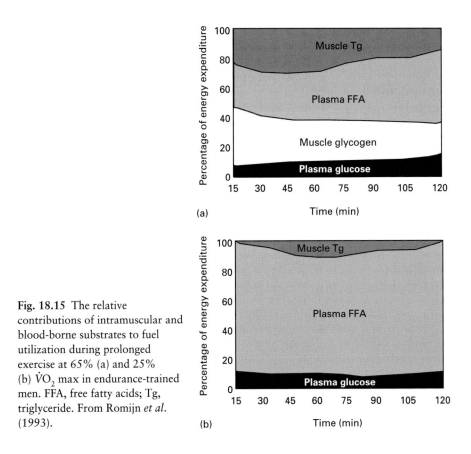

Fig. 18.15 The relative contributions of intramuscular and blood-borne substrates to fuel utilization during prolonged exercise at 65% (a) and 25% (b) $\dot{V}O_2$ max in endurance-trained men. FFA, free fatty acids; Tg, triglyceride. From Romijn *et al.* (1993).

of the subject. At very low exercise intensity (25% $\dot{V}O_2$ max, comparable to walking) plasma NEFAs are the main energy source. As intensity increases, the absolute contribution of plasma glucose and muscle glycogen increases, that of plasma NEFA decreases (Romijn *et al.*, 1993) (Fig. 18.16). The contribution of intramuscular triglycerides is largest at moderate exercise intensity (65% $\dot{V}O_2$ max). At this exercise intensity all four major substrates (plasma NEFA, plasma glucose, muscle glycogen and triglycerides) contribute substantially to energy production. This is the exercise intensity generally chosen to improve fitness. At the high intensity of 85% $\dot{V}O_2$ max the absolute oxidation of fat is reduced and muscle glycogen becomes the most important substrate. This appears to be due not only to reduced fatty acid availability, but also to a limited capacity for fat oxidation in the muscle (Coyle, 1995).

It should be realized that these data have been collected in endurance-trained male subjects under fasting circumstances. Although the general pattern of substrate utilization will be similar, less well trained people will oxidize less fat and will utilize more muscle glycogen at a given percentage of $\dot{V}O_2$ max compared

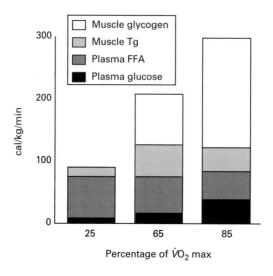

Fig. 18.16 Maximal contribution to energy expenditure derived from glucose and free fatty acids (FFA) taken up from blood and minimal contribution of muscle triglyceride (Tg) and glycogen stored after 30 minutes of exercise, expressed as function of exercise intensity. Total amount of calories derived from the plasma does not change in relation to exercise intensity. From Romijn *et al.* (1993).

with endurance-trained subjects. Pre-exercise carbohydrate-containing meals reduce fat oxidation and increase carbohydrate oxidation during exercise (Coyle, 1995). Women demonstrate greater fat oxidation than equally trained men (Tarnapolsky *et al.*, 1990; Ruby & Robergs, 1994).

Substrate utilization during exercise in obesity

Evidence has accumulated that individuals predisposed to obesity are characterized by a reduced capacity to use fat as an energy substrate when their body mass is still normal. It has also been shown that the β-adrenergically mediated increase in energy expenditure and fat oxidation is reduced in obese men (Blaak *et al.*, 1994). The question therefore arises whether the adaptations in energy metabolism during exercise, which are also partly mediated by the increase in sympathetic activity, are different in lean and obese individuals.

There is surprisingly little information about the substrate utilization of obese compared with lean individuals during exercise. Swan and Howley (1993) showed that the utilization of fat as an energy substrate increased with time during prolonged exercise in upper and lower body obese women, as in lean subjects. Fat utilization percentages in this study corresponded to values reported by other investigators in normal-weight women at approximately the same exercise intensity. Kanaley *et al.* (1993) compared the plasma NEFAs rate of appearance and fat oxidation during exercise in non-obese, upper body obese and lower body obese women. At a comparable relative exercise intensity (45% $\dot{V}O_2$ max) total exercise NEFA availability and oxidation did not differ among groups (Fig. 18.17).

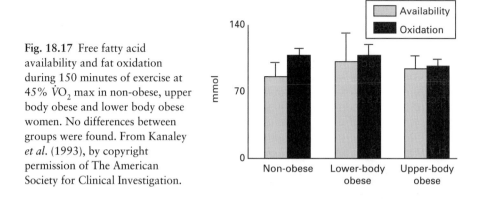

Fig. 18.17 Free fatty acid availability and fat oxidation during 150 minutes of exercise at 45% $\dot{V}O_2$ max in non-obese, upper body obese and lower body obese women. No differences between groups were found. From Kanaley *et al.* (1993), by copyright permission of The American Society for Clinical Investigation.

A study by Wade *et al.* (1990) showed that fatter men, who had a relatively low percentage of slow (type 1) muscle fibres, oxidized less fat at an absolute workload of 100 W than leaner men, with a higher percentage of type I muscle fibres. Type 1 muscle fibres have a greater capacity for fat oxidation than type 2 fibres. However, other studies have failed to reproduce these findings. Geerling *et al.* (1994) found no correlation between percentage body fat and respiratory exchange ratio during exercise in sedentary men with a larger variation in body fat than in Wade's study. Simoneau and Bouchard (1995) could not demonstrate a difference in percentage type 1 muscle fibres in men with low and high subcutaneous fat, matched for $\dot{V}O_2$ max. These results suggest that fat utilization during exercise is similar in obese and lean individuals at the same relative exercise intensity. However, from this finding it is difficult to conclude whether this apparently normal substrate utilization during exercise in the obese is dependent on a high body fat mass. To answer this question, substrate utilization needs to be studied in the pre-obese or in the post-obese state. At the moment these data are not available.

Training and substrate utilization during exercise

Training reduces utilization of both muscle glycogen and blood glucose during exercise at a given absolute submaximal exercise intensity. This training-induced reduction in carbohydrate oxidation during exercise is compensated for by an increase in fat oxidation (Fig. 18.18). A study by Klein *et al.* (1994) has shown that the rate of appearance of glycerol, as a measure of whole-body lipolysis, did not differ between trained and untrained subjects exercising at the same absolute intensity. Another study by Klein *et al.* (1996) showed that at the same relative exercise intensity (70% $\dot{V}O_2$ max) whole-body lipolytic rate is greater in endurance-trained athletes than in sedentary controls. Studies indicate that the main source of increased fat oxidation at a certain absolute exercise intensity

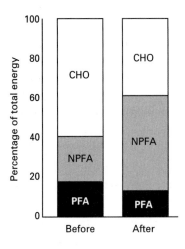

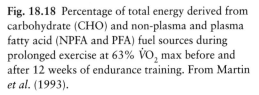

Fig. 18.18 Percentage of total energy derived from carbohydrate (CHO) and non-plasma and plasma fatty acid (NPFA and PFA) fuel sources during prolonged exercise at 63% $\dot{V}O_2$ max before and after 12 weeks of endurance training. From Martin *et al.* (1993).

may not be adipose tissue lipolysis, but rather intramuscular triglyceride stores (Hurley *et al.*, 1986; Martin *et al.*, 1993; Coyle, 1995; Phillips *et al.*, 1996a, b) (Fig. 18.18).

The underlying mechanisms for these training-induced adaptations probably involve changes in muscle respiratory capacity and hormonal adaptations. Increases in the skeletal muscle content of mitochondria, enzymes involved in activation, transfer into mitochondria and beta-oxidation of fatty acids, increases in cytosolic fatty acid-binding protein, and change in activity of regulatory molecules such as malonyl CoA occur with training (Henriksson, 1995; Simoneau, 1995). Training also increases the capacity to store triglycerides in muscle in humans (Morgan *et al.*, 1969). The effects of endurance exercise on the glycolytic capacity of the skeletal muscle is modest, although high-intensity intermittent exercise training can induce increases in the enzymes of the glycolytic pathways. Training generally reduces the magnitude of the hormonal response to a standard exercise load. This is associated with improved target tissue sensitivity and/or responsiveness to a given quantity of hormone.

An interesting and practically very important question is what exercise intensity, duration and frequency are needed to attain the positive effects on fat oxidation. Virtually all training studies used relatively intense exercise (>60% $\dot{V}O_2$ max), 3–6 times per week, >30 minutes' duration. The effectiveness of less intense and/or less frequent and/or shorter duration programmes has not been studied.

Training and non-exercise substrate utilization

Because exercise training is associated with structural and enzymatic adaptations, training may not only affect substrate utilization during exercise but also in the non-exercising state. Many studies have shown that fat oxidation is increased during the first hours after exercise (Bielinski *et al.*, 1985; Bahr *et al.*, 1990). Cross-sectional studies where substrate oxidation has been measured at least 24 hours after the last exercise bout give ambiguous results: similar and increased fasting RQs have been found comparing trained and untrained subjects (Tremblay & Buemann, 1995). Poehlman *et al.* (1994) showed that 8 weeks of endurance training increased basal fat oxidation in elderly persons, without change in fatty acids rate of appearance. The enhanced basal fat oxidation was associated with increased activity of the sympathetic nervous system and increases in FFM. Calles-Escandon *et al.* (1996) demonstrated that endurance training increased fat oxidation at rest independent of changes in body composition. Strength training also increases 24-hour fat oxidation independent of a change in 24-hour EE (Treuth *et al.*, 1995).

Training and substrate utilization in obesity

Data on the effects of exercise training on substrate utilization in the obese are scarce. Training increased muscle fibre area and muscle oxidative capacity in obese women (Krotkiewski *et al.*, 1983, Svendsen *et al.*, 1996). Exercise respiratory exchange ratio was reduced (Svendsen *et al.*, 1996). Buemann *et al.* (1992), on the other hand, found no change in sedentary 24-hour RQ (measured in a respiration chamber) after a training programme in postobese women.

In conclusion, exercise training has the potential to increase fat oxidation at rest and during exercise. At present it is unclear whether training also has these effects in the obese. If exercise does increase fat oxidation in the obese, this may be an important contributing factor in the prevention and treatment of obesity (Flatt, 1987, 1995; Tremblay & Buemann, 1995).

Exercise and risk factors in obesity

Obesity, especially visceral obesity, is associated with an increased risk for type 2 (non-insulin-dependent) diabetes mellitus (NIDDM) and cardiovascular disease, due to hyperlipidaemia and hypertension, and thus with increased mortality and morbidity (Després *et al.*, 1990; Sjöström, 1992; Barlow *et al.*, 1995). Regular exercise has beneficial effects on these risk factors, independent of changes in body mass or body composition. Moreover, exercise may reduce visceral fat, which is likely to be important in the reduction of risk for diabetes and cardiovascular diseases.

Insulin resistance

Regular exercise reduces the insulin resistance that is characteristic of NIDDM. Euglycemic hyperinsulinaemic clamp studies show an increase in insulin sensitivity after training (Bogardus *et al.*, 1984; Krotkiewski *et al.*, 1985). Furthermore, the muscle glucose transporter protein GLUT4 increases with training in patients with NIDDM (Dela *et al.*, 1994). In subjects with visceral obesity, which are characterized by hyperinsulinaemia and insulin resistance, the improvement of insulin sensitivity after training is independent of changes in body-weight (Lamarche *et al.*, 1992; Dengel *et al.*, 1996).

Blood lipids

Individuals with visceral obesity are characterized by elevated plasma triglyceride levels, increased apolipoprotein B concentrations and reduced concentrations of plasma high-density lipoprotein (HDL)-cholesterol (Després *et al.*, 1995). Endurance exercise training induces significant and potentially beneficial changes in plasma lipoprotein levels (reduced plasma triglycerides, increased HDL-cholesterol) (Wood *et al.*, 1988; Williams *et al.*, 1990). These changes are strongly associated with weight change, but may also occur independent of changes in body mass (Lamarche *et al.*, 1992).

Blood pressure

Regular exercise reduces high blood pressure, which is also frequent in obesity. Paffenbarger *et al.* (1983) showed that Harvard alumni who were engaged in regular vigorous exercise had a lower risk of developing hypertension to those who reported no vigorous physical activity. The protective effect of vigorous exercise was greater in subjects with increased BMI.

A meta-analysis of experimental studies on the blood pressure lowering potential of exercise training by Fagard (1995) showed that exercise training reduced blood pressure by on average −10/−8 mmHg in subjects with high blood pressure (≥160/95 mmHg) and −3/−3 mmHg in normotensive individuals (blood pressure ≤140/90 mmHg). These changes were independent of changes in body mass.

Epidemiological data from the Aerobics Center Longitudinal Study by Blair *et al.* (1996) suggest that moderate and high levels of cardiorespiratory fitness provide protection against the force of other mortality predictors, such as smoking, elevated blood pressure, high cholesterol and high BMI in men as well as women. Figure 18.19 shows the risk reduction per minute of greater

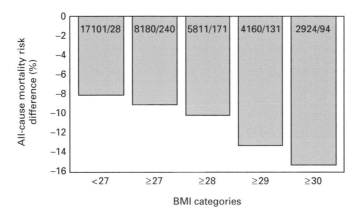

Fig. 18.19 Differences (%) in all-cause mortality risk per minute of greater treadmill time in five BMI categories. Numbers along the top are the number of men/number of deaths. Differences in risk were adjusted for age, physical fitness, resting systolic blood pressure, total cholesterol, BMI, fasting blood glucose, cigarette smoking and health status. All $P < 0.0001$. From Barlow *et al.* (1995).

treadmill time (as a measure of higher fitness) in five BMI categories in the men from this study. Blair therefore concludes that physicians should counsel all their sedentary patients to become more physically active and improve their cardiorespiratory fitness, even though in some patients, despite good adherence to exercise, the clinical variables may fail to improve.

Psychological aspects

Regular exercise produces many different metabolic as well as psychological effects. Therefore, there is a large number of possible explanations why people who exercise are more likely to lose weight and keep it off. Improved psychological functioning may be one of them (Brownell, 1995). Brownell (1995) suggests that a much larger proportion of the variance in energy balance may be explained by energy intake than by metabolic processes. Since psychological processes are clearly involved in the regulation of energy intake, the influence of exercise on weight loss and weight maintenance may be through its impact on psychological variables. Likely candidates are modulation of mood, stress reduction, improved self-efficacy, self-esteem and cognitive schemas responsible for factors such as optimism vs pessimism (Morgan & Goldston, 1987; Plante & Rodin, 1990; Brownell, 1995). Exercise has been shown to improve satisfaction with body shape and weight (King *et al.*, 1989), and has the potential for improving body image in women (Salusso-Deonier & Schwarzkopf, 1991).

Summary of benefits of exercise in obesity

Based on the research that has been described in the previous sections, Table 18.4 summarizes the (potential) benefits of exercise and exercise training for the obese individual.

Training recommendations

Exercise training can be performed at various intensities. Usually training intensities are categorized as (very) low, moderate or (very) high (Table 18.5). According to guidelines of the American College of Sports Medicine, published in 1990, the minimal training intensity threshold for improvement in $\dot{V}O_2$ max is approximately 50% $\dot{V}O_2$ max or heart rate (HR) reserve (or 60% of maximal heart rate). Most beneficial effects of physical activity on cardiovascular disease mortality can be attained through daily low- to moderate-intensity activity

Table 18.4 (Potential) benefits of exercise in obesity.

Increased energy expenditure during exercise
Increased postexercise energy expenditure
Increased non-exercise-training physical activity
Increased resting metabolic rate
Increased TEF
No full compensation of energy expended (on low-fat diet)
Increased preference for carbohydrates
Less reduction of FFM during dieting
Less reduction of RMR during dieting
Increased fat oxidation
Positive psychological effects (mood, self-esteem, self-efficacy, body image)
Protection against increased mortality and morbidity associated with obesity

Table 18.5 Classifcation of intensity of exercise based on 20–60 minutes endurance training. Adapted from American College of Sports Medicine (1990).

Classification of intensity	% $\dot{V}O_2$ max or %HRR	%HR max
Very light (very low)	<30%	<35%
Light (low)	30–49%	35–59%
Moderate	50–74%	60–79%
Heavy (high)	75–84%	80–89%
Very heavy (very high)	≥85%	≥90%

HRR, heart rate reserve (maximal heart rate–resting heart rate); HR max, maximal heart rate.

(40–60% of maximal oxygen uptake) (Fletcher *et al.*, 1996). Activities such as walking for pleasure, gardening, house work and dancing fall in this category. The American Heart Association recommends dynamic exercise with large muscle groups for extended periods of time (30–60 minutes, three to six times weekly) for optimal health promotion (Fletcher *et al.*, 1995). This may include short periods (5–10 minutes) of moderate exercise intensities (60–75% of $\dot{V}O_2$ max). With respect to weight control, training programmes that are conducted at least 3 days per week, of at least 20 minutes duration, and of sufficient intensity to expend approximately 300 kcal per session, are suggested as a threshold level for total body mass and fat mass loss by the American College of Sports Medicine (1990). If the exercise frequency is increased to 4 days per week the expenditure per session may be reduced to 200 kcal. A high frequency and long duration of exercise sessions for effective weight control is stressed. A minimal level of intensity appears less important. Several studies have shown a dissociation between the adaptation of cardiorespiratory fitness and the metabolic improvements which can be induced by endurance training programmes (Duncan *et al.*, 1991; Després & Lamarche, 1994). This has led to the introduction of the concept of 'metabolic fitness', indicating that clinically important metabolic improvements can be obtained with prolonged endurance exercise at low exercise intensities (50% $\dot{V}O_2$ max), which may have a minor effect on $\dot{V}O_2$ max. Tsetsonis and Hardman (1996), for instance, showed that a 3-hour walk at regular walking speed (5–6 km/hr) reduced postprandial lipaemia and increased fat oxidation after a high-fat meal the next day (Fig. 18.20).

On the other hand, there are also studies suggesting that a minimal level of training intensity may be required to attain certain training effects that are considered beneficial for the obese individual. Tremblay *et al.* (1994a) showed

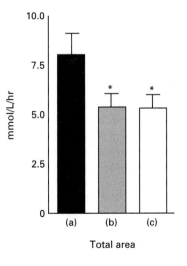

Fig. 18.20 Total area under the 6-hour serum triacylglycerol concentration–time curves after an oral fat load in the morning of day 2 (mean ± SEM). Three trials: control, preceded by a day of minimal physical activity (day 1) (a); preceded by a 3-hour walk at 30% $\dot{V}O_2$ max in the afternoon of day 1 (b); preceded by a 1.5-hour walk at 60% $\dot{V}O_2$ max in the afternoon of day 1 (c). * Significantly different from control, $P < 0.05$. From Tsetsonis and Hardman (1996).

that when part of the sessions in a moderately intense endurance training programme were replaced with high-intensity interval training sessions fat mass decreased more despite a lower total energy cost of this training programme. Moreover, skeletal muscle glycolytic enzymes and 3-hydroxyacyl coenzyme A dehydrogenase, a marker of the activity of the beta oxidation of fat, increased more.

Almost all studies that demonstrated a beneficial effect of exercise training on insulin resistance used fairly vigorous exercise protocols of moderate to high exercise intensities (70–85% $\dot{V}O_2$ max). Kang et al. (1996) showed that a 7-day exercise training programme at an intensity of 50% $\dot{V}O_2$ max did not change

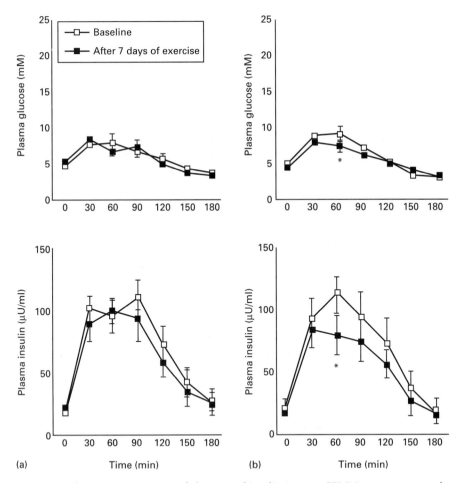

Fig. 18.21 Plasma concentrations of glucose and insulin (mean ± SEM) in response to oral glucose ingestion at baseline and after 7 days of isocaloric exercise at (a) 50% and (b) 70% $\dot{V}O_2$ max in obese subjects. * Significantly decreased ($P < 0.05$) compared with baseline. From Kang et al. (1996).

Table 18.6 Estimation of kilocalories used from fat and carbohydrates for a low- and high-intensity aerobic training bout. Adapted from Wilmore and Costill (1994).

	Low intensity (50% $\dot{V}O_2$ max)	High intensity (75% $\dot{V}O_2$ max)
Average $\dot{V}O_2$ (L/min)	1.50	2.25
Average RER	0.85	0.90
% kcal from CHO	50	67
% kcal from fat	50	33
kcal/30min from CHO	110	222
kcal/30 min from fat	110	110
kcal/30 min total	220	332

RER, respiratory exchange ratio; CHO, carbohydrate.

insulin sensitivity in obese men with normal glucose tolerance, while a training intensity of 70% $\dot{V}O_2$ max (with the same total energy expenditure) improved insulin sensitivity (measured at 23 hours after the last exercise bout) (Fig. 18.21). The authors therefore concluded that if an exercise programme is prescribed with a goal of rapidly improving insulin sensitivity, then this programme should entail at least some component of vigorous exercise. On the other hand, Lamarche *et al.* (1992) showed that a 6-month low-intensity training programme at 55% $\dot{V}O_2$ max improved insulin sensitivity in obese women.

In the late 1980s the idea was introduced that low-intensity training allows the body to use more fat as the energy source, thus quickening the loss of body fat. Since then low-intensity exercise training has been widely advocated for the obese. Although indeed a higher percentage of the energy expended during low-intensity exercise is derived from fat, the total amount of calories derived from fat is not necessarily larger than with moderate-intensity training (Table 18.6).

Thus, the question of which type of exercise training is optimal for the obese probably does not have one single answer. The answer depends on the ultimate goal(s) of the training programme: is it body-weight reduction, fat mass reduction, increased fat oxidation, risk factor reduction or improvement of general fitness, psychological well-being and health? How fast does one want to attain a certain goal? Interindividual differences in response to training programmes are also likely.

Training mode

Dynamic exercise with large muscle groups is usually recommended to improve cardiorespiratory fitness and health, and in weight-control programmes. For the obese especially, non-weight bearing activities, such as swimming or cycling, may be appropriate. For healthy adults, rhythmical resistance exercise, performed at a moderate to slow speed, through the full range of motion, not impeding normal breathing, is recommended for improvement of muscular strength and endurance (American College of Sports Medicine, 1990). This type of dynamic resistance or strength training may be less effective in reducing body-weight and fat mass than endurance training, but has the advantage of increasing FFM (and thereby resting energy expenditure) (Ballor & Keesey, 1991; Ballor et al., 1996). Increased fat oxidation has been reported after strength training in older women (Treuth et al., 1995).

Exercise prescription

Prescriptions of frequency and duration of exercise sessions are simple and straightforward. The intensity of exercise is usually prescribed as a percentage of the maximal oxygen uptake ($\dot{V}O_2$ max). Since $\dot{V}O_2$ (max) is difficult to measure in non-laboratory exercise settings, prescription of exercise intensity is usually based on heart rate or subjective feelings of exertion (RPE, rating of perceived exertion). This is based on the linear relationship between %HR max (%maximal heart rate) or %HRR (%heart rate reserve = (maximal heart rate–resting heart rate)/maximal heart rate) and RPE on one hand and % $\dot{V}O_2$ max on the other hand.

The relationship between %HR max or %HRR and % $\dot{V}O_2$ max has been found to be similar in lean and obese adults (Miller et al., 1991). However, HR max was lower in obese than in lean subjects: in normal-weight subjects HR max can be predicted by 220–age, in obese subjects the equation 200 – 0.5 × age was found to be more accurate (Miller et al., 1991). On the other hand, Jakicic et al. (1995a) showed that the relationship between %HRR and % $\dot{V}O_2$ max in obese women changed with weight loss and that following weight loss the same %HRR represented a higher level of intensity than before. This discrepancy may be due to the fact that subjects in Jakicic's study were more severely obese than the obese in Miller's study.

Jakicic et al. (1995a) also showed that a certain RPE corresponded with the same % $\dot{V}O_2$ max before and after weight loss consistent with existing guidelines (70% = 13–14 RPE). RPE can therefore be used as a subjective marker of exercise intensity in obese individuals.

Exercise adherence

Drop-out rates from exercise programmes are relatively high and the degree of overweight is one of the most consistent predictors of drop-out from exercise

Table 18.7 Exercise adherence (number of days and total duration), predicted $\dot{V}O_2$ max and weight loss (mean ± SD) in overweight women in a 20-week behavioural weight-control programme. Exercise was performed either as multiple short bouts per day (SB) or as one long exercise bout per day (LB). Adapted from Jakicic et al. (1995).

	SB group	LB group
Exercise adherence (days)	87.3 ± 29.5	69.1 ± 28.9 (P < 0.05)
Exercise adherence (min/week)	223.8 ± 69.5	188.2 ± 58.4 (P = 0.08)
Increase in $\dot{V}O_2$ max (%)	5.0	5.6
Weight loss (kg)	−8.9 ± 5.3	−6.4 ± 4.5 (P < 0.07)

programmes (Dishman et al., 1985). It is, therefore, important to develop strategies to improve exercise adherence, especially in the obese.

Brownell (1995) stresses that cognitive factors regarding exercise are of critical importance for success of exercise in weight management. Analysis of prevailing cognitive rules and schemas and, if necessary, intervention should be components of exercise prescription (Brownell, 1995).

Wing and colleagues performed several studies in order to identify factors that might improve exercise adherence in the obese. Short bouts of exercise (multiple 10-minute exercise bouts per day) improved adherence and weight loss, without significantly affecting the changes in cardiorespiratory fitness, compared with a single daily long exercise bout (Jakicic et al., 1995b) (Table 18.7). A personal trainer or financial incentives did not result in enhanced exercise adherence in obese women, although the authors suggest that this may have been in part due to the limited statistical power of the studies (Wing et al., 1996).

Exercise risk

Apart from the benefits, exercise may also have risks. The most serious, but relatively infrequent risk, is that of sudden cardiac death (0–2 per 100 000 hours of vigorous exercise in the general population) (Fletcher et al., 1995). Although less serious, the risk of falls and joint injuries is much larger. The risks associated with exercise are lower in those participating in low-impact activities such as walking. There are no data available on the magnitude of these risks in the obese population.

In the context of risk reduction, obese (and other) individuals with known or suspected cardiovascular, respiratory, metabolic, orthopaedic or neurological disorders are advised to consult their physician before beginning or significantly increasing physical activity, especially when activities with a higher intensity than walking are chosen.

Summary

Exercise is recommended as an important strategy for prevention of obesity and as an effective adjunct to its treatment. It has become clear that not only the extra energy cost of exercise is important in this respect, but that regular exercise has additional beneficial effects in obesity.

• Several large epidemiological studies (NHANES-1, MRFIT, Finnish population studies) support the notion that a high level of physical activity protects against increases in weight and obesity.

• Endurance exercise training alone induces moderate weight and fat loss, which may be slightly more pronounced in overweight than in lean subjects. Resistance training has little effect on weight, but increases FFM. In combination with an energy-restricted diet, endurance exercise training results in additional weight loss, which is small compared with the diet-induced weight loss. However, FFM is reduced less than with diet alone. Resistance exercise training may preserve FFM more effectively during dietary restriction than endurance training.

• Regular exercise is an important predictor of successful weight maintenance after a period of weight loss. Long-term randomized weight reduction studies show that a larger proportion of initial weight loss is maintained in subjects who exercise regularly than in non-exercising subjects.

• Energy expenditure is increased above resting levels during and after the exercise bout. Energy expended during exercise depends on the type, intensity and duration of the exercise bout and the weight of the individual. The net energy cost of exercise may vary roughly between 2 and 20 kcal/kg/hr. The magnitude of the EPOC also depends on duration and intensity. EPOC is small in comparison with the energy expended during the exercise bout itself.

• Although cross-sectional studies indicate that RMR may be increased in highly trained subjects compared to untrained subjects, exercise training programmes generally do not lead to an increase in RMR in lean or obese individuals. The addition of a training programme during a period of dietary restriction in obese individuals, on the other hand, may reduce the decrease in RMR accompanying a negative energy balance.

• The TEF is not affected by exercise training in lean subjects, neither at rest nor after an acute bout of exercise. In the obese, training may increase TEF after acute exercise. However, the absolute increment of total energy expenditure due to this effect is small.

• Exercise training increases average daily energy expenditure. Part of the increase may be due to an increase in non-exercise-training activities, especially in men.

• Lean subjects compensate the energy expended during exercise to a larger extent by increasing energy intake than obese. A larger compensation and even over-compensation takes place on a high-fat diet compared to a high-carbohydrate diet.

- The composition of the substrate mix utilized during exercise depends on the intensity and duration of the exercise and the training status of the subject. At moderate exercise intensity (65% $\dot{V}O_2$ max) utilization of fatty acids increases and that of carbohydrates decreases with time. At very low exercise intensity (25% $\dot{V}O_2$ max) plasma free fatty acids are the main energy source. As intensity increases, the contribution of plasma glucose and muscle glycogen increases, and that of plasma fatty acids decreases. The contribution of intramuscular triglycerides is most pronounced at moderate exercise intensity.

- Endurance exercise training increases fat oxidation during exercise in lean subjects. The main source of the increased fat oxidation are the intramuscular triglyceride stores. The effect of training on substrate utilization in obese individuals has not been studied. Training also increases postexercise and basal fat oxidation.

- Epidemiological data suggest that moderate and high levels of cardio-respiratory fitness provide protection against the force of other mortality predictors, such as smoking, elevated blood pressure and high BMI in men as well as women.

- Since psychological processes are involved in the regulation of energy intake, the influence of exercise on weight loss and weight maintenance may be through its beneficial impact on psychological variables.

- The question of which type of exercise training is optimal for the obese probably does not have a single answer. It will depend on the goal(s) of the training programme: weight reduction, fat mass reduction, increased fat oxidation, risk factor reduction or improvement of general fitness, psychological well-being and health. Frequent exercise sessions (3–6 times per week) of sufficient duration and intensity to expend approximately 300 kcal per session have been recommended for weight loss. Most beneficial effects of exercise training can be attained through regular low- to moderate-intensity (40–60% $\dot{V}O_2$ max) exercise. Some, such as improved insulin sensitivity, however, may require periods of higher intensity exercise (60–75% $\dot{V}O_2$ max).

- Dynamic exercise with large muscle groups is recommended to improve cardiorespiratory fitness and health, and in weight-control programmes. Resistance training is recommended for improvement of muscular strength and endurance, but is less effective in reducing body-weight.

- The degree of overweight is an important predictor of drop-out from exercise programmes. Strategies to improve exercise adherence in the obese need to be developed.

References

Ainsworth, B.E., Haskell, W.L., Leon, A.S. *et al.* (1993) Compendium of physical activities: classification of energy costs of human physical activities. *Medicine and Science in Sports and Exercise* 25, 71–80.

Alméras, N., Lavallée, N., Després, J., Bouchard, C. & Tremblay, A. (1995) Exercise and energy intake: effect of substrate oxidation. *Physiology and Behavior* 57, 995–1000.

American College of Sports Medicine. (1990) The recommended quantity and quality of exercise for developing and maintaining cardiorespiratory and muscular fitness in healthy adults. *Medicine and Science in Sports and Exercise* 22, 265–274.

Andersson, B., Xu, X., Rebuffé-Scrive, M., Terning, K., Krotkiewski, M. & Björntorp, P. (1991) The effects of exercise training on body composition and metabolism in men and women. *International Journal of Obesity* 15, 75–81.

Bahr, R. & Sejersted, O.M. (1991) Effect of feeding and fasting on excess post exercise oxygen consumption. *Journal of Applied Physiology* 71, 2088–2093.

Bahr, R., Ingnis, I., Vaage, O., Sejersted, O.M. & Newsholme, E.A. (1987) Effect of duration of exercise on post exercise O_2 consumption. *Journal of Applied Physiology* 62, 485–490.

Bahr, R., Hansson, P. & Sejersted, O.M. (1990) Triglyceride/fatty acid cycling is increased after exercise. *Metabolism* 39, 993–999.

Ballor, D.L. & Keesey, R.E. (1991) A meta-analysis of the factors affecting exercise-induced changes in body mass, fat mass and fat-free mass in males and females. *International Journal of Obesity* 15, 717–726.

Ballor, D.L. & Poehlman, E.T. (1994) Exercise-training enhances fat-free mass preservation during diet-induced weight loss: a meta-analytical finding. *International Journal of Obesity* 18, 35–40.

Ballor, D.L., Harvey-Berino, J.R., Ades, P.A., Cryan, J. & Calles-Escandon, J. (1996) Contrasting effect of resistance and aerobic training on body composition and metabolism after diet-induced weight loss. *Metabolism* 45, 179–183.

Barlow, C.E., Kohl, H.W., Gibbons, L.W. & Blair, S.N. (1995) Physical fitness, mortality and obesity. *International Journal of Obesity* 19 (suppl. 4), S41–S44.

Berry, M.J., Storsteen, J.A. & Woodard, C.M. (1993) Effects of body mass on exercise efficiency and VO_2 during steady-state cycling. *Medicine and Science in Sports and Exercise* 25, 1031–1037.

Bielinski, R., Schutz, Y. & Jéquier, E. (1985) Energy metabolism during the postexercise recovery. *American Journal of Clinical Nutrition* 42, 69–82.

Bingham, S.A., Goldberg, G.R., Coward, W.A., Prentice, A.M. & Cummings, J.H. (1989) The effect of exercise and improved physical fitness on basal metabolic rate. *British Journal of Nutrition* 61, 155–173.

Blaak, E.E., Westerterp, K.R., Bar-Or, O., Wouters, L.J.M. & Saris, W.H.M. (1992) Effect of training on total energy expenditure and spontaneous activity in obese boys. *American Journal of Clinical Nutrition* 55, 777–782.

Blaak, E.E., van Baak, M.A., Kemerink, G.J., Pakbiers, M.T.W., Heidendal, G.A.K. & Saris, W.H.M. (1994) β-Adrenergic stimulation of energy expenditure and forearm skeletal muscle metabolism in lean and obese men. *American Journal of Physiology* 267, E306–E315.

Blair, S.N. (1993) Evidence for success of exercise in weight loss and control. *Archives of Internal Medicine* 119, 702–706.

Blair, S.N., Kampert, J.B., Kohl, H.W. *et al.* (1996) Influences of cardiorespiratory fitness and other precursors on cardiovascular disease and all-cause mortality in men and women. *Journal of the American Medical Association* 276, 205–210.

Bogardus, C., Ravussin, E., Robbins, D.C., Wolfe, R.R., Horton, E.S. & Sims, E.A.H. (1984) Effects of physical training and diet therapy on carbohydrate metabolism in patients with glucose intolerance and non-insulin-dependent diabetes mellitus. *Diabetes* 33, 311–318.

Brownell, K.D. (1995) Exercise and obesity treatment: Psychological aspects. *International Journal of Obesity* 19 (suppl. 4), S122–S125.

Buemann, B., Astrup, A. & Christensen, N.J. (1992) Three months aerobic training fails to affect

24-hour energy expenditure in weight-stable, post-obese women. *International Journal of Obesity* **16**, 809–816.

Calles-Escandón, J., Goran, M.I., O'Connell, M., Nair, K.S. & Danforth, E. (1996) Exercise increases fat oxidation at rest unrelated to changes in energy balance or lipolysis. *American Journal of Physiology* **270**, E1009–E1014.

Costill, D.L. (1986) *Inside Running: Basics of Sports Physiology*. Benchmark Press, Indianapolis.

Coyle, E.F. (1995) Substrate utilization during exercise in active people. *American Journal of Clinical Nutrition* **61** (suppl.), 968S–979S.

Davis, J.R., Tagliaferro, A.R., Kertzer, R., Gerardo, T., Nichols, J. & Wheeler, J. (1983) Variations in diet-induced thermogenesis and body fatness with aerobic capacity. *European Journal of Applied Physiology and Occupational Physiology* **50**, 319–329.

Dela, F., Ploug, T., Handberg, A. *et al.* (1994) Physical training increases muscle GLUT4 protein and mRNA in patients with NIDDM. *Diabetes* **43**, 862–865.

Dengel, D.R., Pratley, R.E., Hagberg, J.M., Rogus, E.M. & Goldberg, A.P. (1996) Distinct effects of aerobic exercise training and weight loss on glucose homeostasis in obese sedentary men. *Journal of Applied Physiology* **81**, 318–325.

DePue, J.D., Clark, M.M., Ruggiero, L., Medeiros, M. & Pera, V. (1995) Maintenance of weight loss: a needs assessment. *Obesity Research* **3**, 241–248.

Després, J.P. & Lamarche, B. (1994) Low-intensity endurance exercise training, plasma lipoproteins and the risk of coronary heart disease. *Journal of Internal Medicine* **236**, 7–22.

Després, J.P., Bouchard, C., Tremblay, A., Savard, R. & Marcotte, M. (1985) Effects of aerobic training on fat distribution in male subjects. *Medicine and Science in Sports and Exercise* **17**, 113–118.

Després, J.P., Moorjani, S., Lupien, P.J., Tremblay, A., Nadeau, A. & Bouchard, C. (1990) Regional distribution of body fat, plasma lipoproteins, and cardiovascular disease. *Arteriosclerosis* **10**, 497–511.

Després, J., Lamarche, B., Bouchard, C., Tremblay, A. & Prud'homme, D. (1995) Exercise and the prevention of dyslipidemia and coronary heart disease. *International Journal of Obesity* **19** (suppl. 4), S45–S51.

Dishman, R.K., Sallis, J.E. & Orenstein, D.R. (1985) The determinants of physical activity and exercise. *Public Health Reports* **100**, 158–171.

Donnelly, J.E., Jakicic, J. & Gunderson, S. (1991) Diet and body composition. *Sports Medicine* **12**, 237–249.

Duncan, J.J., Gordon, N.F. & Scott, C.B. (1991) Women walking for health and fitness. How much is enough? *Journal of the American Medical Association* **266**, 3295–3299.

Durrant, M.L., Royston, J.P. & Wloch, R.T. (1982) Effect of exercise on energy intake and eating patterns in lean and obese humans. *Physiology and Behavior* **29**, 449–454.

Fagard, R.H. (1995) Prescription and results of physical activity. *Journal of Cardiovascular Pharmacology* **25** (suppl. 1), S20–S27.

Flatt, J.P. (1987) Dietary fat, carbohydrate balance, and weight maintenance: effects of exercise. *American Journal of Clinical Nutrition* **45**, 296–306.

Flatt, J. (1995) Integration of the overall response to exercise. *International Journal of Obesity* **19** (suppl. 4), S31–S40.

Fletcher, G.F., Balady, G., Froelicher, V.F., Hartley, L.H., Haskell, W.L. & Pollock, M.L. (1995) Exercise standards. A statement for healthcare professionals from the American Heart Association. *Circulation* **91**, 580–615.

Fletcher, G.F., Balady, G., Blair, S.N. *et al.* (1996) Statement on exercise: benefits and recommendations for physical activity programs for all Americans. *Circulation* **94**, 857–862.

Foster, G.D., Wadden, T.A., Kendrick, Z.V., Letizia, K.A., Lander, D.P. & Conill, A.M. (1995) The energy cost of walking before and after significant weight loss. *Medicine and Science in Sports and Exercise* **27**, 888–894.

Frayn, K.N. (1996) *Metabolic Regulation. A Human Perspective*. London: Portland Press.

Frey-Hewitt, B., Vrauizan, K.M., Dreon, D.M.Z., Wood, P.D. (1990) The effect of weight loss by dieting or exercise on resting metabolic rate in overweight men. *International Journal of Obesity* **14**, 327–334.

Garrow, J.S. & Summerbell, C.D. (1995) Meta-analysis: effect of exercise, with or without dieting, on the body composition of overweight subjects. *European Journal of Clinical Nutrition* **49**, 1–10.

Geerling, B.J., Alles, M.S., Murgatroyd, P.R., Goldberg, G.R., Harding, M. & Prentice, A.M. (1994) Fatness in relation to substrate oxidation during exercise. *International Journal of Obesity* **18**, 453–459.

Goran, M.I. & Poehlman, E.T. (1992) Endurance training does not enhance total energy expenditure in healthy elderly persons. *American Journal of Physiology* **263**, E950–E957.

Gore, C.J. & Withers, R.T. (1990) The effect of exercise intensity and duration on the oxygen deficit and excess post-exercise oxygen consumption. *European Journal of Applied Physiology* **60**, 169–174.

Haapanen, N., Miilunpalo, S., Pasanen, M., Oja, P. & Vuori, I. (1997) Association between leisure time physical activity and 10-year body mass change among working-aged men and women. *International Journal of Obesity* **21**, 288–296.

Henriksson, J. (1995) Muscle fuel selection: effect of exercise and training. *Proceedings of the Nutrition Society* **54**, 125–138.

Hensrud, D.D., Weinsier, R.L., Darnell, B.E. & Hunter, G.R. (1995) Relationship of co-morbidities of obesity to weight loss and four-year weight maintenance/rebound. *Obesity Research* **3** (suppl. 2), 217s–222s.

Hill, J.O., Heymsfield, S.B., McMannus III, C. & DiGirolamo, M. (1984) Meal size and thermic response to food in male subjects as a function of maximum aerobic capacity. *Metabolism* **33**, 743–749.

Holden, J.H., Darga, L.L., Olson, S.M., Stettner, D.C., Ardito, E.A. & Lucas, C.P. (1992) Long-term follow-up of patients attending a combination very-low calorie diet and behaviour therapy weight loss programme. *International Journal of Obesity* **16**, 605–613.

Holmér, I. (1974) Physiology of swimming man. *Acta Physiologica Scandinavica* (suppl. **407**), 7–55.

Horber, F.F., Kohler, S.A., Lippuner, K. & Jaeger, P. (1996) Effect of regular physical training on age-associated alteration of body composition in men. *European Journal of Clinical Investigation* **26**, 279–285.

Hurley, B.F., Nemeth, P.M., Martin III, W.H., Hagberg, J.M., Dalsky, G.P. & Holloszy, J.O. (1986) Muscle triglyceride utilization during exercise: effect of training. *Journal of Applied Physiology* **60**, 562–567.

Jakicic, J.M., Donnelly, J.E., Pronk, N.P., Jawad, A.F. & Jacobsen, D.J. (1995a) Prescription of exercise intensity for the obese patient: the relationship between heart rate, VO_2 and perceived exertion. *International Journal of Obesity* **19**, 382–387.

Jakicic, J.M., Wing, R.R., Butler, B.A. & Robertson, R.J. (1995b) Prescribing exercise in multiple short bouts versus one continuous bout: effects on adherence, cardiorespiratory fitness, and weight loss in overweight women. *International Journal of Obesity* **19**, 893–901.

Kannaley, J.A., Cryer, P.E. & Jensen, M.D. (1993) Fatty acid kinetic responses to exercise. Effects of obesity, body fat distribution, and energy-restricted diet. *Journal of Clinical Investigation* **92**, 225–261.

Kang, J., Robertson, R.J., Hagberg, J.M. *et al.* (1996) Effect of exercise intensity on glucose and insulin metabolism in obese individuals and obese NIDDM patients. *Diabetes Care* **19**, 341–349.

Kayman, S., Bruvold, W. & Stern, J.S. (1990) Maintenance and relapse after weight loss in women: behavioral aspects. *American Journal of Clinical Nutrition* **52**, 800–807.

Keim, N.L., Barbieri, T.F. & Belko, A.Z. (1990) The effect of exercise on energy intake and body composition in overweight women. *International Journal of Obesity* **14**, 335–346.

Kempen, K.P.G. (1996) Metabolic effects of weight cycling in obesity. Maastrict: Universitaire Pers Maastrict.

King, A.C., Taylor, C.B., Haskell, W.L. & DeBusk, R.F. (1989) Influence of regular aerobic exercise on psychological health: A randomized controlled trial of healthy middle-aged adults. *Health Psychology* **8**, 305–324.

King, N.A. & Blundell, J.E. (1995) High-fat foods overcome the energy expenditure due to exercise after cycling and running. *European Journal of Clinical Nutrition* **49**, 114–123.

King, N.A., Burley, V.J. & Blundell, J.E. (1994) Exercise-induced suppression of appetite: effects on food intake and implications for energy balance. *European Journal of Clinical Nutrition* 48, 715–724.

King, N.A., Snell, L., Smith, R.D. & Blundell, J.E. (1996) Effects of short-term exercise on appetite responses in unrestrained females. *European Journal of Clinical Nutrition* 50, 663–667.

Klein, S., Coyle, E.F. & Wolfe, R.R. (1994) Fat metabolism during low-intensity exercise in endurance-trained and untrained men. *American Journal of Physiology* 267, E934–E940.

Klein, S., Weber, J., Coyle, E.F. & Wolfe, R.R. (1996) Effect of endurance training on glycerol kinetics during strenuous exercise in humans. *Metabolism* 45, 357–361.

Kohrt, W.M., Obert, K.A. & Holloszy, J.O. (1992) Exercise training improves fat distribution patterns in 60- to 70-year-old men and women. *Journal of Gerontology* 47, M99–M105.

Kohrt, W.M., Landt, M. & Birge, S.J. (1996) Serum leptin levels are reduced in response to exercise training, but not hormone replacement therapy, in older women. *Journal of Clinical Endocrinology and Metabolism* 81, 3980–3985.

Krotkiewski, M., Bylund-Fallenius, A., Holm, J., Björntorp, P., Grimby, G. & Mandroukas, K. (1983) Relationship between muscle morphology and metabolism in obese women: the effects of long-term physical training. *European Journal of Clinical Investigation* 13, 5–12.

Krotkiewski, M., Lönnroth, P., Mandroukas, K. *et al.* (1985) The effects of physical training on insulin secretion and effectiveness and on glucose metabolism in obesity and Type 2 (non-insulin-dependent) diabetes mellitus. *Diabetologia* 28, 881–890.

Lamarche, B., Deprés, J.P., Pouliot, M.C. *et al.* (1992) Is body fat loss a determinant factor in the improvement of carbohydrate and lipid metabolism following aerobic exercise training in obese women? *Metabolism* 41, 1249–1256.

Leijssen, D.P.C., van Baak, M.A., Campfield, L.A. & Saris, W.H.M. (1997) The influence of energy balance and exercise on 24 hour plasma leptin profile. *International Journal of Obesity* 21 (suppl. 2), S102.

Martin III, W.H., Dalsky, G.P., Hurley, B.F. *et al.* (1993) Effect of endurance training on plasma free fatty acid turnover and oxidation during exercise. *American Journal of Physiology* 265, E708–E714.

Mayer, J., Roy, P. & Mitra, K.P. (1956) Relation between caloric intake, body weight, and physical work: studies in an industrial male population in West Bengal. *American Journal of Clinical Nutrition* 4, 169–175.

McArdle, W.D., Katch, F.I. & Katch, V.L. (1996) *Exercise Physiology, Energy, Nutrition and Human Performance*. Baltimore: Williams & Wilkins.

Meijer, G.A.L., Janssen, G.M.E., Westerterp, K.R., Verhoeven, F., Saris, W.H.M. & Ten Hoor, F. (1991a) The effect of a 5-month training programme on physical activity: evidence for a sex difference in the metabolic response to exercise. *European Journal of Applied Physiology* 62, 11–17.

Meijer, G.A.L., Westerterp, K.R., Seyts, G.H.P., Janssen, G.M.E., Saris, W.H.M. & Ten Hoor, F. (1991b) Body composition and sleeping metabolic rate in response to a 5-month endurance-training programme in adults. *European Journal of Applied Physiology* 62, 18–21.

Miller, W.C., Wallace, J.P. & Eggert, K.E. (1991) Predicting max HR and the HR-VO$_2$ relationship for exercise prescription in obesity. *Medicine and Science in Sports and Exercise* 25, 1077–1081.

Morgan, T.E., Short, F.A. & Cobb, L.A. (1969) Effect of long-term exercise on skeletal muscle lipid composition. *American Journal of Physiology* 216, 82–86.

Morgan, W.P. & Goldston, S.E. (eds) (1987) *Exercise and Mental Health*. New York: Hemisphere.

Oscai, L.B. (1973) The role of exercise in weight control. *Exercise and Sport Sciences Reviews* 1, 103–123.

Paffenbarger, R.S., Wing, A.L., Hyde, R.T. *et al.* (1983) Physical activity and incidence of hypertension in college alumni. *American Journal of Epidemiology* 117, 245–257.

Pavlou, K.N., Krey, S. & Steffee, W. (1989) Exercise as an adjunct to weight loss and maintenance in moderately obese subjects. *American Journal of Clinical Nutrition* 49, 1115–1123.

Phillips, S.M., Green, H.J., Tarnapolsky, M.A., Heigenhauser, G.J.F. & Grant, S.M. (1996a) Progressive effect of endurance training on metabolic adaptations in working skeletal muscle. *American Journal of Physiology* 270, E265–E272.

Phillips, S.M., Green, H.J., Tarnapolsky, M.A.M, Heigenhauser, G.J.F., Hill, R.E. & Grant, S.M. (1996b) Effects of training duration on substrate turnover and oxidation during exercise. *Journal of Applied Physiology* **81**, 2182–2191.

Plante, T.G. & Rodin, J. (1990) Physical fitness and enhanced psychological health. *Current Psychology: Research Review* **9**, 3–24.

Poehlman, E.T., Tremblay, A., Nadeau, A., Dussault, J., Thériault, G. & Bouchard, C. (1986) Heredity and changes in hormones and metabolic rates with short-term training. *American Journal of Physiology* **250**, E711–E717.

Poehlman, E.T., Melby, C.L., Badylak, S.F. & Calles, J. (1989) Aerobic fitness and resting energy expenditure in young adult males. *Metabolism* **38**, 85–90.

Poehlman, E.T., Melby, C.L. & Goran, M.I. (1991) The impact of exercise and diet restriction on daily energy expenditure. *Sports Medicine* **11**, 78–101.

Poehlman, E.T., Gardner, A.W., Arciero, P.J., Goran, M.I. & Calles-Escandon, J. (1994) Effects of endurance training on total fat oxidation in elderly persons. *Journal of Applied Physiology* **76**, 2281–2287.

Prentice, A.M., Goldberg, G.R., Jebb, S.A., Black, A.E., Murgatroyd, P. & Diaz, E.O. (1991) Physiological responses to slimming. *Proceedings of the Nutrition Society* **50**, 441–458.

Racette, S.B., Schoeller, D.A., Kushner, R.F. & Neil, K.M. (1995) Exercise enhances dietary compliance during moderate energy restriction in obese women. *American Journal of Clinical Nutrition* **62**, 345–349.

Ravussin, E. & Bogardus, C. (1989) Relationship of genetics, age, and physical fitness to daily energy expenditure and fuel utilization. *American Journal of Clinical Nutrition* **49**, 968–975.

Richard, D. (1995) Exercise and the neurobiological control of food intake and energy expenditure. *International Journal of Obesity* **19** (suppl. 4), S73–S79.

Rissanen, A.M., Heliövaara, M., Knekt, P., Reunanen, A. & Aromaa, A. (1991) Determinants of weight gain and overweight in adult Finns. *European Journal of Clinical Nutrition* **45**, 419–430.

Romijn, J.A., Coyle, E.F., Sidossis, L.S. *et al.* (1993) Regulation of endogenous fat and carbohydrate metabolism in relation to exercise intensity and duration. *American Journal of Physiology* **265**, E380–E391.

Ruby, B.C. & Roberts, R.A. (1994) Gender differences in substrate utilisation during exercise. *Sports Medicine* **17**, 393–410.

Salusso-Deonier, C.J. & Schwarzkopf, R.J. (1991) Sex differences in body cathexis associated with exercise involvement. *Perceptual Motor Skills* **73**, 139–145.

Saris, W.H.M. (1989) Physiological aspects of exercise in weight cycling. *American Journal of Clinical Nutrition* **49**, 1099–1104.

Saris, W.H.M. (1993) The role of exercise in the dietary treatment of obesity. *International Journal of Obesity* **17** (suppl. 1), S17–S21.

Saris, W.H.M. (1995) Exercise with or without dietary restriction and obesity treatment. *International Journal of Obesity* **19** (suppl. 4), S113–S116.

Saris, W.H.M. & van Baak, M.A. (1994) Consequences of exercise on energy expenditure. In: Hills, A.P. & Wahlqvist, M.L. (eds) *Exercise and Obesity*, pp. 85–102. London: Smith-Gordon.

Saris, W.H.M., van Erp-Baart, M.A., Brouns, F.J.P.H., Westerterp, K.R. & Ten Hoor, F. (1989) Study on food intake and energy expenditure during extreme sustained exercise: the Tour de France. *International Journal of Sports Medicine* **10** (suppl. 1), S26–S31.

Schulz, L.O., Nyomba, B.L., Alger, S., Anderson, T.E. & Ravussin, E. (1991) Effect of endurance training on sedentary energy expenditure measured in a respiratory chamber. *American Journal of Physiology* **260**, E257–E261.

Schwartz, R.S., Shuman, W.P., Larson, V. *et al.* (1991) The effect of intensive endurance exercise training on body fat distribution in young and older men. *Metabolism* **40**, 545–551.

Segal, K.R. (1995) Exercise and thermogenesis in obesity. *International Journal of Obesity* **19** (suppl. 4), S80–S87.

Segal, K.R., Gutin, B., Albu, J. & Pi-Sunyer, X.F. (1987) Thermic effects of food and exercise in lean and obese men of similar lean body mass. *American Journal of Physiology* **252**, E110–E117.

Segal, K.R., Blando, L., Ginsberg-Fellner, F. & Edano, A. (1992) Postprandial thermogenesis at rest and postexercise before and after physical training in lean, obese and mildly diabetic men. *Metabolism* 41, 868–878.

Simoes, E.J., Byers, T., Coates, R.J., Serdula, M.K., Mokdad, A.H. & Heath, G.W. (1995) The association between leisure-time physical activity and dietary fat in American adults. *American Journal of Public Health* 85, 240–244.

Simoneau, J. (1995) Adaptation of human skeletal muscle to exercise-training. *International Journal of Obesity* 19 (suppl. 4), S9–S13.

Simoneau, J. & Bouchard, C. (1995) Skeletal muscle metabolism and body fat content in men and women. *Obesity Research* 3, 23–29.

Sjöström, L.V. (1992) Morbidity in severely obese subjects. *American Journal of Clinical Nutrition* 55, 508S–515S.

Skinner, J.S., Hutsler, R., Bergteinova, V. & Buskirk, E.R. (1973) Perception of effort during different types of exercise and under different environmental conditions. *Medicine and Science in Sports and Exercise* 5, 110–115.

Staten, M. (1991) The effect of exercise on food intake in men and women. *American Journal of Clinical Nutrition* 53, 27–31.

Svendsen, O.L., Hassager, C. & Christiansen, C. (1994) Six months' follow-up on exercise added to a short-term diet in overweight postmenopausal women—effects on body composition, resting metabolic rate, cardiovascular risk factors and bone. *International Journal of Obesity* 18, 692–698.

Svendsen, O.L., Krotkiewski, M., Hassager, C. & Christiansen, C. (1996) Effects on muscles of dieting with or without exercise in overweight postmenopausal women. *Journal of Applied Physiology* 80, 1365–1370.

Swan, P.D. & Howley, E.T. (1993) Substrate utilization during prolonged exercise in obese women differing in body fat distribution. *International Journal of Obesity* 18, 263–268.

Tarnopolsky, L.J., MacDougall, J.D., Atkinson, S.A., Tarnopolsky, M.A. & Sutton, J.R. (1990) Gender differences in substrate for endurance exercise. *Journal of Applied Physiology* 68, 302–308.

Thompson, D.A., Wolfe, L.A. & Eikelboom, R. (1988) Acute effects of exercise intensity on appetite in young men. *Medicine and Science in Sports and Exercise* 20, 222–227.

Thörne, A. & Wahren, J. (1989) Diet-induced thermogenesis in well-trained subjects. *Clinical Physiology* 9, 295–305.

Toth, M.J. & Poehlman, E.T. (1996) Effects of exercise on daily energy expenditure. *Nutrition Reviews* 54, S140–S148.

Tremblay, A. & Buemann, B. (1995) Exercise-training, macronutrient balance and body weight control. *International Journal of Obesity* 19, 79–86.

Tremblay, A., Fontaine, E., Poehlman, E.T., Mitchell, D., Perron, L. & Bouchard, C. (1986) The effect of exercise-training on resting metabolic rate in lean and moderately obese individuals. *International Journal of Obesity* 10, 511–517.

Tremblay, A., Nadeau, A., Després, J.P., St-Jean, L., Thériault, G. & Bouchard, C. (1990a) Long-term exercise training with constant energy intake. 2: Effect on glucose metabolism and resting energy expenditure. *International Journal of Obesity* 14, 75–84.

Tremblay, A., Després, J.P., Leblanc, C. *et al.* (1990b) Effect of intensity of physical activity on body fatness and fat distribution. *American Journal of Clinical Nutrition* 51, 153–157.

Tremblay, A., Coveney, S., Després, J., Nadeau, A. & Prud'homme, D. (1992) Increased resting metabolic rate and lipid oxidation in exercise-trained individuals: evidence for a role of β-adrenergic stimulation. *Canadian Journal of Physiology and Pharmacology* 70, S1342–1347.

Tremblay, A., Simoneau, J. & Bouchard, C. (1994a) Impact of exercise intensity on body fatness and skeletal muscle metabolism. *Metabolism* 43, 814–818.

Tremblay, A., Alméras, N., Boer, J., Kranenbarg, E.K. & Després, J.P. (1994b) Diet composition and postexercise energy balance. *American Journal of Clinical Nutrition* 59, 975–979.

Treuth, M.S., Hunter, G.R., Weinsier, R.L. & Kell, S.H. (1995) Energy expenditure and substrate utilization in older women after strength training: 24-h calorimeter results. *Journal of Applied Physiology* 78, 2140–2146.

Tsetsonis, N.V. & Hardman, A.E. (1996) Reduction in postprandial lipemia after walking: influence of exercise intensity. *Medicine and Science in Sports and Exercise* **28**, 1235–1242.

van Baak, M.A. (1979) *The Physiological Load during Walking, Cycling, Running and Swimming, and the Cooper Exercise Programs.* Meppel: Krips Repro.

van Dale, D., Saris, W.H.M. & Ten Hoor, F. (1990) Weight maintenance and resting metabolic rate 18–40 months after a diet/exercise treatment. *International Journal of Obesity* **14**, 347–359.

Wade, A.J., Marbut, M.M. & Round, J.M. (1990) Muscle fibre type and aetiology of obesity. *Lancet* **335**, 805–808.

Weigle, D.S., Sande, K.J., Iverius, P.H., Monsen, E.R. & Brunzell, J.D. (1988) Weight loss leads to a marked decrease in nonresting energy expenditure in ambulatory subjects. *Metabolism* **37**, 930–938.

Williams, P.T., Krauss, R.M., Vranizan, K.M., & Wood, P.D. (1990) Changes in lipoprotein subfractions during diet-induced and exercise-induced weight loss in moderately overweight men. *Circulation* **81**, 1293–1304.

Williamson, D.F., Madans, J., Anda, R.F., Kleinman, J.C., Kahn, H.S. & Byers, T. (1993) Recreational physical activity and ten-year weight change in a US national cohort. *International Journal of Obesity* **17**, 279–286.

Wilmore, J.H. (1995) Variations in physical activity habits and body composition. *International Journal of Obesity* **19** (suppl. 4), S107–S112.

Wilmore, J.H. & Costill, D.L. (1994) *Physiology of Sport and Exercise.* Champaign: Human Kinetics.

Wing, R.R., Jeffery, R.W., Pronk, N. & Hellerstedt, W.L. (1996) Effects of a personal trainer and financial incentives on exercise adherence in overweight women in a behavioral weight loss program. *Obesity Research* **4**, 457–462.

Woo, R. & Pi-Sunyer, F.X. (1985) Effect of increased physical activity on voluntary intake in lean women. *Metabolism* **34**, 836–841.

Woo, R., Garrow, J.S. & Pi-Sunyer, F.X. (1982) Effect of exercise on spontaneous calorie intake in obesity. *American Journal of Clinical Nutrition* **36**, 470–477.

Wood, P.D. (1996) Clinical applications of diet and physical activity in weight loss. *Nutrition Reviews* **54**, S131–S135.

Wood, P.D., Stefanick, M.L., Dreon, D.M. *et al.* (1988) Changes in plasma lipids and lipoproteins in overweight men during weight loss through dieting as compared with exercise. *New England Journal of Medicine* **319**, 1173–1179.

Young, J.C., Treadway, J.L., Balon, T.W., Gavras, H.P. & Ruderman, N.B. (1986) Prior exercise potentiates the thermic effect of a carbohydrate load. *Metabolism* **35**, 1048–1053.

Zahorska-Markiewicz, B. (1980) Thermic effect of food and exercise in obesity. *European Journal of Applied Physiology* **44**, 231–235.

CHAPTER 19

Drug Treatment of Obesity: General Principles and Current Therapies

ROLAND T. JUNG

The ideal weight-reducing drug

Despite the health benefits and social incentives for weight reduction, obese subjects are often unsuccessful in achieving, and then maintaining, weight loss with diet restriction even when combined with behavioural therapy and increased exercise. Because of this, pharmacological agents have been used to promote weight loss or to increase compliance with a weight-loss programme. The ideal drug treatment should produce dose-related weight loss, permit the user to achieve and maintain their weight-loss goal, be safe when used chronically and have no tolerance and addictive potential. To date, no such drug has been devised but the potential is there for research to lead the way forward. Nevertheless, the present concept for the use of such drugs for the treatment of obesity will require adjustment. Restrictions for the pharmacological treatment of obesity presently differs from that advised for all other chronic diseases. When treating hypertension, diabetes, cardiovascular disease or hyperlipidaemia, clinicians accept the need for continued drug usage to improve the situation and in so doing accept that this may not necessarily normalize parameters. Clinicians also accept that the drug has to be maintained if the abnormal condition is to be controlled. This is quite unlike the present policy as applied to the obese person where weight-reducing agents are often expected to promote normal weight within the regulation imposed period of treatment, often 12 weeks, and then patients are expected to maintain their weight loss indefinitely after discontinuation of therapy; such expectation is unreasonable. Obesity is no different from say diabetes where the glycaemic condition is rigorously treated long term, and yet despite obesity being a major determinant in many, vigorous weight-reduction therapy is often ignored in most long-term diabetic therapy plans. Weight-reducing drugs need to be given long term and therefore must be safe to do so. Most importantly they need to be effective although the concept that the agent needs to have the ability to reduce weight to the ideal is unnecessary as a reduction of 5–10% of body-weight is now known to have a profound effect on disease parameters and if this modest reduction is maintained can be effective on the body's health economy.

Weight-reducing drugs appear to be effective in some but not others even when compliance is not a problem. The most likely explanation is that there are subsets of patients who do not respond to a particular drug agent as their obesity problem may not be related to that agent's corrective action. This is not surprising if one considers the polygenic nature of the genetic influence on body-weight where over 20 genes may be implicated with one or more in dominance in one patient compared to another. This implies that different individual drugs or combinations may be required in the future somewhat akin to the experience in hypertension, hyperlipidaemia and non-insulin-dependent diabetes mellitus (NIDDM). Another difficulty with the presently available anorectic drugs is that they tend to lose their effect after 3–6 months. This plateau effect is not due to a compliance problem, or to tolerance, or to a lessening in support from health-care professionals. Some have conjectured whether this is due to some influence of cortical centres which overcome the hypothalamic effects of such agents or to the control of acute and chronic weight loss being under different physiological influences (Goldstein & Potvin, 1994). This requires further detailed research but has the implication that drugs used for acute weight loss may be different from those that might have to be used for long-term control.

Guidelines for usage

Guidelines for the use of weight-reducing drugs have been recently issued in the U.K. by the Scottish Intercollegiate Guidelines Network (Obesity in Scotland: integrating prevention with weight management, 1996) and expanded by a report from the Royal College of Physicians of London (Overweight and the obese patients: principles of management with particular reference to the use of drugs, 1997). The advice given mainly concerned dexfenfluramine, but with the withdrawal of fenfluramine and dexfenfluramine both reports have been revised and no specific drug for use in obesity has been advocated in U.K. This situation is to be reconsidered as and when new drugs are licensed (e.g., orlistat and sibutramine). Nevertheless, the principles for use of such agents still require consideration. Both reports advise use of anorectic or other obesity-reducing drugs only when weight loss achieved by a weight management programme consisting of diet with behavioural modification and an exercise plan, did not achieve a 10% weight loss over 3 months. The patients recommended for such therapy should have a body mass index (BMI) of $30 kg/m^2$ or more. The guidelines recommended that the drug be given at the prescribed dosage for up to 12 weeks in the first instance with the goal of achieving at least a 10% weight loss from the outset of the management plan. If not achieved the drug should cease

Table 19.1 FDA guidance on the development of drugs for treating obesity. From Finer (1997).

- Encourage new drugs that will be efficacious, safe, for specific aetiology
- Foster development for long-term or indefinite use
- Demonstrate benefit that is greater than with diet, exercise, behavioural modification alone
- Weight loss on drug treatment at 1 year should exceed placebo by at least 5% of baseline weight
- Significant improvement in co-morbidity and/or quality of life
- Exhibit safety commensurate with efficacy and projected duration of use

but if successful may be continued for as long as its licence allows with careful monitoring for adverse events.

An important use of such agents may be their ability to directly influence other co-morbid risk factors independent of weight loss, such as lipid profile and glycaemic control in NIDDM patients (O'Kane *et al.*, 1994). Such duality of action on both weight and a co-morbid risk factor and the use of clear guidelines with strict monitoring for adverse events might encourage acceptance for long-term usage of newer agents amongst the many physicians who up to now have not favoured their prescription. In the U.S.A., the Food and Drugs Administration (FDA) have issued guidance concerning the standards of clinical efficacy necessary for registering new anti-obesity treatments as shown in Table 19.1

The need for properly constructed evidence-based trials

There is also a need to improve the evidence basis for the efficacy and long-term safety of such drugs by properly executed trials of sufficient numbers to give meaningful results. Small inadequate trials have hindered the interpretation of the effectiveness or otherwise of weight-reduction agents. Such trials should be carried out according to Good Clinical Practice and have appropriate pretrial statistical evaluation of the population size required for valid statistical results (Table 19.2). Trials have often been conducted over too short a time, such as 8 weeks, were often in the past not placebo controlled, were not done in a double-blind manner, were not clearly randomized and had no run-in period of assessment. Drug compliance must be rigorously secured by at least counting the pills given and returned, with possibly some other blood or urine check. Adjuvant therapy is often ignored but is vital in assessing trials. For instance one needs to know the diet used, the quality of care provided by the therapist, whether the groups visited more than one therapist and if so the method used to control for this and whether behavioural therapy and exercise were included.

Table 19.2 Checklist for a weight-reduction drug trial.

- Ethical approval
- Good Clinical Practice procedure
- Pretrial statistical evaluation of trial size
- Patient selection criteria
  Age
  Sex
  Assessment for eating disorders
  Psychological assessment
  Types; persistent diet failures or otherwise
  Motivation
  Insight by patients
- Study characteristics
  Run-in time
  Length of study
  Randomized
  Double blind
  Placebo controlled
  Compliance checks
  Adjuvant therapy
     Quality of care provided by the therapist
     Frequency of visits throughout trial consistency
     Group vs individual therapy
     Diet type
     Behavioural therapy
     Exercise regimen
     Therapy for co-morbid conditions
  Post-trial follow-up
- Analysis
  Intention to treat
  Completion basis
- Use of standards for evaluating the 'success' of the trial

One also needs to know the frequency of visits, whether in a group or individual session, whether there is pretrial assessment of motivation and psychological indicators, and the influence of co-morbid conditions and their treatment.

Patient selection is often not well described and yet is crucial for interpretation of the final results in comparison with trials reported by others. For instance, was the number of binge eaters and those with eating disorders controlled in the trial? Was the state of the pretrial psychological pattern assessed in each patient especially for those with significant depression such that the groups had similar representation? Often trials consist of patients who had failed all previous attempts to lose weight which is not representative of the population at large where the drug is likely to be marketed and may differ in effectiveness.

There is also a tendency for negative results not to be published or unavailable to those conducting meta-analysis often resulting in a skewed interpretation of a drug's potential and side-effect profile resulting in subsequent prescriber indifference if not hostility. Long-term data beyond 1 year is often lacking and is essential for any clinical recommendation for chronic usage. Similarly long-term post-trial follow-up is necessary especially for weight regain. Studies on patients with significant co-morbid diseases such as hypertension and hyperlipidaemia are required although studies in diabetes are now becoming available. Statistical analysis of the results of such trials are often confusing with some analysed on an 'intention to treat' basis whereas others by 'completion'. It is not surprising, therefore, that the popularity and acceptance of drug therapy for obesity management is poor amongst doctors in general.

Standards for evaluating a weight-reduction trial

In recent years clinicians and the FDA have begun to set some standard evaluating criteria (see Table 19.1) for the effectiveness of such weight-reducing drugs. Sayler *et al.* (1994) have suggested criteria for the evaluation of a weight-reduction clinical trial. The first requirement sets out three follow-up periods to adjudicate on success designated 'minimum' (6 months), 'intermediate' (24 months) and 'full' (60 months). Each period has a differing set of endpoints. Briefly a 'minimum' endpoint would expect a 5–10%, 'intermediate' a 50% and 'full' a 100% improvement in the parameters measured. Weight alone or BMI would not be sufficient for there is a need to assess obesity-related co-morbid risk factors such as systolic blood pressure, diastolic pressure, HbA_{1c}, blood glucose, total cholesterol, low-density lipoprotein (LDL) to high-density lipoprotein (HDL) cholesterol ratio and triglycerides; all biochemistry measured in the fasting state. Categorization of overall success of the trial would be defined by evaluating changes across factors simultaneously. A potential definition of overall success of the trial would be based on success in at least one weight-related factor (such as kilogram weight or BMI) and at least one of the above designated obesity-related risk factors (see the section on fluoxetine for an example). They also suggest restricting analysis to those patients who complete the trial. Alternatively, they suggest all randomized patients could be included and any patient who discontinues early considered a failure and designated as such. However, if the discontinuation rates are similar between treatments, then all could be included on an 'intention to treat' basis as treatment differences in success rates using any of the above criteria would be approximately the same. Finally, the need to assess that a patient does not worsen during a trial is covered by specific definitions applied across all three levels of success (Sayler *et al.*, 1994). Another checklist for 'success' in a trial is given in Table 19.3 from

Table 19.3 Indicators of success. Based on suggested outcome indicators in *Management of Obesity in Scotland* (1996).

- Weight loss
  Success > 5 kg
  Excellence > 10 kg
  Exceptional > 20 kg
- Weight maintenance
  Weight regain limited to <3 kg over 2 years' follow-up
  Maintain waist circumference reduction of > 4 cm
- Co-morbidity
  Reduction in:
  Systolic pressure
  Diastolic pressure
  Cholesterol
  HDL-cholesterol
  LDL/HDL cholesterol
  Triglycerides
  Fasting blood glucose
  HbA_{1c}

Management of Obesity in Scotland (1996). The potential abuse of weight-reducing drugs is also a limitation on licensing and widespread usage but this could be controlled in medical circles by proper physician-derived guidelines strictly adhered to in all sectors whether public or private possibly as a condition of the drug licence and individual prescribing, with the necessary audit and commercial clinic licence to ensure adherence.

General classification

In a review of data from weight-reduction trials in 7725 patients, the available pharmacological agents were found to produce weight loss on average of 0.23 kg/week greater than placebo in the short term with very little available information on long-term usage (Goldstein & Potvin, 1994). The main classes of drugs available or about to be available operate by either inducing malabsorption or through appetite suppression or via thermogenesis to increase energy expenditure. They will be now discussed under these three headings.

Gastro-intestinal acting agents

Attempts have been made to reduce caloric intake by producing feelings of satiety with the use of bulk-forming agents such as bran or methylcellulose. There is little evidence to support this claim. Cimetidine has been reported to promote weight loss. In one trial of cimetidine 200 mg or placebo with a 5 MJ (1200 kcal)/day diet, weight loss was reported 7.3 kg greater on the drug than on placebo (Stoa-Birketvedt, 1993). Waist/hip ratio and perceived hunger were reduced on cimetidine. The mechanism of action is speculative but was suggested to be a reduction in hunger brought about by a decrease in gastric acid output. Nevertheless, another trial similarly conducted failed to confirm these findings, with no significant difference in weight loss on cimetidine vs placebo (Rasmussen *et al.*, 1993). Another strategy is to restrict the bioavailability of dietary energy intake. Cholestyramine has been used but gastro-intestinal side-effects have made it unpopular. Diethyl aminoethyl dextran (DEAED) which acts in a similar fashion to cholestyramine by binding bile acids, has been tried in obese humans (Cairella, 1987). Weight loss over 6 weeks averaged 0.83 kg/week compared with 0.41 kg/week on placebo. Side-effects of flatulence, loose stools and abdominal borborygmus and fullness are disadvantages.

Orlistat (tetrahydrolipstatin)

Orlistat is a chemically synthesized hydrogenated derivative of lipstatin, itself produced by *Streptomyces toxytricini*. This substance is a potent inhibitor of gastric, pancreatic and carboxylester lipase (Hogan *et al.*, 1987). Orlistat acts by binding covalently to the serine residue of the active site of gastric and pancreatic lipases. Given orally it operates within the lumen of the gut reducing ingested triglyceride hydrolysis. It produces a dose-dependent reduction in dietary fat absorption, which is near maximal at a dose of 120 mg thrice daily. This produces a 30% inhibition of dietary fat absorption which can contribute to an additional caloric deficit of approximately 0.8 MJ (200 kcal)/24 hours (Guerciolini, 1997). Orlistat is only minimally absorbed with carbon-14-labelled studies indicating faecal recovery of 96.4% and urinary excretion of 1.13% (Zhi *et al.*, 1996a). Two major metabolites have been reported one with a 2-hour half-life, the other somewhat longer, with a plasma t_{max} of 6.8 hours. The timing of dosage need not be mid-meal, as administration at 0.5, 1 and 2 hours postprandial is equally effective as measured by faecal fat excretion (Hussain *et al.*, 1994).

A short-term five-centre trial (Drent *et al.*, 1995a) showed that weight loss was dose dependent. After 12 weeks orlistat produced an additional weight loss compared to placebo of 0.63 kg with 30 mg, 0.71 kg with 180 mg and 1.75 kg with 360 mg/day. A 1-year single-centre study of orlistat 360 mg/day on a diet containing 30% of calories as fat and designed to produce an energy deficit of 2.5 MJ (600 kcal)/day, resulted in a weight reduction of 8.6 kg (8.4%) compared to placebo of 5.5 kg (5.7%) at 6 months out (James *et al.*, 1997). Thereafter the placebo group regained weight whereas the orlistat group maintained their loss with a 2.6% weight loss at 1 year on placebo compared to 8.4% on orlistat. A multicentre 1-year U.K. trial of 267 patients given orlistat 360 mg/day showed a weight loss of 8.5% compared to 5.4% on placebo (Finer, 1997). Some 28% of those on orlistat lost more than 10% of initial body-weight compared to 17% of the placebo group based on intention to treat basis. Weight loss involved fat with little change in lean body mass. Further 1 year and 2 year studies are underway but have yet to report.

Orlistat has also been investigated in patients with hyperlipidaemia unresponsive to dietary change (Tonstad et al., 1994). In a multicentre, randomized double-blind study of 173 patients (BMI 25 kg/m^2) orlistat was given at variable dosages over 8 weeks with a weight maintenance diet. Weight decreased significantly (1.2 kg) only on the 360-mg dosage. Total cholesterol was reduced by 4–11% and LDL-cholesterol by 5–10% depending on dosage. HDL-cholesterol was unaltered except on the highest dosage where it decreased 8%. Triglyceride was unchanged but there was a reduction in apolipoprotein AI and B (up to 10%) on all dosages but not on placebo. Postprandial triglyceridaemia has been reported to be reduced by 27% (Reitsma et al., 1994) with 19% decrease in chylomicrons. The most likely mechanism involves a decrease in chylomicron formation by a reduced absorption of intestinal triglyceride due to the action of orlistat. The reduced delivery of dietary lipid and fatty acids to the liver is associated with up-regulation of hepatic LDL receptors resulting in a decrease in LDL-cholesterol. Trials in patients with diabetes have been completed and are awaiting full evaluation but do indicate a significant improvement in glycaemic control in both established diabetes and in those with impaired glucose handling. Over 1 year HbA$_{1c}$ decreased by 0.5%.

Orlistat does not appear on single dosage studies to affect to a clinical significant extent the absorption and pharmacokinetics of drugs with a narrow therapeutic index such as phenytoin (Melia et al., 1996), warfarin (Zhi et al., 1996b), digoxin (Melia et al., 1995), or compounds frequently used by obese patients, e.g., oral contraceptives (Hartmann et al., 1996), glyburide (Zhi et al., 1995), pravastatin, atenolol, captopril, frusemide and slow-release nifedipine (Weber et al., 1996). Orlistat has been reported not to produce significant disturbance to gastric emptying, gastric acidity, gallbladder motility, bile composition and lithogenicity (Guerciolini, 1997). Others, however, have shown increased gastric emptying when using the double-indicator technique with a triple-lumen duodenal tube (Schwizer et al., 1997). Release of cholecystokinin has been reported either decreased or unchanged (Froehlich et al., 1996; Schwizer et al., 1997). No differences have been noted in the response of thyroid hormones, catecholamines, insulin-like growth factor-1 (IGF-1) and insulin-like growth-factor binding protein-3 (IGFBP-3) between orlistat and placebo treated groups in a 12-week trial (Drent et al., 1995b).

Adverse events have involved the gastro-intestinal tract with soft or liquid stools, abdominal pain, colic, flatus with discharge and faecal urgency or incontinence (3–15%). In all, 38% on 30 mg, 73% on 90 mg and 86% on 360 mg reported one or more gastro-intestinal adverse events (Drent *et al.*, 1995a). In a 12-week trial in 52 subjects (Drent & Van der Veen, 1993) adverse events were described as mild and transient with only one patient having to drop out due to faecal incontinence. Overall, some 5% have to withdraw because of side-effects in trials. Vitamin A was unaltered (Drent & Van der Veen, 1993), vitamin E decreased 3–14% with increasing dosages whereas vitamin D was reduced on 360 mg (Tonstad *et al.*, 1994). Absorption of supplementary vitamin E is reduced by 43–60% by orlistat but not that of vitamin A. Short-term treatment (3–6 days) with orlistat does not alter endogeneous profiles of β-carotene in plasma but when β-carotene was given during orlistat treatment, its absorption was reduced by one-third (Zhi *et al.*, 1996c). Hence two-thirds of a supplemental dose of β-carotene would be absorbed.

Acarbose

Acarbose in an α-glucosidase inhibitor used in diabetes mellitus to reduce carbohydrate absorption. Chronic usage indicates that it does not have any significant weight-reducing potential. Following conventional dietary weight reduction in 24 obese (116 kg to 88 kg), subjects were divided into two groups (William-Olsen *et al.*, 1985). One group was given acarbose (1500 mg/day) for the first year followed by placebo for a second year. Weight increased by 3.7 kg on acarbose during the first year and increased further by 4.0 kg in the second year on placebo. The other group were given placebo in the first year and showed an increase in weight of 10 kg with no increase (0.16 kg) in the second year. This suggests that acarbose might limit weight regain but gastro-intestinal side-effects at the dosage used (some 10-fold higher than now recommended for use in diabetes) would limit its acceptance.

Appetite suppressants

The currently available anorectic drugs belong to one of two groups, namely those that act on the catecholaminergic pathway and those that act on the serotonergic system. Diethylpropion, phentermine and mazindol which act on the catecholaminergic system cause some cerebral activation which may interfere with sleep, although there is a wide individual variability in response. These drugs should be used with care because of the danger of psychological dependence, although most patients do not experience this difficulty on cessation of therapy if the manufacturers' recommended dosages are followed. The clinical use of these agents has been severely curtailed in the U.K. by the General Medical Council due to dependency, potential for abuse and side-effects. In U.S.A. these drugs are classified by the U.S. Drug Enforcement Administration Schedule as class 4 where class 1 represents the most addictive drugs (amphetamine, for example, is classified class 2).

Phentermine

Munro *et al.* (1968) reported a double-blind 36-week trial of continuous and intermittent use of phentermine in 108 obese women. There were three comparable groups, one given placebo, another continuous phentermine (30 mg/ day) and the third given cyclical 4-weekly drug therapy alternating with placebo. All were instructed on a 4.2 MJ/day diet. At 36 weeks those on placebo had lost 4.8 kg, those on continuous phentermine 12.2 kg and the third group on intermittent therapy 13 kg. The overall anorectic effect lasted throughout the study but was more efficacious in the first 5 months of treatment. This trial clearly indicated that intermittent therapy was as effective as continuous medication. Side-effects consisted of central nervous system stimulation namely insomnia, irritability, agitation, tension and anxiety and were severe enough for discontinuance in 8% of patients treated with phentermine (Fig. 19.1).

In another paper from this group (Steel *et al.*, 1973), 175 women on 4.2 MJ/ day diet were given various combinations of fenfluramine or phentermine over a 9-week period. Those on continuous fenfluramine lost 11.9 kg whereas those on intermittent phentermine (week about with placebo) lost a similar weight namely 12.0 kg. Intermittent fenfluramine on a week on and off basis was less efficacious with a 7.9-kg weight loss and was associated with a high default rate and also a high incidence of depression developing several days after the weekly cessation of fenfluramine. Such led to the recommendation that fenfluramine should not be given intermittently, should be contraindicated in those with a history of depression or with active depression and should be tailed off gradually at the end of therapy. This is in contrast to phentermine where intermittent therapy is both effective and advisable to reduce dependence. Steel *et al.* (1973) also reported no benefit by alternating fenfluramine with phentermine on a weekly basis as weight loss was 12.0 kg, similar to continuous fenfluramine or intermittent phentermine therapy but the side-effects were greater and phentermine did not prevent the postfenfluramine depression.

Weintraub *et al.* (1992) has evaluated phentermine (15 mg) combined with fenfluramine (60 mg) in a 4-year study. Initially the study involved 121 subjects over 34 weeks; the combined therapy resulted in a weight loss of 14.2 kg

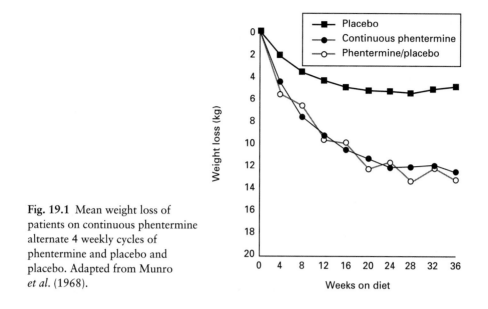

Fig. 19.1 Mean weight loss of patients on continuous phentermine alternate 4 weekly cycles of phentermine and placebo and placebo. Adapted from Munro *et al.* (1968).

(15.9% of initial weight) compared to 4.6 kg loss with placebo. Both groups had instruction on diet, exercise and behavioural therapy with a 6-week run-in before drug therapy began. Weintraub *et al.* (1992) then reported on extensions to this study with various combinations of phentermine and fenfluramine. By week 104, those given continuous combined therapy had lost 11.6 kg from the outset of the trial. Fifty-nine subjects completed a third year of the trial gaining 2.7 kg during this third year but were still on average 9.4 kg below outset. Overall combined therapy in conjunction with behavioural modification, exercise and diet continued to help participants maintain weight loss for up to 3 years. Fewer subjects continued into fourth year, namely 27 on combined therapy and 24 on placebo. By week 190, those on combined therapy were 5.0 kg below their outset weight compared to a loss of 2.1 kg on placebo. Then drug therapy ceased and the subjects were monitored until week 210. The participants had difficulty maintaining their weight loss without anorexiant agents, as by week 210 weight was on average only 1.4 kg below outset. Some in the trial had intermittent therapy and this group did not appear to do as well as those who had continuous treatment. Lipid profiles were also analysed (Weintraub *et al.*, 1992). By week 139, HDL-cholesterol had increased by 27%, total cholesterol to HDL ratio increased by 25% and triglyceride had decreased by 29%. Even after therapy had ceased and most of the weight regrettably regained (week 210), HDL-cholesterol was still 15% above and triglyceride 16% below outset levels. Total cholesterol and LDL-cholesterol showed less dramatic shifts.

The conclusion was that overall this change in lipid profile should have decreased their risk of coronary heart disease but this was not proven. Interestingly only 15.7% of participants left the study due to adverse events.

This most extensive study illustrates the difficulty of weight loss and then maintenance in obesity and indicates the need to consider life-long drug therapy if weight loss and its beneficial effects on health are to be maintained. The authors commented on some salient points noted during this 4-year study. The first was the need to create individual and realistic goals for weight loss and the maintenance. Rebound weight regain was a problem in those who were set too strict a goal and who ironically lost a lot of weight. Success should be measured by a modest weight loss and then the maintenance of this loss. The behavioural programme should not be too ambitious or rigid. The most successful patients did not follow the entire behavioural programme but simply tried to avoid clearly aberrant behaviour, such as bingeing. It was also clear that the behavioural groups should be kept together as any breakup or mixing was detrimental for the patients achieved much support from other members of their group. The exercise programme also should not be too ambitious, as some attempted too much thereby undertaking unsustainable programmes. Subjects did best with consistent, modest exercise programmes. Finally, mention was made that the participants often resented, and even objected to, dealing with dietitians who had never had a weight problem. Of course, not all dietitians treating the obese need to have or have had a weight problem but do need to develop greater empathy and understand more about the stresses and struggles of obese people. The combination of centrally acting anorectic agents cannot now be recommended following the report by Connolly and colleagues in 1997 (see p. 489).

Diethylpropion

McKay (1973) reported a 24-week trial in 20 overweight patients given either placebo or diethylpropion 75 mg/day. On the drug the overall weight loss was 11.7 kg/week compared to 2.5 kg on placebo. On average those receiving diethylpropion lost 0.49 kg/week compared to 0.1 kg/week on placebo. Systolic and diastolic pressures and pulse rate decreased more in the diethyl-propion group and the former was correlated with the weight lost. Side-effects were described as minimal and mainly due to central nervous system stimulation. Hypertensive crises may occur if given during treatment with or within 14 days of a monoamine oxidase inhibitor. Care should be taken with driving during usage due to possible over-stimulation or rebound sedation during and after discontinuation of the drug. The manufacturers suggest that this drug may be used intermittently such as 6 weeks on and off to reduce the risk of dependency. They also emphasize that long-term safety has not been established. In a short-term trial (8 weeks) by Silverstone *et al.* (1970) in 26 subjects it was suggested that diethylpropion was more effective than fenfluramine with twice as many losing more weight on diethylpropion than on fenfluramine, although overall weight losses were disappointing (2.0 vs 1.27 kg).

Mazindol

Mazindol is an imadazo-isoindole anorectic agent which possibly has been best evaluated in the work of Enzi *et al.* (1976) conducted in 102 obese subjects. In their complex analytical evaluations three groups of patients were each treated for 15 weeks continuously but subdivided into five treatment periods each of 3 weeks' duration. The first group (26 subjects) were given diet alone (3–5 MJ/day) for 9 weeks then mazindol for the final 6 weeks. This group lost 6 kg on diet alone and a further 4.2 kg on mazindol making total weight loss 10.2 kg. The second group (26 subjects) were given diet with placebo for 6 weeks then diet alone for 3 weeks and finally mazindol for 6 weeks. Hence this group were similar to the first except for placebo effect. Weight loss was similar namely 6.2 kg in first 9 weeks and then 4.3 kg on mazindol; total weight loss 10.5 kg. The third group of 50 subjects were given mazindol for the initial 6 weeks followed by diet alone for 3 weeks and then diet and placebo for the final 6 weeks. Weight loss on mazindol was 6.2 kg and on diet with or without placebo 0.7 kg; total weight loss 7.0 kg. The weight loss on mazindol for the initial 6 weeks (6.2 kg) was similar statistically to the 4.7 kg lost on diet alone (group 1) or the 5.4 kg lost on diet and placebo (group 2). However, the weight loss with mazindol given in the final 6 weeks (4.2 kg in groups 1 and 2) was significantly greater ($P = 0.001$) than the 0.96 kg lost on diet alone. The conclusion was that mazindol was effective once diet compliance had reduced, namely after 9 weeks of energy restriction.

In another trial (Enzi *et al.*, 1976), 47 women were given mazindol inter-mittently (40–60 days at 1 mg/day) with similar periods on diet alone. Fifteen patients achieved on average 380 days (280–480 days) with 230 days on mazindol and 150 days on diet alone. Controls consisted of 10 patients on diet alone for 400 days. Weight loss in the mazindol group was 14.2 kg compared to 10.2 kg in the controls. Side-effects were frequent consisting of nervousness, insomnia, dizziness, dry mouth, constipation, polyuria and 'goose flesh' with 'chills'. These side-effects attenuated in the long term. Higher dosages of mazindol are associated with a greater prevalence of central nervous system side-effects; 30% on 6 mg/day.

Phenylpropanolamine

This racemic mixture of norephedrine esters is the component of many 'cold cures'. The major action is to stimulate hypothalamic adrenoceptors to decrease appetite rather than alter thermogenesis (Alger *et al.*, 1993). This drug has a low abuse potential and is superior to placebo on weight loss although modest, 0.7–1.8 kg over 4–12 weeks (Morgan & Funderburk, 1990).

Sibutramine

This new drug received U.S. approval for registration in 1997. Sibutramine is a serotonin and noradrenalin re-uptake inhibitor (SRNI) which decreases food intake through β_1- and $5HT_{2A/2C}$-receptor agonist activity and enhances metabolic rate via stimulation of peripheral β_3-receptors. Sibutramine's effects are predominantly mediated by two pharmacologically active metabolites, its primary and secondary amines (Stock, 1997). Sibutramine and its active metabolites do not cause the release of monoamine neurotransmitters and do not have affinity for their receptors. In rodents sibutramine dose dependently inhibits food intake by enhancing the natural physiological process of satiety. It also stimulates thermogenesis in rats producing sustained increases of oxygen consumption of up to 30% as a result of central activation of efferent sympathetic activity which, in turn, activates β_3-adrenoceptors in brown adipose tissue (Stock, 1997). This is considered the cause of the 18-fold increase in brown adipose tissue glucose utilization induced by sibutramine in rats.

In obese individuals sibutramine produces dose-related weight loss when given in the range 5–30 mg/day, with optimal weight loss at 10 and 15 mg/day. In a 12-week trial (Weintraub *et al.*, 1991), 5 mg/day resulted in a 2.9-kg loss whereas 20 mg/day produced a 5.0-kg loss; placebo group lost 1.4 kg. In a double-blind placebo-controlled trial (Bray *et al.*, 1995), sibutramine (30 mg/day) resulted in a 6.1-kg weight reduction over 12 weeks compared to 0.9-kg loss on placebo. A meta-analysis of such data suggests that the percentage of patients losing 5% of baseline weight after 12 weeks is 19% on placebo, 49% for sibutramine 10 mg, and 55% for sibutramine 15 mg (Finer, 1997). In 3-month studies, weight reduction with sibutramine 10 mg/day was similar to dexfenfluramine 15 mg twice daily, or ephedrine/caffeine 20/20 mg 3 times daily or fluoxetine 60 mg/day (Davis & Faulds, 1996).

A large-scale randomized study in 12 U.K. general practices involving 485 patients has been reported by Jones and Heath (1996). Out of the 255 patients who completed treatment for 12 months, 8.3 kg weight loss was achieved with placebo, 10.2 kg on sibutramine 10 mg/day and 10.5 kg on the 15-mg dosage. Over 5% loss of body-weight was achieved in 20% of those on placebo, in

40% on 10 mg of sibutramine and in 57% on 15-mg dosage. Sibutramine-induced weight loss is associated with a reduction in waist/hip ratio, decreases in plasma triglyceride, total cholesterol and low-density lipoprotein (LDL) cholesterol; with increase of high-density lipoprotein (HDL) cholesterol (Lean, 1997). A 12-week study in patients with NIDDM showed a weight loss of 2.4 kg compared to 0.1 kg on placebo with an insignificant 0.4% reduction of glycated haemoglobin (Griffiths *et al.*, 1995). Adverse events include dry mouth, constipation, insomnia, irritability, unusual impatience or excitation, headache, rhinitis and nausea (Weintraub *et al.*, 1991). The noradrenergic effects of sibutramine can cause an increase in heart rate and blood pressure in some, or prevent the expected decrease in blood pressure with weight loss (Finer, 1997).

Dexfenfluramine

Dexfenfluramine is the dextrorotatory isomer of the racemic compound DL-fenfluramine. Although both were withdrawn in 1997 (see later) the extensive world-wide use for decades of fenfluramine and dexfenfluramine necessitates a description of its pharmacology, efficacy and adverse events, as both are often used as baseline comparison in evaluating newer agents. Both these drugs released serotonin from nerve endings and prevented re-uptake, with DL-fenfluramine the first clinically useful appetite suppressant of this type. Possibly the best known study of DL-fenfluramine was reported by Stunkard *et al.* (1980). In an open-label 6-month study in 134 obese patients, DL-fenfluramine at a dosage up to 120 mg/day resulted in a 14.5-kg weight loss; behavioural programme produced 10.9-kg loss, whereas the drug combined with the behavioural education enhanced weight loss to 15.3 kg. Weight regain over 6 months post therapy was the least for the behavioural therapy group. In a study by Hudson (1977) weight loss on 80–120 mg DL-fenfluramine over 1 year was 7.6 kg but much of the weight lost occurred in the first 3 months with a plateau between the eighth and 12th month of therapy. Regain over the second year on placebo was disappointing with all but 1 kg regained. Although this drug is chemically related to amphetamine, the introduction of a CF_3 group into the molecule altered the pharmacological character with a low risk of abuse or dependence. Dependence had been rarely reported and was said to have occurred very seldom in subjects without a history of drug abuse. The UN Commission on Narcotic Drugs had endorsed the WHO recommendation that 'fenfluramine did not have amphetamine-like abuse potential nor was there evidence of significant health or social problems arising from its use'. To improve the specificity on weight reduction at a lower dosage dexfenfluramine had become the preferred choice in U.K. and further discussion will concern this drug alone.

Dexfenfluramine had a terminal half life of 18 hours with a clearance approaching 44 hours in the obese (Cheymol *et al.*, 1995). An international trial from 24 centres (Guy-Grand *et al.*, 1989) of dexfenfluramine (30 mg/day) in 822 obese patients resulted in a 1-year weight loss of 9.8 kg on the drug but 7.2 kg on placebo (Table 19.4). In this trial a variety of diets were used with at least one site using a very-low-calorie diet (VLCD). Review of the weight loss in those who completed the study (Fig. 19.2) indicated that most of the weight loss occurred in the first 6 months, both on the drug and also on placebo, with a slight regain in the final 6 months. Closer scrutiny indicated that twice as many on the drug as on placebo achieved a weight loss of more than 10% of initial weight (35 vs 17%). In another large study involving 819 patients cared for by 243 practising physicians in Austria (Geyer *et al.*, 1995), weight loss over 3 months on dexfenfluramine was 7.7 kg in females and 9.3 kg in males (not placebo controlled). In a detailed study by Mathus-Vliegen *et al.* (1992) in 75 patients with average BMI of 39, on a diet of 4.2 MJ/day and monthly

Table 19.4 Significant adverse events in obesity trials vs placebo using dexfenfluramine. Adapted from Guy-Grand *et al.* (1989).

Adverse event	Dexfenfluramine % ($n = 404$)	Placebo % ($n = 418$)
Tiredness	28	20
Diarrhoea	15	9
Dry mouth	12	4
Polyuria	7	3
Drowsiness	5	2

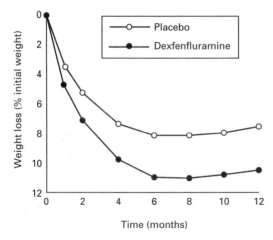

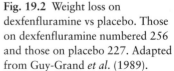

Fig. 19.2 Weight loss on dexfenfluramine vs placebo. Those on dexfenfluramine numbered 256 and those on placebo 227. Adapted from Guy-Grand *et al.* (1989).

follow-up, the patients randomized to dexfenfluramine lost 10.7 kg compared to 8.0 kg on placebo after 12 months. Once again the weight loss was initially rapid on both the drug and placebo with the lowest weight on dexfenfluramine (16.4 kg lost) observed at 7.4 months and at 7.0 months on placebo (12.9 kg). Thereafter there was an increase in weight with a further sharp rise during the final 2 months discontination of the drug or placebo (increased 2.8 kg and 1.0 kg, respectively) between the 12th and 14th months of the study. Of those on dexfenfluramine 39.5% lost more than 10% of their weight compared to 30% on placebo. This study was also one of the centres in the international trial reported by Guy-Grand *et al.* (1989).

Mathus-Vliegen *et al.* (1992) also investigated the effect of dexfenfluramine on cardiovascular risk factors in the above trial. Over the year systolic blood pressure decreased 27.8 and 27.3 mmHg and the diastolic pressure decreased by 17.4 and 14.8 mmHg in the drug and placebo groups, respectively. Total cholesterol showed no significant reduction whereas triglyceride decreased 0.5 mmol/L on dexfenfluramine and 0.22 mmol/L on placebo. Fasting glucose reduced 0.75 mmol/L on the drug compared to 0.14 mmol/L on placebo. Most of the reductions in blood pressure and biochemistry occurred in the first 6 months with a plateau effect parallel to the weight-loss plateau thereafter. Others have also described improvement in cardiovascular risk factors. Pfohl *et al.* (1994) followed 48 patients for 1 year and then 22 for a further 3 years. Dexfenfluramine was given for 1 year only with a 11.2% (10.8 kg) weight loss compared to a 9.1% (8.7 kg) loss on placebo. Systolic pressure declined by 7.3 and 9.9 mmHg on the drug and placebo, respectively, with once again no change in total cholesterol and none in triglyceride or glucose. During the subsequent 3-year follow-up of a subgroup, the previous dexfenfluramine-treated group regained more than the entire weight lost (+1.5 kg) whereas the placebo group regained less and managed to maintain a 2.1-kg weight loss compared to their initial body-weight. Three of the placebo group, but only one of the drug group, maintained a loss of more than 10% of their body-weight. Systolic pressure, cholesterol, triglyceride and glucose all increased to a level greater than at the onset of the study except for diastolic pressure which returned to baseline levels (Table 19.5). This emphasized the need for appropriate preventive measures to hinder weight regain or cardiovascular risk factor deterioration. Whereas most studies report no change in total cholesterol, Holdaway *et al.* (1995) have reported a decrease in cholesterol on dexfenfluramine (−0.38 mmol/L) compared to placebo (−0.06 mmol/L) over 3 months therapy with also improved insulin sensitivity of +11% on the drug and +4% on placebo (weight loss 3.8 vs 1.1 kg on placebo).

The weight lost on dexfenfluramine would appear to involve fat although surprisingly few studies report this parameter. O'Connor *et al.* (1995) studied

Table 19.5 Weight and cardiovascular risk factors at the beginning of the study, after 6 and 12 months on dexfenfluramine and then at 48 months after cessation of the drug at 12 months into the trial. Note the deterioration of all risk factors other than diastolic pressure which returned to baseline. Mean levels only shown with significance based on two way variance of months 12 and 48 compared. Adapted from Pfohl *et al.* (1994).

Parameter	Beginning	6 months	12 months	48 months	Variance 12/48
Weight (kg)	94.5	—	Lost 10.9	Gained 1.5	—
Cholesterol (mmol/L)	5.55	5.59	5.34	6.19	0.0102
Triglycerides (mmol/L)	1.17	1.30	1.27	1.91	0.0019
Glucose (mmol/L)	4.30	3.82	4.17	4.86	0.0002
Systolic pressure (mmHg)	134.1	131.4	126.8	139.1	0.0041
Diastolic pressure (mmHg)	86.4	84.1	80.9	87.3	0.0599

60 subjects over 6 months. Those on dexfenfluramine lost 9.7 kg of which 5 kg was calculated as fat; waist circumference decreased 10.5 cm. On placebo weight loss was 4.9 kg of which only 1 kg was fat and waist decrease was only 5.7 cm. In this study an increase in HDL-cholesterol was reported. Five months after the cessation of dexfenfluramine this same group had regained weight while the placebo group continued weight loss, such that at the 11th month from the outset of the trial both groups had lost similar weight (6.0 kg vs 6.2 kg on placebo). In the study of Pfohl *et al.* (1994) reviewed above, waist/hip ratio decreased 0.08 on dexfenfluramine and 0.04 on placebo which indicates that possibly visceral fat might be reduced but precise measurements for this are needed.

The mechanism of weight loss on dexfenfluramine appears to be mainly by appetite suppression and not by any significant increase in thermogenesis. In one study where no caloric restriction was imposed, caloric intake decreased on dexfenfluramine from 6.7 to 5.6 MJ/day (Lafreniere *et al.*, 1993) with no change in the resting metabolic rate (RMR) or diet-induced thermogenesis (DIT). In another (Van Gaal *et al.*, 1995), RMR expressed per kilogram fat-free mass decreased on placebo but not on dexfenfluramine with a slight increase in the DIT to a glucose load compared to a decrease in the placebo group. However, in this study the diet was a 3.1 MJ/day protein sparing modified fast. Schutz *et al.* (1992) reviewed the literature and came to the conclusion that weight loss on dexfenfluramine above that of placebo was not due to its putative thermogenic effect but directly attributable to its anorectic action. This was further supported by the finding that energy expenditure measured by 24-hour direct heat sink calorimetry did not alter 1 month after cessation of a 13-month trial of dexfenfluramine whether expressed in kilojoules per kilogram body-weight or kilojoules per kilogram per lean mass; this held even when energy expenditure was subdivided into day and night periods.

Dexfenfluramine has also been used as an adjuvant to a very-low-energy restricted diet. Andersen *et al.* (1992) studied 42 subjects on a 1.6 MJ/day formula diet with an additional free intake allowance of up to 2.6 MJ/day in a trial conducted over 1 year. The subjects were randomized to dexfenfluramine or placebo. Weight loss was considerable in both groups (about 14 kg) but in kilogram weight loss both groups were practically identical. The authors then compared the weight lost to the outset weight, as the placebo group were initially heavier. They reported that dexfenfluramine group did better up to 6 months, thereafter weight was regained by both groups such that at 12 months any weight loss difference was lost. Therefore, the advantage of dexfenfluramine taken while on a VLCD would appear minimal. Another use of dexfenfluramine had been to maintain a reduced weight once rapid weight loss has been achieved using VLCD. Over a 6-month surveillance those given dexfenfluramine lost a further 5.9 kg (lost 14.9 kg on VLCD) whereas those on placebo regained 2.9 kg of the 13.5 kg lost during VLCD (Finer, 1989). Dexfenfluramine had been used to prevent weight gain following cessation of smoking. In normal-weight subjects those on placebo gained 3.5 kg over 3 months whereas those on dexfenfluramine gained just 1.0 kg (Spring *et al.*, 1995).

Dexfenfluramine was also beneficial in diabetic patients, a group who are particularly resistant to weight loss except in the immediate postdiagnostic period. In a study from Australia reported by Willey *et al.* (1992), 34 diabetic patients were randomly assigned to dexfenfluramine or placebo for 12 weeks while maintaining their existing regimens of metformin with or without sulphonylurea. Those on the dexfenfluramine lost 3.9 kg whereas on placebo the loss was only 0.6 kg. Such a small reduction of weight (4%) from the drug was beneficial for glycaemic control with a reduction of HbA_{1c} from 7.5 to 6.3% and fructosamine from 313 to 274 µmol/L. Systolic pressure reduced 9 mmHg and diastolic pressure 12 mmHg. The improvement in glycaemic control did not correlate with the weight lost suggesting that dexfenfluramine had a direct effect on glycaemic management. This is in keeping with the effect of acute dexfenfluramine in non-diabetic obese subjects where an 8-day course decreased fasting plasma glucose by 0.5 mmol/L, serum insulin by 18%, reduced glucose oxidation by 36% and increased non-oxidative glucose disposal by 41% (measured by clamp studies), indicating increased insulin sensitivity by a direct effect of the drug but not by weight reduction, as weight remained stable throughout (Andersen *et al.*, 1993). In type 2 diabetic patients dexfenfluramine given as one 30-mg dose increased free fatty acid turnover (7.8–10.7 μmol/kg/min) and oxidation (9.5–11.5%), with a 24% reduction in serum glucose (Greco *et al.*, 1995) again emphasizing its direct role on glucose and fat metabolism.

In another trial in 48 patients with type 2 diabetes (Stewart *et al.*, 1993) conducted over 3 months the placebo group gained 0.3 kg whereas those on dexfenfluramine lost 3.8 kg. Fasting blood glucose decreased 1.0 mmol/L and HbA$_{1c}$ decreased 1.4% on the drug; the figures for the placebo group being +0.6 mmol/L and +0.2%, respectively. Another trial in patients with long-standing diabetes conducted in Scotland showed similar weight losses with those on 3 months dexfenfluramine losing 3.4 kg compared to 1.6 kg on diet alone (Manning *et al.*, 1995). In this trial glycaemic control did not improve. Although the drug was only given for 3 months to comply with statutory regulations in the U.K., the trial of diet was continued for 1 year. The above groups were then compared with a group given diet plus behavioural therapy and another who received dietary advice at home on a one to one basis. The 'control' group consisted of those patients who were not given any specific advice other than that available in a routine diabetic clinic. This latter group gained 1.2 kg, those given behavioural therapy lost 3.1 kg, the home teaching group lost 1.0 kg, clinic visit group lost 2.0 kg whereas the dexfenfluramine group maintained a 3.0 kg loss. Some 3 years after the trial ended the dexfenfluramine group still maintained their weight loss advantage with all other groups having regained most of the weight lost (Table 19.6).

In the largest multicentre trial reported (Guy-Grand *et al.*, 1989), the most often reported side-effects included tiredness, diarrhoea, dry mouth, polyuria and drowsiness (see Table 19.4). There had been reports of isolated cases of fits

Table 19.6 Weight loss or gain in diabetic patients on four different weight reduction treatment programmes compared to a control group. After 1 year the most weight was lost by the dexfenfluramine treated group but closely followed by the behavioural group. Then the patients were seen at the diabetic clinic with the same structure as offered to the control group. At the end of the fourth year both the home visit and dexfenfluramine group had maintained their weight loss. From Manning *et al.* (1995a).

	Clinic	Dexfenfluramine	Behavioural	Home visits	Control
12 months	−1.88 kg	−3.01 kg	−2.76 kg	−1.71 kg	+1.0 kg
48 months	−0.48kg	−2.46kg	−0.95kg	−1.92kg	+0.35 kg

with dexfenfluramine and so it was not recommended for use in epileptic patients. Depression had been reported both whilst taking but also on abrupt cessation of this drug, although less so on the d isomer. Dexfenfluramine, was generally not advisable in the depressed patient. The most controversial danger of usage beyond 3 months was the risk of pulmonary hypertension. In 1996 Abenhaim *et al.* reported a case-control study of 95 patients with pulmonary hypertension from 35 centres in four European countries. In this study some 30 cases (31.6%) reported the use of appetite suppressants with 80% of these having taken dexfenfluramine (18 cases) or fenfluramine (6 cases). The odds ratio associated with use in the last year before diagnosis was 10.1 and with past use 2.4. The odds ratio increased with the duration of exposure namely 1.8 if taken for less than 3 months and 23.1 for longer durations. The odds ratio with obesity alone was 1.6 only. Therefore the risk of developing pulmonary hypertension associated with appetite suppressant drugs was given as 28 cases per million person-years or 14 deaths per million person-years of treatment (Manson & Faich, 1996). This is said to be close to the risk of death from penicillin-induced anaphylaxis or oral contraceptive associated venous thrombosis.

In 1997, Connolly *et al.* reported on echocardiological and surgical findings in 24 women on a combination of phentermine and fenfluramine, many taking the combination for 1 year. Echocardiography demonstrated an unusual heart condition involving both left and right sided heart valves producing regurgitation. Of these some eight women also had newly documented pulmonary hypertension. Five of the women required cardiac surgical intervention. These valves at surgery had a glistening white appearance with plaque-like encasement of the leaflets and chordae: histopathological features identical to those seen in carcinoid syndrome or ergotamine induced valve disease, all conditions associated with raised serotonin. Subsequently, further cases were reported to the FDA. The majority were reported in patients on the combination of fenfluramine and phentermine, with some 14% on dexfenfluramine alone and possibly just one case on phentermine alone. Over 95% of cases are in females with a duration of usage of 9 months, although usage of less than 1 month has also been reported. Obviously a reliable case controlled evaluation is required with evaluation of reversibility on drug cessation. While this is awaited both fenfluramine and dexfenfluramine have been withdrawn by the manufacturer.

Fluoxetine

Fluoxetine is a highly specific inhibitor of serotonin re-uptake into presynaptic nerve endings in the brain and was initially introduced as an antidepressant (Fig. 19.3). Its action is quite unlike that of the tricyclic antidepressants which

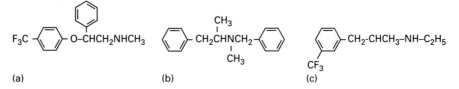

Fig. 19.3 Structure of (a) fluoxetine, (b) benzphetamine and (c) dexfenfluramine.

can cause weight gain possibly by their effects on noradrenalin in the medial hypothalamus. Both fluoxetine and norfluoxetine, an active metabolite, have a long plasma half life, the former 2–3 days, the latter 7–9 days. The drug is extensively metabolized and undergoes renal elimination. Impairment of renal function, increasing age and the degree of obesity do not appear to alter the clearance of fluoxetine although this is decreased by hepatic impairment. Fluoxetine is an inhibitor of cytochrome P450-II-D6 in humans and has been shown to inhibit the metabolism of those drugs which are substrates for this enzyme. It does not affect the elimination of alcohol and has no direct effect on blood pressure although mean heart rate can be reduced (Lucas, 1992). Although there is psychometric and EEG evidence to suggest a vigilance enhancing property, fluoxetine does not exhibit amphetamine-like stimulant activity.

Fluoxetine has a dose-dependent effect on weight loss. Levine *et al.* (1989) have reported on a dose–response study of 655 non-depressed obese adults randomized to placebo or four dosage levels of fluoxetine (10, 20, 40 or 60 mg). The patients were mainly female with a mean age of 40 years and mean weight of 94 kg. All groups except the 10 mg fluoxetine group had a significantly greater weight loss at 8 weeks than the placebo. The mean weight losses at 8 weeks were 0.9, 1.9, 2.2, 3.9 kg on 10, 20, 40, 60 mg fluoxetine, respectively, compared to a loss of only 0.5 kg on placebo. The important point to note is that the subjects were given no specific dietary or exercise instructions and were seen weekly. In such short-term studies the average weight loss was 0.5 kg/week compared to less than 0.1 kg on placebo.

In a long-term 1-year trial reported by Darga *et al.* (1991), 45 obese subjects (BMI mean 37.6) were randomly allocated to either fluoxetine 60 mg/day or placebo. Both groups were counselled on a diet with a caloric content reduction intended to produce a weight loss theoretically of 0.5 kg/week. There was no behavioural therapy or exercise specifically recommended. Drop-out rate was 39% on fluoxetine and 27% on placebo. Weight loss at 1 year averaged 8.2 kg on the drug and 4.5 kg on placebo. Further analysis indicated that at week 29 those on fluoxetine who eventually completed the study had lost 12.4 kg compared to 4.5 kg on placebo. Thereafter the fluoxetine group showed a weight regain averaging 4.2 kg whereas the placebo group did not. The regain on fluoxetine was inversely related to the initial weight loss. The reason for this regain after 6 months is unknown but was not due to lack of compliance, but a reduction in frequency of visits may have been involved although this had no effect on the placebo group. Tolerance was thought unlikely as this should have developed earlier on in the trial but could not be disproven.

In another 1-year trial reported by Marcus *et al.* (1990), 45 patients were recommended dietary restriction as well as behavioural therapy and exercise. The patients were also stratified as binge and non-binge eaters. On 60 mg fluoxetine per day mean weight loss at week 52 was 13.9 kg compared to a weight regain of 0.6 kg on placebo. Most of the weight on fluoxetine was lost during the first 5 months of therapy (11.2 kg) with little change thereafter. The drug did not appear to have a differential benefit for binge eaters.

Goldstein *et al.* (1994) have reported on the ten-site study of 458 patients conducted over 52 weeks in which the above two studies formed two of the sites; those two sites were reported separately as they appeared to do better than the others (Fig. 19.4). The patients were mainly Caucasian had a mean age of 43 years and a mean BMI of 36 kg/m². Overall the fluoxetine group (60 mg/ day) showed the most weight loss compared to placebo at week 20 (5.1 kg on fluoxetine compared to 2.4 kg on placebo). Although some patients continued to lose weight for 1 year on fluoxetine, overall this was not sustained and the

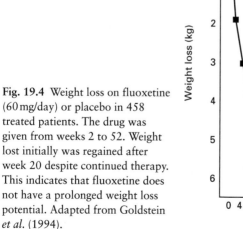
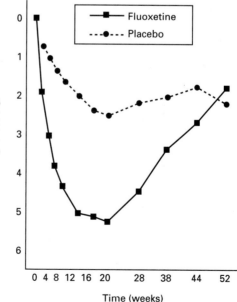

Fig. 19.4 Weight loss on fluoxetine (60 mg/day) or placebo in 458 treated patients. The drug was given from weeks 2 to 52. Weight lost initially was regained after week 20 despite continued therapy. This indicates that fluoxetine does not have a prolonged weight loss potential. Adapted from Goldstein *et al.* (1994).

final analysis showed that there was no treatment difference at 52 weeks (1.7 kg loss on drug vs 2.1 kg loss on placebo). Once again the reason for this was unclear. Patients with a baseline BMI of greater than 40 appeared to do better than those who were less obese. The only reason suggested for the better results in the two specific sites above was nutrition counselling in one and behavioural therapy in another.

Sayler et al. (1994) evaluated fluoxetine in a re-analysis of eight randomized, double-blind, controlled trials involving 522 subjects on fluoxetine compared with 504 on placebo lasting at least 36 weeks. The drug showed an 8% improvement in BMI, a 10% reduction in systolic blood pressure and a 10% improvement in total cholesterol and fasting glucose. Using the definition of success based on at least one weight-related factor and at least one obesity-related risk factor (see p. 469) Sayler et al. (1994) concluded that fluoxetine was successful at the 'minimum' defined level in 28.3% of patients taking the drug compared to 22.5% on placebo ($P=0.058$). At the 'intermediate' level success was only achieved by 3.7% of those on fluoxetine and just 1.6% on placebo. The corresponding values for the 'full' success level were 0.2 and 0%, respectively.

Adverse events (Table 19.7) accounted for one-third of the drop-out rate in the above reported study by Darga et al. (1991). An overall comparison of

Table 19.7 Significant side-effects of fluoxetine therapy in obesity trials vs placebo. Adapted from Levine et al. (1989).

Event	Fluoxetine % ($n = 1174$)	Placebo % ($n = 590$)
Headache	26	19
Nausea	15	7
Asthenia	12	5
Diarrhoea	12	7
Nervousness	12	6
Somnolence	11	4
Insomnia	9	4
Sweating	6	2
Dyspepsia	6	3
Dry mouth	5	3
Constipation	4	2
Tremor	3	1
Decreased libido	3	< 1
Anorexia	2	1
Vomiting	2	1
Urinary frequency	2	1
Thirst	1	< 1

1174 subjects on fluoxetine with 590 on placebo indicated that side-effects were minimal with headache, nausea, asthenia, sweating, diarrhoea, nervousness and somnolence being most prominent (Wise, 1992). Asthenia, somnolence and sweating were dose dependent (Levine *et al.*, 1989). Fluoxetine does not appear to increase suicidal intent in those obese with depression. Goldstein *et al.* (1993) reported suicidal ideation during obesity clinical trials as 0.23% on fluoxetine and 0.27% on placebo. In another report (Heiligenstein *et al.*, 1993), a comprehensive meta-analysis indicated that fewer patients (0.15%) on fluoxetine exhibited events suggestive of aggression (hostility, personality disorders, antisocial reaction) than on placebo (0.65%). Sleep-related eating disorders such as nightly sleep-related binge eating, have also been reported improved on fluoxetine (Schenck *et al.*, 1993). Fluoxetine also increases the minimum sleep oxygen saturation (73% to 81%) by reducing or abolishing rapid eye movement (REM) sleep (Kopelman *et al.*, 1992). Total apnoea and hypoapnoea indices also decrease especially in those worst affected. Pituitary hormone fuction studies were unaltered by fluoxetine except for a slight reduction in the thyroid-stimulating hormone (TSH) response to thyrotrophin-releasing hormone (TRH) by about 23% in obese (and lean) with a restoration of basal prolactin levels if depressed in the obese; prolactin responses to TRH was unaltered (Pijl *et al.*, 1993).

Visser *et al.* (1993) have reported on the effect of fluoxetine on body composition and visceral fat assessed using magnetic resonance imaging scans. In this study, 38 abdominally obese males (mean BMI 28, waist/hip ratio 0.97) were randomly allocated to placebo or 60 mg/day of fluoxetine for 12 weeks after a placebo run in of 2 weeks. Weight loss was 5.9 kg in the fluoxetine group and 2.4 kg on placebo. The reduction in fat mass was 3.5 kg on fluoxetine and 2.2 kg on placebo which were statistically similar. The reduction in lean mass was, however, proportionally greater on fluoxetine (2.4 kg) than placebo (0.2 kg) indicating a lack of protein sparing with this drug. The absolute and proportional changes in the subcutaneous fat area were greater than the change in visceral fat and also significantly greater on fluoxetine. For subcutaneous fat there was a 13% reduction on fluoxetine but a 4% reduction on placebo. Visceral fat reduced 3% on fluoxetine but increased 1% on placebo. It would appear that fluoxetine decreases fat mass mainly by reducing subcutaneous rather than visceral fat during modest weight loss.

The mechanism of weight reduction would appear to be mainly by a reduction in intake. In a study by Lawton *et al.* (1995), mean daily intakes calculated from food diary records indicated an intake of 7.7 MJ on placebo and 6.0 MJ when the same subjects were on fluoxetine. In another report based on food records while subjects were on no specific diet, intake was also reduced in those on fluoxetine (4.6 MJ) compared to placebo (7.6 MJ). In this report the authors calculated that the reduction in intake accounted entirely for the weight lost over the 6 weeks of their study (Pijl *et al.*, 1991). These findings are in keeping with the viewpoint of Stinson *et al.* (1992) who found that fluoxetine did not stimulate metabolism over a 14-day study. In this study there were two treatment periods each of 2 weeks separated by a 6-week out phase. Thirty obese subjects underwent a double-blind randomized crossover of placebo or fluoxetine (60 mg/day). No difference was found between the two stages with regard to RMR, total dietary induced thermogenesis (DIT), peak DIT and the time taken to reach peak DIT. This contrasts to the work of Bross and Hoffer (1995) whose study involved 20 obese women on a very-low-caloric formula diet of just 1.76 MJ/day for 3 weeks. Those assigned to placebo showed a decline of RMR below prediet after 5.6 days of energy restriction whereas those on fluoxetine had an increase of RMR by 4.4% within 3 days, which then decreased below prediet after 9.8 days. Basal body temperature increased by 0.28°C within 3 days of fluoxetine, a feature not observed on placebo. Urinary noradrenalin and serum triiodothyronine decreased equally in both groups.

Fluoxetine has also been compared with benzphetamine or placebo (Ferguson & Feighner, 1987), in 150 non-depressed subjects over an 8-week study, weight loss averaged 4.8 kg on fluoxetine, 4.0 kg on benzphetamine and 1.7 kg on placebo. Subjects who reported carbohydrate craving lost more weight (5.5 kg) than those who did not (3.2 kg) suggesting that fluoxetine suppresses carbohydrate intake. In another study, fluoxetine was used to prevent weight gain on cessation of smoking (Spring *et al.*, 1995). Normal-weight women (144 subjects) were randomly assigned to fluoxetine 40 mg/day or dexfenfluramine 30 mg/day or placebo for 14 weeks. The drop-out rate was highest for fluoxetine at 57% whereas with dexfenfluramine it was 36% and on placebo 44%. All groups gained weight on cigarette cessation, least on the dexfenfluramine (1.0 kg) which was significantly less than either fluoxetine (2.7 kg) or placebo (3.5 kg).

Studies have also been conducted in patients with diabetes mellitus. Effectiveness has been demonstrated in 19 obese type 2 diabetic patients, seven of whom were on diet alone for glycaemic control and 12 on oral hypoglycaemic agents (O'Kane *et al.*, 1994). Weight loss averaged 4.6 kg on fluoxetine (60 mg/day) at 3 months (placebo −0.8 kg), 6.3 kg at 6 months (placebo +0.2 kg), 6.3 kg at 9 months (placebo +0.8 kg) and 4.3 kg at 1 year (placebo +1.5 kg). Once again some regain was apparent, as previously reported, in non-diabetic subjects. Median fasting blood glucose and HbA_{1c} levels decreased significantly after 3 months (1.9 mmol/L and 1.7% absolute, respectively) and at 6 months (1.8 mmol/L and 1.7%) but neither showed a significant difference to placebo at 9 and 12 months of therapy with fluoxetine. There was no significant change in total serum cholesterol in the year but patients on fluoxetine did exhibit a 0.5 mmol/L decrease in serum triglyceride at 3 months' therapy but not thereafter.

Energy and nutrient intake was assessed at the outset and every 3 months of this study using 7-day food diaries. These indicated that fluoxetine was associated with a decrease in energy intake of 1.1 MJ/day at 3 months and 0.8 MJ/day at 6 months compared to the placebo group, but no difference was noted at 9 and 12 months. This decrease in energy intake was associated with a fall in carbohydrate intake of 30 g/day at 3 months and 23 g/day at 6 months compared to placebo. Also, the authors noted that there was a decrease in the carbohydrate intake as a percentage of the total daily energy intake of 5.9% at 3 months, 6.1% at 6 months and 4.0% at 9 months. There were no changes in fat and protein intake until 6 months when the intake of fat expressed as a percentage of daily energy intake rose to 5.9%. Once again the conclusion would appear that in the short term fluoxetine is useful in diabetic patients but does not appear to have a role long term where other methods or drugs are required.

Fluoxetine would also appear safe in the elderly diabetic patient as shown by a 6-month study of 30 obese elderly (mean 67 years) patients with type 2 diabetes (Connolly et al., 1995) given a 5–6.6 MJ diet alone with no hypoglycaemic medication. Weight loss with fluoxetine (60 mg/day) was 3.3 kg at 2 months and 3.9 kg at 6 months which compared most favourably with the placebo group who lost no weight. The authors also reported that weight loss plateaued at 2 months and then maintained for a further 4 months. Non-compliance with the diet was suggested as the reason for the smaller weight losses in the elderly. HbA_1 decreased by 0.9% at 3 months with a similar reduction at 6 months if on fluoxetine but a rise of 0.1% on placebo. Side-effects were not worse in the elderly and only three patients withdrew for this reason from the fluoxetine group. Fluoxetine has also been tested in insulin-treated type 2 diabetic patients. In a trial of 48 obese type 2 insulin-treated patients (Gray et al., 1992) randomized to fluoxetine 60 mg/day or placebo for 24 weeks, the drug resulted in a 9.3-kg weight loss compared to 1.9 kg on placebo. HbA_{1c} was also reduced more on fluoxetine (1.7%) than on placebo (0.8%). In addition those on fluoxetine required less insulin with a 47% decrease in dosage (placebo 19% decrease).

Fluoxetine has a slight direct effect on glucose handling but confined to those with marked insulin resistance. Clamp studies (Potter van Loon et al., 1992) in diabetic patients after 14 days of treatment with fluoxetine showed no alteration in maximal peripheral glucose uptake although half-maximal peripheral glucose uptake was achieved at a lower insulin level (180 mU/L vs 225 mU/L on placebo). There was also no significant reduction in basal hepatic glucose output in the diabetic patients. In non-diabetic subjects half maximal glucose uptake was unchanged in the presence of fluoxetine although basal hepatic glucose output was reduced (8.6 vs 9.2 μmol/kg/min). When the authors studied the diabetics and non-diabetics together it was apparent that only individuals with the most insulin resistance demonstrated a decrease in the half maximal glucose uptake. The same applied for hepatic insulin resistance.

Fluoxetine has also been used in Prader–Willi syndrome with beneficial effect on weight control and both skin-pricking and hair-pulling self-mutilating behaviour (Dech & Budow, 1991).

Thermogenic drugs

Thyroid hormones

Thyroid hormones in pharmaceutical dosages have the disadvantages of rapidly reducing lean body mass (Abraham et al., 1987) and affect cardiac function with arrhythmic potential; hence, they are not recommended for the treatment of obesity. Many patients are under the misapprehension that thyroxine replacement therapy for hypothyroidism will result in significant weight loss without the need to reduce energy intake. A recent study of 28 treated hypothyroid patients showed an average weight loss of only 0.6 kg after 1 year of therapy (Pears et al., 1990).

Ephedrine and caffeine

Ephedrine has been used in the treatment of obesity but is more efficacious when combined with caffeine. Ephedrine is a sympathomimetic agent acting on both α- and β-adrenoceptors releasing noradrenalin from nerve endings. Although considered a thermogenic drug 75% of the fat loss on ephedrine is due to its anorectic activity and only 25% due to an increase in energy expenditure (Astrup et al., 1992a). Astrup and colleagues (1992b) investigated the weight losing potential of ephedrine alone, ephedrine with caffeine, caffeine alone and placebo in 180 obese patients advised a 4.2-MJ diet over 24 weeks. On ephedrine (60 mg/day) average weight loss was 16.6 kg, on caffeine (600 mg/day) 11.5 kg, on ephedrine with caffeine (60 and 600 mg, respectively) 16.6 kg whereas weight loss on placebo was 13.2 kg. Their conclusion was that ephedrine or caffeine alone were no better than placebo but that ephedrine combined with caffeine was efficacious. Earlier studies had suggested that ephedrine alone was effective but in those studies the groups were small and so the risk of statistical type 2 errors high. Often these early studies involved much higher dosages of ephedrine of up to 150 mg/day with consequent unwelcome side-effects such as a substantive acute rises in blood pressure, tremor and glucose intolerance, hence the need to potentiate a lower dose of ephedrine with caffeine.

The investigators in the above study (Astrup *et al.*, 1992b) also noted that the weight loss stabilized out at 20 weeks in all groups with more weight loss in the first 12 weeks on ephedrine and caffeine (11.7 kg) than in the second half of the study (4.9 kg). Waist/hip ratio decreased in all groups with no significant differences. Systolic and diastolic blood pressure decreased equally in all groups. However, there was a transient rise in blood pressure at 4 weeks in those on ephedrine with caffeine of just 0.2 mmHg systolic and 0.5 mmHg diastolic compared to reductions of 4.6 mmHg systolic and 1.0 mmHg diastolic on placebo. By 24 weeks, systolic pressure had decreased by 4.8 and 6.7 mmHg on ephedrine/caffeine or placebo, respectively, and diastolic pressure had decreased 0.9 and 4.9 mmHg, respectively (non-significant difference). Heart rate also decreased with again no group differences.

These findings are of importance, as acute dose administration of ephedrine with caffeine to normal-weight subjects has been reported to raise heart rate by 7 beats per minute and to increase systolic pressure by 5–7 mmHg with diastolic pressure unaffected (Astrup *et al.*, 1991). The fall in blood pressure during dieting may therefore be due to the well recognized hypotensive effect of energy restriction and weight loss over-riding the slight hypertensive action of the drugs. In the above study, patients with blood pressures up to 110 mmHg were included and only one patient had to be withdrawn due to severe hypertension (185/125). Consequently moderate hypertension should not contraindicate treatment with ephedrine and caffeine at the above dosages but blood pressure should be carefully monitored especially in the early stages of dieting. Experience in severe hypertensive patients is lacking.

Breum *et al.* (1994) have compared weight loss and blood pressure changes between dexfenfluramine and ephedrine combined with caffeine. In their study, 103 subjects were advised to follow a 5-MJ diet and randomly given double blind either dexfenfluramine (30 mg/day) or ephedrine and caffeine (60/600 mg/day). After 15 weeks both groups lost similar weight, those on dexfenfluramine lost 6.9 kg and those on ephedrine/caffeine 8.3 kg. The reduction in systolic pressure was similar at 15 weeks namely 7.8 mmHg on dexfenfluramine and 10.6 mmHg on ephedrine/caffeine. The values for the reduction in diastolic pressure were 4.6 and 3.5 mmHg, respectively. Heart rate decreased 2.7 beats per minute on dexfenfluramine but increased 1.1 beats per minute on ephedrine/caffeine. Total cholesterol was reported to have decreased equally in both groups. After cessation of this 15-week double-blind study the patients were offered a further 15 weeks of treatment with ephedrine and caffeine. Fifty-seven patients agreed to this. Those who were originally treated with ephedrine/caffeine lost a further 2.3 kg whereas those previously given dexfenfluramine lost 1.6 kg (not significantly different). Blood pressure was reported unchanged. Interestingly during the first 15-week trial side-effects were reported in 43% on dexfenfluramine and in 54% on ephedrine/caffeine, with central nervous system side-effects, especially agitation, more pronounced on ephedrine/caffeine, but gut reactions more frequent on dexfenfluramine. In both groups the side-effects subsided after 1 month of therapy.

Ephedrine/caffeine acutely increases plasma glucose, insulin and C-peptide which subside on chronic therapy. During ephedrine therapy alone given for 3 months there is a 10% sustained rise in RMR and a sustained increase by about 9% in glucose-induced thermogenesis (Astrup et al., 1986). The respiratory quotient (RQ) indicated that relatively more lipid was oxidized (13–15 g/day) during chronic ephedrine treatment than observed in the controls and this oxidation of fat accounted for the observed raised energy expenditure averaging 0.76 MJ/24 hours. It was from such measurements that it was possible to estimate that 20–25% of the weight loss caused by ephedrine/caffeine was due to the stimulation of energy expenditure, the remaining 75–80% due to a decrease in energy intake (Astrup et al., 1992a). One might expect that raised fat oxidation might influence lipid profiles. These were investigated in an 8-week study of 32 women given 4.2 MJ/day diet (Buemann et al., 1994). Weight loss was 8.4 kg with ephedrine/caffeine (60/600 mg/day) and 7.1 kg on placebo. Total cholesterol decreased equally in both groups. HDL-cholesterol decreased by 0.14 mmol/L on placebo but remained unaltered on ephedrine/caffeine. The latter were associated with a significant decrease in plasma triglyceride (0.25 mmol/L) but no change was noted on placebo. During this study body fat was measured by impedance and found to decrease by 6.5 kg compared to a weight loss of 8.4 kg on ephedrine/caffeine (77% of weight loss). This compared to a fat loss of 5.8 kg and a weight loss of 7.1 kg on placebo (82%).

The maintenance of lean mass on ephedrine/caffeine is important, for this would preserve energy expenditure especially when dieting and drug therapy ceased. A specific study to investigate such a protein sparing effect was conducted in 14 obese women on 4.2-MJ diet over 8 weeks (Astrup et al., 1992a). Those on ephedrine/caffeine lost 4.5 kg more body fat and 2.8 kg less lean mass than on placebo for the same total body-weight loss. Those on placebo lost 8.4 kg composed of 4.5 kg fat and 3.9 kg lean mass whereas ephedrine/caffeine group lost 10.1 kg composed of 9.0 kg fat and 1.1 kg lean mass. This suggested a protein sparing effect due to repartitioning. Mention needs to be made of plasma glucose which decreases on chronic therapy at modest ephedrine dosages of 60 mg/day, as higher dosages have been associated with acute deterioration in glycaemic control. In the above study (Buemann et al., 1994) of the comparison of ephedrine/caffeine and dexfenfluramine plasma glucose decreased to a similar extent on both drugs. Significant studies on the use of ephedrine/caffeine in diabetes are not available.

Long-term trials on obese non-diabetic patients are also limited. In one such study of ephedrine/caffeine/aspirin (75–150/150/330 mg), 24 obese subjects were given no energy restrictive diet (Daly *et al.*, 1993). Initially the first stage of the study involved 8 weeks' therapy, with weight loss on the combination therapy of 2.2 vs 0.7 kg on placebo. Thirteen of the placebo-treated subjects returned 5 months later and received combination drug therapy or placebo for a further 8 weeks with loss of 3.2 kg on the former and just 1.3 kg on the placebo. Six of these subjects continued their combination therapy. After a further 5 months, weight loss in five of these subjects averaged 5.2 kg (compared to no loss when off therapy previously). The sixth subject lost 66 kg over 13 months by self-imposed caloric restriction. In a continuation of the study reported above by Astrup *et al.* (1992b) of the use of various combinations of ephedrine, ephedrine/caffeine or placebo, all the patients were continued from week 24 on the most efficacious therapy namely ephedrine/caffeine (Toubro *et al.*, 1993) (Fig. 19.5). This was given until week 52 while maintaining a 5-MJ diet. Those previously on ephedrine/caffeine lost just 0.2 kg, those previously on ephedrine gained 0.1 kg, but those on caffeine lost 2.5 kg and those previously given placebo lost 1.7 kg. The important practical point is that unlike fluoxetine continued use of ephedrine/

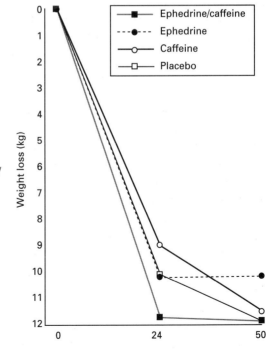

Fig. 19.5 Weight loss on ephedrine/caffeine, ephedrine, caffeine and placebo given until week 24 and then diet alone (5 MJ) continued to week 50 with ephedrine/caffeine given to all groups from weeks 26 to 50. Note that this combination therapy which produced effective weight reduction in the first 6 months did not produce further weight loss but prevented weight regain. Adapted from Toubro *et al.* (1993). Note that weight is not regained on diet.

caffeine appears to maintain the weight lost even if weight loss shows a nadir at 20 weeks.

Side-effects of ephedrine/caffeine occur in 50–60% of patients mainly at the outset and are transient. The most common side-effects reported are dizziness, insomnia, tremor, agitation, nausea, palpitations and dry mouth. In rodent studies aspirin, administered with ephedrine and caffeine in combination, increases its thermogenic and weight-reducing potency. This does not appear to be the case in humans where aspirin does not further potentiate the acute thermic effect of ephedrine/caffeine with a meal.

Atypical β-adrenergic agonists

In 1984 a new family of thermogenic atypical adrenergic agonists was reported (Fig. 19.6). In genetic obese rodents, this type of drug produced marked weight loss with protein sparing, by stimulating preferentially brown fat thermogenesis. Trials in humans have involved two agents namely BRL 26830A (Connacher *et al.*, 1988, 1992) and BRL 35135 (Smith *et al.*, 1989). Acute ingestion of 100 mg raised metabolic rate by an average 11.5% in obese women (Connacher *et al.*, 1988). Weight loss over 18 weeks using 400 mg BRL 26830A in 40 subjects averaged 15.4 kg on BRL 26830A compared to 10 kg on placebo; diet consisted of 3.3 MJ/day (Connacher *et al.*, 1988). Nitrogen balance studies confirmed that, like ephedrine, BRL 26830A also had a protein sparing effect. Systolic and diastolic pressures reduced to a similar extent on drug and placebo. There was also no difference in the decline in cholesterol, triglyceride or glucose between the groups. In a second 12-week study, BRL 26830A had no beneficial result on weight although in this study previously refractory hospital referred patients were chosen (Chapman *et al.*, 1988). When both studies were pooled for those who completed 12 weeks of therapy the results indicated that BRL 26830A had an appreciable anti-obesity effect (Cawthorne, 1992). A smaller study of 16 patients (Zed *et al.*, 1985) on a low-calorie liquid formula diet for 6 weeks has also indicated that BRL 26830A promoted weight loss (9.3 vs 6.6 kg on placebo). Work with BRL 35135 has been less successful as regards weight loss although this drug enhances glycaemic control in obese NIDDM patients by reducing insulin resistance by as much as 30% in acute 10-day studies (Smith

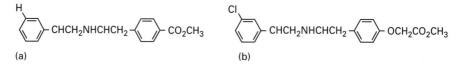

(a)   (b)

Fig. 19.6 Structure of two thermogenic β-adrenoceptor drugs (a) BRL 26830A and (b) BRL 35135.

et al., 1989). Tremor is observed on BRL 26830A but is dose dependent and short lived in many (Connacher *et al.*, 1992).

Growth hormone

The recent advent of genetically engineered supplies of growth hormone has stimulated interest in its possible use in obesity. Growth hormone enhances fat oxidation during energy restriction and also promotes nitrogen retention. Synder *et al.* (1988) in an 11-week study of obese diet-restricted subjects found no advantage with growth hormone on either body-weight or lean mass lost. As has been reported with its use in children, nitrogen conservation in the obese was improved by growth hormone but only for the initial 33 days of the trial. Serum triiodothyronine also increased during the initial 45 days despite energy restriction but thereafter declined to levels below that observed at the outset. Increases in energy expenditure of as much as 25% have been reported during the first month of therapy in growth hormone treated hypopituitary adult patients (Chong *et al.*, 1994). This study indicated that after 6 months' treatment weight remained unchanged although fat mass decreased by 5.8 kg whereas lean mass increased by 6.2 kg. Others have reported a decrease in body-weight in hypopituitary adults given growth hormone with a loss in abdominal fat and a gain in lean mass (Salomon *et al.*, 1989). What is not clear is whether with time fat mass reaccumulates due to increased energy intake. In the elderly with low IGF-1, growth hormone therapy for 6 months has also been reported to increase lean mass by 8.8% with a 14.4% decrease in fat mass but a body-weight increase of 1 kg (Rudman *et al.*, 1990). Growth hormone therapy would not appear to be a feasible proposition either clinically or financially for the treatment of the obese.

Conclusion

There is a need for a pharmacological approach to the management of obesity but one which can be safely and effectively prescribed for the long term. As obesity is associated with considerable co-morbidity, drug therapies which reduce weight and alleviate co-morbid disease are most likely to receive acceptance. The introduction of newer agents such as orlistat and sibutramine should achieve an advance towards this goal.

References

Abenhaim, I., Moride, Y., Brenot, F. *et al.* (1996) Appetite suppressant drugs and the risk of primary pulmonary hypertension. *New England Journal of Medicine* **335**, 609–616.

Abraham, R., Zed, C., Mitchell, T. *et al.* (1987) The effect of a novel B-agonist BRL 26830A on weight and protein loss in obese patients. *International Journal of Obesity* **11**, 306A (abstract).

Alger, S., Larson, K., Boyce, V.L. (1993) Effect of phenylpropanolamine on energy expenditure and weight loss in overweight women. *American Journal of Clinical Nutrition* **57**, 120–126.

Andersen, P.H., Richelsen, E., Bak, J. *et al.* (1993) Influence of short term dexfenfluramine therapy on glucose and lipid metabolism in obese non-diabetic patients. *Acta Endocrinologica Copenhagen* **128**, 251–258.

Andersen, T., Astrup, A., Quaade, F. *et al.* (1992) Dexfenfluramine as adjuvant to a low calorie formula diet in the treatment of obesity; a randomised trial. *International Journal of Obesity and Related Metabolic Disorders* **16**, 35–40.

Astrup, A., Madsen, J., Holst, J.J. & Christensen, N.J. (1986) The effects of chronic ephedrine treatment on substrate utilisation, the sympathoadrenal activity, and energy expenditure during glucose induced thermogenesis in man. *Metabolism* **35**, 260–265.

Astrup, A., Toubro, S., Cannon, S., Hein, P. & Madsen, J. (1991) Thermogenic synergism between ephedrine and caffeine in healthy volunteers: a double-blind, placebo controlled study. *Metabolism* **40**, 323–329.

Astrup, A., Buemann, B., Christensen, N.J. *et al.* (1992a) The effect of ephedrine/caffeine mixture on energy expenditure and body composition in obese women. *Metabolism* **41**, 686–688.

Astrup, A., Breum, L., Toubro, S., Hein, P. & Quaade, F. (1992b) The effect and safety of an ephedrine/caffeine compound compared to ephedrine, caffeine and placebo in obese subjects on an energy restricted diet. A double blind trial. *International Journal of Obesity and Related Metabolic Disorders* **16**, 269–277.

Bray, G.A., Ryan, D.H., Gordon *et al.* (1995) Double blind trial of sibutramine in overweight subjects. *International Journal of Obesity and Related Metabolic Disorders* **19** (suppl. 2), 393 (abstract).

Breum, L., Pedersen, J.K., Ahlstrom, F. & Frimodt-Moller, J. (1994) A comparison of an ephedrine/caffeine combination and dexfenfluramine in the treatment of obesity. A double blind multicenter trial in general practice. *International Journal of Obesity and Related Metabolic Disorders* **18**, 99–103.

Bross, R. & Hoffer, L.J. (1995) Fluoxetine increases resting energy expenditure and basal body temperature in humans. *American Journal of Clinical Nutrition* **61**, 1020–1025.

Buemann, B., Marckmann, P., Christensen, N.J. & Astrup, A. (1994) The effect of ephedrine plus caffeine on plasma lipids and lipoproteins during a 4.2 Mj/day diet. *International Journal of Obesity and Related Metabolic Disorders* **18**, 329–332.

Cairella, M. (1987) Use of DEAE-D in the treatment of obesity. *International Journal of Obesity* **11** (suppl. 3), 221–224.

Cawthorne, M.A. (1992) Thermogenic drugs. In: Björntorp, P. & Brodoff, B.N. (eds) *Obesity*, pp. 762–777. Philadelphia: Lippincott.

Chapman, B.J., Farquahar, D.L., Galloway, S., Simpson, G.K. & Munro, J.F. (1988) The effects of a new β-adrenoceptor agonist BRL 26830A in refractory obesity. *International Journal of Obesity* **12**, 119–123.

Connacher, A.A., Mitchell, P.E.G. & Jung, R.T. (1988) Weight loss in obese subjects on a restricted diet given BRL 26830A, a new atypical β-adrenoceptor agonist. *British Medical Journal* **26**, 1217–1220.

Connacher, A.A., Bennet, W.M. & Jung, R.T. (1992) Clinical studies with the β-adrenoceptor agonist BRL 26830A. *American Journal of Clinical Nutrition* **55**, 258S–261S.

Chong, P.K.K., Jung, R.T., Scrimgeour, C.M., Rennie, M.J. & Paterson, C.R. (1994) Energy expenditure and body composition in growth hormone deficient adults on exogenous growth hormone. *Clinical Endocrinology* **40**, 103–110.

Cheymol, G., Weissenburger, J., Poirier, J.M. & Gellee, C. (1995) The pharmacokinetics of dexfenfluramine in obese and non-obese subjects. *British Journal of Clinical Pharmacology* **39**, 684–687.

Connolly, V.M., Gallagher, A. & Kesson, C.M. (1995) A study of fluoxetine in obese elderly patients with type 2 diabetes. *Diabetic Medicine* 12, 416–418.

Connolly, H.M., Crary, J.L., McGoon, M.D. *et al.* (1997) Valvular heart disease associated with fenfluramine-phentermine. *New England Journal of Medicine* 337, 581–588.

Daly, P.A., Krieger, D.R., Dulloo, A.G., Young, J.B. & Landsberg, L. (1993) Ephedrine, caffeine and aspirin: safety and efficacy for treatment of human obesity. *International Journal of Obesity and Related Metabolic Disorders* 17 (suppl. 1), S73–S78.

Darga, L.L., Carroll-Michals, L., Botsford, S.L. & Lucas, C.P. (1991) Fluoxetine's effect on weight loss in obese subjects. *American Journal of Clinical Nutrition* 54, 321–325.

Davis, R. & Faulds, D. (1996) Dexfenfluramine. An updated review of its therapeutic use in the management of obesity. *Drugs* 52, 696–724.

Dech, B. & Budow, L. (1991) The use of fluoxetine in an adolescent with Prader–Willi syndrome. *Journal of the American Academy of Child and Adolescent Psychiatry* 30, 298–302.

Drent, M. & Van der Veen, E. (1993) Lipase inhibition: a novel concept in the treatment of obesity. *International Journal of Obesity and Related Metabolic Disorders* 17, 241–244.

Drent, M.L., Larsson, I., William-Olsson, T. *et al.* (1995a) Orlistat (RO-18-0647), a lipase inhibitor in the treatment of human obesity; a multiple dose study. *International Journl of Obesity and Related Metabolic Disorders* 19, 221–226.

Drent, M.L., Popp-Snijders, C., Ader, H.J., Jansen, Z.B. & van-der-Veen, E.A. (1995b) Lipase inhibition and hormonal status, body composition and gastrointestinal processing of a liquid high fat mixed meal in moderately obese subjects. *Obesity Research* 3, 573–581.

Enzi, G., Baritussio, A., Marchiori, E. & Crepaldi, G. (1976) Short term and long term clinical evaluation of a non-amphetamine anorexiant (mazindol) in the treatment of obesity. *Journal of International Medical Research* 4, 305–318.

Finer, N., Finer, S. & Naoumova, R.P. (1992) Drug therapy after very low calorie diets. *American Journal of Clinical Nutrition* 56, 195s–198s.

Finer, N. (1997) Present and future pharmacological approaches. In: Finer, N. (ed.) *British Medical Bulletin* 53, 409–432.

Ferguson, J.M. & Fleighner, J.P. (1987) Fluoxetine induced weight loss in overweight non-depressed humans. *International Journal of Obesity* 11 (suppl. 3), 163–170.

Froehlich, F., Hartmann, D., Guezelhan, C., Gonvers, J.J., Jansen, J.B. & Fried, M. (1996) Influence of orlistat on the regulation of gallbladder contraction in man: a randomised double-blind placebo controlled crossover study. *Digestive Disease Science* 41, 2404–2408.

Geyer, G., Haidinger, G., Francesconi, M. *et al.* (1995) Effect of dexfenfluramine on eating behaviour and body weight of obese patients: results of a field study of Isomeride in Austrian general practice. *Acta Medica Austriaca* 22, 95–109.

Goldstein, D. & Potvin, J. (1994) Long-term weight loss: the effect of pharmacologic agents. *American Journal of Clinical Nutrition* 60, 647–657.

Goldstein, D.J., Rampey, A.H., Potvin, J.H., Masica, D.N. & Beasley, C.M. (1993) Analysis of suicidality in double blind placebo controlled trials of pharmacotherapy for weight reduction. *Journal of Clinical Psychiatry* 54, 309–316.

Goldstein, D.J., Rampey, A.H., Enas, G.G., Potvin, J.H., Fludzinski, L.A. & Levine, I.R. (1994) Fluoxetine: a randomised clinical trial in the treatment of obesity. *International Journal of Obesity and Related Metabolic Disorders* 18, 129–135.

Gray, D.S., Fujioka, K., Devine, W. & Bray, G.A. (1992) Fluoxetine treatment of the obese diabetic. *International Journal of Obesity and Related Metabolic Disorders* 16, 193–198.

Greco, A.V., Mingrone, G., Capristo, E., De-Gaetano, A., Ghirlanda, G. & Castagneto, M. (1995) Effects of dexfenfluramine on free fatty acid turnover and oxidation in obese patients with type 2 diabetes mellitus. *Metabolism* 44 (suppl. 2), 57–61.

Griffiths, J., Byrnes, A.E. & Frost, G. (1995) Sibutramine in the treatment of overweight non-insulin dependent diabetics. *International Journal of Obesity* 19 (suppl. 2), 41 (abstract).

Guerciolini, R. (1997) Mode of action of Orlistat. *International Journal of Obesity* 21 (suppl. 3), S12–S23.

Guy-Grand, B., Apfelbaum, M., Crepaldi, G., Gries, A., Lefebvre, P. & Turner, P. (1989) International trial of long-term dexfenfluramine in obesity. *Lancet* 2, 1142–1145.

Hartmann, D., Guzelhan, C., Zuiderwijk, P.B. & Odink, J. (1996) Lack of interaction between orlistat and the oral contraceptives. *European Journal of Clinical Pharmacology* **50**, 421–424.

Hogan, S., Fileury, A., Hadvary, P. *et al.* (1987) Studies on the anti-obesity activity of tetrahydro-lipstatin, a potent and selective inhibitor of pancreatic lipase. *International Journal of Obesity* **11** (suppl. 3), 35–42.

Heiligenstein, J.H., Beasley, C.M. & Potvin, J.H. (1993) Fluoxetine not associated with increased aggression in controlled clinical trials. *International Clinical Psychopharmacology* **8**, 277–280.

Holdaway, I.M., Wallace, E., Westbrooke, L. & Gamble, G. (1995) Effect of dexfenfluramine on body weight, blood pressure, insulin resistance and serum cholesterol in obese individuals. *International Journal of Obesity and Related Metabolic Disorders* **19**, 749–751.

Hudson, K.D. (1977) The anorectic and hypotensive effect of fenfluramine in obesity. *Journal of the Royal College of General Practitioners* **27**, 497–501.

Hussain, Y., Guzelhan, C., Odink, J., van-der-Beek, E.J., Hartmann, D. (1994) Comparison of the inhibition of dietary fat absorption by full versus divided doses of orlistat. *Journal of Clinical Pharmacology* **34**, 1121–1125.

James, W.P.T., Avenell, A., Broom, J. & Whitehead, J. (1997) A one-year trial to assess the value of orlistat in the management of obesity. *International Journal of Obesity* **21** (suppl. 3), 524–530.

Jones, S.P. & Heath, M.J. (1996) Long term weight loss with sibutramine; 5% responders. *International Journal of Obesity* **20** (suppl. 4), abstract 20-521-FP3; 157.

Kopelman, P.G., Elliott, M.W., Simonds, A., Cramer, D., Ward, S. & Wedzicha, J.A. (1992) Short term use of fluoxetine in asymptomatic obese subjects with sleep related hypoventilation. *International Journal of Obesity and Related Metabolic Disorders* **16**, 825–830.

Lucas, R.A. (1992) The human pharmacology of fluoxetine. *International Journal of Obesity and Related Metabolic Disorders* **16** (suppl. 4), S49–S54.

Lafreniere, F., Lambert, J., Rasio, E. & Serri, I. (1993) Effects of dexfenfluramine on body weight and post-prandial thermogenesis in obese subjects. A double-blind placebo controlled study. *International Journal of Obesity and Related Metabolic Disorders* **17**, 25–30.

Lawton, C.L., Wales, J.K., Hill, A.J. & Blundell, J.E. (1995) Serotonergic manipulation, meal induced stiety and eating pattern: effect of fluoxetine in obese female subjects. *Obesity Research* **3**, 345–356.

Lean, M.E. (1997) Sibutramine—a review of clinical efficacy. *International Journal of Obesity* **21** (suppl. 1), S30–36.

Levine, L.R., Thompson, R.G. & Bosomworth, J.C. (1989) Fluoxetine, a serotonergic drug for obesity control. In: Björntorp, P. & Rossner, S. (eds) *Obesity in Europe 88*, pp. 319–321. London: Libbey.

Levine, L.R., Enas, G.G., Thompson, I.W. *et al.* (1989) Use of fluoxetine, a selective serotonin-uptake inhibitor, in the treatment of obesity: a dose response study. *International Journal of Obesity* **13**, 635–645.

Management of Obesity in Scotland (1996) Published by the Scottish Intercollegiate Guidelines Network (SIGN), Royal College of Physicians Edinburgh.

Manson, J.E. & Faich, G.A. (1996) Pharmocotherapy for obesity—Do the benefits outweigh the risks? *New England Journal of Medicine* **335**, 659–660.

Manning, R.M., Jung, R.T., Leese, G.P. & Newton, R.W. (1995) The comparison of four weight reduction strategies aimed at overweight diabetic patients. *Diabetic Medicine* **12**, 409–415.

Marcus, M.D., Wing, R.R., Ewing, L., Kern, E., McDermott, M. & Gooding, W. (1990) A double blind placebo controlled trial of fluoxetine plus behavior modification in the treatment of obese binge-eaters and non-binge-eaters. *American Journal of Psychiatry* **147**, 876–881.

Mathus-Vliegen, E.M.H., Van de Voorde, K., Kok, A.M.E. & Res, A.M.A. (1992) Dexfenfluramine in the treatment of severe obesity: a placebo controlled investigation of the effects on weight loss, cardiovascular risk factors, food intake and eating behaviour. *Journal of Internal Medicine* **232**, 119–127.

McKay, R.H.G. (1973) Long term use of diethylpropion in obesity. *Current Medical Research and Opinion* **1**, 489–493.

Melia, A.T., Zhi, J., Koss-Twardy, S.G. *et al.* (1995) The influence of reduced dietary fat absorption induced by orlistat on the pharmacokinetics of digoxin in healthy volunteers. *Journal of Clinical Pharmacology* 35, 840–843.

Melia, A.T., Mulligan, T.E. & Zhi, J. (1996) The effect of orlistat on the pharmacokinetics of phenytoin in healthy volunteers. *Journal of Clinical Pharmacology* 36, 654–658.

Morgan, J.P. & Funderburk, F.R. (1990) Invited commentary: phenylpropanolamine and the medical literature: a thorough reading is required. *International Journal of Obesity* 14, 569–574.

Munro, J.F., MacCuish, A.C., Wilson, E.M. & Duncan, L.J.P. (1968) Comparison of continuous and intermittent anorectic therapy in obesity. *British Medical Journal* 1, 352–354.

O'Connor, H.T., Richman, R.M., Steinbeck, K.S. & Caterson, I.D. (1995) Dexfenfluramine treatment of obesity: a double blind trial with post trial follow-up. *International Journal of Obesity and Related Metabolic Disorders* 19, 181–189.

O'Kane, M., Wiles, P.G. & Wales, J.K. (1994) Fluoxetine in the treatment of obese type 2 diabetic patients. *Diabetic Medicine* 11, 105–110.

Pears, J., Jung, R.T. & Gunn, A. (1990) Long term weight changes in related hyperthyroid and hypothyroid patients. *Scottish Medical Journal* 35, 180–182.

Pfohl, M., Luft, D., Blomberg, I. & Schmulling, R.M. (1994) Long term changes of body weight and cardiovascular risk factors after weight reduction with group therapy and dexfenfluramine. *International Journal of Obesity and Related Metabolic Disorders* 18, 391–395.

Pijl, H., Koppeschaar, H.P., Willekens, F.L., Op-de-Kamp, I., Veldhuis, H.D. & Meinders, A.E. (1991) Effect of serotonin re-uptake inhibition by fluoxetine on body weight and spontaneous food choice in obesity. *International Journal of Obesity* 15, 237–242.

Pijl, H., Koppeschaar, H.P.F., Willekens, F.L.A., Frolich, M. & Meinders, A.E. (1993) The influence of serotonergic neurotransmission on pituitary hormone release in obese and non-obese females. *Acta Endocrinologica* 128, 319–324.

Munro, J.F., MacCuish, A.C., Wilson, E.M. & Duncan, L.J.P. (1968) Comparison of continuous and intermittent anorectic therapy in obesity. *British Medical Journal* 1, 352–354.

Potter van Loon, B.J., Radder, J.K., Frolich, M., Krans, H.M., Zwinderman, A.H. & Meinders, A.E. (1992) Fluoxetine increases insulin action in obese type 2 diabetic patients. *International Journal of Obesity and Related Metabolic Disorders* 16 (suppl. 4), S55–S61.

Rasmussen, M.H., Anderson, T., Breum, L., Gotzche, P.C. & Hilsted, J. (1993) Cimetidine suspension as adjuvant to energy restricted diet in treating obesity. *British Medical Journal* 306, 1093–1096.

Reitsma, J.B., Castro-Cabezas, M., De-Bruin, T.W., Erkelens, D.W. (1994) Relationship between improved postprandial lipemia and low density lipoprotein metabolism during treatment with tetrahydrolipstatin, a pancreatic lipase inhibitor. *Metabolism* 43, 293–298.

Rudman, D., Feller, A.G., Nairaj, H.S. *et al.* (1990) Effects of human growth hormone in men over 60 years old. *New England Journal of Medicine* 323, 1–6.

Salomon, F., Cuneo, R.C., Hesp, R. & Sonksen, P.H. (1989) Effect of body composition of six months replacement with recombinant human growth hormone in adults with growth hormone deficiency. *Journal of Endocrinology* 321, 1797–1803.

Sayler, M., Goldstein, D., Roback, P. & Atkinson, R. (1994) Evaluating success of weight loss programs with an application to fluoxetine weight reduction clinical trial data. *International Journal of Obesity and Related Metabolic Disorders* 18, 742–751.

Schenk, C.H., Hurwitz, T.D., O'Connor, K.A. & Mahowald, M.W. (1993) Additional categories of sleep related eating disorders and the current status of treatment. *Sleep* 16, 457–466.

Schutz, Y., Munger, R., Deriaz, O. & Jequier, E. (1992) Effect of dexfenfluramine on energy expenditure in man. *International Journal of Obesity and Related Metabolic Disorders* 16 (suppl. 3), S61–S66.

Schwizer, W., Asal, K., Kreiss, C. *et al.* (1997) Role of lipase in the regulation of upper gastrointestinal function in humans. *American Journal of Physiology* 273, G612–G620.

Silverstone, J.T., Cooper, R.M. & Begg, R.R. (1970) A comparative trial of fenfluramine and diethylpropion in obesity. *The British Journal of Clinical Practice* 24, 423–425.

Smith, S.A., Zed, C., McCullough, D. *et al.* (1989) Thermogenic activity in man of BRL 35135: a potent and selective atypical β-adrenoceptor agonist. *International Journal of Obesity* 13 (suppl. 1), 133 (abstract).

Spring, B., Wurtman, J., Wurtman, R. *et al.* (1995) Efficacies of dexfenfluramine and fluoxetine in preventing weight gain after smoking cessation. *American Journal of Clinical Nutrition* **62**, 1181–1187.

Steel, J.M., Munro, J.F. & Duncan, L.J.P. (1973) A comparative trial of different regimens of fenfluramine and phentermine in obesity. *The Practitioner* **211**, 232–236.

Stewart, G.O., Stein, G.R., Davis, T.M. & Findlater, P. (1993) Dexfenfluramine in type 2 Diabetes; effect on weight and diabetes control. *Medical Journal of Australia* **158**, 167–169.

Stinson, J.C., Murphy, C.M., Andrews, J.F. & Tomkin, G.H. (1992) An assessment of the thermogenic effects of fluoxetine in obese subjects. *International Journal of Obesity and Related Metabolic Disorders* **16**, 391–395.

Stoa-Birketvedt, G. (1993) Effect of cimetidine suspension on appetite and weight in overweight subjects. *British Medical Journal* **306**, 1091–1093.

Stock, M.J. (1997) Sibutramine: a review of the pharmacology of a novel anti-obesity agent. *International Journal of Obesity* **21** (suppl. 1), S25–29.

Synder, D.K., Clemmons, D.R. & Underwood, L.E. (1988) Treatment of obese, diet restricted subjects with growth hormone for 11 weeks. Effects on anabolism, lipolysis and body composition. *Journal of Clinical Endocrinology and Metabolism* **67**, 54–61.

Stunkard, A.J., Craighead, L.W. & O'Brien, R. (1980) Controlled trial of behavioural therapy, pharmacotherapy and their combination in the treatment of obesity. *Lancet* ii, 1045–1047.

Tonstad, S., Pometta, D., Erkelens, D.W. *et al.* (1994) The effect of the gastrointestinal lipase inhibitor, orlistat, on serum lipids and lipoproteins in patients with primary hyperlipidaemia. *European Journal of Clinical Pharmacology* **46**, 405–410.

Toubro, S., Astrup, A., Breum, L. & Quaade, F. (1993) The acute and chronic effects of ephedrine/caffeine mixtures on energy expenditure and glucose metabolism in humans. *International Journal of Obesity and Related Metabolic Disorders* **17** (suppl. 3), S73–S77.

Van Gaal, L.F., Vansant, G.A., Steijaert, M.C. & De-Leeuw, I.H. (1995) Effects of dexfenfluramine on resting metabolic rate and thermogenesis in premenopausal obese women during therapeutic weight reduction. *Metabolism* **44** (suppl. 2), 42–45.

Visser, M., Seidell, J.C., Koppeschaar, H.P.F. & Smits, P. (1993) The effect of fluoxetine on body weight, body composition and visceral fat accumulation. *International Journal of Obesity and Related Metabolic Disorders* **17**, 247–253.

Weber, C., Tam, Y.K., Schmidte, K.E., Schrezenmeier, G., Jonkmann, J.H. & van Brummelen, P. (1996) Effect of lipase inhibitor orlistat on the pharmacokinetics of four different antihypertensive drugs in healthy volunteers. *European Journal of Clinical Pharmacology* **51**, 87–90.

Weintraub, M., Rubio, A., Golik, A., Byrne, L. & Scheinbaum, M.L. (1991) Sibutramine in weight control: a dose ranging, efficacy study. *Clinical Pharmacology and Therapeutics* **50**, 330–337.

Weintraub, M., Sundaresan, P.R., Schuster, B. *et al.* (1992) Long term weight control. *Clinical Pharmacology and Therapeutics* **51**, 586–645.

Willey, K.A., Molyneaux, L.M., Overland, J.E. & Yue, D.K. (1992) The effects of dexfenfluramine on blood glucose control in patients with type 2 diabetes. *Diabetic Medicine* **9**, 341–343.

William-Olsson, T., Krotkiewski, M. & Sjostrom, L. (1985) Relapse reducing effects of acarbose after weight reduction in severely obese subjects. *Journal of Obesity and Weight Regulation* **4**, 20–32.

Wise, S.D. (1992) Clinical studies with fluoxetine in obesity. *American Journal of Clinical Nutrition* **55**, 181S–184S.

Zed, C.A., Harris, G.S., Harrison, P.J. & Robb, G.H. (1985) Anti-obesity activity of a novel β-adrenoceptor agonist (BRL 26830A) in diet-restricted obese subjects. *International Journal of Obesity* **9**, 231 (abstract).

Zhi, J., Melia, A.T., Koss-Twardy, S.G. *et al.* (1995) The influence of orlistat on the pharmacokinetics and pharmacodynamics of glyburide in healthy volunteers. *Journal of Clinical Pharmacology* **35**, 521–525.

Zhi, J., Melia, A.T., Funk, C. *et al.* (1996a) Metabolic profiles of minimally absorbed orlistat in obese/overweight volunteers. *Journal of Clinical Pharmacology* **36**, 1006–1011.

Zhi, J., Melia, A.T., Guerciolini, R. *et al.* (1996b) The effect of orlistat on the pharmacokinetics and pharmacodynamics of warfarin in healthy volunteers. *Journal of Clinical Pharmacology* **36**, 659–666.

Zhi, J., Melia, A.T., Koss-Twardy, S.G., Arora, S. & Patel, I.H. (1996c) The effect of orlistat, an inhibitor of dietary fat absorption, on the pharmacokinetics of beta-carotene in healthy volunteers. *Journal of Clinical Pharmacology* **36**, 152–159.

CHAPTER 20

Strategies for Discovering Drugs to Treat Obesity

GEORGE A. BRAY

Introduction

Following the discovery of leptin in 1994 (Zhang *et al.*, 1994) and the report by Weintraub *et al.* (1992) using a combination of drugs to treat obesity effectively, interest in new approaches for the treatment of obesity has increased rapidly. This chapter will provide an overview of potential mechanisms which might frame these new approaches. A rational approach to drug discovery requires an assessment of the importance of various components of the system or systems which control body fat distribution. Figure 20.1 presents a schematic showing the basic mechanisms underlying an increase in total body fat, and the mechanisms involved in altering the distribution of the fat which is stored. The shift from one fat level to another without shifting the distribution of fat between visceral and non-visceral compartments can be presented by a greater intake of nutrient energy than the amount of energy that is being expended. That is, the individual or animal is in positive energy balance. The mechanisms involved in the control of energy balance and how they may relate to the development of new drugs will be described. In addition, the mechanisms involved in the altered distribution of body fat will be reviewed since these mechanisms may be quite different from those determining levels of total body fat.

Obesity and hypertension have a number of features in common that may guide the future of drug development. Both body-weight and blood pressure are feedback systems which regulate vascular tone. These involve both the sympathetic nervous system (SNS) and the angiotensin system. The efferent systems for regulation of body fat might be viewed as the sympathetic system and the secretion of insulin. The controlled system for blood pressure includes the level of body fluids, the tone of the vessels and the function of the heart. By analogy, the controlled system for body fat includes the gut where food is digested and absorbed, the circulatory system which transports nutrients for storage or oxidation, the adipose tissue where fat is stored and the tissues which oxidize fatty acids.

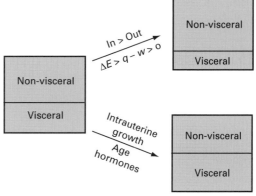

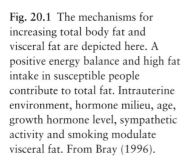

Fig. 20.1 The mechanisms for increasing total body fat and visceral fat are depicted here. A positive energy balance and high fat intake in susceptible people contribute to total fat. Intrauterine environment, hormone milieu, age, growth hormone level, sympathetic activity and smoking modulate visceral fat. From Bray (1996).

Afferent blood pressure signals are generated from the baroceptors and from atrial natriuretic peptide (ANP). The afferent messages in the weight regulating system include leptin and the afferent vagal system from gut and liver.

Prior to the introduction of chlorthiazide in 1958, hypertension had three major treatments: diet, drugs and surgery. A low-salt diet was the dietary mainstay. If begun early enough a very-low-salt diet could be beneficial in treating hypertension. Effective pharmacological therapy was introduced in 1958 and later the use of very-low-salt diets was abandoned. Drug treatment for hypertension prior to 1958 included reserpine, hydralazine and ganglionic blockers. The side-effects of these drugs were substantial and limited their use. Finally, surgical sympathectomy was a drastic method used effectively in some people. The analogy with treatment of obesity are the low- and very-low-calorie diets, the use of drugs which, regrettably, have significant side-effects, and the use of gastric and intestinal bypass surgery.

In 1958 chlorothiazide was introduced. By producing a diuresis, sodium was reduced and the first effective treatment for hypertension appeared. Orlistat, a pancreatic lipase inhibitor, might be viewed as the analogue to the diuretic. The loss of calories as undigested triglycerides would be like the loss of sodium with diuretics. The current centrally active noradrenergic and serotonergic drugs described elsewhere may be analogous to the early drugs used to treat hypertension. Finally, sympathectomy for treating hypertension is analogous to gastric surgery for obesity.

If today for obesity is analogous to 1958 for hypertension, then we can expect a variety of new and effective drugs. Some of these will act at the level of the controller to modulate feeding. Others will work at the level of the afferent signalling system to modulate feeding. Other drugs are likely to control obesity by modulating metabolic processes in the controlled system like the drugs which affect the angiotensin system or the nitric oxide system. Finally, there will be drugs which modulate afferent signals and those which regulate food intake.

Pharmacological approaches to treat obesity

Pharmacological approaches to reduce food intake

Peripherally acting agents

The nutrients, monoamines, and peptides which alter food intake peripherally generally do so by decreasing food intake. The peptides are summarized in Table 20.1

NUTRIENTS

Glucose and hexose analogues

Peripheral injections of glucose decrease food intake in experimental animals (Russek, 1963). Both gastro-intestinal and hepatic sites have been postulated for the inhibitory effects of glucose on food intake, and the vagus nerve may be

Table 20.1 Peptides which affect food intake.

Peptides which increase food intake	Peptides which decrease food intake
Galanin	Apoprotein IV
Growth hormone releasing hormone	Bombesin
β-Casomorphin	Calcitonin (CGRP)
Insulin	Cholecystokinin (CCK)
Melanocyte concentrating hormone	Corticotrophin-releasing hormone (CRH)
Neuropeptide-Y	Cytokines/leptin
Opioids	Enterostatin
Somatostatin	Glucagon
	Glucagon like peptide-1 (GLP-1)
	Insulin
	Leptin
	α-Melanocyte-stimulating hormone
	Neuromedin B
	Neurotensin
	Oxytocin
	Thyrotropin-releasing hormone (TRH)
	Urocortin
	Vasopressin

the connection between the peripheral receptors and the brain (Niijima, 1984). When glucose is infused into the portal circulation, vagal afferent firing is reduced as a function of glucose concentration. Infusion of either glucose or arginine will lower vagal firing and increase sympathetic efferent firing of nerves to brown adipose tissue (Inoue *et al.*, 1991).

5,7-Anhydro-mannitol or deoxy-fructose is an analogue of fructose. Peripheral injection of this compound stimulates food intake (Tordoff *et al.*, 1991). One mode of action which has been proposed is a decrease in hepatic adenosine triphosphate (ATP) concentrations. Pyruvate and lactate, two metabolites of glucose, also decrease food intake when injected peripherally (Langhans, 1996; Nagase *et al.*, 1996). Analogues of these various metabolite might pose interesting molecules to test for anti-obesity effects.

Lipoproteins, fatty acids and ketones

Inhibition of fatty acid oxidation with 2-mercaptoacetate (Ritter *et al.*, 1992), an inhibitor of acetyl-CoA dehydrogenase, or with methyl palmoxirate (Friedman, 1995), an inhibitor of carnitine acyltransferase I will increase food intake. Studies in animals indicate that this increased food intake is predominately carbohydrate and/or protein but not fat, even when fat is the only available nutrient (L. Singer, D.A. York and G.A. Bray unpublished observations). The peripheral effects of 2-mercaptoacetate are blocked by hepatic vagotomy but the effects of methyl palmoxirate are not (Ritter & Taylor, 1989, 1990).

Administration of 3-hydroxybutyric acid, a key end product of fatty acid oxidation, decreases food intake (Langhans, 1996). This inhibition of food intake is dependent on an intact vagus nerve since both vagotomy and capsaicin treatment which destroys afferent vagal nerve fibres, block the inhibitory effects of 3-hydroxybutyric acid. Several lactone derivatives produced from glucose and fatty acids have been shown by Sakata and his colleagues to reduce food intake (Sakata & Kurokawa, 1992). The physiological role of these metabolic products is at present unclear.

Apoprotein IV (Apo IV) is a peptide produced by the intestine which is incorporated into lipoproteins and chylomicrons. When this peptide is injected either peripherally or into the brain there is a significant decrease in food intake. The release of Apo IV during the hydrolysis of lipoproteins by lipoprotein lipase in the periphery has been hypothesized to be a satiety signal related to fat digestion (Fujimoto *et al.*, 1993; Okumura *et al.*, 1995). The components of this peptide which produces the effect will provide new clues for a peripherally acting agent that can reduce food intake.

PERIPHERAL MONOAMINES

Noradrenalin

Treatment with β_2-agonists will reduce food intake with little effect or thermogenesis. Clenbuterol was 10–30 times as potent as a β_1-agonist (dobutamine) or a β_3-agonist (ICI D-7114) in reducing food intake (Yamashita *et al.*, 1994). However, β_3-agonists do reduce food intake in lean and obese rats (Tsujii & Bray, 1992) and in lean mice (K. Okuma, G.A. Bray and D.A. York unpublished observations). This has been extended by Flier and his colleagues (Mantzoros *et al.*, 1996) using knockouts of the β_3-adrenergic receptors in mice. In such animals, the peripheral injection of β_3-agonists which normally reduces food intake is obliterated, indicating that there are peripheral β_3-adrenergic receptors involved in the modulation of food intake which act as inhibitory signals for feeding.

Destruction of brown adipose tissue in mice with a diphtheria toxin suicide gene is associated with reduced thermogenesis, increased food intake and increased body fat, particularly in the males (Lowell *et al.*, 1993). In animals maintained at elevated ambient temperatures, these effects are eliminated, suggesting that the loss of the heat-producing system related to loss of the uncoupling protein in brown adipose tissue may play a role in the peripheral feedback on food intake (Melnyk *et al.*, 1995).

Serotonin

Peripheral injection of serotonin reduces food intake and specifically decreases fat intake (Bray & York, 1972; Orthen-Gambill & Kanarek, 1982). Since the majority of serotonin is located in the gastro-intestinal track, it may be that serotonin receptors in this tissue play an important role in the modulation of food intake, in response to enteral signals or to the rate of gastric emptying.

PEPTIDES

A number of peptides modulate feeding (see Table 20.1) (Morley, 1987; Lee *et al.*, 1994). This discussion will deal first with those peptides which act peripherally. In a later section (Pepride neurotransmitters and neuromodulators) I will discuss the centrally acting peptide neuromodulators.

Cholecystokinin

The octapeptide of cholecystokinin (CCK_8) as well as the full-length cholecystokinin molecule (CCK_{33}) are produced in the gastro-intestinal track. When injected parentally, cholecystokinin produces a dose-related reduction in sham-feeding in experimental animals and in lean and obese humans but the doses are near those that cause gastro-intestinal cramping and nausea (Kissileff *et al.*, 1981; Stracher *et al.*, 1982; Baile & Della Ferra, 1984; Boosalis *et al.*, 1992; Smith & Gibbs, 1994; Gutzwiler *et al.*, 1994). CCK acts on CCK_A receptors in the pyloric channel of the stomach to cause constriction of the pylorus and to slow gastric emptying (Corwin *et al.*, 1991). Peptide analogues of CCK provide one avenue for drug development (Moran *et al.*, 1992). The recently described benzodiazepines which are CCK agonists are a second way to use this strategy (Henke *et al.*, 1996). Antagonists to CCK breakdown is a third approach to enhancing the effect of CCK and to altering gastric emptying, gastric distention and food intake.

Vagotomy blocks the reduction in food intake produced by the peripheral injection of CCK suggesting that afferent messages are generated in the gastroduodenal/hepatic circuit and relayed to the brain by the vagus nerve (Geary & Smith, 1983). These vagal messages initiated by the intraperitoneal injection of CCK activate several neuronal complexes in the brain including the nucleus of the tractus solitarius (NTS), the lateral parabrachial nucleus and the amygdala, as assessed by expression of the c-*fos* gene product (Hamamura *et al.*, 1991). The production of early satiety by CCK does not require an intact medial hypothalamus because it occurs in human beings with hypothalamic injury and obesity (Boosalis *et al.*, 1992).

Bombesin

Bombesin (BBS) is a tetradecapeptide which was isolated from amphibian skin and is similar in structure to mammalian gastrin-releasing peptide (GRP) (Lee *et al.*, 1994). Peripheral administration of BBS to experimental animals and humans (Lieverse *et al.*, 1993; Muurhainen *et al.*, 1993) will reduce food intake but in contrast to CCK this is not blocked by vagotomy although it can be blocked by combined cord section and vagotomy (Gibbs *et al.*, 1979). The effects of BBS are independent of CCK since blockers of the effects of CCK do not impair the effects of BBS. Both BBS and GRP will decrease food intake in humans making the development of receptor agonists a potential therapeutic strategy.

Glucagon and glucagon-like peptide-1

Glucagon is a 29 amino acid peptide which depresses food intake after peripheral administration (Geary & Smith, 1983; Geary, 1990). It produces a dose-dependent inhibition of food intake following portal vein administration in experimental animals. Antibodies which bind glucagon increase food intake suggesting that the signals generated by pancreatic glucagon act in the liver and may be physiologically relevant in modulating feeding. Glucagon depresses food intake in men, but this does not occur if glucagon and CCK are given simultaneously (Geary *et al.*, 1992). Glucagon-like peptide-1 (GLP-1; glucagon 6-29), which results from post-translutunal processing of pro-glucagon, is an alternative peptide for anti-obesity development because it works peripherally and possibly centrally as well (Kreyman *et al.*, 1989; Shughrue & Lane, 1996; Turton *et al.*, 1996).

Insulin and insulin secretion

The effects of insulin on food intake depend on dose and route of administration (Brief & Davis, 1984; Arase *et al.*, 1988a). In doses which will lower blood glucose, insulin is hyperphagic probably because it produces hypoglycaemia. In contrast, chronic infusion of low doses of insulin (Vander Weele *et al.*, 1982) or injection of insulin antibodies into the portal circulation increases food intake suggesting that portal and/or peripheral insulin concentrations may serve as an inhibitory signal for feeding. Schwartz *et al.* (1992) have shown that cerebrospinal fluid (CSF) insulin reflects integrated plasma levels and that insulin enters the brain by a carrier mediated process. They have proposed that it may be the central insulin rather than the peripheral insulin which is serving as the feedback signal. A low level of insulin secretion and enhanced insulin sensitivity both predict weight gain in Pima Indians (Ravussin & Swinburn, 1992; Schwartz *et al.*, 1995).

Hyperinsulinaemia and insulin resistance are characteristic of obesity. Blockade of insulin release by vagotomy (Inoue & Bray, 1977; Cox & Powley, 1981) destruction of the β-cells by streptozotocin (York & Bray, 1972) or by islet transplants (Inoue *et al.*, 1978) reduce or prevent weight gain following ventromedial hypothalamus (VMH) lesions. Diazoxide is one approach to lowering insulin clinically and may be successful in slowing weight gain. An agent which reduces insulin secretion and obesity in experimental animals has been reported by Campfield *et al.* (1995) and opens the field to new potential agents.

Insulin resistance is associated with reduced GLUT4 and glucokinase levels in experimental animals. A peroxisome proliferator activated receptor (PPAR-γ) located upstream of the genes for these enzymes appears to modulate the insulin induction of these enzymes. The thiozoladinedione drugs such as troglitazone binds to this PPAR-γ and 'sensitize' these receptors to allow glucokinase and GLUT4 to be expressed. Whether this type of pharmacological manipulation of insulin resistance will affect body fat stores is still unclear.

Enterostatin

Enterostatin (Val-Pro-Gly-Pro-Arg) is a pentapeptide produced by cleavage of a pancreatic enzyme, procolipase, by trypsin in the intestine (Lin *et al.*, 1994). Procolipase is secreted in response to dietary fat and its signal peptide, enterostatin, is highly conserved across a number of species (Erlansen-Albertsson *et al.*, 1991). Enterostatin decreases food intake whether given centrally or peripherally (Shargill *et al.*, 1991). Injection of enterostatin peripherally selectively reduces fat intake by nearly 50% in animals which prefer dietary fat (Okada *et al.*, 1991). The peripheral effects of enterostatin are blocked by vagotomy or capsaicin treatment indicating the importance of afferent vagal information (Lin *et al.*, 1995). This afferent information activates c-fos expression in the NTS in the lateral parabrachial nucleus, the amygdala and the supraoptic nucleus (Tian *et al.*, 1994). Injection of enterostatin also enhances serotonin turnover in the central nervous system (CNS). The dose–response curve for enterostatin is U-shaped with an optimal inhibitory effect at 1 nmol peripherally. Higher and lower doses are less effective and at high doses enterostatin actually stimulates food intake. Enterostatin stimulates the SNS at doses which decrease food intake (Nagase *et al.*, 1996).

β-casomorphin

β-casomorphin is a cleavage product of milk casein (Lin *et al.*, 1997). It has seven amino acids with the sequence Y-P-F-P-G-P-I (Tyr-Pro-Phe-Pro-Gly-Pro-Ile) in contrast to the V-P-G-P-R (Val-Pro-Gly-Pro-Arg) sequences for enterostatin. Because of the P-X-P similarities between enterostatin and β-casomorphin, β-casomorphin and its 4 and 5 amino acid N-terminal fragments were tested on food intake. β-casomorphin 1-7 stimulates food intake when injected peripherally. This effect is completely lost if G-H-I, the three carboxy-terminal amino acids, are removed. β-casomorphin 1-4, however, still retains its morphine-like properties. Thus, the G-H-I (Gly-His-Ile) carboxy-terminal tripeptide contains important information for modulating feeding.

Leptin and cytokines

Leptin is a 167 amino acid peptide whose receptor is a member of the gp 130 cytokine super family (see above). Leptin clearly has a physiological role in maintaining the tonic responsiveness of a variety of steroid-mediated pathways including glucocorticoids, oestrogens, aldosterone and androgens (Bray, 1996).

In addition to leptin, a variety of other cytokines will decrease food intake (Plata-Salaman, 1991). Among these are interleukin-1β (IL-1β), interleukin-

6, tumour necrosis factor (TNF-α) and cachetin. The role of the cytokine molecules, except leptin, in the physiological control systems for feeding has not been established. Leptin and the cytokine signalling systems provide novel leads for drug development, particularly because of their modulation of steroid action. The gene products of the *ob/ob, db/db* or *fa/fa* rat were conceived as modulators of steroid action by reducing the transcription of GR–steroid complexes.

Centrally acting agents

NUTRIENTS

Glucose and glucose analogues

Glucose receptors have been identified in the brain. The injection of glucose into the ventricular system in doses ranging from 2 to 30 μmol has been shown to reduce food intake in some experiments (Kurata *et al.*, 1986; Tsujii & Bray, 1990) but others have shown no effect (Berthoud & Baetig, 1974). The presence of glucoreceptors in the hypothalamus (Oomura *et al.*, 1969) and the fact that injection of phlorizin, a competitor for glucose transport into the third ventricle, will increase food intake in experimental animals (Pankseep & Meeker, 1976) suggest that glucose in the CNS probably plays a role in modulation of feeding. Glucose injected into the third cerebral ventricle increases sympathetic firing rate to brown adipose tissue showing a functional role for hypothalamic glucoreceptors in the reciprocal relationship of food intake and the activity of the SNS (Sakaguchi & Bray, 1987).

Several analogues of glucose have been used to explore further the role of glucose in feeding (Table 20.2). 2-deoxy-D-glucose (2DG) is an analogue of glucose which is transported into cells and phosphorylated but not further metabolized. This metabolite blocks metabolism of glucose-6-phosphate and

Table 20.2 Metabolites which affect food intake.

Increase	Decrease
2-deoxy-D-glucose	Glucose
5,7-anhydromannitol	3-hydroxybutyrate
2-mercaptoacetate	Lactate
Methylpalmoxirate	Pyruvate
	β_2-adrenergic agonists
	β_3-adrenergic agonists

produces intracellular glucopenia which stimulates food intake in experimental animals and human beings.

2-DG increase in food intake inhibits sympathetic activity to brown adipose tissue and increases the firing rate of the adrenal nerves which increase adrenalin secretion (Thompson & Campbell, 1977; Egawa et al., 1989). The hyperglycaemia produced by 2-DG can be obliterated by adrenodemodulation indicating that it is the adrenalin release and hepatic glycogenolysis that provides the glucose. Using the expression of the gene product c-fos peripheral injection of 2-DG has been shown to activate a number of neuronal groups in the brain including the NTS, the lateral parabrachial nucleus and the amygdala. Selective peripheral hepatic vagotomy does not block this activation sequence by 2-DG, suggesting that the major site for action for 2-DG may be in the hindbrain (Ritter & Taylor, 1989, 1990).

A second glucose analogue is 5-thioglucose which will impair the metabolism of central or peripheral glucose. This analogue has been used by Ritter et al. (1992) to show the presence of glucose receptors in the hindbrain. Like 2-DG, 5-thioglucose will stimulate food intake. Gold thioglucose is a third glucose analogue. It is transported into the hypothalamus where the gold deposits damage neuronal tissue and lead to obesity (Debons et al., 1982). Phlorizin, a drug which blocks glucose transport, increases food intake when injected into the cerebro-ventricular system (Glick & Mayer, 1968).

This effect of 2-DG may involve γ-aminobutyric acid (GABA) receptors since injection of picrotoxin, an antagonist of GABA receptors, will block the stimulation of food intake by 2-deoxyglucose (Tsujii & Bray, 1990).

Fatty acids and ketones

Infusion of 3-hydroxybutyrate into the brain's ventricular system will depress food intake in lean animals independent of diet (Davis et al., 1981; Arase et al., 1988a). Infusion of 3-hydroxybutyrate significantly reduces food intake and body-weight and increases sympathetic activity (Sakaguchi & Bray, 1988b). These effects of ketones in the CNS are consistent with the observations of Oomura et al. (1975) showing the presence of fatty acid responsive neurons in the lateral hypothalamus.

Amino acids

Administration of tryptophan in high doses orally will decrease food intake by enhancing brain tryptophan which is converted to serotonin, a neurotransmitter known to reduce food intake. Tryptophan is transported across the blood–brain barrier by a transporter which also transports other large neutral amino acids. When these other amino acids are increased, tryptophan entry is reduced by competition for the transporter.

Amino acids in the CNS can be excitatory or inhibitory. Glutamic acid serves as a general neuronal excitatory agent and GABA and glycine serve as general inhibitory amino acids. Glutamate infusion into the periformical area increases food intake and body-weight (Stanley *et al.*, 1993b). GABA may also have a role in modulating food intake. Microinjection of GABA can increase food intake in the medial hypothalamus and inhibit food intake when given into the lateral hypothalamus. Antagonists of GABA, such as picrotoxin or bicucculine can block the stimulation of feeding produced by 2-deoxyglucose (Tsujii & Bray, 1991). Monosodium glutamate, a flavour enhancer, will damage hypothalamic neurons when injected into neonatal rats. This is followed by an obesity which develops without significant hyperphagia but with a decrease in sympathetic activity (Yoshida *et al.*, 1984).

MONOAMINE NEUROTRANSMITTERS

Receptors on which monoamines act to reduce food intake

Noradrenalin

Three noradrenergic receptors mediate the effects of noradrenalin to increase or decrease food intake (Leibowitz & Brown, 1980; Leibowitz, 1986). This allows two strategies for drug discoveries. The first is to design agonists that are specific for the desired receptor. The second is to block reuptake of noradrenalin in regions where the increased noradrenalin pool will have the desired effect on food intake.

α_1-*adrenergic receptors*. Noradrenalin acting on α_1-adrenergic receptors in the paraventricular nucleus decreases food intake. Adrenergic agonists such as phenylpropanolamine or metaraminol will also reduce food intake. This effect is blocked by injection of α_1-adrenergic antagonists (Wellman, 1990). Evidence for the α_1-adrenergic system being involved in human beings is suggested by the fact that the α_1-adrenergic antagonist terazosin, which is used to treat hypertension, is associated with small weight gains relative to placebo in double-blind randomized controlled trials (Physicians Desk Reference, 1997).

α_2-*adrenergic receptors*. Activation of α_2-adrenergic receptors in the paraventricular nucleus by noradrenalin or by clonidine (Leibowitz, 1986; Tsujii & Bray, 1992) will stimulate food intake in experimental animals. This effect can be blocked by α_2-adrenergic antagonists such as yohimbine or idazoxan.

Clinically, neither clonidine nor yohimbine have significant effects on body-weight.

β_1-*adrenergic receptors*. Noradrenalin stimulation of β_1-adrenergic receptors located in the perifornical area will decrease food intake (Leibowitz, 1986). This can be accomplished pharmacologically by blockade of noradrenalin reuptake as seen with mazindol or by enhancing noradrenalin release as seen with phentermine or diethylpropion. Similarly β_2-agonists such as clenbuterol and salbutamol will decrease food intake. The importance of noradrenalin in regulation of food intake is suggested by three observations. First, lesions of the ventral noradrenergic bundle which abolishes noradrenalin release in the perifornical area is associated with weight gain (Ahlskog & Hoebel, 1973). Second, injection of a tyrosine hydroxylase blocker, α-methyl-*p*-tyrosine into the perifornical area increases feeding by blocking noradrenalin synthesis. Finally, infusion of noradrenalin into the ventromedial nucleus (VMN) can increase food intake, decrease sympathetic activity and produce obesity (Shimazu *et al.*, 1986).

Serotonin

There are seven different families of serotonin receptors (5-hydroxytryptamine (5HT)) with several receptor subtypes in some of these families (Baez *et al.*, 1995). Most of these subtypes are in the $5HT_1$ and $5H_2$ series. The signal transduction system for most of the serotonin receptors involves G-coupled activation or inhibition of adenylate cyclase.

Serotonin is clearly involved in regulation of food intake (Leibowitz *et al.*, 1988; Blundell *et al.*, 1995). Several serotonin receptors have been implicated in feeding systems. Activation of the $5HT_{1A}$ receptor, an autocrine receptor in the dorsal raphe nuclei, stimulates food intake acutely (Dourish, 1995). Chronic administration of a $5HT_{1A}$ receptor agonist down-regulates $5HT_{1A}$ receptors and no longer stimulates feeding. Stimulation of the $5\text{-}HT_{1B}$, $5\text{-}HT_{2A}$ or $5\text{-}HT_{2C}$ will reduce food intake. The $5\text{-}HT_3$ receptor may be involved in the anorectic response to diets which are deficient in single amino acids (Hammer *et al.*, 1990).

Drugs which block serotonin reuptake such as fluoxetine and sertraline significantly decrease food intake (Goldstein *et al.*, 1995). The effect of fluoxetine on food intake is not inhibited by metergoline suggesting that this effect may be by some other mechanism than serotonin. Drugs which release serotonin and act as partial reuptake inhibitors such as dexfenfluramine also decrease food intake (Garattini, 1995). These inhibitory effects of dexfenfluramine are blocked by metergoline and methysergide, two broad-spectrum serotonin antagonists. Reduction of food intake by dexfenfluramine is also blocked by lesions in the lateral parabrachial nucleus (Li *et al.*, 1994). In double-blind clinical studies dexfenfluramine significantly reduced fat intake (Goodall *et al.*, 1993). Ritanserin, a $5HT_{2C}$ antagonist, blocked this effect suggesting that $5HT_{2C}$ receptors may mediate the effects of serotonin on feeding.

Drugs which block serotonin and noradrenalin uptake have an interesting spectrum of actions and suggest that the serotonin/noradrenalin system is involved in both food intake and mood states. Two highly specific serotonin reuptake inhibitors, fluoxetine and sertraline, are very effective antidepressants and produce modest weight loss which fades after 12–20 weeks of treatment (Darga *et al.*, 1991; Wadden *et al.*, 1995). Two drugs developed as antidepressants (mazindol and sibutramine) are inhibitors of noradrenalin reuptake (mazindol) and in the case of sibutramine, serotonin reuptake as well. They appear to be better appetite suppressants than antidepressants. Venlafaxine, a drug which also blocks reuptake of serotonin and noradrenalin, is an antidepressant but like fluoxetine and sertraline has only weak effects on food intake. The spectrum of activities on the cardiovascular system associated with these drugs also varies considerably. Mazindol shows very little cardiovascular effect whereas sibutramine and venlafaxine which inhibit the reuptake of both noradrenalin and serotonin are associated with slight increases in heart rate and blood pressure (Ryan *et al.*, 1995). There is clearly more to learn about the relation of serotonin and noradrenalin in the control of food intake and mood.

The importance of serotonin receptors in regulation of human feeding is further demonstrated by the weight increase associated with use of cyproheptidine. This drug is a serotonin antagonist which is used in the treatment of pruritus in allergic conditions. It is also claimed to reduce adrenocorticotrophic hormone (ACTH) secretion and has been used in treating Cushing's disease.

Dopamine

Two dopamine receptors, D_1 and D_2, have been identified (Terry *et al.*, 1995). Drugs acting on either of these receptors can alter food intake but may also be associated with a variety of effects on mood. Bromocriptine, a specific D_2-agonist, has been associated with suggestive decreases in food intake (Parada *et al.*, 1989). Sulpuride, an antagonist of the dopamine D_1-receptors, can increase food intake. NMI-8731, another dopamine antagonist, has also been associated with decreased food intake.

Bromocriptine, a dopamine agonist, has been used for treatment of prolactin-secreting adenomas without noticable changes in body-weight. Based on studies on experimental animals in which prolactin secretion was associated with fat storage in migratory and prehibernating animals, a clinical trial was conducted.

Bromocriptine, administered in appropriately timed doses was claimed to reduce skinfold thickness. Its role in clinical treatment of obesity is currently being assessed (Cincotta & Meier, 1996).

Histamine

Experimentally, histamine H-3 receptors in the CNS has been implicated in the modulation of food intake (Sakata *et al.*, 1994; Sakata, 1995). Destruction of histidine decarboxylase with α-fluoromethylhistidine or blockade of histamine receptors with chlorpheneramine or meperamine can decrease food intake in experimental animals. In humans cimetidine suspension has been shown to reduce appetite and body-weight in obese subjects (Stoa-Birketvedt, 1993). Some of the weak neuroleptics such as chlorpromazine, thioridazine and mesoridazine may increase body-weight by acting on histamine receptors as well as serotonin receptors.

MECHANISMS BY WHICH DRUGS MODULATE
MONOAMINE RECEPTORS

There are several mechanisms by which the receptors described above can be activated, and these represent most of the currently available drugs.

Agonists

Direct receptor agonists are one approach. Phenylpropanolamine is an agonist for the α_1-receptor (Wellman, 1990). When injected into the paraventricular nucleus (PVN) food intake is reduced. Injection of α_1-antagonists into the PVN increases feeding suggesting that there may be a tonic inhibitory system involving this receptor.

Clonidine is a prototype α_2-adrenergic agonist which increases feeding in rats (Leibowitz *et al.*, 1985). Review of the clinical literature does not show any effect on human weight status suggesting that this receptor may not be important in human beings.

β_2-adrenergic agonists such as salbutamol and clenbuterol will decrease food intake when injected into the cerebral ventricular system or peripherally (Bray & Tsujii, 1992; Yamashita *et al.*, 1994), indicating that the central receptors mediating noradrenalin may be β_2-receptors.

Several serotoninergic agonists have been identified. 8-OHDPAT (8-hydroxy-2-diphenyl amino tetraline) is an agonist for the $5HT_{1A}$ receptor which increases food intake (Dourish, 1995). Quipazine is a serotonin agonist which decreases food intake. The D-norfenfluramine metabolite of dexfenfluramine also appears to be an agonist for the 5HT receptor in the PVN where it will decrease food intake.

Antagonists

Antagonists to the monoamine receptors noted above have effects opposite to those of the agonists. Clinically used antagonists to the α_1-receptor are used to treat hypertension. Terasozin has been reported to produce a significant weight gain compared to placebo, suggesting that the α_1-receptor is tonically involved in modulating human body-weight. Antagonists to the α_2-receptors do not affect weight in experimental animals (Idazoxan). Antagonists to serotonin receptors, like those to α_1-receptors, do increase food intake. Cyproheptidine is a serotonin antagonist noted for its weight gain.

Reuptake inhibitors

Several drugs which cause weight loss fall in this category. Mazindol is a tricyclic drug which is sympathominetic and which is associated with weight loss by blocking reuptake of noradrenalin.

Fluoxetine and sertraline are serotonin reuptake inhibitors that decrease food intake and body-weight. In clinical trials fluoxetine produces significantly greater weight loss for the first 20–24 weeks. Thereafter, fluoxetine loses its effectiveness and most subjects regain weight to levels not significantly different by 10–12 months. The reason for this tachyphylaxis is unknown.

Drugs which block reuptake of both serotonin and noradrenalin also reduce body-weight. In animals fluoxetine and nisoxetine, individual blockers of serotonin and noradrenalin uptake, produce weight loss comparable to sibutramine. Venlafaxine, a serotonin norepinephrine reuptake inhibitor (SNRI) antidepressant, produces weight loss in many patients. Sibutramine, another SNRI, has been evaluated for its effect on body-weight in trials lasting 2–6 months. In these studies there is a dose–response effect which lasts for up to 12 months (Bray *et al.*, 1996).

Drugs releasing monoamines

Most noradrenergic drugs which lower body-weight including benzphetamine, phendimetrazine, diethylpropion and phentermine are thought to release noradrenalin from the preganglionic storage vesicle. The released noradrenalin activates β-adrenergic receptors to reduce food intake. Most of the published mechanistic studies on these drugs were done more than 20 years ago. It is possible that reuptake mechanisms may also be involved.

Fenfluramine is a β-phenethylamine which is structurally similar to the drugs listed above, but differs pharmacologically. Fenfluramine is thought to release serotonin and to block its reuptake. Patients treated with fenfluramine do not regain weight with long-term treatment as is observed with fluoxetine. This difference may be due to the release of serotonin by fenfluramine which does not occur with fluoxetine.

PEPTIDE NEUROTRANSMITTERS AND NEUROMODULATORS

The peptides which are involved in the transduction of afferent messages into efferent signals for the motor pattern generator which drives the systems for food seeking and food selection and for the metabolic processes which handle the ingested food can be divided into two groups (see Table 20.1). One group of peptides increase food seeking and may selectively affect nutrient preferences (Table 20.3). A second and larger group of peptides decrease food intake and may likewise have macronutrient specificity in the nutrients they decrease.

Peptides which increase feeding

Neuropeptide-Y

Neuropeptide-Y (NPY) is a 36 amino acid peptide which is one of the most potent stimulators of food intake known (Clark *et al.*, 1984; Kalra & Crowley, 1992). It also produces a dose-dependent decrease in sympathetic activity to brown adipose tissue (Egawa *et al.*, 1990a, 1991; Billington *et al.*, 1994). NPY primarily stimulates the intake of carbohydrate and accomplishes this effect mainly through its action on the Y_5 receptors in the PVN (Gerald *et al.*, 1996). These effects of NPY are blocked by antibodies to NPY or by anti-sense olionucleotides to NPY synthesis (Akabayashi *et al.*, 1994).

Table 20.3 Macronutrient specificity of neurotransmitters.

	Effect on macronutrient intake	
	Increase	Decrease
Fat	Dynorphin	Enterostatin Serotonin
Protein	Growth hormone releasing hormone	
Carbohydrate	Neuropeptide-Y Noradrenalin (α_2-receptor)	
Salt	Angiotensin	

The NPY circuit involved in feeding originates in the arcuate nucleus with its first relays in the paraventricular nucleus and perifornical area (Stanley et al., 1993a). The level of NPY in the arcuate nucleus is decreased by treatment with leptin (Stephens et al., 1995) and increased by a starvation and diabetes (Schwartz et al., 1992). The perifornical area of the medial hypothalamus appears to be most responsive to NPY. NPY is located in many regions of the brain as well as in peripheral tissues and it is cosecreted with noradrenalin in many, but not all, circumstances. Antagonists to the effect of NPY have been identified (Kanatani et al., 1996) and offer promise for therapeutic treatment of obesity. NPY produces reciprocal effects on food intake and gonadotropin secretion and reproductive function (Kalra & Kalra, 1996).

Stimulation of food intake by injection of NPY into the paraventricular nucleus is blocked by parenteral injection of naloxone but not by injection of naloxone into the PVN. On the other hand, when naloxone is injected into the hindbrain, the stimulation of food intake by NPY injected into the PVN is blocked, suggesting that there is an opioid receptor system activated by NPY in the PVN which has opioid receptors in the hindbrain (Kotz et al., 1995).

A transgenic mouse which is deficient in NPY does not show any alteration in body fat or feeding suggesting that the NPY system may be sufficient to modify feeding but it is not essential (Erickson et al., 1996; Kanatani et al., 1996). However, mice with the NPY-knockout are more susceptible to convulsions.

Opioids

Both dynorphin (Hamilton & Bozarth, 1988) and β-endorphin (Grandison & Guidotti, 1977) stimulate food intake when injected into the ventricular system

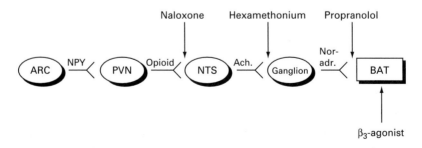

Fig. 20.2 Connections between arcuate nucleus and brown adipose tissue (BAT). Nor-adr., noradrenalin; Ach, acetylcholine; PUN, paraventricular nucleus; NTS, nucleus of the traetus solitarius.

of the brain. These effects can be blocked by antagonists to κ-opioid receptors. Stimulation of κ-opioid receptors increases fat intake which can be blocked by κ-opioid antagonists (Barton et al., 1995b). Nalaxone, an antagonist to opioid receptors, reduces food fat intake (Holtzman, 1979) and interferes with the effects of NPY (Kotz et al., 1995).

Galanin

Galanin is a 29 amino acid peptide isolated from both the gastro-intestinal tract and brain (Merchenthaler et al., 1993). Injection of galanin into the third ventricle of the brain or into the PVN will increase food intake (Kyrkouli et al., 1990; Beck et al., 1993). Some studies have suggested that this peptide preferentially stimulates fat intake (Tempel et al., 1988; Leibowitz, 1995) but others show that these effects on fat intake were because animals were fat-preferring animals and that galanin merely stimulated the underlying food preference of the animal (Smith et al., 1996). Galanin stimulates feeding when injected into the hindbrain as well as the PVN and these effects of galanin in both the third ventricle and hindbrain can be blocked by M_{40}, a peptide antagonist to galanin (Koegler & Ritter, 1996). Galanin antagonists are thus potential targets for therapeutic agents.

Growth hormone releasing hormone and somatostatin

Growth hormone releasing hormone (GHRH) and somatostatin (SRIF) are both released into the hypothalamic portal vein system and stimulate (GHRH) or inhibit (SRIF) growth hormone release from the pituitary. At low doses, each of these peptides has been claimed to increase food intake and GHRH has been claimed to selectively increase protein intake (Vaccarino & Hayward, 1988; Dickson & Vaccarino, 1994; Okada et al., 1996).

Melanocyte concentrating hormone

Melanocyte concentrating hormone (MCH) is a cyclic 19 amino acid peptide whose mRNA is exclusively expressed in the zona incerta and lateral hypothalamus (Bittencourt et al., 1992). Two other peptides are processed from the MCH precursor and have similarities to CRH and to GHRH. Injection of 5 µg of MCH into the lateral ventricle significantly increased food intake of experimental animals. The location of the peptide in the lateral hypothalamus (LH) suggests that the reduced food intake and increased sympathetic activity of LH-lesioned animals may be due to loss of MCH (Presse & Nahon, 1993; Deray et al., 1994; Presse et al., 1996).

Peptides which decrease feeding

Cholecystokinin

CCK injected into the CNS will decrease food intake (Crawley & Corwin, 1994) and increase sympathetic activity (Yoshimatsu *et al.*, 1992) by acting through CCK$_B$-receptors. A biological role for CCK is suggested by the fact that food in the stomach is associated with a release of CCK in the hypothalamus and that blockade of CCK in the brain with anti-CCK antibodies can increase food intake. The use of specific CCK antagonists also suggest an important physiological role for this peptide since these antagonists can increase basal food intake. Benzodiazepine derivatives which are CCK agonists may work in the CNS to decrease feeding (Henke *et al.*, 1996).

Corticotrophin-releasing hormone and urocortin

Corticotrophin-releasing hormone (CRH) is involved in three important functional roles (Rothwell, 1990; Glowa *et al.*, 1992). First, it is the peptide which is secreted from the PVN into the hypothalamic portal system to enhance adrenocorticotrophic hormone (ACTH) release from the pituitary gland. Second, CRH modulates the function of the autonomic nervous system, including inhibition of the parasympathetic nervous system and activation of the peripheral components of the SNS which increase thermogenesis (Arase *et al.*, 1988b; Egawa *et al.*, 1990b; De Souza, 1995). Third, CRH has a variety of effects on exploratory and other behaviours. Chronic infusion of CRH will reduce weight gain in both obese and lean experimental animals (Arase *et al.*, 1988a, 1989). Overexpression of CRH in a transgenic mouse increases food intake (Stenzel-Poore *et al.*, 1992).

Urocortin is a member of the CRH family, but its location in the lateral hypothalamus and several other brain regions is different from CRH. It has a higher affinity for the CRH$_2$-receptors and its distribution corresponds to the distribution of these receptors. Urocortin produces a dose-dependent decrease in food intake and is considerably more potent than CRH. At doses which depress food intake, urocortin does not produce the anxiogenic effects seen with CRH (Spina *et al.*, 1996).

α-melanocyte-stimulating hormone and the melanocortin receptor

The methylation of melanocyte-stimulating hormone (MSH), a 13 amino acid peptide produced by the post-translational processing of propriomelanocortin (POMC), dramatically modifies its central function (Tsujii & Bray, 1989). Injection of the non-acetylated form of MSH into the third ventricle has no effect on food intake whereas the acetylated form, α-MSH, reduces food intake. It probably does this by acting on melanocortin receptors in the brain. The agouti signalling protein probably produces obesity by competing with the α-MSH (Lu *et al.*, 1994). Endorphin, another peptide formed from POMC, stimulates food intake in the non-acetylated form but with acetylation, endorphin no longer stimulates feeding. Thus, modulation of acetylation can modulate the effects of central neurotransmitters and may provide a strategy for drug development. The importance of the melanocortin receptors in control of food intake has been supported by two recent studies. An agonist to the melanocortin receptor will inhibit food intake in several mouse models of hyperphagia including the *ob/ob* (Lep^{ob}) mouse, mice injected with NPY, overnight fasted mice and in the yellow (A^{vy}) mouse (Fan *et al.*, 1997). This is similar to the effects of α-MSH noted above. A second approach used gene targeting to disrupt the melanocortin-4 receptor in the brain of mice which resulted in significant weight gain (Huszar *et al.*, 1997). All of these data suggest that this system may be a productive one for pharmacological intervention.

Leptin and cytokines

A variety of cytokines, including leptin, will decrease food intake when injected into the CNS. Of particular interest is that leptin will not reduce food intake in *db/db* mice and *fa/fa* rats which lack the leptin receptor for these cytokines. The inhibitory effects of interleukin-1β may be modulated by α-MSH.

Calcitonin and its gene-related peptide

Modulation of calcium can affect food intake. Calcium availability can be manipulated by injecting calcium, altering calmodulin or by injecting calcitonin. Calcitonin and its gene-related peptide (CGRP) both decrease food intake (Krahn *et al.*, 1986) presumably by making calcium more available and thus possibly modulating ion channels.

Glucagon-like peptide-1

GLP-1 is a fragment of the 6-29 segment of glucagon. Injection of GLP-1 into the CNS has been reported to decrease food intake whereas exendin, an antagonist to GLP-1 receptor, increases food intake and weight gain. The importance of the finding has been questioned by the finding that GLP-1 is aversive (van Dijk *et al.*, 1997) and that knock-out of the GLP-1 receptor does not affect food intake or body-weight of mice (Scrocchi *et al.*, 1996), but does impair the incretin function of GLP-1.

Insulin

Infusion of insulin into the ventricular system decreases food intake and body-weight of baboons (Woods *et al.*, 1979) and rodents (Brief & Davis, 1984; Arase *et al.*, 1988a; McGowan *et al.*, 1990; Schwartz *et al.*, 1992). This occurs in animals eating a high-carbohydrate diet but not those eating a high-fat diet (Arase *et al.*, 1988a). Schwartz and colleagues have demonstrated that changes in CSF insulin reflect blood levels and are related to food intake. They showed that the entry of insulin is a facilitated process and that it may be a negative feedback for regulating fat stores.

Bombesin and neuromedin B

Central injection of BBS reduces food intake (Gibbs *et al.*, 1979) and activates the SNS (Barton *et al.*, 1995a). In animals that have been starved or have VMH lesions, BBS produces a profound drop in temperature because SNS cannot be activated (Barton *et al.*, 1995a). In intact animals, BBS will reduce body temperature if a ganglionic blocking drug or the β-antagonist, propranolol, is given which will eliminate the sympathetic activation of the thermogenic system in brown adipose tissue by BBS.

Oxytocin and vasopressin

An oxytocin pathway modulating food intake under stressful circumstances has been identified (Olson *et al.*, 1991). Activation of this pathway can also reduce sodium intake. A possible role in the normal control of feeding is suggested by the increase in oxytocin following treatment with fenfluramine. Arginine vasopressin will also reduce food intake and may be related to stimulation of the SNS (Langhans *et al.*, 1991). Whether these peptides whose major role is in lactation and control of renal water excretion are viable targets for pharmacological development is doubtful.

Thyrotropin-releasing hormone and cyclo-His-Pro

Thyrotropin-releasing hormone (TRH) is a tripeptide with the amino acid sequence, pyro-Glu-His-Pro (p-Glu-His-Pro), and was the first hypothalamic peptide to be identified. As its name implies, it is released from the hypothalamic neurons into the hypothalamic portal system and stimulates thyroid-stimulating hormone (TSH) release from the pituitary. When TRH is injected into the ventricular system of the brain it reduces food intake. Cyclo-His-Pro, the terminal two amino acids of TRH, are also effective in reducing food intake (Prasad, 1989; Prasad *et al.*, 1995). It was initially thought that cyclo-His-Pro was formed from TRH, but its distribution in the brain and gut suggests that it is formed separately. A variety of derivatives of cyclo-His-Pro have been synthesized but are less potent than the dipeptide (Kow & Pfaff, 1991). Cyclo-His-Pro and cyclo-Asp-Pro, derived from enterostatin, both decrease food intake peripherally and centrally, but cyclo-Asp-Pro is more potent and is more specific in suppressing fat intake.

Neurotensin

Neurotensin (NT) injected into the ventricular system of the brain has only weak effects on feeding (Stanley *et al.*, 1983). However, the rise of neurotensin in the circulation after a meal suggests that it may have some peripheral involvement in satiety. Injections of NT into the ventral tegmental area of rats results in feeding. The colocalization of NT with dopamine suggests that it may play a role in modulating mesolimbic messages from dopaminergic signals (Kalivas & Taylor, 1985; Sandoval & Kulkosky, 1992).

Pharmacological approaches to altering metabolism or shifting nutrient partitioning

Preabsorptive gastro-intestinal agents

Drugs or chemicals which inhibit nutrient digestion or absorption reduce the availability of nutrients and thus the energy supplied to the organism. Koopmans *et al.* (1994) have made use of this concept by doing various kinds of short-circuit intestinal operations in parabiotic animals. In one model, food flows from one animal into a second animal shortly after entering the duodenum requiring a marked increase in food intake in the first animal with the short intestine and a marked reduction of oral food intake in the animal with the added food supply in order to provide nutrient balance. The important question about drugs which modify intestinal absorption of nutrients is whether compensation will occur similar to that observed in the Koopmans studies. Among the agents which have been studied experimentally are inhibitors of amylase and disaccharidases, which inhibit the digestion of starches and disaccharides, and lipase inhibitors, which inhibit the digestion of fat. No protease inhibitors have been evaluated clinically.

ORLISTAT

This product (originally called tetrahydrolipstatin) is the partially hydrogenated derivative of the naturally-occurring bacterial lipase inhibitor lipstatin. This small molecule is a potent inhibitor of pancreatic lipase and has been developed for human use (Hauptman *et al.*, 1992) because of its local activity within the GI tract (see Chapter 19).

OLESTRA

Olestra is a sucrose polyester with 5.6 or 7 fatty acids per molecule of sucrose. The characteristics of the resulting 'fat-like' molecule depend on the fatty acids to which it is esterified. Since the fat has the bulk and feel of normal fat the volume of food eaten with olestra substitution will remain normal. Substitution of olestra for normal fat in a single meal is followed by complete caloric compensation within 24 hours (Rolls *et al.*, 1992) when all of the meals have olestra, studies for 2 weeks (Sparti *et al.*, 1995) and 3 months (H. Roy, J. Lovejoy, G.A. Bray, unpublished observations) do not show compensation and there is a small but significant loss of body-weight.

Postabsorptive mechanisms for altering metabolism or nutrient partitioning

Hydroxycitrate and chlorocitrate

The central role of the citrate ATP-lyase in fat synthesis led to the evaluation of inhibitors of this enzyme. Hydroxycitrate was the initial drug developed by Hoffman La Roche (Sullivan *et al.*, 1983). This drug decreases food intake in a variety of experimental animals, but during early development it was replaced by chlorocitrate, which has been used in clinical trials. In one weight-loss study there was a small but significant difference in weight loss (Triscari & Sullivan, 1984).

Steroid hormones

Gonadal steroids. Androgens and oestrogens have potent effects on body composition (Forbes *et al.*, 1992). At the onset of puberty, androgens rise in males and lead to the reduction in percentage of body fat and an increase in musculature along with masculinization. The low levels of androgens and the rise of oestrogens during puberty in females are associated with the appearance of increased subcutaneous body fat and the development of mammary tissue and ovulatory cycles. Androgens and oestrogens also play a key role in formation and enlargement of visceral fat. The level of visceral fat is higher in men than premenopausal women (Sjöstrom, 1988; Kotani *et al.*, 1994). In women the total quantity of fat to produce similar changes in blood pressure and lipids is about 20 kg more than in men (Krotkiewski *et al.*, 1983). During mid-life, visceral fat increases in men, but does not rise much in women until after the menopause (Sjöstrom, 1988; Kotani *et al.*, 1994). Part of this change may be due to the declining growth hormone levels with ageing. The increasing quantity of visceral fat and the decline in testosterone in men with advancing age suggested that treatment with testosterone might lower visceral fat.

Clinical trials using testosterone undeconate orally or testosterone cream topically by Marin and colleagues (Marin *et al.*, 1992; 1993) have shown that in men with visceral fat, testosterone can significantly reduce visceral fat over a 9-month period of treatment. In a second study by Lovejoy *et al.* (1995, 1996), the anabolic steroid oxandralone orally was also shown to reduce visceral fat at 3 months but injected nandrolone did not maintain this effect over the next 6 months.

Adrenal steroids. Adrenal glucocorticoids also play an important role in distribution of altered nutrient stores and body fat. At higher doses, glucocorticoids produce the clinical syndrome of Cushing's disease with a central pattern of fat distribution (Orth, 1995). The clinical syndrome of adrenal insufficiency called Addison's disease is associated with marked loss of body-weight and body fat.

Excess glucocorticoids are associated with increased catabolism of muscle tissue and increased fat stores particularly in the central regions of the body. Studies of fat storage and distribution following treatment of patients with Cushing's disease (Lonn *et al.*, 1994) have shown a decrease in visceral fat when glucocorticoids are lowered. As noted above, the presence of glucocorticoids is essential for the development of all forms of experimental obesity (Bray *et al.*, 1990). Adrenalectomy in genetically obese mice, which are deficient in leptin (see Table 20.1) or which have an absent or abnormal leptin receptor, will prevent the development of obesity. In addition, adrenalectomy will reduce food intake to normal and increase sympathetic activity, increase muscle mass, enhance insulin sensitivity and restore all defects except the reproductive system in the *ob/ob* mouse to normal (Ohshima *et al.*, 1984; Saito & Bray, 1984; Shargill *et al.*, 1991; Shimizu *et al.*, 1993). Thus, the genetic defects of leptin deficiency or non-functional leptin receptors require glucocorticoids for their phenotypic expression.

The only clinically useful steroid agonist which modifies body fat is megestrol acetate, a progestational agent which works in humans (Tchekmedyian *et al.*, 1992) and animals (McCarthy *et al.*, 1994). In clinical trials in women with breast cancer, and subjects with AIDS this progestational agent has been shown to increase food intake and body fat.

Dehydroepiandrosterone (DHEA) and its sulphated derivative are the most abundant adrenal steroids. More than a gram per day is produced. DHEA is low in obesity and for this reason has been studied in detail (Clore, 1995). In obese mice (Yen et al., 1977; Berdanier & McIntosh, 1989), rats (Clear, 1989) and dogs (MacEwen et al., 1989) the addition of DHEA to the diet will reduce body fat.

DHEA has been tried for its effect on body-weight in several clinical trials but with the exception of one trial (see Clore, 1995) has not shown any significant effects. A steroid derivative of DHEA called etiocholandione has been suggested to reduce body-weight in one preliminary study (Zumoff et al., 1994).

Growth hormone

Growth hormone is an essential agent for nutrient partitioning in at least two circumstances. The first is during growth. In its absence, growth slows dramatically or ceases altogether. Treatment of growth hormone deficient children with human growth hormone restores growth and decreases subcutaneous body fat. The presence of excess growth hormone before the epiphyses fuse increases height and gigantism is the result. Gigantism and non-fusion of the epiphyses is also the result of aromatase deficiency which blocks conversion of steroids to oestrogen. After fusion of the epiphysial plates when linear growth is no longer possible excess growth hormone produces acromegaly which is associated with an increase in soft tissue, and a decrease in body fat. Removal of excess growth hormone is associated with an increase of subcutaneous fat and an increase in visceral fat (Lonn et al., 1996). Growth hormone secretion declines with age and may play a role in the increase in visceral fat. Treatment of adults with growth hormone will decrease visceral fat and clinical trials to test this effect in subjects with increased visceral fat are underway.

A second setting in which growth hormone has a major role on nutrient partitioning is in the lactating animal. In cows, treatment with bovine somatotropin markedly increases the production of milk.

β-adrenergic receptors

The stimulation of β_2-adrenergic receptors by agonists such as clenbuterol or ractopamine will increase the mass of muscle tissue and decrease fat tissue in a variety of large and small animals (Rothwell & Stock, 1987). Not all β_2-adrenergic agonists are equally effective in this process suggesting that there is a component of the β_2-adrenergic receptor system which is associated with tissue growth and nutrient partitioning where other components are less involved.

Insulin

Hyperinsulinaemia is characteristic of obesity. Injection of excess doses of insulin in diabetics increases body-weight, predominantly as fat. Insulinomas which produce insulin will also increase body fat but only to a small extent. These higher levels of insulin make it much more difficult to lose body fat.

Pharmacological approaches to modulating thermogenesis

Thyroid hormones

Thyroid hormone was the earliest drug used for treatment of obesity (see Bray, 1976). We now know that this class of hormones produce their effects by acting on receptors which are members of the superfamily of steroid receptors. There is a log-dose effect of thyroid hormone on energy expenditure. One early hypothesis for the effects on energy expenditure was that it worked through uncoupling of oxidative phosphorylation. A more recent hypothesis suggests that it enhances the turnover of ions at cell membranes, which increases ATP utilization for activation transport. In addition to its effects on thermogenesis and increasing fat metabolism, thyroid hormone also increases metabolism of lean body tissue and bone. In addition, thyroid hormone increases cardiac irritability and in clinical trials using D-thyroxine to reduce heart attacks, D-thyroxine was associated with increased death rates. Thus, the use of thyroid hormone other than as hormone replacement in hypothyroid individuals is not indicated.

Uncoupling of oxidative phosphorylation

One mechanism originally proposed for thyroid hormone was to uncouple oxidative phosphorylation. This was based on the demonstration that dinitrophenol, a drug developed by the dye industry, produced weight loss by uncoupling oxidative phosphorylation. Dinitrophenol was used to treat obesity in the 1930s until the untoward side-effects such as cataracts and neuropathy made it unacceptable (see Bray, 1976 and UCP-2 and UCP-3, below).

Catecholamines

Infusion of noradrenalin into animals or humans increases energy expenditure.

This effect results from stimulation of β_3- or β_2-adrenergic receptors. In small rodents control of energy expenditure for thermogenesis to maintain body temperature is critical (Himms-Hagan, 1989). This is accomplished by activation of β_3-adrenergic receptors on brown adipose tissue, which activates uncoupling protein. The uncoupling protein (UCP) increases heat production by opening a proton leak pathway in the mitochondria in brown adipose tissue. Although there is only a small amount of brown adipose tissue in adult humans, its mass can be increased by stimulation with noradrenalin which occurs in patients with phaeochromocytomas, a disease which is associated with the production of excess quantities of noradrenalin. The UCP is activated through the β_3-receptors where stimulation increases the hydrolysis of triglycerides with release of fatty acids that interact with UCP to open paths for the proton leak (Ricquier et al., 1991). In young animals a cafeteria-style diet will increase activity of this noradrenergically mediated UCP suggesting the possibility that drugs, which increase β_3-adrenergic activity, might be valuable therapeutic agents (Arch et al., 1984; Yen, 1994; Yoshida et al., 1994; Himms-Hagan & Ghorbani, 1995). When the β_3-adrenergic receptor has been eliminated by knock-out techniques in transgenic animals, there is little effect on body-weight presumably because β_2- and β_3-receptors can replace much of the function of β_3-receptors. However, the decrease in food intake by stimulation of β_3-receptors is eliminated in these animals. These agents may be of value for obesity and diabetes. Two additional UCPs have been identified and are called UCP-2 and UCP-3. There is presently few data on these mitochondrial peptides but they offer an additional glimmer of hope.

Summary and conclusions

From the preceding discussion it is clear that many different mechanisms can be called on to alter the state of body fat and fat distribution. These have led to a number of new concepts for drug development (Table 20.4). The important question is which one(s) of these will be the most effective from a clinical perspective.

Reviewing the anti-obesity drugs it may be possible to divide them into three groups. The first would be those which act through the medial hypothalamus and have effects similar to VMH or PVN lesions. These would include NPY antagonists, galanin antagonists, α_1-adrenergic agonists, β_2-adrenergic agonists and leptin. A second site of action might be the system in the NTS which integrates peripheral taste with information from the hypothalamus to alter afferent signals from the hepatic vagus and the medial hypothalamus which affect food intake. The mediation of these signals might be through serotonin, opioid receptors, MSH receptors, glucose receptors or CRH/urocortin receptors. The third

Table 20.4 New drugs for obesity. Adapted from Bray (1993).

Mechanism of action	Drugs
Reduce food intake or shift nutrient preferences	Serotonin-like drugs Opioid antagonists α_2-antagonists α_1-agonists CCK NPY antagonists Enterostatin Galanin antagonists Leptin GLP-1
Inhibit gastric emptying or shift nutrient partitioning	Chlorocitrate Acrabose Orlistat Olestra β-adrenergic agonists Androgens/oestrogens Glucocorticoids
Stimulate thermogenesis	β_3-agonists Thyroid analogues Uncoupling agents

system would be the systems modulated by steroids, including glucocorticoids, androgens and oestrogens. Since adrenalectomy blocks the obesities produced by hypothalamic lesions, oestrogen deficiency and leptin deficiency, they must act downstream from the VMH system. Tapping into this system pharmacologically could provide long-term potential benefits. The peripheral β_3-adrenergic agonist would seem to be a very strong potential strategy to accomplish this.

References

Ahlskog, J.E. & Hoebel, B.E. (1973) Overeating and obesity from damage to a noradrenergic system in the brain. *Science* 182, 166–169.

Akabayashi, A., Wahlestedt, C., Alexander, J.T. & Leibowitz, S.F. (1994) Specific inhibition of endogenous neuropeptide Y synthesis in arcuate nucleus by antisense oligonucleotides suppresses feeding behaviour and insulin secretion. *Brain Research, Molecular Brain Research* 21, 55–61.

Arase, K., Fisler, J.S., Shargill, N.S., York, D.A. & Bray, G.A. (1988a) Intracerebroventricular infusions of 3-OH-butyrate and insulin in a rat model of dietary obesity. *American Journal of Physiology* 255, R974–R982.

Arase, K., York, D.A., Shimizu, H., Shargill, N. & Bray, G.A. (1988b) Effects of corticotrophin releasing factor on food intake and brown adipose tissue. *American Journal of Physiology* **255**, E255–E259.

Arase, K., Shargill, N.S. & Bray, G.A. (1989) Effects of corticotropin releasing factor on genetically obese (fatty) rats. *Physiology and Behaviour* **45**, 565-570.

Arch, J.R.S., Ainsworth, A.T., Cawthorne, M.A. *et al.* (1984) Atypical beta-adrenoceptor on brown adipocytes as target for anti-obesity drugs. *Nature* **309**, 163–165.

Baez, M., Kursar, J.D., Helton, L.A., Wainscott, D.B. & Nelson, D.L.G. (1995) Molecular biology of serotonin receptors. *Obesity Research* **3**, 441–447.

Baile, C.A. & Della-Fera, M.A. (1984) Peptidergic control of food intake in food-producing animals. *Federation Proceedings* **43**, 2898–2902.

Barton, C., York, D.A. & Bray, G.A. (1995a) Bombesin-induced hypothermia in rats tested at normal ambient temperatures: Contribution of the sympathetic nervous system. *Brain Research Bulletin* **37**, 163–168.

Barton, C., Lin, L., York, D.A. & Bray, G.A. (1995b) Differential effects of enterostatin, galanin and opioids on high-fat diet consumption. *Brain Research* **702**, 55–60.

Beck, B.B., Nicolas, J.P. & Burlet, C. (1993) Galanin in the hypothalamus of fed and fasted lean and obese zucker rats. *Brain Research* **623**, 124–130.

Berdanier, C.D. & McIntosh, M.K. (1989) Genotypic differences in metabolic responses to DHEA. In: Lardy, H. & Stratmen, F. (eds) *Hormones, Thermogenesis and Obesity. Proceedings of the Eighteenth Steenbock Symposium*. Madison: *University of Wisconsin*, 385–397.

Berthoud, H.R. & Baettig, K. (1974) Effects of insulin and 2-deoxy-D-glucose on plasma glucose level and lateral hypothalamic eating threshold in the rat. *Physiology and Behaviour* **12**, 547–556.

Billington, C.J., Briggs, J.E., Harker, S., Grace, M. & Levine, A.S. (1994) Neuropeptide-Y in hypothalamic paraventricular nucleus — A center coordinating energy metabolism. *American Journal of Physiology* **266**, 1765–1770.

Bittencourt, J.C., Presse, F., Arias, C. *et al.* (1992) The melanin-concentrating hormone system of the rat brain: an immuno- and hybridization histochemical characterization. *Journal of Comparative Neurology* **319**, 218–245.

Blundell, J.E., Lawton, C.L. & Halford, J.C.G. (1995) Serotonin, eating behaviour, and fat intake. *Obesity Research* **3**, 471-476.

Boosalis, M.G., Gemayel, N., Lee, A., Bray, G.A., Laine, L. & Cohen, H. (1992) Cholecystokinin and the satiety: effect of hypothalamic obesity and gastric bubble insertion. *American Journal of Physiology* **262**, R241–R244.

Bray, G.A. (1976) *The Obese Patient: Major Problems in Internal Medicine*. Philadelphia: W.B. Saunders.

Bray, G.A. (1993) Use and abuse of apetite-suppressant drugs in the treatment of obesity. *Annals of Internal Medicine* **119** (Pt 2), 707–713.

Bray, G.A. (1996) Leptin and leptomania. *Lancet* **348**, 140–141.

Bray, G.A. & York, D.A. (1972) Studies on food intake of genetically obese rats. *American Journal of Physiology* **223**, 176–179.

Bray, G.A., Fisler, J.S. & York, D.A. (1990) Neuroendocrine control of the development of obesity: Understanding gained from studies of experimental animal models. *Frontiers in Neuroendocrinology* **11**, 128–181.

Brief, D.J. & Davis, J.D. (1984) Reduction of food intake and body weight by chronic intraventricular insulin infusion. *Brain Research Bulletin* **12**, 571–575.

Campfield, L.A., Smith, F.J., Mackie, G. *et al.* (1995) Insulin normalization as an approach to the pharmacological treatment of obesity. *Obesity Research* **3** (suppl. 4), 591S–603S.

Cincotta, A.H. & Meier, A.H. (1996) Bromocriptine (Ergoset) reduces body weight and improves glucose tolerance in obese subjects. *Diabetes Care* **19**, 667–670.

Clark, J.T., Kalra, P.S., Crowly, W.R. & Kalra, S.P. (1984) Neuropeptide Y and human pancreatic polypeptide stimulate feeding behavior in rats. *Endocrinology* **115**, 427–429.

Cleary, M.P. (1989) Antiobesity effect of dehydroepiandrosterone in the zucker rat. In: Lardy, H. & Stratman, F. (eds) *Hormones, Thermogenesis and Obesity. Proceedings of the Eighteenth Steenbock Symposium*. Madison: University of Wisconsin, 365–376.

Clore, J.N. (1995) Dehydroepiandrosterone and body fat. *Obesity Research* 3 (suppl. 4), 613–616.

Corwin, R.L., Gibbs, J. & Smith, G.P. (1991) Increased food intake after type A but not type B cholecystokinin receptor blockade. *Physiology Behaviour* 50, 255–258.

Cox, J.E. & Powley, T.L. (1981) Intragastric pair feeding fails to prevent VMH obesity or hyperinsulinemia. *American Journal of Physiology* 240, E566–E572.

Crawley, J.N. & Corwin, R.L. (1994) Biological actions of cholecystokinin. *Peptides* 15, 731–755.

Darga, L.L., Carroll-Michals, L., Botsford, S.J. & Lucas, C.P. (1991) Fluoxetine's effect on weight loss in obese subjects 1–3. *American Journal of Clinical Nutrition* 54, 321–325.

Davis, J.D., Wirtshafter, D., Asin, K.E. & Brief, D. (1981) Sustained intracerebroventricular infusion of brain fuels reduces body weight and food intake in rats. *Science* 212, 81–83.

Debons, A.F., Siclari, E., Das, K.C. & Fuhr, B. (1982) Gold thioglucose-induced hypothalamic damage, hyperphagia, and obesity: dependence on the adrenal gland. *Endocrinology* 110, 2024–2029.

Deray, A., Griffond, B., Colard, C., Jacquemard, C., Bugnon, C. & Fellmann, D. (1994) Activation of the rat melanin-concentrating hormone neurons by ventromedial hypothalamic lesions. *Neuroscience* 27, 185–194.

De Souza, E.B. (1995) Corticotropin-releasing factor receptors: Physiology, pharmacology, biochemistry and role in central nervous system and immune disorders. *Psychoneuroendocrinology* 20, 789–819.

Dickson, P.R. & Vaccarino, F.J. (1994) GRF-induced feeding: Evidence for protein selectivity and opiate involvement. *Peptides* 15, 1343–1352.

Dourish, C.T. (1995) Multiple serotonin receptors: opportunities for new treatments for obesity? *Obesity Research* 3 (suppl. 4), 449S–462S.

Drent, M.L. & van der Veen, E.A. (1995) First clinical studies with orlistat: A short review. *Obesity Research* 3, 623S–625S.

Egawa, M., Yoshimatsu, H. & Bray, G.A. (1989) Effects of 2-deoxy-D-glucose on sympathetic nerve activity to interscapular brown adipose tissue. *American Journal of Physiology* 257, R1377–R1385.

Egawa, M., Yoshimatsu, H. & Bray, G.A. (1990a) Effect of corticotrophin releasing hormone and neuropeptide Y on electrophysiological activity of sympathetic nerves to interscapular brown adipose tissue. *Neuroscience* 34, 771–775.

Egawa, M., Yoshimatsu, H. & Bray, G.A. (1990b) Preoptic area injection of corticotrophin-releasing hormone stimulates sympathetic activity. *American Journal of Physiology* 259, R799–R806.

Egawa, M., Yoshimatsu, H. & Bray, G.A. (1991) Neuropeptide-Y suppresses sympathetic activity to interscapular brown adipose tissue in rats. *American Journal of Physiology* 260, R328–R334.

Erickson, J.C., Clegg, K.E. & Palmiter, R.D. (1996) Sensitivity to leptin and susceptibility to seizures of mice lacking neuropeptide Y (see comments). *Nature* 381, 415–421.

Erlanson-Albertsson, C., Mei, J., Okada, S., York, D. & Bray, G.A. (1991) Pancreatic procolipase propeptide, enterostatin, specifically inhibits fat intake. *Physiology and Behaviour* 49, 1191–1194.

Fan, W., Boston, B.A., Kesterson, R.A., Hruby, V.J. & Cone, R.D. (1997) Role of melanocortinergic neurons in feeding and the agouti obesity syndrome. *Nature* 385, 165–168.

Forbes, G.B., Porta, C.R., Herr, B.E. & Griggs, R.C. (1992) Sequence of changes in body composition induced by testosterone and reversal of changes after drug is stopped (technical note). *Journal of the American Medical Association* 267, 397–399.

Friedman, M.I. (1995) Control of energy intake by energy metabolism. *American Journal of Clinical Nutrition* 62, 1096S–1100S.

Fujimoto, K., Machidori, H., Iwakiri, R., Yamamoto, K., Fujisaki, J. & Tso, P. (1993) Effect of intravenous administration of apolipoprotein A-IV on patterns of feeding, drinking and ambulatory activity of rats. *Brain Research* 608, 233–237.

Garattini, S. (1995) Biological actions of drugs affecting serotonin and eating. *Obesity Research* 3, 463–470.

Geary, N. (1990) Pancreatic glucagon signals postprandial satiety. *Neuroscience and Biobehavioural Reviews* 14, 323–338.

Geary, N. & Smith, G. (1983) Selective hepatic vagotomy blocks pancreatic glucagon's satiety effect. *Physiology and Behaviour* **31**, 391–394.

Geary, N., Kissileff, H.R., Pi-Sunyer, F.X. & Hinton, V. (1992) Individual, but not simultaneous, glucagon and cholecystokinin infusions inhibit feeding in men. *American Journal of Physiology* **262**, R975–R980.

Gerald, C., Walker, M.W., Criscione, L. *et al.* (1996) A receptor subtype involved in neuropeptide-Y-induced food intake (see comments). *Nature* **382**, 168–171.

Gibbs, J., Fauser, D., Rowe, E., Rolls, B., Rolls, E. & Madison, S. (1979) Bombesin suppresses feeding in rats. *Nature* **282**, 208–210.

Glick, Z. & Mayer, J. (1968) Hyperphagia caused by cerebral ventricular infusion of phloridzin. *Nature* **219**, 1374.

Glowa, J.R., Barrett, J.E., Russell, J. & Gold, P.W. (1992) Effects of corticotrophin releasing hormone on appetitive behaviors. *Peptides* **13**, 609–621.

Goldstein, D.J., Rampey, A.H. Jr, Roback, P.J. *et al.* (1995) Efficacy and safety of long-term fluoxetine treatment of obesity—maximizing success. *Obesity Research* **3** (suppl. 4), 481S–490S.

Goodall, E.M., Cowen, P.J., Franklin, M. & Silverstone, T. (1993) Ritanserin attenuates anorectic, endocrine and thermic responses to d-funfluramine in human volunteers. *Psychopharmacology (Berlin)* **112**, 461–466.

Grandison, L. & Guidotti, A. (1977) Stimulation of food intake by muscimol and beta endorphin. *Neuropharmacology* **16**, 533–536.

Gutzwiller, J.P., Ketterer, S., Hildebrand, P. *et al.* (1994) Peripheral CCKa receptor blockade increases food intake in man. *Gastroenterology* **106**, A813.

Hamamura, M., Leng, G., Emson, P.C. & Kiyama, H. (1991) Electrical activation and c-fos mRNA expression in rat neurosecretory neurons after systemic administration of cholecystokinin. *Journal of Physiology (London)* **444**, 51–63.

Hamilton, M.E. & Bozarth, M.A. (1988) Feeding elicited by dynorphin (1–13) microinjections into the ventral tegmental area in rats. *Life Science* **43**, 941–946.

Hammer, V.A., Gietzen, D.W., Beverly, J.L. & Rogers, Q.R. (1990) Serotonin 3 receptor antagonists block anorectic responses to amino acid imbalance. *American Journal of Physiology* **259**, R627–R636.

Hauptman, J.D., Jeunet, F.S. & Hartmann, D. (1992) Initial studies in humans with the novel gastrointestinal lipase inhibitor Ro 18-0647 (tetrahydrolipstatin). *American Journal of Clinical Nutrition* **55**, 309S–313S.

Henke, B.R., Willson, T.M., Sugg, E.E. *et al.* (1996) 3-(1H-indazol-3-ylmethyl)-1, 5-benzodiazepines: CCK-A agonists that demonstrate oral activity as satiety agents. *Journal of Medicine Chemistry* **39**, 2655–2658.

Himms-Hagen, J. (1989) Brown adipose tissue theromogenesis and obesity. *Progress in Lipid Research* **28**, 67–115.

Himms-Hagen, J. & Ghorbani, M. (1995) Reversal of obesity in *fa/fa* rats by treatment with a β_3-adrenoceptor agonist, CL 316,243: cellularity and biochemical characteristics of white and brown adipose tissues. *Obesity Research* **3**, 406.

Holtzman, S.G. (1979) Suppression of appetitive behavior in the rat by naloxone: lack of effect of prior morphine dependence. *Life Sciences* **24**, 219–226.

Huszar, D., Lynch, C.A., Fairchild-Huntress, V. *et al.* (1977) Targeted disruption of the melanocortin-4 receptor results in obesity in mice. *Cell* **88**, 131–141.

Inoue, S. & Bray, G.A. (1977) The effect by subdiaphragmatic vagotomy in rats with ventromedial hypothalamic obesity. *Endocrinology* **100**, 108–114.

Inoue, S., Bray, G.A. & Mullen, Y. (1978) Transplantation of pancreatic beta cells prevents the development of hypothalamic obesity in rats. *American Journal of Physiology* **235**, E266–E271.

Inoue, S., Nagase, H., Satoh, S. *et al.* (1991) Role of the efferent and afferent vagus nerve in the development of ventromedial hypothalamic (VMH) obesity. *Brain Research Bulletin* **27**, 511–515.

Kalivas, P.W. & Taylor, S. (1985) Behavioral and neurochemical effect of daily injection with neurotensin into the ventral tegmental area. *Brain Research* **358**, 70–76.

Kalra, S.P. & Crowley, W.R. (1992) Neuropeptide Y: a novel neuroendocrine peptide in the control of pituitary hormone secretion, and its relation to luteinizing hormone. *Frontiers in Neuroendocrinology* **13**, 1–46.

Kalra, S.P., Sahu, A., Dube, M.G., Buonavera, J.J. & Kalva, P.S. (1996) Neuropeptide-Y and its neutral connections in the etiology of obesity and associated neuroendocrine and behavioral disorders. In: Bray, G.A. & Ryan, D.H. (eds), *Molecular and Genetic Aspects of Obesity*, Vol. 5, pp. 219–232. Baton Rouge: Louisianna State University Press.

Kanatani, A., Ishihara, A., Asahi, S., Tanaka, T., Ozaki, S. & Ihara, M. (1996) Potent neuropeptide Y Y_1 receptor antagonist, 1229U91: blockade of neuropeptide Y-induced and physiological food intake. *Endocrinology* **137**, 3177–3182.

Kissileff, H.R., Pi-Sunyer, F.X., Thornton, J. & Smith, G.P. (1981) C terminal octapeptide of cholecystokinin decreases food intake in man. *American Journal of Clinical Nutrition* **34**, 154–160.

Koegler, F.H. & Ritter, S. (1996) Feeding induced by pharmacological blockade of fatty acid metabolism is selectively attenuated by hindbrain injections of the galanin receptor antagonist, M40. *Obesity Research* **4**, 329–336.

Koopmans, H.S., Wang, D.M., Koslowsky, I. & Kloiber, R. (1994) The effect of cross-circulation on food intake. *Obesity Research* **3**, 331S.

Kotani, K., Tokunaga, K., Fujioka, S. *et al.* (1994) Sexual dimorphism of age-related changes in whole-body fat distribution in the obese. *International Journal of Obesity* **18**, 207–212.

Kotz, C.M., Grace, M.K., Briggs, J., Levine, A.S. & Billington, C.J. (1995) Effects of opioid antagonists naloxone and naltrexone on neuropeptide-Y induced feeding and brown fat thermogenesis in the rat. *Journal of Clinical Investigation* **96**, 163–170.

Kow, L.M. & Pfaff, D.W. (1991) The effects of the TRH metabolite cyclo (His-Pro) and its analogs on feeding. *Pharmacology, Biochemistry and Behaviour* **38**, 359–364.

Krahn, D.D., Gosnell, B.A., Levine, A.S. & Morley, J.E. (1986) The effect of calcitonin gene-related peptide on food intake involves aversive mechanisms. *Pharmacology, Biochemistry and Behaviour* **24**, 5.

Kreyman, B., Ghatei, M.A., Burnet, P. *et al.* (1989) Characterization of glucagon-like peptide-1-(7-36) amide in the hypothalamus. *Brain Research* **502**, 325–331.

Krotkiewski, M., Björntorp, P., Sjöstrom, L. & Smith, U. (1983) Impact of obesity on metabolism in men and women. Importance of regional adipose tissue distribution. *Journaal of Clinical Investigation* **72**, 1150–1162.

Kurata, K., Fujimoto, K., Sakata, T., Etou, H. & Fukagawa, K. (1986) D-glucose suppression of eating after intra third ventricle infusion in rat. *Physiology and Behaviour* **37**, 615–620.

Kyrkouli, S.E., Stanley, B.G., Hutchins, R., Seirafi, R.D. & Leibowit, S.F. (1990) Peptide amine interactions in the hypothalamic paraventricular nucleus — analysis of galanin and neuropeptide-Y in relation to feeding. *Brain Research* **521**, 185–191.

Langhans, W. (1996) Role of the liver in the metabolic control of eating: what we know and what we do not know. *Neuroscience Bulletin* **20**, 145–153.

Langhans, W., Delprete, E. & Scharrer, E. (1991) Mechanisms of vasopressins anorectic effect. *Physiology and Behaviour* **49**, 169–176.

Lee, M.C., Schiffman, S.S. & Pappas, T.N. (1994) Role of neuropeptides in the regulation of feeding behavior: a review of cholecystokinin, bombesin, neuropeptide Y, and galanin. *Neuroscience Biobehavioral Reviews* **18**, 313–323.

Leibowitz, S.F. (1995) Brain peptides and obesity: pharmacological treatment. *Obesity Research* **3**, 573S–589S.

Leibowitz, S.F. (1986) Brain monoamines and peptides: role in the control of eating behavior. *Federation Proceedings* **45**, 1396–1403.

Leibowitz, S.F. & Brown, L.L. (1980) Histochemical and pharmacological analysis of catecholaminergic projections to the perifornical hypothalamus in relation to feeding inhibition. *Brain Research* **201**, 315–345.

Leibowitz, S.F., Brown, J, Tretter, J.R. & Kirchgessner, A. (1985) Norepinephrine, clonidine and tricylic antidepressants selectively stimulate carbohydrate ingestion through the adrenergic system of the paraventricular nucleus. *Pharmacology Biochemistry and Behavior* **23**, 541–550.

Leibowitz, S.F., Weiss, G.F. & Shor-Posner, G. (1988) Hypothalamic serotonin: pharmacological, biochemical, and behavioral analyses of its feeding–suppressive action. *Clinical Neuropharmacology* **11** (suppl. 1), 51–71.

Li, B.H., Spector, A.C. & Rowland, N.E. (1994) Reversal of dexfenfluramine-induced anorexia and c-Fos/c-Jun expression by lesion in the lateral parabrachial nucleus. *Brain Research* **640**, 255–267.

Lieverse, R.J., Jansen, J.B.M.J., van de Zwan, A. *et al.* (1993) Bombesin reduces food intake in lean man by a cholecystokinin-independent mechanism. *Journal of Clinical Endocrinology and Metabolism* **76**, 1495–1498.

Lin, L., Okada, S., York, D.A. & Bray, G.A. (1994) Structural requirements for the biological activity of enterostatin. *Peptides* **15**, 849–854.

Lin, L., York, D.A. & Bray, G.A. (1997) B-casomorphins stimulate and enterostatin inhibitis the intake of dietary fat in rats. *American Journal of Physiology* **19**, 325–331.

Lonn, L., Kvist, H., Ernest, I. & Sjostrom, L. (1994) Volume determinations by computed tomography before and after treatment of women with Cushing's syndrome. *Metabolism* **43**, 1517–1522.

Lonn, L., Johansson, G., Sjostrom, L., Kvist, H., Oden, A. & Bengtsson, B.A. (1996) Body composition and tissue distributions in growth hormone deficient adults before and after growth hormone treatment. *Obesity Research* **4**, 45–54.

Lovejoy, J.C., Bray, G.A., Greeson, C.S. *et al.* (1995) Oral anabolic steroid treatment, but not parenteral androgen treatment, decreases abdominal fat in obese, older men. *International Journal of Obesity* **19**, 614–624.

Lovejoy, J.C., Bray, G.A., Bourgeois, M.O. *et al.* (1996) Exogenous androgens influence body composition and regional body fat distribution in obese postmenopausal women—a Clinical Research Center Study. *Journal of Clinical Endocrinology and Metabolism* **81**, 2198–2203.

Lowell, B.B., Susulic, V.S., Hamann, A. *et al.* (1993) Development of morbid obesity in transgenic mice following the genetic ablation of brown adipose tissue. *Clinical Research* **41**, A260.

Lu, D., Willard, D., Patel, I.R. *et al.* (1994) Agouti protein is an antagonist of the melanocyte-stimulating-hormone receptor. *Nature* **371**, 799–802.

MacEwen, E.G., Kurzman, I.D. & Haffa, A.L.M. (1989) Antiobesity and hypocholesterolemic activity of dehydroepiandrosterone (DHEA) in the dog. In: Lardy, H. & Stratman, F. (eds) *Hormones, Thermogenesis and Obesity. Proceedings of the Eighteenth Steenbock Symposium.* Madison, WI: University of Wisconsin, 399–414.

Mantzoros, C.S., Frederich, R.C., Susulic, V.S., Lowell, B.D., Maratos-Flier, E. & Flier, J.S. (1996) Activation of beta (3) adrenergic receptors suppresses leptin expression and mediates a leptin-independent inhibition of food intake in mice. *Diabetes* **45**, 909–914.

Marin, P., Holmang, S., Jonsson, L. *et al.* (1992) The effects of testosterone treatment on body composition and metabolism in middle-aged obese men. *International Journal of Obesity* **16**, 991–997.

Marin, P., Holmang, S., Gustafsson, C. *et al.* (1993) Androgen treatment of abdominally obese men. *Obesity Research* **1**, 245–251.

McCarthy, H.D., Crowder, R.E., Dryden, S. & Williams, G. (1994) Megestrol acetate stimulates food and water intake in the rat: Effects on regional hypothalamic neuropeptide Y concentrations. *European Journal of Pharmacology* **265**, 99–102.

McGowan, M.K., Andrews, K.M., Kelly, J. & Grossman, S.P. (1990) Effects of chronic intra-hypothalamic infusion of insulin on food intake and diurnal meal patterning in the rat. *Behavioral Neuroscience* **104**, 373–385.

Melnyk, A., Harper, M.E., Triandafillou, J. & Himms-Hagen, J. (1995) Raising at thermoneutrality prevents obesity in brown adipose tissue (BAT)-ablated mice. *Obesity Research* **3**, 407.

Merchenthaler, I., Lopez, F.J. & Negro-Vilar, A. (1993) Anatomy and physiology of central-galanin containing pathways. *Progress in Neurobiology* **40**, 711–769.

Moran, T.H., Sawyer, T.K., Seeb, D.H., Ameglio, P.J., Lombard, M.A. & McHugh, P.R. (1992) Potent and sustained satiety actions of a cholecystokinin octapeptide analogue. *American Journal of Clinical Nutrition* **55**, 286S–290S.

Morley, J.E. (1987) Neuropeptide regulation of appetite and weight. *Endocrine Reviews* **8**, 256–287.

Muurahainen, N.E., Kissileff, H.R. & Pi-Sunyer, F.X. (1993) Intravenous infusion of bombesin reduces food intake in humans. *American Journal of Physiology* **264**, R350–R354.

Nagase, H., Bray, G.A. & York, D.A. (1996) Effect of galanin and enterostatin on sympathetic-nerve activity to interscapular brown adipose-tissue. *Brain Research* **709**, 44–50.

Niijima, A. (1984) Reflex control of the autonomic nervous system activity from the glucose sensors in the liver in normal and midpontine-transected animals. *Journal of the Autonomic Nervous System* **10**, 279–285.

Niijima, A., Rohner-Jeanrenaud F. & Jeanrenaud B. (1984) Role of ventromedial hypothalamus on sympathetic efferents of brown adipose tissue. *American Journal of Physiology* **247**, R650–R654.

Ohshima, K., Shargill, N.S., Chan, T.M. & Bray, G.A. (1984) Adrenalectomy reverses insulin resistance in muscle from obese (*ob/ob*) mice. *American Journal of Physiology* **246**, E193–E207.

Okada, S., York, D.A., Bray, G.A. & Erlanson-Albertsson, C. (1991) Enterostatin, (Val-Pro-Asp-Pro-Arg), the activation peptide of procolipase selectivity reduces fat intake. *Physiology and Behaviour* **49**, 1185–1189.

Okada, K., Ishi, S., Minami, S., Sugihara, H., Shibasaki, T. & Wakabayashi, T. (1996) Intra-cerebroventricular administration of the growth hormone releasing peptide KP-102 increases food intake in free-feeding rats. *Endocrinology* **137**, 5155.

Okumura, T., Fukagawa, K., Tso, P., Taylor, I.L. & Pappas, T.N. (1995) Mechanism of action of intracisternal apolipoprotein A-IV in inhibiting gastric acid secretion in rats. *Gastroenterology* **109**, 1583–1588.

Olson, B.R., Drutaros, M.D., Chow, M.S., Hruby, V.J., Stricker, E.M. & Verbalis, J.G. (1991) Oxytocin and an oxytocin agonist administered centrally decrease food intake in rats. *Peptides* **12**, 113–118.

Oomura, Y., Ono, T., Ooyama, H. & Wayner, M.J. (1969) Glucose and osmosensitive neurons of the rat hypothalamus. *Nature* **222**, 282–284.

Oomura, Y., Nakamura, T., Sugimori, M. & Yamada, Y. (1975) Effect of fatty acid on the rat lateral hypothalamic neurons. *Physiology and Behavior* **14**, 483–486.

Orth, D.N. (1995) Cushing's Syndrome. *New England Journal of Medicine* **332**, 791–803.

Orthen-Gambill, N. & Kanarek, R.B. (1982) Differential effects of amphetamine and fenfluramine on dietary self-selection in rats. *Pharmacology, Biochemistry and Behaviour* **16**, 303–309.

Panksepp, J. & Meeker, R. (1976) Suppression of food intake in diabetic rats by voluntary consumption and intrahypothalamic injection of glucose. *Physiology and Behavior* **16**, 763–770.

Parada, M.A., Hernandez, L., Paez, X., Baptista, T., De Parada, M.P. & De Quidada, M. (1989) Mechanism of the body weight increase induced by systemic sulpuride. *Pharmacology, Biochemistry and Behavior* **33**, 45–50.

Physicians Desk Reference, 51st edn, p. 435. Montvale, N.J.: Medical Economics Co, 1997.

Plata-Salaman, C.R. (1991) Immunoregulators in the nervous system. *Neuroscience and Bio-behavioral Reviews* **15**, 185–215.

Prasad, C. (1989) Neurobiology of cyclo-(His-Pro). *Annals of the New York Academy of Sciences* **553**, 232–251.

Prasad, C., Mizuma, H., Brock, J.W., Porter, J.R., Svec, F. & Hilton, C. (1995) A paradoxical elevation of brain cyclo(his-pro) levels in hyperphagic obese Zucker rats. *Brain Research* **699**, 149–153.

Presse, F. & Nahon, J.L. (1993) Differential regulation of melanin-concentrating hormone gene expression in distinct hypothalamic areas under osmotic stimulation in rat. *Neuroscience* **55**, 709–720.

Presse, F., Sorokovsky, I., Max, J.P., Nicolaidis, S. & Nahon, J.L. (1996) Melanin-concentrating hormone is a potent anorectic peptide regulated by food-deprivation and glucopenia in the rat. *Neuroscience* **71**, 735–745.

Ravussin, E. & Swinburn, B.A. (1992) Pathophysiology of obesity. *Lancet* **340**, 404–408.

Ricquier, D., Casteilla, L. & Bouillaud, F. (1991) Molecular studies of the uncoupling protein. *FASEB Journal* **5**, 2237–2242.

Ritter, S. & Taylor, J.S. (1989) Capsaicin abolishes lipoprivic but not glucoprivic feeding in rats.

American Journal of Physiology 256, R1232–R1239.

Ritter, S. & Taylor, J.S. (1990) Vagal sensory neurons are required for lipoprivic but not glucoprivic feeding in rats. *American Journal of Physiology* 258, R1395–R1401.

Ritter, S., Calingasan, N.Y., Hutton, B. & Dinh, T.T. (1992) Cooperation of vagal and central neural systems in monitoring metabolic events controlling feeding behavior in neuroanatomy and physiology of abdominal vagal afferents. In: Ritter, S., Ritter R.C., Barnes, C.D. (eds) *Neuroanatomy and Physiology of Abdominal Vagal Afferents*, pp. 249–277. Boca Raton: CRC Press.

Rolls, B.J., Pirraglia, P.A., Jones, M.B. & Peters, J.C. (1992) Effects of olestra, a noncaloric fat substitute, on daily energy and fat intakes in lean men. *American Journal of Clinical Nutrition* 56, 84–92.

Rothwell, N.J. (1990) Central effects of CRF on metabolism and energy-balance (Review). *Neuroscience and Biobehavioral Reviews B* 14, 263–271.

Rothwell, N.J. & Stock, M.J. (1987) Influence of clenbuterol on energy balance, thermogenesis and body composition in lean and genetically obese Zucker rats. *International Journal of Obesity* 11, 641–647.

Russek, M. (1963) A hypothesis on the participation of hepatic glucoreceptors in the control of food intake. *Nature* 197, 79–80.

Ryan, D.H., Kaiser, P. & Bray, G.A. (1995) Sibutramine: a novel new agent for obesity treatment. *Obesity Research* 3, 553S–559S.

Saito, M. & Bray, G.A. (1984) Adrenalectomy and food restriction in the genetically obese (*ob/ob*) mouse. *American Journal of Physiology* 246, R20–R25.

Sakaguchi, T. & Bray, G. (1987) The effect of intrahypothalamic injections of glucose on sympathetic efferent firing rate. *Brain Research Bulletin* 18, 591–595.

Sakaguchi, T., Arase, K. & Bray, G.A. (1988a) Sympathetic activity and food intake of rats with ventromedial hypothalamic lesions. *International Journal of Obesity* 12, 43–49.

Sakaguchi, T., Arase, K. & Bray, G.A. (1988b) Effect of intrahypothalamic hydroxybutyrate on sympathetic firing rate. *Metabolism* 37, 732-735.

Sakata, T. (1995) Histamine receptor and its regulation of energy metabolism. *Obesity Research* 3 (suppl. 4), 541S–548S.

Sakata, T. & Kurokawa, M. (1992) Feeding modulation by pentose and hexose analogues. *American Journal of Clinical Nutrition* 55, 272S–277S.

Sakata, T., Kurokawa, M., Oohara, A. & Yoshimatsu, H. (1994) A physiological role of brain histamine during energy deficiency. *Brain Research Bulletin* 35, 135–139.

Sandoval, S.L. & Kulkosky, P.J. (1992) Effects of peripheral neurotensin on behavior of the rat. *Pharmacology Biochemistry and Behavior* 41, 385–390.

Schwartz, M.W., Figlewicz, D.P., Baskin, D.G., Woods, S.C. & Porte, D. Jr (1992) Insulin in the brain: a hormonal regulator of energy balance. *Endocrine Reviews* 13, 387–414.

Schwartz, M.W., Boyko, E.J., Kahn, S.E., Ravussin, E. & Bogardus, C. (1995) Reduced insulin-secretion: an independent predictor of body weight gain. *Journal of Clinical Endocrinology and Metabolism* 80, 1571–1576.

Scrocchi, L.A., Brown, T.J., Maclusky, N. *et al.* (1996) Glucose intolerance but normal satiety in mice with a null mutation in the glucagon-like peptide 1 receptor gene. *Nature Medicine* 2, 1254–1258.

Shargill, N.S., Tsujii, S., Bray, G.A. & Erlanson-Albertsson, C. (1991) Enterostatin suppresses food intake following injection into the third ventricle of rats. *Brain Research* 544, 137–140.

Shimazu, T., Noma, M. & Saito, M. (1986) Chronic infusion of norepinephrine into the ventromedial hypothalamus induces obesity in rats. *Brain Research* 369, 215–223.

Shimizu, H., Ohshima, K., Bray, G.A., Peterson, M. & Swerdloff, R.S. (1993) Adrenalectomy and castration in the genetically obese (*ob/ob*) mouse. *Obesity Research* 1, 377–383.

Shughrue, P.J. & Lane, M.V. (1996) Merchenthaler I. Glucagon-like peptide-1 receptor (GLP1-R) mRNA in the rat hypothalamus. *Endocrinology* 137, 5159.

Sjöström, L. (1988) Measurement of fat distribution. In: Bouchard, C. & Johnson, F.L. (eds) *Fat Distribution During Growth and Later Health Outcomes*, pp. 43–61. New York: Alan R. Liss.

Smith, G.P. & Gibbs, J. (1994) Satiating effect of cholecystokinin. *Annals of the New York Academy of Sciences* **713**, 236–241.

Smith, B.K., York, D.A. & Bray, G.A. (1996) Effects of dietary preference and galanin administration in the paraventricular or amygdaloid nucleus on diet self-selection. *Brain Research Bulletin* **39**, 149–154.

Sparti, A., Windhauser, M., Lovejoy, J. & Bray, G. (1995) Subjects eat for carbohydrate not calories after dietary fat replacement with olestra. *American Journal of Clinical Nutrition* **61** (suppl.), 902 (abstract).

Spina, M., Merlo-Pich, E., Chan, R.K. *et al.* (1996) Appetite-suppressing effects of urocortin, a CRF-related neuropeptide. *Science* **273**, 1561–1564.

Stacher, G., Steinringer, H., Schnierer, G. & Winklehner, S. (1982) Cholecystokinin octapeptide decreases intake of solid food in man. *Peptides* **3**, 133.

Stanley, B.G., Hoebel, B.G. & Leibowitz, S.F. (1983) Neurotensin: Effects of hypothalamic and intravenous injections on eating and drinking in rats. *Peptides* **4**, 493–500.

Stanley, B.G., Magdalin, W., Seirafi, A., Thomas, W.J. & Leibowitz, S.F. (1993a) The perifornical area: the major focus of (a) patchily distributed hypothalamic neuropeptide Y-sensitive feeding system(s). *Brain Research* **604**, 304–317.

Stanley, B.G., Willett, V.L., Donias, H.W., Ha, L.H. & Spears, L.C. (1993b) The lateral hypothalamus: a primary site mediating excitatory amino acid-elicited eating. *Brain Research* **630**, 41–49.

Stenzel-Poore, M.P., Cameron, V.A., Vaughan, J., Sawchenko, P.E. & Vale, W. (1992) Development of Cushing's syndrome in corticotrophin-releasing factor transgenic mice. *Endocrinology* **130**, 3378–3386.

Stephens, T.W., Basinski, M., Bristow, P.K. *et al.* (1995) The role of neuropeptide Y in the antiobesity action of the obese gene product. *Nature* **377**, 530–532.

Stoa-Birketvedt, G. (1993) Effect of cimetidine suspension on appetite and weight in overweight subjects. *British Medical Journal* **306**, 1091–1093.

Sullivan, A.C., Hamilton, J.G. & Triscari, J. (1983) Metabolic inhibitors of lipid biosynthesis as anti-obesity agents. In: Curtis-Prior, P.B. (ed.) *Biochemical Pharmacology of Obesity*, pp. 311–37. Amsterdam: Elsevier Science Publishers.

Tchekmedyian, N.S., Hickman, M., Siau, J. *et al.* (1992) Megestrol acetate in cancer anorexia and weight loss. *Cancer* **69**, 1268–1274.

Tempel, D.L., Leibowitz, K.J. & Leibowitz, S.F. (1988) Effects of PVN galanin on macronutrient selection. *Peptides* **9**, 309–314.

Terry, P., Gilbert, D.B. & Cooper, S.J. (1995) Dopamine receptor subtype agonists and feeding behavior. *Obesity Research* **3** (suppl. 4), 515S–523S.

Thompson, D.A. & Campbell, R.G. (1977) Hunger in man induced by 2-deoxy-D-glucose: glucoprivic control of taste preference and food intake. *Science* **198**, 1065–1068.

Tian, Q., Nagase, H., York, D.A. & Bray, G.A. (1994) Vagal–central nervous system interactions modulate the feeding responses to peripheral enterostatin. *Obesity Research* **2**, 527–534.

Tordoff, M.G., Rawson, N. & Friedman, M.I. (1991) 2,5-anhydro-D-mannitol acts in liver to initiate feeding. *American Journal of Physiology* **261**, R283–R288.

Triscari, J. & Sullivan, A.C. (1984) Antiobesity effects of a novel lipid synthesis inhibitor (Ro 22-0654). *Life Sciences* **34**, 2433–2442.

Tsujii, S. & Bray, G.A. (1989) Acetylation alters the feeding response to MSH and beta-endorphin. *Brain Research Bulletin* **23**, 165–169.

Tsujii, S. & Bray, G.A. (1990) Effects of glucose, 2-deoxyglucose, phlorizin, and insulin on food intake of lean and fatty rats. *American Journal of Physiology* **258**, E476–E481.

Tsujii, S. & Bray, G.A. (1991) GABA-related feeding control in genetically obese rats. *Brain Research* **540**, 48–54.

Tsujii, S. & Bray, G.A. (1992) Food intake of lean and obese zucker rats following ventricular infusions of adrenergic agonists. *Brain Research* **587**, 226–232.

Turton, M.D., O'Shea, D., Gunn, I. *et al.* (1996) A role for glucagon-like peptide-1 in the central regulation of feeding. *Nature* **379**, 69–72.

Vaccarino, F.J. & Hayward, M. (1988) Microinjections of growth hormone-releasing factor into the medial preoptic area/suprachiasmatic nucleus region of the hypothalamus stimulate food intake in rats. *Regulatory Peptides* **21**, 21–28.

van Dijk, G., Thiele, T.E., Seeley, R.J., Woods, S.C. & Bernstein, I.L. (1997) Glucagon-like peptide-1 and satiety. *Nature* **385**, 214.

Vander Weele, D.A., Haraczkiewicz, E. & Van Itallie, T.B. (1982) Elevated insulin and satiety in obese and normal weight rats. *Appetite* **3**, 99–109.

Wadden, T.A. Bartlett, S.J., Foster, G.D. *et al.* (1995) Sertraline and relapse prevention training following treatment by very-low-calorie diet: a controlled clinical trial. *Obesity Research* **3**, 549–557.

Weintraub, M., Sundaresan, P.R., Schuster, B. *et al.* (1992) Long term weight control: the National Heart, Lung and Blood Institute funded multimodal intervention study. I–VII. *Clinical Pharmacology and Therapeutics* **51**, 581–646.

Wellman, P.J. (1990) A review of the physiological bases of the anorexic action of phenyl-propanolamine (d,l-norephedrine). *Neuroscience and Biobehavioral Reviews* **14**, 339–355.

Woods, S.C., Lotter, E.C., McKay, D. & Porte, D. (1979) Chronic intracerebroventricular infusion of insulin reduces food intake and body weight of baboons. *Nature* **282**, 503–505.

Yamashita, J., Onai, T., York, D.A. & Bray, G.A. (1994) Relationship between food intake and metabolic rate in rats treated with β-adrenoceptor agonists. *International Journal of Obesity* **18**, 429–433.

Yen, T.T. (1994) Antiobesity and antidiabetic b-agonists: lessons learned and questions to be answered. *Obesity Research* **2**, 472–480.

Yen, T.T., Allan, J.A., Pearson, D.V., Acton, J.M. & Greenberg, M.M. (1977) Prevention of obesity in A^{vy}/a mice by dehydroepiandrosterone. *Lipids* **12**, 409–413.

York, D.A. & Bray, G.A. (1972) Dependence of hypothalamic obesity on insulin, the pituitary and the adrenal gland. *Endocrinology* **90**, 885–894.

Yoshida, T., Nishioka, H., Nakamura, Y. & Kondo, M. (1984) Reduced norepinephrine turnover in mice with monosodium glutamate-induced obesity. *Metabolism* **33**, 1060–1063.

Yoshimatsu, H., Egawa, M. & Bray, G.A. (1992) Effects of cholecystokinin on sympathetic activity to interscapular brown adipose tissue. *Brain Research* **597**, 298–303.

Yoshida, T., Sakane, N., Wakabayashi, Y., Umekawa, T. & Kondo, M. (1994) Anti-obesity effect of CL 316,243, a highly specific beta 3-adrenoceptor agonist, in mice with monosodium-L-glutamate-induced obesity. *European Journal of Endocrinology* **131**, 97–102.

Zhang, Y.Y., Proenca, R., Maffei, M., Barone, M., Leopold, L. & Friedman, J.M. (1994) Positional cloning of the mouse obese gene and its human homologue. *Nature* **372**, 425–432.

Zumoff, B., Strain, G.E., Heymsfield, S.B. & Lichtman, S. (1994) A randomized double-blind crossover study of the antiobesity effect of etiocholanedione. *Obesity Research* **2**, 13–18.

CHAPTER 21

....

Surgical Treatment of Obesity

JOHN G. KRAL

....

Introduction

Since obesity finally has been recognized as a *disease* requiring medical treatment to ameliorate or prevent disability or premature death, and obesity also has been recognized as being *chronic*, requiring life-long management, it follows that outcome evaluation of treatment for obesity should assess long-term changes in morbidity and mortality. Weight loss *per se* is a useless end-point of treatment of obesity even though it is correlated with improvements in co-morbidity and increases in quality-adjusted life years (QUALYs).

Regardless of the genetics or molecular biology underlying obesity, the poor results of dietary, behavioural or drug treatment reflect the failure on the part of the obese patient, to change eating behaviour either because of volitional breakdown or inability to substitute other activity for eating or reflect the absence of sufficiently effective drugs for long-term use. Surgery provides the most powerful, if not the only methods for altering behaviour. Thus, it is not surprising that surgical approaches to treating obesity are the only methods that have had any success in achieving sustained medically significant weight loss. No non-surgical method has been demonstrated to achieve a medically significant degree of weight loss sustained for a meaningful period of time (>5 years) in the majority of patients with body mass index (BMI) >30kg/m². These poor results doubtlessly underlie the therapeutic nihilism, lack of interest in obesity on the part of physicians and unwillingness of third party payers to reimburse hospitalization or outpatient services for treatment of obesity alone.

It is more than 5 years since an NIH Consensus Development Conference on Gastrointestinal Surgery for Severe Obesity in the U.S.A., based on follow-up data of a minimum of 5 years, concluded that gastric restrictive or bypass procedures are justified and that the immediate operative mortality rates are relatively low (NIH Consensus Development Conference Panel, 1991). During the 5 years since this statement, safety has improved and substantial additional long-term data have accrued, demonstrating the safety and durability of various anti-obesity operations.

The following is a summary of recent developments and data after the publication of the proceedings of the conference, to which the interested reader is referred (Foster, W.R., Burton, B.T. & Hubbard, V.S. (eds) (1992) Gastrointestinal Surgery for Severe Obesity. *American Journal of Clinical Nutrition* 55, 487S–619S). This chapter covers indications, methods, results and future needs.

Indications

'Established' indications

Because of the high prevalence of co-morbid conditions, though sometimes clinically occult, and the poor prognosis *quoad vitam*, a BMI of 40 kg/m^2 or higher is an absolute indication for surgery in a fully informed, consenting adult in optimal medical condition to tolerate general anaesthesia. There have been several attempts on the part of internists and, more frequently, insurance carriers to require documented failure of previous non-operative treatment before accepting surgical treatment. With or without documentation, it is exceedingly rare if even possible that any patient at this level of weight would request surgery without multiple such failures. According to one estimate surgical candidates have undergone a mean of five prior non-surgical treatment trials before presenting for operative treatment.

Patients with BMI of 35–40 kg/m^2 and the existence of one or more serious obesity-related conditions ameliorated by weight loss, such as hypertension, pulmonary insufficiency, non-insulin-dependent diabetes mellitus (NIDDM), thromboembolism, etc., are also candidates for surgical treatment. Once again, informed or preferably *educated* consent is a prerequisite.

Evolving indications

Since the safety of the surgical procedures has improved significantly with the introduction of minimally invasive laparoscopic anti-obesity operations, it is reasonable to expect a widening of indications to lower levels of BMI in the face of serious co-morbidity and failure of other treatment to effectively control co-morbidity. With the recent development of promising drugs it will become necessary to demonstrate a more favourable cost/benefit ratio for life-long medication compared to operative treatment. According to one comparison of costs in the U.S.A., the cost per kilogram of weight loss was less for surgical than medical treatment already after 5 years (Martin *et al.*, 1995b) even though the surgical patients weighed more (133 vs 116 kg) and their gross cost was eight times that of the medical patients (U.S. $24 000 vs $3000). The costs did not include chronic anti-obesity drugs, which were not available at the time.

Table 21.1 The obesity severity index (Kral, 1996). Maximum = 20 points.

Male sex	1	Neck/thigh >0.70	2
Age >40 years	1	Cardiomegaly	2
Smoker	2	Uncontrolled blood pressure	2
Sleep apnoea history	1	Haemoglobin >15 g/litre	1
Thromboembolism	1	P_{CO_2} > 45 mmHg	1
Diabetes	1	Hyperinsulinaemia	2

BMI: 28–31 = 1; 32–40 = 2; >40 = 3.

Recognition of sensitive markers of disease severity in obesity such as body fat distribution, impaired glucose disposal, family history or coexistence of traditional risk factors allows a more rational risk stratification for selection of surgical candidates. The Obesity Severity Index is one such attempt to identify patients at higher risk and to allow prospective comparison of different clinical series among investigators (Table 21.1) (Kral, 1996). The index is analogous to Child's classification of liver cirrhosis, Imrie's or Ranson's criteria in acute pancreatitis or the American Surgeon's Association preoperative classification of anaesthesia risk, to name a few. Adoption of a method for risk stratification would do away with the insensitive measure of relative or absolute weight as an indication for surgery.

Methods

Gastric restriction

Gastric restriction is achieved by vertical stapling creating a small-capacity (<20 ml) compartment emptying into the rest of the stomach through a constrictive banded opening (diameter: 0.9 cm) (vertical banded gastroplasty; Fig. 21.1) (Mason, 1987). Restriction can also be achieved by circumgastric banding, pinching off a small proximal pouch limited by an obstructive banded stoma (gastric banding; Fig. 21.2a). Over the long term (years) patients may 'out-eat' the operation by consuming high caloric density liquid or liquifying foods or by constantly (over-) distending the pouch so it stretches.

An ingenious modification of circumgastric banding uses an inflatable band attached to a subcutaneous reservoir, accessible for hypodermic injection or fluid withdrawal to adjust the size of the opening (Fig. 21.2b) (Kuzmak, 1992).

Malabsorption

The first widely performed anti-obesity operations were intestinal bypasses of

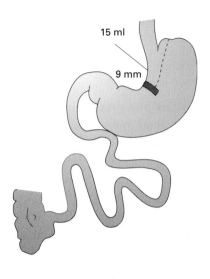

Fig. 21.1 Vertical stapled gastroplasty with a banded outlet. Pouch size: 15 ml.

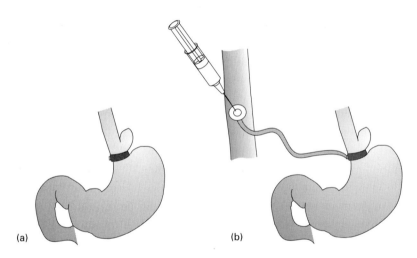

Fig. 21.2 (a) Gastric banding. (b) Adjustable gastric band attached to a subcutaneous port.

varying dimensions and configurations (Kral, 1987). The rationale was to create sufficient malabsorption to cause weight loss without jeopardizing the health of the patient through serious deficiencies or frank malnutrition. Small bowel resection had originally been performed in a few patients but there was understandable reluctance to perform irreversible procedures for a disease that essentially was considered cosmetic and/or self-inflicted. Short-circuiting more than 90% of the small intestine was thought to achieve the same goal while leaving the option of reconnecting the bowel as needed.

It is both interesting and ironic that the intestinal bypass operation had initially unrecognized appetitive effects that potentiated the weight loss from malabsorption and created a more dangerous operation than simple small bowel resection. These appetitive effects are still poorly understood but have been utilized in recently developed anti-obesity procedures described later. Intestinal bypass surgically creates a 'blind loop' of intestine that is prone to bacterial overgrowth, the cause of serious complications of these operations. They have largely been discontinued because of difficulties in management leading to unacceptable complication rates.

Combinations

Gastric bypass operations, which combine gastric restriction by partitioning the stomach, with malabsorption or strictly speaking, maldigestion, were introduced around the same time as intestinal bypass but were not widely performed until stapling instruments facilitated the performance of these technically more demanding procedures. In its current version, standard gastric bypass is performed by stapling shut a < 20-ml vertically oriented pouch (similar to that of vertical banded gastroplasty), separating the pouch from the rest of the stomach and connecting the pouch to jejunum transected 50 cm from the ligament of Treitz (Roux-en-Y gastric bypass; Fig. 21.3) (Cucchi *et al.*, 1995). This arrangement limits ingestion because of the small pouch and then, through a poorly understood feedback mechanism elicited by undigested nutrients reaching (and distending?) the jejunum, causes nimiety.

Modifications of gastric bypass experiment with varying lengths of bypassed small intestine similar to intestinal bypass, with the objective of increasing the

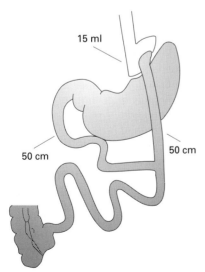

15 ml

50 cm

50 cm

Fig. 21.3 Gastric bypass with a separated pouch draining through a Roux-en-Y gastrojejunostomy.

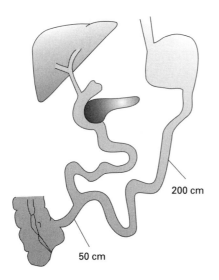

200 cm

50 cm

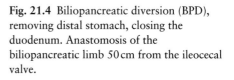

Fig. 21.4 Biliopancreatic diversion (BPD), removing distal stomach, closing the duodenum. Anastomosis of the biliopancreatic limb 50 cm from the ileocecal valve.

amount of malabsorption. Foremost among these operations is biliopancreatic diversion (or bypass) (BPD) originated in 1976. It consists of (irreversible) resection of most of the distal stomach and attachment of the first 150 cm of small bowel just 50 cm short of the ileocecal valve (Fig. 21.4). The operation causes restriction of intake, maldigestion and malabsorption by diversion of biliopancreatic juices to the terminal ileum (Scopinaro *et al.*, 1996). Other, similar operations leave the stomach stapled off creating a so-called distal gastric bypass (Sugerman *et al.*, 1996) or 'long-limb' Roux-en-Y gastric bypass (Brolin *et al.*, 1992).

Appetitive approaches

The goal of anti-obesity surgery is to alter eating behaviour and/or energy balance. Some of the mechanisms are summarized in Table 21.2. The primary objectives of the procedures mentioned above have been to physically or mechanically limit ingestion and/or absorption of food. Any appetitive effect of those methods is mainly aversive conditioning. Other, less common surgical techniques have focussed on physiological regulation of appetite. In distinction to several of the other methods, these operations have always been preceded by animal experiments before being employed in humans. For example, stereotactic electrolytic lesions of hypothalamic 'hunger' centres had been demonstrated to cause weight loss in rats. However, this method was only temporarily effective in a small clinical study reported in 1974. Such studies do not seem to have been repeated.

Truncal vagotomy was effective in reducing weight in several species and obesity models and was demonstrated to have different modes of action including

Table 21.2 Effects of anti-obesity surgery on eating behaviour and energy balance.

Decreased energy intake via satiety or aversive nimiety
Stimulation of esophagus/upper stomach
    Distention
        Small gastric pouch
        Narrow outlet of pouch
        Delayed emptying of stomach ('barostat')
Stimulation of small intestine
    Distention
    Nutrients
Central effects
    Peptides released by:
        Distention
        Nutrients
    Toxins
        Bacterial overgrowth
        Toxic bile acids
    Substrate
        Free fatty acid mobilization
        Hepatic gluconeogenesis

Increased output via malabsorption/maldigestion
Rapid small intestinal transit
Diversion of digestive juices
Increased thermogenesis

delayed gastric emptying, disrupted eating pattern and altered food preferences before being used in humans. The long-term clinical weight-loss experience was modest and unable to compete with gastroplasty or gastric bypass. However, the addition of vagotomy to gastroplasty potentiates the loss induced by restriction alone (Kral *et al.*, 1993).

As alluded to earlier, intestinal bypass operations have appetitive effects separate from the malabsorption. The exact mechanism(s) is not known but there is evidence that undigested food in the distal small bowel elicits satiety signals via release of gut neuropeptides (Koopmans & Sclafani, 1981). Several candidate peptides have been implicated such as cholecystokinin, enteroglucagon, gastrin, neurotensin or motilin, but it is likely that the appetitive effects emanate from complex interactions of multiple factors.

Attempts have been made to use the putative satiety-inducing effects of lower gut signals in surgical procedures. Intestinal interposition, by transposing a segment of terminal ileum to the proximal jejunum, had originally been tested in rats (Koopmans & Sclafani, 1981) before clinical use in only five patients, with inconsistent and transitory results. The principle was more successful when incorporated into an intestinal bypass operation connecting the first 5 cm of jejunum to 50 cm of terminal ileum (so-called duodeno-ileal bypass; Kral, 1989a).

A more recent version of BPD described above among the combined procedures, the duodenal switch operation, transects the duodenum proximally and interposes a limb of small bowel between the stomach with retained pylorus and the terminal ileum in an attempt to add satiety-inducing effects to the malabsorption created by the bypass (DeMeester et al., 1987). Reportedly the weight-loss experience is comparable to BPD but the patients have fewer postprandial symptoms in the form of nausea, vomiting or dumping (P. Marceau, personal communication, 1997).

Laparoscopic anti-obesity surgery

Laparoscopic techniques have become quite common in most types of surgery through an explosive evolution during the 1990s. The most prevalent operation performed laparoscopically, and the procedure to start this trend was cholecystectomy. It became clear early on that this minimally invasive technique (no large incision) was particularly well suited to severely obese patients (Schirmer et al., 1992). Exposure was significantly better with the laparoscopic image projected on the video monitor and the instruments could easily be manipulated in the large insufflated peritoneal cavity. Thus, it is not surprising that virtually all of the anti-obesity procedures have been successfully performed laparoscopically (Belachew & Monami, 1995; Lönroth et al., 1996; Wittgrove et al., 1996). An added advantage in the severely obese is the significant reduction in sedating pain medication and the greater ease of prompt postoperative ambulation, an important component of the perioperative management of obese patients (Kral, 1995).

Laparoscopic adjustable banding (LAB) has been performed in many centers, primarily in Europe, with series of hundreds of patients (Belachew & Monami, 1995). So far the observation time is not adequate to fully evaluate this approach, but it is quite obvious that this restrictive technique can never match the weight loss of combined malabsorptive procedures such as gastric bypass or BPD in the heavier patients. A major benefit, however, is the availability of a safer, less invasive procedure for lighter patients with milder co-morbidity and a less aggressive eating disorder.

Results

Co-morbidity reduction

Reduction of mortality would seem to be an unassailable end-point for outcome evaluation of treatment for severe obesity. Unfortunately, the quality of data on the natural history of severe obesity is poor and omissions in hospital discharge statistics complicate the interpretation of this outcome measure. The most appropriate medically assessable end-point of treatment of obesity is reduction of (co-)morbidity. It accompanies patients' perceptions of improvement in quality of life though the two measures are not totally congruent. Even with respect to mortality, some patients actually prefer death to continued life-long suffering as severely obese.

Surgical anti-obesity procedures have been demonstrated to ameliorate or cure most co-morbid conditions in the majority of patients followed for 5 years or more (Table 21.3). This confirms the pathogenetic importance of obesity in these many conditions and in some instances sheds light on pathophysiological mechanisms. In the case of NIDDM there is an immediate correction post-operatively before any weight loss has occurred (Pories *et al.*, 1995) thus showing that insensitivity to insulin action in muscle, liver or adipocytes is of less importance than previously assumed. A cluster of co-morbid conditions have traditionally been linked to increased intra-abdominal pressure. A recent study in 84 severely obese surgical candidates (BMI = 52) demonstrated correlations between intra-abdominal pressure and sagittal abdominal diameter ($r = 0.67$) and obesity co-morbidity (Sugerman *et al.*, 1997). With substantial postoperative

Table 21.3 Conditions cured or ameliorated by gastro-intestinal anti-obesity surgery compiled from the literature.

Cardiopulmonary
  Hypertension
  Heart failure
  Oedema
  Respiratory insufficiency
  Asthma
Diabetes
Dyslipidaemia
Oesophagitis
Gynaecological
  Infertility
  Delivery
  Urinary incontinence
Liver cirrhosis and fibrosis
Operative risk
Osteoarthritis
Pseudotumour cerebri
Quality of life
Sleep disorder
Thromboembolism

weight loss there were remarkably high correlations between decreases in pressure and improvement in the various co-morbidities supporting the aetiological importance of increased intra-abdominal pressure (Sugerman & Windsor, 1995).

Best documented among conditions cured or improved by surgically induced weight loss is NIDDM. Because of its own array of serious co-morbidities including blindness, kidney failure and stroke and its increasing prevalence, effective treatment or better, prevention of NIDDM is one of the most important contributions of anti-obesity surgery. In one meticulously followed series of hundreds of operated patients, gastric bypass was demonstrated to prevent the progression of impaired glucose tolerance to diabetes more than 30-fold (Pories *et al.*, 1995). In a recent follow-up comparing 154 NIDDM patients with gastric bypass to 72 matched NIDDM patients choosing not to be operated, there was a fivefold reduction in mortality (MacDonald *et al.*, 1997). Only 7.1% of the operated patients required treatment for NIDDM compared to 81.5% of non-operated 'controls' under chronic medical supervision.

Similarly, given the effectiveness of anti-obesity surgery in treating hypertension (Foley *et al.*, 1992; Carson *et al.*, 1994), dyslipidaemia (Barakat *et al.*, 1992; Gleysteen, 1992), cardiopulmonary failure (Alpert *et al.*, 1985; Sugerman *et al.*, 1992) and numerous other serious complications (see Table 21.3) it is reasonable to expect surgically induced weight loss to prevent premature death from stroke, myocardial infarction or sudden death. Such data are being collected in the Swedish national registry and intervention study of obese subjects (SOS) (Sjöström *et al.*, 1992).

It has been suggested that weight loss can prevent obesity-related cancers such as breast (Schapira *et al.*, 1994), prostate or colon cancer though there are no epidemiological intervention studies to prove it. Potentially anti-obesity surgery could provide the means for demonstrating this concept, though large (multi-centre) long-term studies will be necessary. In the U.S.A. a consortium of 'bariatric' surgeons have created a central registry, the National Bariatric Surgery Registry (NBSR) (Mason *et al.*, 1992) which ultimately should facilitate studies of this nature.

Complications and side-effects

Side-effects are common after any gastro-intestinal surgery and it is not surprising that anti-obesity operations designed to alter gastro-intestinal physiology cause numerous side-effects, some of them desired. Vomiting or regurgitation tops the list in the early postoperative period after gastroplasty and gastric bypass. As a side-effect, this symptom is readily amenable to patient education, as is the case with many of the side-effects of this type of surgery (Kral, 1996). It is important to recognize that vomiting may be a sign that the patient is unable to adapt eating behaviour to the restrictions of the operation (the 'gastroplasty diet'; Kral & Kissileff, 1987). Alternatively it may be a symptom of a stricture of the stoma requiring endoscopic dilatation or rarely, surgical intervention. In this circumstance vomiting must be classified as a *complication* of the operation. In general, vomiting after gastroplasty is more often from eating behaviour than from technical problems.

Gastric bypass causes 'dumping', well-known from ulcer surgery (Van Der Kleij *et al.*, 1996), with a prevalence varying between 20 and 70% depending on the vigilance of the investigator. It is considered a side-effect because it seems desirable as a means to modify the high-caloric, high-fat, soft diet foiling purely gastric restrictive operations (the 'soft calorie syndrome'; Kral & Kissileff, 1987) and thus leads to greater sustained weight loss. A recent retrospective report using questionnaire data, however, implies that some other (unknown) mechanism than dumping is responsible for superior weight loss (Mallory *et al.*, 1996). Obviously dumping, desirable or not, responds to dietary counselling. Complications of gastric bypass include deficiencies, anaemia, diarrhoea and abdominal distention with pain (Table 21.4). Once again, the prevalence is highly dependent on the diligence of the investigator and the level of education of the patients. As with the operations discussed below, meticulous follow-up is necessary to prevent the complications of gastric bypass.

The more aggressive malabsorptive combined operations such as BPD and extended gastric bypass by design cause greater weight loss and thus greater potential for malnutrition. Intestinal bypass operations were abandoned in some centres because of the excessive demands of managing patients with these operations (McFarland *et al.*, 1985). Thus, it is crucially important to recognize and implement vigorous follow-up routines for patients with BPD and similar operations. Provision of the necessary quality of care is rather expensive regardless of who bears the cost, not factoring in the benefits of managing

Table 21.4 Side-effects and complications of standard gastric bypass pooled from peer-reviewed publications.

Side-effects		Complications	
Dumping	70%	B_{12} deficiency	25%
Dairy intolerance	50%	Abdominal	15%
Constipation	40%	Vomiting	15%
Headache	40%	Diarrhoea	15%
Hair loss	33%	Incisional hernia	15%
Depression	15%	Anaemia	15%
		Arrhythmia	10%
		Vitamin deficiency (non-B_{12})	10%

the obesity and its co-morbidity, and must be included in the informed consent. The most important complications of BPD, protein malnutrition (Gianetta *et al.*, 1987) and deficiencies of fat-soluble vitamins with secondary hyper-parathyroidism (Chapin *et al.*, 1996), are preventable with a meticulous follow-up regimen (Kral, 1994) including mandatory life-long taking of supplements.

Failure to lose weight or weight regain must be included among complications of anti-obesity operations as must all reoperations for any indication. Indeed, the actuarial revision rate has been proposed as one measure of the success of an operation. Reoperations regardless of indication seem to be more common after gastric restrictive operations such as the vertical banded gastroplasty, though the commonest indication for reoperation after these procedures is weight regain. Revision rates vary between 5% and as much as 25% depending on procedure, patient population and setting. Some of the reasons for reoperations have been identified as purely technical and have led to modifications and improvements. It is important to keep in mind that revisional bariatric surgery has a higher complication rate even in the best of hands and should be performed at centres dedicated to this type of surgery.

Mortality

The surgical mortality rate has rapidly decreased since the late 1970s when it varied between 2% to as much as 5% in some centres. According to the Bariatric Surgery Registry mentioned earlier mortality is currently around 0.2%. This figure is actually lower than the 'natural history' of patients on waiting-lists for operations, and considerably lower than that of obese patients undergoing operations for other diseases than obesity. With the increasing adoption of laparoscopic techniques, operative mortality is expected to decrease further.

Future needs

Patient selection

Though important discoveries of genetic bases for severe obesity have been made through linkage studies and using molecular techniques they have not yet translated into therapeutic advances. The enthusiasm and focus on molecular biology, albeit understandable, seems to have diverted attention from the crucial task of identifying and characterizing subtypes of human obesity in order to optimize therapeutic and preventive strategies. It is widely acknowledged that obesity is polygenic and multifactorial, yet very little progress, if any, has been made toward studying differences in treatment outcome based on pretreatment characteristics or attempting selective assignment to improve results.

Most surgeons engaged in anti-obesity surgery have adopted (and sometimes adapted) one particular operation which they use exclusively, seeking to identify a 'procedure of choice' for all obese patients with no regard to individualization. Many of the failures of surgery are not solely technical but as much based on poor patient selection and inability to identify outcome predictors.

Numerous studies have sought to identify common psychological or psycho-pathological traits among obese subjects. Profiles have been described and used to characterize responders to dietary and behavioural interventions with very little success. Similarly a few such studies have been performed in patients undergoing various types of obesity surgery. These studies have mostly used the Minnesota Multiphasic Personality Inventory (MMPI) and have been limited to short-term follow-up (Blankmeyer et al., 1989). The data are discordant. In studies of non-surgical populations greater amounts of psychopathology are generally associated with poorer weight loss. One study of surgical patients also found that those with more personality disorders preoperative lost less weight after being operated (Larsen, 1990). A more recent study investigating preoperative dieting, interestingly found more psychopathology among successful dieters. There were, however, no differences in weight loss between the two groups (Martin et al., 1995a) in agreement with an earlier study investigating the ability of weight lost on diet to predict postoperative weight loss (Charles, 1985). Most studies quite consistently, however, reveal that preoperative psychopathology predicts postoperative *medical* complications (e.g., Valley & Grace, 1986).

A few reports have indicated that race (Sugerman et al., 1989; Martin et al., 1991) and socio-economic status influence weight loss as well as postoperative complication rates, as does smoking (Martin et al., 1991). These various indicators have helped to identify patients at risk but have not had any impact on weight loss or co-morbidity reduction.

In the search for predictors of outcome after gastro-intestinal surgery for obesity it would seem intuitively obvious that some aspect of eating behaviour prior to undergoing surgery would be an effective prognosticator of weight loss. One attempt, based on food preferences, identified classification as so-called sweets-eaters as opposed to non-sweets-eaters as a predictor of less weight loss after gastric restriction (Sugerman et al., 1989). Sweets-eaters, it was suggested, should be allocated to gastric bypass operations. More recent data, using a survey covering 3 months of food intake before and 6, 12 and 24 months after gastric restrictive or gastric bypass operations, refutes selective assignment by these criteria, actually finding that high consumers of carbohydrate lost more weight than those in the lowest quartile after gastroplasty (Lindroos et al., 1996). Interestingly, the study on dumping cited above (Mallory et al., 1996) had selected non-sweets-eaters for gastroplasty. At follow-up, however,

60% of the gastric bypass patients and only 25% of gastroplasty patients were classified as non-sweets-eaters. This demonstrates shifts in eating behavior induced by the different procedures in agreement with one published study (Brolin *et al.*, 1994).

In studies of candidates for obesity surgery using the Universal Eating Monitor (UEM) for covert assessment of eating behaviour (Kissileff *et al.*, 1980) we found that eating rate and volume consumed predicted short-term (18 months) weight loss after gastric restrictive operations (Kral, 1986). However, the results did not stand up over the long term (4–8 years). Subsequently others have identified that postoperative binge eating is associated with weight regain after gastroplasty (Hsu *et al.*, 1996) but there are no published prospective studies of the outcome of patients with diagnosed binge-eating disorder (BED) having different kinds of anti-obesity operations. One retrospective analysis suggests that BPD might correct binge eating (Adami *et al.*, 1996). This is plausible, given the mechanical constraints of all gastric operations, but does not yet conclusively address this important issue.

Though there is considerable information on the importance of psycho-social and environmental factors for the development of eating disorders (Kanter *et al.*, 1992), obesity (Felitti, 1993), digestive diseases (Leserman *et al.*, 1996) and metabolic disturbances (Surwit & Schneider, 1993), this information does not seem to have been used in the design of outcome studies of treatment of these conditions, particularly not obesity. During the last 5 years increasing attention has been paid to the roles of childhood sexual and physical abuse and parental alcohol abuse in the aetiology of adult obesity (Felitti, 1993), gastro-intestinal health status (Leserman *et al.*, 1996) and binge eating (Kanter *et al.*, 1992). The prevalence of BED is high in severe obesity, varying between 40 and 90% in different populations. Several studies have indicated that BED predicts poor outcome of behavioural treatment of obesity. Thus, it is important to diagnose BED and its antecedents in future prospective studies allocating patients to different types of anti-obesity treatment, particularly operations with different modes of action. If the preliminary report that BPD might correct binge eating (Adami *et al.*, 1996) is verified in a prospective trial, it would support selective assignment of BED patients.

As I have pointed out earlier, anti-obesity operations rely to varying degrees on the cooperation or ability of the patient to modify eating behaviour (Kral, 1992). Purely gastric restrictive operations require the most cognitive restraint in adhering to the 'gastroplasty diet'. Malabsorptive operations and those with appetitive effects place different demands on the patients, instead requiring the taking of vitamin and mineral supplements and keeping appointments for follow-up monitoring.

Staged surgery and multimodality treatment

The absence of sensitive outcome predictors and the hazards associated with a substantial recurrence rate in the heaviest patients, between 5–25% after gastric bypass and 10–35% after gastroplasty (Benotti & Forse, 1996), creates a need for a staged or step-care approach to severely obese patients (Kral, 1984). Reasonable criteria for reoperations for weight loss are recurrence of serious co-morbidity, weight regain to within 20% of original excess weight or persistence of co-morbidity responsive to additional weight loss. Availability of the minimally invasive laparoscopic techniques, particularly the adjustable silicone band which causes minimal adhesions and disruption of the normal anatomy permits a staged approach to anti-obesity surgery. It will allow identification of a subgroup of obese patients who will only require this relatively benign intervention, as discussed earlier in this chapter.

Patients for whom this gastric restrictive operation is insufficient will require more aggressive procedures which are likely to include a malabsorptive component. Even after patient selection methods have been perfected there will always be a subgroup of patients with particularly severe forms of obesity who might ultimately require additional surgery.

Multimodality treatment has so far only included dietary and behavioural methods in conjunction with surgery and the results have been disappointing. The development of new gastro-intestinally active drugs such as acarbose and tetrahydrolipstatin might provide a 'rescue' strategy for patients with failure of gastric restriction. So far, no such trials have been published.

Clinical research on anti-obesity surgery

From the foregoing there would seem to be a great need for prospective randomized controlled trials comparing different treatment modalities and strategies. However, there are serious scientific and ethical obstacles to such studies in severely obese subjects. Fully informed subjects as well as the investigator must be convinced of the equivalency of two treatment arms for the subject to agree to randomization and for the investigator to ethically portray them as being equivalent. Persons agreeing to enter a randomized study differ from those refusing (Kral, 1984), just as obese people seeking treatment are different from those abstaining (Fitzgibbon et al., 1993). The consent process must guarantee the subjects' right to self-selection which implicitly flaws the randomization process.

In studies comparing surgery to other treatment the appearance of differences in risk or danger, whether real or not, automatically imposes a selection bias. With serious disease such as obesity there is a therapeutic imperative. However, the documented failure of all non-surgical treatment in severely obese patients in fact creates a dilemma in designing any study comparing with surgical treatment. Indeed, many studies have been designed but not completed because of difficulties in recruiting patients to the non-operative group and for inability to provide sufficient numbers of patients completing the study. Unequal numbers of drop-outs invariably flaw such trials.

Controls for studies like these can never be scientifically valid. Obviously sham or placebo surgery is not an option, nor is blinding. Some studies have used patients on waiting lists, though the validity of such controls have been called into question from a methodological viewpoint (Wilson, 1978). Non-equivalency, if not total ineffectiveness of non-surgical options, invalidates the control process just as it does randomization as mentioned above. Surgical trials of obesity surgery, thus must be limited to observational studies as has generally been recognized for surgical clinical research (Hu *et al.*, 1996).

Summary

- Surgical methods for treating severe obesity include gastric restriction, malabsorption, appetitive procedures and combinations of these.
- Gastroplasty and standard gastric bypass are most common, but increasingly malabsorptive versions of gastric bypass are being used for heavier patients (BMI $\geq 50 \, kg/m^2$).
- Laparoscopic methods and improvements in technique and management have decreased mortality below 0.5% in experienced centres, less than actuarial mortality in the severely obese.
- Candidates for anti-obesity surgery have BMI $\geq 35 \, kg/m^2$, but indications for surgery are expected to widen by including patients with serious obesity-related co-morbidity with BMI $< 35 \, kg/m^2$.
- Standardized disease severity assessment should replace traditional weight criteria in all clinical research on obesity.
- Because of the lack of outcome predictors and valid methods for patient selection, a staged surgical approach is suggested.
- Operations can prevent disease progression, particularly diabetes, and can effectively improve serious co-morbidity for > 5 years.
- Preoperative teaching and meticulous postoperative follow-up are vital components of an anti-obesity surgery programme since most complications are preventable.

References

Adami, G.F., Gandolfo, P. & Scopinaro, N. (1996) Binge eating in obesity. *International Journal of Obesity* 20, 793–794.

Alpert, M.A., Terry, B.E. & Kelly, D.L. (1985) Effect of weight loss on cardiac chamber size, wall thickness and left ventricular function in morbid obesity. *American Journal of Cardiology* **56**, 783–786.

Barakat, H.A., McLendon, V.D., Marks, R. *et al.* (1992) Influence of morbid obesity and non-insulin-dependent diabetes mellitus on high-density lipoprotein composition and subpopulation distribution. *Metabolism* **41**, 37–41.

Belachew, M. & Monami, B. (1995) Laparoscopic adjustable Silicone gastric banding: technique and preliminary results. *Obesity Surgery* **5**, 258.

Benotti, F.N. & Forse, R.A. (1996) Safety and long-term efficacy of revisional surgery in severe obesity. *American Journal of Surgery* **172**, 232–235.

Blankmeyer, B.L., Smylie, K.D., Price, D.C., Costello, R.H., McFee, A.S. & Fuller, D.S. (1989) A replicated five cluster MMPI typology of morbidly obese female candidates for gastric bypass. *International Journal of Obesity* **14**, 235–247.

Brolin, R.E., Kenler, H.A., Gorman, J. *et al.* (1992) Long-limb gastric bypass in the superobese. *Annals of Surgery* **215**, 387–395.

Brolin, R.E., Robertson, L.B., Kenler, H.A. & Cody, R.P. (1994) Weight loss and dietary intake after vertical banded gastroplasty and Roux-en-Y gastric bypass. *Annals of Surgery* **220**, 782–790.

Carson, J.L., Ruddy, M.E., Duff, A.E., Holmes, N.J., Cody, R.P. & Brolin, R.E. (1994) The effect of gastric bypass surgery on hypertension in morbidly obese patients. *Archives of Internal Medicine* **154**, 193–200.

Chapin, B.L., LeMar, H.J., Knodel, D.H. & Carter, F.L. (1996) Secondary hyperparathyroidism following biliopancreatic diversion. *Archives of Surgery* **131**, 1048–1053.

Charles, S.C. (1985) Psychological predictors of obesity surgery outcome. In: Hirsch, J. & Van Itallie, T.B. (eds) *Recent Advances in Obesity Research: IV. Proceedings of the Fourth International Congress Obesity*, pp. 254–259. London: John Libbey.

Cucchi, S.G., Pories, W.J., MacDonald, K.G. & Morgan, E.J. (1995) Gastro-gastric fistulas, a complication of divided gastric bypass surgery. *Annals of Surgery* **221**, 387–391.

DeMeester, T.R., Fuchs, K.H., Ball, C.S., Albertucci, M., Smyrk, T.C. & Marcus, J.N. (1987) Experimental and clinical results with proximal end-to-end duodenojejunostomy for pathologic duodenogastric reflux. *Annals of Surgery* **206**, 414–426.

Felitti, V.J. (1993) Childhood sexual abuse, depression and family dysfunction in adult obese patients: a case control study. *Southern Medical Journal* **86**, 732–736.

Fitzgibbon, M.L., Stolley, M.R. & Kirschenbaum, D.S. (1993) Obese people who seek treatment have different characteristics than those who do not seek treatment. *Health Psychology* **12**, 342–345.

Foster, W.R., Burton, B.T. & Hubbard, V.S. (1992) Gastrointestinal surgery for severe obesity. *American Journal of Clinical Nutrition* **55**, 487S–619S.

Foley, E.F., Benotti, P.N., Borlase, B.C. *et al.* (1992) Impact of gastric restrictive surgery on hypertension in the morbidly obese. *American Journal of Surgery* **163**, 294–297.

Gianetta, E., Friedman, D., Adami, G.F. *et al.* (1987) Etiological factors of protein malnutrition after biliopancreatic diversion. *Clinical Gastroenterology* **16**, 503–504.

Gleysteen, J.J. (1992) Results of surgery: long-term effects on hyperlipidemia. *American Journal of Clinical Nutrition* **55**, 591S–596S.

Hsu, L.K.G., Betancourt, S., Sullivan, S.P. (1996) Eating disturbances before and after vertical banded gastroplasty: a pilot study. *International Journal of Eating Disorders* **19**, 23–34.

Hu, X., Wright, J.G., McLeod, R.S., Lossing, A. & Walters, B.C. (1996) Observational studies as alternatives to randomized clinical trials in surgical clinical research. *Surgery* **119**, 473–475.

Kanter, R.A., Williams, B.E. & Cummings, C. (1992) Personal and parental alcohol abuse and victimization in obese binge eaters and nonbingeing obese. *Addictive Behaviors* **17**, 439–445.

Kissileff, H.R., Klingsberg, G., Van Itallie, T.B. (1980) Universal eating monitor for continuous recording of solid or liquid consumption in man. *American Journal of Physiology* **238**, R14–R22.

Koopmans, H.S. & Sclafani, A. (1981) Control of body weight by lower gut signals. *International Journal of Obesity* **5**, 491–495.

Kral, J.G. (1984) Gastroplasty and diet in morbid obesity. *New England Journal of Medicine* 310, 1743.

Kral, J.G. (1986) The current status of obesity surgery: constructive criticism. *Surgery Annual* 18, 165–180.

Kral, J.G. (1987) Malabsorptive procedures in surgical treatment of morbid obesity. *Clinical Gastroenterology* 16, 293–305.

Kral, J.G. (1989a) Duodeno-ileal bypass. In: Deitel, M. (ed.) *Surgery for the Morbidly Obese Patient*, pp. 99–103. Philadelphia, PA: Lea & Febiger.

Kral, J.G. (1989b) Surgical treatment of obesity. *Medical Clinics of North America* 73, 251–264.

Kral, J.G. (1992) Surgical treatment of obesity. In: Wadden, T.A. & Van Itallie, T.B. (eds) *Treatment of Obesity by Diet and Lifestyle Change*, pp. 496–506. New York: Guilford Publications.

Kral, J.G. (1994) Therapy of severe obesity. In: Haubrich, W., Schaffner, F. & Berk, J.E. (eds) *Bockus Gastroenterology*, 5th edn, pp. 3231–3239. Philadelphia, PA: W.B. Saunders.

Kral, J.G. (1995) Obesity. In: Lubin, M.F., Walker, H.K. & Smith III, R.B. (eds) *Medical Management of the Surgical Patient*, 3rd edn, pp. 415–423. Philadelphia, PA: Lippincott.

Kral, J.G. (1996) Side-effects, complications and problems in anti-obesity surgery: Introduction of the obesity severity index. In: Angel, A., Anderson, H. & Bouchard, C. *et al. Progress in Obesity Research*, Vol. 7, pp. 655–661. London: John Libbey.

Kral, J.G. & Kisseleff, H.R. (1987) Surgical approaches to the treatment of obesity. *Annals of Behavioral Medicine* 9, 15–19.

Kral, J.G., Görtz, L., Hermanson, G. & Wallin, G.S. (1993) Gastroplasty for obesity: Long-term weight loss improved by vagotomy. *World Journal of Surgery* 17, 75–79.

Kuzmak, L.I. (1992) Stoma adjustable silicone gastric banding. *Probl Gen Surgery* 9, 298–317.

Larsen, F. (1990) Psychosocial function before and after gastric banding surgery for morbid obesity. A prospective psychiatric study. *Acta Psychiatrica Scandinavica* 82 (suppl. 359), 1–54.

Leserman, J., Drossman, D.A., Li, Z., Tommey, T.C., Nachman, G. & Glogau, L. (1996) Sexual and physical abuse history in gastroenterology practice: how types of abuse impact health status. *Psychosomatic Medicine* 58, 4–15.

Lindroos, A.-K., Lissner, L. & Sjöström, L. (1996) Weight change in relation to intake of sugar and sweet foods before and after weight reducing gastric surgery. *International Journal of Obesity* 20, 634–643.

Lönroth, H., Dalenbäck, J., Haglind, E. *et al.* (1996) Vertical banded gastroplasty by laparoscopic technique in the treatment of morbid obesity. *Surgical Laparoscopy and Endoscopy* 6, 102–107.

MacDonald, K.G., Long, S.D., Swanson, M.S. *et al.* (1997) The gastric bypass operation reduces the progression and mortality of non-insulin dependent-diabetes mellitus. *Journal of Gastrointestinal Surgery* 1, 213–220.

Mallory, G.N., Macgregor, A.M.C. & Rand, C.S.W. (1996) The influence of dumping on weight loss after gastric restrictive surgery for morbid obesity. *Obesity Surgery* 6, 474–478.

Martin, L.F., Tan, T.L., Holmes, P.A. *et al.* (1991) Preoperative insurance status influences postoperative complication rates for gastric bypass. *American Journal of Surgery* 161, 625–634.

Martin, L.F., Tan, T.L., Holmes, P.A., Becker, D.A., Horn, J. & Bixler, E.O. (1995a) Can morbidly obese patients safely lose weight preoperatively. *American Journal of Surgery* 169, 245–253.

Martin, L.F., Tan, T.-L., Horn, J.R. *et al.* (1995b) Comparison of the costs associated with medical and surgical treatment of obesity. *Surgery* 118, 599–607.

Mason, E.E. (1987) Morbid obesity: Use of vertical banded gastroplasty. *Surgical Clinics of North America* 67, 521–537.

Mason, E.E., Renquist, K.E. & Jiang, D. (1992) Perioperative risks and safety of surgery for severe obesity. *American Journal of Clinical Nutrition* 55, 573S–576S.

McFarland, R.J., Gazet, J.-C. & Pilkington, T.R.E. (1985) A 13-year review of jejunoileal bypass. *British Journal of Surgery* 72, 81–87.

NIH Consensus Development Conference Panel (1991) Gastrointestinal surgery for severe obesity. *Annals of Internal Medicine* 115, 956–961.

Pories, W.J., Swanson, M.S., MacDonald, K.G. *et al.* (1995) Who would have thought it? An operation proves to be the most effective therapy for adult-onset diabetes mellitus. *Annals of Surgery* 222, 339–352.

Schapira, D., Clark, R., Wolff, P. *et al.* (1994) Visceral obesity and breast cancer risk. *Cancer* 74, 632–639.

Schirmer, B.D., Dix, J., Stephen, P.A.C. *et al.* (992) Laparoscopic cholecystectomy in the obese patient. *Annals of Surgery* 216, 146–152.

Scopinaro, N., Gianetta, E., Adami, G.F. *et al.* (1996) Biliopancreatic diversion for obesity at eighteen years. *Surgery* 119, 261–268.

Sjöström, L.V., Larsson, B., Backman, L. *et al.* (1992) Swedish obese subjects (SOS): Recruitment for an intervention study and a selected description of the obese state. *International Journal of Obesity* 16, 465–479.

Sugerman, H.J. & Windsor, A.C.J. (1995) Increased sagittal abdominal diameter increases abdominal pressure and obesity co-morbidity: all improved with surgically-induced weight loss. *Obesity Surgery* 5, 262.

Sugerman, H.J., Londrey, G.L., Kellum, J.M. *et al.* (1989) Weight loss with vertical banded gastroplasty and Roux-Y bypass for morbid obesity with selective versus random assignment. *American Journal of Surgery* 157, 93–102.

Sugerman, H.J., Fairman, R.P., Sood, R.K. *et al.* (1992) Long-term effects of gastric surgery for treating respiratory insufficiency of obesity. *American Journal of Clinical Nutrition* 55, 597S–601S.

Sugerman, H.J., Kellum, J.M. & DeMaria, E.J. (1996) Conversion to distal gastric bypass for failed standard gastric bypass for morbid obesity. *Gastroenterology* 110, A1421.

Sugerman, H.J., Windsor, A., Bessos, M. *et al.* (1997) Intraabdominal pressure, sagittal abdominal diameter and obesity comorbidity. *Journal of Internal Medicine* 241, 71–79.

Surwit, R.S. & Schneider, M.S. (1993) The role of stress in the etiology and treatment of diabetes mellitus. *Psychosomatic Medicine* 55, 380–393.

Valley, V. & Grace, D.M. (1986) Psychosocial risk factors in gastric surgery for obesity: identifying guidelines for screening. *International Journal of Obesity* 11, 105–113.

Van Der Kleij, F.G.H., Vecht, J., Lamers, C.B.H.W. & Masclee, A.A.M. (1996) Diagnostic value of dumping provocation in patients after gastric surgery. *Scandinavian Journal of Gastroenterology* 31, 1162–1166.

Wilson, T.G. (1978) Methodological considerations in treatment outcome research on obesity. *Journal of Consulting and Clinical Psychology* 46, 687–702.

Wittgrove, A.C., Clark, W. & Schubert, K.R. (1996) Laparoscopic gastric bypass, Roux-en-Y: technique and results in 75 patients with 3–30 months follow-up. *Obesity Surgery* 6, 500–504.

CHAPTER 22

Benefits and Risks of Weight Loss: Obesity and Weight Cycling

MICHAEL E.J. LEAN AND CATHERINE R. HANKEY

Background level of health risks attached to overweight: the potential for benefit from weight loss

Both cross-sectional and longitudinal studies demonstrate strong and consistent associations between overweight, indicated by either body mass index (BMI) or waist circumference, and a range of conditions affecting most systems of the body (see Chapter 1). Whether or not the associations indicate causal relationships, there is potential for weight loss to reduce disease burdens, both acutely and over a long time course of disease development.

Debate about the health hazards of overweight, and the benefits of weight loss have been dominated by consideration of coronary heart disease although the symptoms and distress of the overweight relate closely to other obesity-related conditions. It is now beyond dispute that obesity is an important factor in cardiovascular disease (CVD). Earlier confusion is likely to have resulted from inappropriate attempts to examine study results with multivariate analyses. These analyses 'controlled' for the influences of the well-established risk factors of hypertension, hyperlipidaemia and impaired glucose tolerance. All these conditions can to a large extent be regarded as being reversible consequences of overweight, which also relate to the influence of a central fat distribution.

The most powerful analyses to demonstrate the effect of overweight on CVD have resulted from large longitudinal studies such as Whitehall, Intersalt, American Cancer Association, Framingham and the Boston Nurses study. The results of these principle studies are similar, but nonetheless there are some aspects of the evidence which prevent the drawing of simple conclusions. The crude relationships between BMI and mortality and morbidity are not linear but follow a J-shaped distribution. Risks increase rapidly when BMI is under 20 (probably related to smoking), but rather gradually as overweight develops above BMI $>25 \, \text{kg/m}^2$, more markedly where BMI exceeds $30 \, \text{kg/m}^2$. This relationship has been interpreted as indicating a lesser problem with CVD risk in the overweight than amongst the underweight. However, since underweight people are less common (BMI $<20 \, \text{kg/m}^2$ in only 6% of the population) and overweight is so frequent (BMI $>25\,kg/m^2$ in 53% of the population) (Bennett *et al.*, 1995) the contribution of overweight to CVD is much greater.

There is a clear diminution in the CVD risk attached to overweight with increasing age (Must *et al.*, 1992) and a difference in age-related risk between the sexes (Barrett-Conner *et al.*, 1984). The development of CVD takes place over a long period of time, and the duration of overweight is likely to be important in determining the degree of reversibility of the disease. However, it is possible that other mechanisms may drive the same disease process, such that being overweight may accelerate it at an early stage, and perhaps less so in older people. It is also possible that different mechanisms for CVD apply at different extremes of BMI. Thus, smoking and presumably thrombophilia dominate the cardiac risk profile of the underweight, while atheroma is likely to be more important in the overweight. In terms of symptoms and total medical burden, the main health hazard of overweight is not CVD, but a range of other related conditions which contribute importantly to ill health and health service costs. This is particularly the case for older people.

Cardiovascular disease and weight loss

There is evidence for health benefits from weight loss on most major CVD risk factors, symptoms and possibly even on atheroma regression. Five principal risk factors for CVD are influenced by overweight:
1 hypertension;
2 impaired glucose tolerance (IGT) or non-insulin-dependent diabetes mellitus (NIDDM);
3 hyperlipidaemias (usually elevations in plasma triglyceride and reduction in HDL cholesterol and elevations of all small dense LDL (LDL_3) cholesterol;
4 altered haemostatic factors;
5 altered rheological factors.
Recent information also links overweight with increased LDL oxidizability, reflecting the increased proportion of LDL_3 (van Gaal *et al.*, 1997). During weight loss all these factors are improved, and there may be additional improvements if the individual is then able to take more exercise.

Weight loss and blood pressure

Weight loss appears to reduce blood pressure in all individuals, thin and obese, normotensive and hypertensive. A retrospective analysis of blood pressure in military recruits to the Danish Armed Forces was carried out (Sonneholm *et al.*, 1989). Those who lost weight for whatever reason showed reductions in blood pressure. The influence of weight change in longitudinal cohort studies were

also examined in the Boston Nurses and Harvard Physician studies (Manson
et al., 1990; Must et al., 1992). In both studies a higher BMI increased risks of
CVD, indicating an effect of mild to moderate overweight in elevating risk.

Virtually all of the studies reporting the effects of weight loss in blood pressure
show a marked and predictable reduction, even with the relatively low weight
losses (2–5 kg) achieved by conventional dietary means. A possible confounding
factor which makes simple analysis of weight loss difficult is the inverse relationship between sphygmomanometer cuff size and blood pressure measurement.
This means some apparent reductions in blood pressure recorded with the same
instrument before and after weight loss might be artefactual. This effect is likely
to be very small, given the trivial changes in upper arm circumference which
will result from weight loss in clinical practice. The effect of weight loss in
upper arm circumference can be predicted from published equations (James
et al., 1994). Each 1 cm of arm circumference is equivalent to about 1.2 BMI
units in both men and women, or about 4 kg for a patient of BMI 30 kg/m².

Practically all dietary approaches to weight loss involve a lowering of sodium
intake, which will also contribute to blood pressure lowering. Meta-analyses
have drawn the very clear conclusion that a decrease in sodium intake of 50 mmol/
day will reduce systolic blood pressure significantly, by about 5 mmHg in
normotensive or 7 mmHg in hypertensive individuals aged 50–59 (Law et al.,
1991a,b). Reductions in diastolic blood pressure are approximately half
these values. The separate effects of weight loss and sodium restriction on blood
pressure have also been studied (Reisin et al., 1978). An 11-kg weight loss
produced a 20% decrease in both systolic and diastolic blood pressure in
hypertensive subjects. This was a fall from a mean initial blood pressure of 160/
90 mmHg. These differences were maintained even when sodium intakes were
kept constant by encouraging high intake of salty foods.

Moderate weight losses achieved using a variety of dietary approaches are
related to blood pressure reductions of approximately 1 mmHg systolic and
2 mmHg diastolic for each 1% reduction in body-weight. These levels of blood
pressure reduction from conventional weight loss are similar to those benefits
obtained from widely used antihypertensive drugs. Possible interactions between
antihypertensive drug therapy and weight loss for blood pressure reduction
were also studied (Oberman et al., 1990) in hypertensive individuals with body-
weight more than 110% ideal. Weight loss of 4.5 kg led to blood pressure
changes of 20 mmHg systolic and of 15 mmHg diastolic in drug-treated patients.
The possible influences of antihypertensive drugs on weight loss were also
studied (Davis et al., 1993). In an atenolol-treated group weight loss was 2.7 kg,
chlorthalidone 6.9 kg and placebo 4.9 kg. Decreases in diastolic blood pressure
were 2, 4 and 2mmHg, respectively. Long-term weight loss after 5 years' monitoring decreased the rate of failure in blood pressure control for those receiving

placebo, low-dose diuretic or beta blockers by 23%. The results were similar in each drug group. This study also reminds us that beta blockers tend to impede weight loss, and can cause weight gain.

The long-term effects on blood pressure were compared in weight and salt reduction programmes using 12-month programmes of weekly/monthly group sessions (Rissanen *et al.*, 1985). These focused on weight reduction, salt restriction or both. Mean weight reductions of 7.0 and 5.0 kg were achieved in the weight reduction, and the weight reduction and salt restriction groups after 3 months and maintained at 12 months. Negligible weight changes were achieved in the sodium restriction group. Systolic and diastolic blood pressure significantly fell in the weight-loss group. These reductions in systolic blood pressure were 159–147 and 150–143 mmHg for the weight loss and the weight loss and sodium restriction groups, respectively. The diastolic changes were 101–94, and 98–93 mmHg. The salt restriction group showed no significant fall in blood pressure, though 24-hour sodium excretion fell by 50–35 mmol.

The practicality of applying weight reduction or salt reduction programmes for hypertension management was studied (Wassertheil-Smoller *et al.*, 1992). The trial of antihypertensive medications study (TAIM) evaluated nine diet drug combinations in 878 mildly hypertensive moderately obese participants. A group given advice to restrict sodium intake reduced sodium excretion significantly, in contrast with the group advised on weight reduction and the usual diet group, who increased their sodium excretion. The greatest changes in blood pressure were observed in the weight reduction/chlorthalidone treated group. A weight loss of 6.8 kg reduced blood pressure by 15 mmHg. In the weight reduction/ atenolol group 3.0 kg loss was accompanied by 14.8 mmHg fall in blood pressure. The diet/placebo groups all exhibited a smaller decrease in blood pressure of 8.9 mmHg with a weight loss of 4.4 kg. The weight reduction intervention lowered blood pressure more than the low-sodium/high-potassium diets. Additional comparisons were made to determine whether diet therapy enhanced the impact of pharmacological therapy. Weight reduction with chlorthalidone yielded a significantly lower diastolic blood pressure (an additional fall of 4.3 mmHg). Weight reduction in combination with atenolol tended to enhance the impact of diet therapy (a difference of 2.4 mmHg). The results of this study confirm the value of weight loss alone on improving hypertension. However, the value of reducing sodium intake is not proven. The additional benefits of antihypertensive medication together with weight reduction are shown.

Conclusion

It is clear that weight loss of an order achievable in clinical practice of 5–10 kg will reduce normal blood pressure by a valuable amount. The expected reduction is around 1.0–1.7 mmHg systolic and 0.8–1.0 mmHg diastolic per kilogram weight loss respectively, or 1.8–2.0 mmHg per 1% weight loss in normotensive overweight subjects. Blood pressure reduction to this degree will confer benefits in reduction of cardiovascular disease, in particular stroke.

In the management of hypertensive individuals, important changes in blood pressure are achieved after weight loss. Weight reduction, sodium restriction and exercise training can add to the blood pressure lowering by non-pharmacological means (without the risk of side-effects). For individuals who remain significantly hypertensive, despite weight loss, the addition of antihypertensive drug therapy will continue to be effective.

Weight loss and impaired glucose tolerance and non-insulin-dependent diabetes mellitus

In all adults, an effect of age is to produce a decline in insulin sensitivity. The reasons are not known in detail, but overweight has a compounding action at any age. Amongst those who are predisposed, presumably for genetic reasons or through acquired pancreatic disease, becoming overweight accelerates the progression to reach the diagnostic criteria for IGT and NIDDM.

The majority of NIDDM patients are overweight, around 75% in most studies (Hadden et al., 1975; Lean et al., 1990) and weight gain seems predominantly to be acquired during adulthood (Holbrook, 1989; Chan et al., 1994). It has been shown that 10 kg body-weight increase since the age of 18 led to increased mortality in middle adulthood (Manson, 1995). Physical inactivity seems to be a key factor in the development of diabetes (Colditz et al., 1995). Exercise training has been shown to improve insulin sensitivity separately from any effect on body-weight (Koivisto & Defronzo, 1984).

An underlying predisposition to IGT and NIDDM is identifiable from a number of relatively simple markers including family history of NIDDM in first-degree relative, impaired glucose tolerance during pregnancy, high waist circumference, and origins in South Asia. The U.K. Prospective Diabetes Study (UKPDS) results have suggested that weight loss of around 18 kg is needed to achieve normoglycaemia, defined as a fasting blood glucose below 6 mmol/L (UKPDS, 1990). However, lesser degrees of weight loss improve glucose tolerance significantly and also other risk factors for people with diabetes, such as elevated lipids and blood pressure (Vessby et al., 1984). A retrospective survival analysis in NIDDM patients with BMI above 25 kg/m^2 suggests that 15–20% weight loss in the first year after diagnosis could reverse the elevated mortality risk of NIDDM. Each kilogram of weight loss extends life expectancy by about 3–4 months in this group which had a mean age of 64 at diagnosis (Lean et al., 1990). This study demonstrates benefit in elderly patients. A similar finding was that weight loss of 9 kg or more led to 30–40% reduction in diabetes-related mortality (Williamson *et al.*, 1995).

The improvement in diabetic control with weight loss can be very marked in newly diagnosed patients who have symptomatic diabetes. For the majority of NIDDM patients weight loss is sufficient to remove symptoms. Hadden *et al.* (1975) demonstrated that a 10% weight loss (8.2 kg) reduced fasting blood glucose from 12 to below 8 mmol/L which represents the diagnostic threshold for diabetes. In a primary care setting a reduction in plasma glucose from 8.2 to 6.5 mmol/L with a 3.2-kg (2%) reduction in body-weight was demonstrated (Bitzen *et al.*, 1988).

Once body-weight is stabilized in a newly diagnosed diabetic patient, insulin sensitivity continues to decline with age (UKPDS, 1995). Attempts to check this progress with further dietary interventions have usually met with limited success in terms of weight loss when conventional dietary interventions are used. The benefits were greatest in subjects categorized as having poorly controlled diabetes, but for patients whose body-weight was greater than 120% ideal body-weight, as little as 4.4% weight loss led to a significant 4.3% decrease in HbA_{1c} and a 15% decrease in fasting blood glucose (Wing *et al.*, 1990).

It has been observed that plasma glucose concentration does not always improve after weight loss (Watts *et al.*, 1990). Amongst NIDDM patients who had each achieved a weight loss of 9.1 kg, 41% showed improvements in metabolic control (responders), but the remainder failed to demonstrate benefits (non-responders). Responders showed a 50% fall in blood glucose from 14.0 to 7.0 mmol/L. The non-responders showed an increase in fasting blood glucose from 14.0 to 18.0 mmol/L (22%). No predictive differences between these groups were seen in the age, body-weight or initial fasting blood glucose. Although the plasma glucose response to weight loss cannot be forecast by initial clinical parameters the success or failure of diet therapy can be predicted from the plasma glucose level after a weight loss of 2.3–4.5 kg. The authors concluded that moderately obese patients with NIDDM who remain hyperglycaemic after a weight loss of 2.3–4.5 kg are unlikely to improve with further weight loss and should be considered swiftly for treatment with either oral hypoglycaemic agents or insulin.

The impacts of diet restriction and of weight loss are separate on glycaemic control, as with lipid changes. Active energy restriction appears to have a marked but transient effect on blood glucose and insulin sensitivity. When active weight loss ceases, then there is a tendency for insulin sensitivity to return gradually towards its starting point, reaching a new point defined by the new body-weight. Diet composition also influences insulin sensitivity and may be changed during weight management. This phenomenon makes interpretation of results from short-term studies e.g. with very-low-calorie diets (VLCD) in NIDDM difficult to interpret. A VLCD was used to achieve 10.5 kg weight loss in 30 subjects over 40 days (Henry *et al.*, 1985). A subgroup of 12 subjects were further evaluated during 40 days of refeeding. Blood glucose fell from 297 to 158 mg/L after 20 days and further to 138 mg/L at day 40, a total decrease of 40%. Refeeding to maintain weight losses resulted in a secondary 80% increase in fasting blood glucose, though this remained markedly lower than before weight loss (254 vs 167 mg/dl glucose).

A comparison between VLCD (400 kcal/day) and a more conventional 1000 kcal reducing diet was made in 93 obese NIDDM subjects (Wing *et al.*, 1994). At the end of the year weight loss of 11 SD 6.5 kg body-weight was achieved by both treatments, with significant benefits on blood pressure, blood lipids and glycaemic control. Glycosylated haemoglobin fell by 0.5% for those with weight loss less than 5 kg, by 1.5% for those who lost 5–15 kg and by 2.2% for those who had lost more than 15 kg. One year after the end of this 12-month study, the mean regain of weight was 6 kg. This was accompanied by a loss of all the benefits that had been demonstrated from weight loss apart from a significant decrease in the use of anti-diabetic medications. In another study intermittent VLCD use, in 3-month phases, significantly improved the weight loss of a 1200 kcal diet over 12 months (Wing *et al.*, 1994).

In practical terms, weight loss of the order 5–7 kg is usually fairly easily achieved in the newly diagnosed patients, with conventional dietary advice in a routine clinic setting. People with NIDDM are not more resistant to weight loss for any metabolic reason, although resting metabolic rate (RMR) tends to fall when diabetic control is improved (Connacher *et al.*, 1988) and the initial weight loss is often better maintained in NIDDM patients who continue to attend an outpatient clinic than in patients with simple obesity. A review of body-weight changes in NIDDM patients with BMI greater than 25 kg/m² in Aberdeen showed that patients with BMI under 25 kg/m² at diagnosis had on average gained 1.3 kg 1 year after diagnosis, those with BMI 25–30 kg/m² at diagnosis had lost 2.6 kg, and those with BMI greater than 30 kg/m² at diagnosis had lost 6.8 kg 1 year after diagnosis. These results indicate that dietary intervention, at least in the first year after diagnosis of diabetes, is relatively rewarding.

Weight loss is less easy to achieve in established NIDDM patients, i.e., on a subsequent occasion (Blonk *et al.*, 1994), but interventions must be evaluated against control patients who tend to gain weight without intervention, and relatively modest losses (e.g., 5%) should be considered very successful. Manning *et al.* (1995) achieved 1 year losses of 2–3 kg by a variety of routine clinic approaches, against a gain of 1–2 kg in control subjects. The best result in this study was from the introduction of dexfenfluramine.

When weight loss is inadequate by conventional lifestyle approaches in NIDDM patients, the high health risks (in young patients especially) can justify more aggressive approaches, such as VLCD followed by long-term pharmaceutical appetite modification (Finer *et al.*, 1992) or surgical interventions which can normalize metabolic status in most cases (Pories *et al.*, 1992).

Conclusion

Avoiding weight gain during adulthood would have a major effect on delaying or avoiding completely the development of IGT and diabetes. The opportunity exists for targeting advice directed at those identified through family history of NIDDM, IGT in pregnancy, high waist circumference or waist/hip ratio, or origins in South Asia. Weight loss of 5% body-weight leads to clinically important improvements in diabetic control. Loss of 10–20% body-weight in overweight NIDDM patients can normalize metabolic control and possibly also life expectancy. Long-term follow-up results do not support the routine use of VLCD alone, but VLCD followed by an effective long-term weight maintenance programme might effectively cure this disease. Physical activity is an important adjunct to diet in the management of NIDDM.

Weight loss and blood lipids

The most characteristic lipid disturbance in obesity is elevated triglycerides and low HDL (Björntorp, 1990). Total cholesterol is clearly also frequently elevated in the overweight (Gregory *et al.*, 1990). Elevated LDL-cholesterol in obesity is common, but probably reflects background lipid profiles in the general population, not a specific effect of overweight (Barrett-Connor, 1985). This pattern points to increased CVD risk. The elevated triglycerides, coupled with an increased ratio of hepatic lipase to lipoprotein lipase in the overweight, leads to an excess of the small dense LDL (LDL_3 cholesterol) particles which are readily oxidized and highly atherogenic (Sattar *et al.*, 1998).

Influence of spontaneous body-weight fluctuation on blood lipids

Data from the Framingham Study suggest that there are small benefits in serum cholesterol as well as blood glucose concentrations in those subjects whose body-weight fell over a 10-year period (Higgins *et al.*, 1988). Long-term data from the Framingham Study indicate a relationship between change in body-weight and cholesterol over the 30-year monitoring period (Garrison *et al.*, 1985). This suggests some long-term improvement in serum cholesterol levels with weight loss from cardiovascular considerations, but some spontaneous weight loss may possibly be linked with cholesterol lowering caused by underlying disease within the population (Higgins *et al.*, 1993).

Studies of weight loss on blood lipids

With weight loss, serum lipids, including total cholesterol as well as plasma insulin all decrease acutely (Wolf & Grundy, 1983). In the longer term after weight re-stabilization there remain important sustained improvements in triglycerides and increases in HDL-cholesterol concentrations. A meta-analysis included 70 published studies which satisfied their inclusion criteria (Dattilo & Kris-Etherton, 1992). Those studies which achieved a mean weight loss < 1.5 kg were excluded but studies with a duration of 1 week or greater were included. Each kilogram of weight loss led to reductions of 0.6–0.8% in total cholesterol, LDL and HDL fractions and triglyceride. An increase of 0.8%/kg weight loss in HDL was seen after weight loss had stabilized. However, in a contrasting study the separate effects of energy restriction and weight loss on serum lipids in postmenopausal women were examined (120–150% > ideal body-weight (IBW)) before and after a 10-kg weight loss in modestly overweight women (BMI 25–30) (Weinsier *et al.*, 1992). Acute energy restriction lowered triglyceride by 32%, total cholesterol by 6%, LDL by 4%, LDL/HDL ratio by 8.0% and increased HDL-cholesterol by 4%. Stable weight loss was associated with lowered triglyceride by 13%, total cholesterol by 8%, LDL cholesterol by 8%, but HDL and the LDL/HDL ratio were unchanged. These findings suggest reduction to a weight-steady non-obese state improves lipid profiles, but illustrates the different effects of active energy restriction and stable weight loss. Results may also depend on the initial BMI.

The combination of physical activity and diet is more effective than either method alone in promoting weight loss (Skender *et al.*, 1996). Physical activity also limits the proportion of lean tissue lost in slimming regimens (Garrow & Summerbell, 1995) and limits weight regain (Wing *et al.*, 1992a; Skender *et al.*, 1996). A weight-loss programme which included subjects being randomized to receive either diet alone or diet and physical activity showed a beneficial effect in maintaining reductions in plasma lipids (Svedsen *et al.*, 1994). A moderate weight loss (8 kg) maintained at 7 kg at 9 months in overweight subjects found plasma triglycerides 20% below initial values and HDL had increased by 10%. However, the initial reductions in total cholesterol and LDL-cholesterol achieved after 12 weeks' weight loss had disappeared. The group who were still current exercisers at follow-up, however, had a significantly greater reduction in body-weight than non-exercisers (10.6 vs 6.6 kg).

A transient hypercholesterolaemia of weight reduction has been described (Phinney *et al.*, 1991) which is thought to reflect the release of stored cholesterol from adipose tissue deposits. Using a VLCD approach they achieved a 30-kg weight loss in overweight subjects. Serum cholesterol initially rose by 8%, but fell to 10% below starting value during weight maintenance.

Weight loss and lipids at different levels of body mass index and waist/hip ratio

A few studies of weight loss have categorized subjects by both BMI and waist/hip ratio (Table 22.1) (Lean *et al.*, 1995). Cut-off values of waist/hip ratio above which health risks increase appreciably, a waist/hip ratio 0.95 in men and 0.80 in women have emerged from prospective studies. Metabolic risk factors particularly serum concentrations of triglycerides and HDL-cholesterol improve most with weight loss in subjects with waist/hip ratio above these values (Den Besten *et al.*, 1988; Sönnichsen *et al.*, 1992; Wing *et al.*, 1992b; Kanaley *et al.*, 1993; Houmard *et al.*, 1994).

With increasing gain there are increases in the risk of morbidity from all causes. The increases take place steadily from BMI of 25–30 and then more rapidly at higher BMIs (Garrow, 1988). Consequently, the benefits of intentional weight loss are greater at higher BMI, especially in those of BMI $>30 \, \text{kg/m}^2$ who are the most frequently studied group (Goldstein, 1992). However, some reduction in the risk of diabetes mellitus has been reported between BMI 25 and 22.5 as part of the Boston Nurses Study (Colditz *et al.*, 1995). The findings concerning weight loss and health require careful interpretation, as some weight changes reported within large epidemiological studies have indicated a negative effect of weight loss on mortality and morbidity, probably due to underlying disease (see pp. 564–5) (Fig. 22.1).

Conclusion

In overweight people acute energy restriction and weight loss leads to rapid, though relatively large short-term reduction in blood lipids particularly triglycerides, but including HDL. These changes are seen in short studies, whose results should not be attributed entirely to weight loss. There may be a paradoxical transient rise in cholesterol with very severe restriction. After about 5 weeks, HDL tends to rise.

In longer-term (>3 months) studies, after stabilization of energy balance at a new lower weight, overall lipid profiles are improved. Each kilogram of weight loss reduces total plasma cholesterol and LDL cholesterol by close to 1%, and increases HDL cholesterol by about 1–2%. The benefits for plasma triglycerides are greater, a 1-kg loss leading to a total reduction of 2–3%. Benefits are greatest where the baseline levels are highest, greatest in men, and in subjects with high waist/hip ratios. Similar benefits are found in diabetic and non-diabetic individuals and in the elderly.

Table 22.1 Studies reporting metabolic benefits of weight loss in groups with differing waist/hip ratios.

| Reference | Mean baseline data | | | | | % Change in outcome measure | | | | | |
	Sex	No. of subjects	Age (years)	Waist/hip ratio	BMI (kg (%))	Weight loss (kg (%))	Triglycerides	Cholesterol Total	LDL	HDL	Treatment
Den Besten et al. (1988)	F	8	37.0	0.74	31.6	9.6 (10.9)	-16.2	-7.4	NA	-7.4	Low-calorie diet
Den Besten et al. (1988)	F	7	36.0	0.82	34.6	10.8 (11.4)	-38.4	-10.8	NA	-13.0	Low-calorie diet
Dennis et al. (1993)	F	18	45.0	0.77	30.0	9.0 (11.0)	-22.5	-6.2	-9.3	+3.7	Low-calorie diet
Dennis et al. (1993)	F	32	44.0	0.87	31.0	9.2 (11.2)	-23.4	-1.0	0.0	+11.4	Low-calorie diet
Kanaley et al. (1993)	F	9	35.3	0.74	32.1	7.7 (8.8)	-8.4	NA	NA	+5.8	Low-calorie diet and exercise
Kanaley et al. (1993)	F	10	36.1	0.89	33.4	9.2 (10.3)	-20.7	NA	NA	+20.0	Low-calorie diet and exercise
Lean et al. *	F	30	51.5	0.75	28.1	6.0 (8.1)	-15.7	-5.6	-6.9	-0.6	Low-calorie diet and slimming capsule†
Lean et al. *	F	16	57.6	0.84	28.9	5.2 (7.1)	-19.8	-3.9	-3.2	+0.7	Low-calorie diet and slimming capsule†
Lean et al. *	F	27	52.0	0.76	33.7	8.2 (9.4)	-8.3	-2.9	-2.7	-2.0	Low-calorie diet and slimming capsule†
Lean et al. *	F	52	53.5	0.85	35.7	6.2 (6.9)	-17.1	-2.9	-1.6	+0.5	Low-calorie diet and slimming capsule†
Sönnichsen et al. (1992)	M	40	49.7	1.02	41.4	6.4 (6.8)	-11.0	-16.5	-21.1	NA	Low-calorie diet
Houmard et al. (1994)	M	13	47.2	0.96	30.4	2.0 (2.1)	-20.3	-0.3	NA	+8.2	Exercise
Wing et al. (1992)	M	101	37.3	0.97	31.0	9.8 (10.2)	-16.2	-9.8	NA	NA	Low-calorie diet

NA, not available.

* Unpublished data.

† Proprietary food-based capsule.

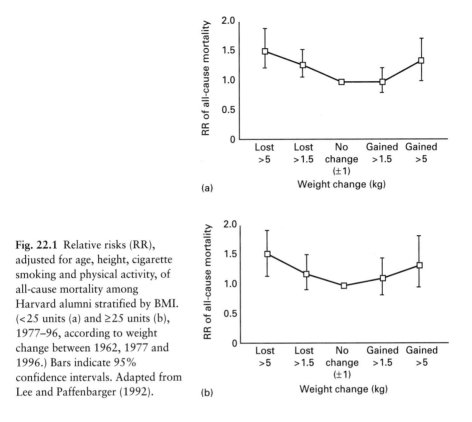

Fig. 22.1 Relative risks (RR), adjusted for age, height, cigarette smoking and physical activity, of all-cause mortality among Harvard alumni stratified by BMI. (<25 units (a) and ≥25 units (b), 1977–96, according to weight change between 1962, 1977 and 1996.) Bars indicate 95% confidence intervals. Adapted from Lee and Paffenbarger (1992).

Weight loss and clotting: haemostasis, rheology and fibrinolysis

A wide range of cardiovascular risks in terms of altered haemostatic, rheological and fibrinolytic factors which influence thrombosis formation (haemostatic and rheological factors). Many have been associated with overweight (Ernst *et al.*, 1989; Ernst, 1990; Meade *et al.*, 1993; DoH, 1994). In particular, the coagulation factors VII and X are directly associated with BMI and relate to thrombosis (Meade *et al.*, 1987) and risk of fatal myocardial infarction (Bottiger & Carlson, 1982).

Blood rheology

Several clinical studies have examined the effect of weight loss on rheological measures. The use of a VLCD (470–514 kcal/day) for 12 weeks with weight loss in obese subjects (mean BMI 37 kg/m²) reduced plasma viscosity by 3.5% (Poggi *et al.*, 1994). A weight loss of close to 16% body-weight decreased the aggregability of the red cells by 16%. However, plasma fibrinogen remained unaffected by the drastic changes in body-weight (Ernst *et al.*, 1989). A 1000kcal/L day diet intervention was used in obese subjects to achieve a 15% weight loss over 3 months (Ernst & Matrai, 1987). The blood and plasma viscosity fell by 27% and 5%, respectively, red cell aggregation by close to 20% and haematocrit by 5.5%. It is possible that acute energy restriction had effects other than simply via weight loss in these changes. One study used a conventional dietary approach over 3 months to reduce body-weight by 5.0 kg in subjects with BMI 35 kg/m². Red cell aggregability fell by 10%, though other measures of blood viscosity were not significantly improved (Hankey *et al.*, 1997).

Haemostatic factors

Coagulation factor VIIc and X were measured in 114 overweight subjects following a weight-reducing diet for 3 months (Baron *et al.*, 1989). Initially, after 1 month of weight reduction (approximately 2.5 kg) the coagulation markers decreased significantly. However, the differences were not maintained when the diet was continued to achieve weight loss of 4.2 kg. Another study has found that weight loss of 5 kg over 3 months on a low-fat diet reduced factor VII activity by 10% (Hankey *et al.*, 1997). Some of this effect may have been related to diet composition: as shown with a 10% decrease in factor VII activity after a reduction in dietary fat to 30% dietary energy, without significant weight loss (Marckmann *et al.*, 1993).

Fibrinolysis

Weight loss in overweight subjects improves fibrinolytic capacity probably by decreasing plasminogen activator inhibitor (PAI) (Andersen *et al.*, 1988). A weight loss of 5% achieved by a regimen of physical activity in young men aged 20–30 years who were moderately overweight (BMI of 26.5 kg/m²) resulted in improvements in PAI of 42% (Gris *et al.*, 1990). Other studies of the effects of body-weight reduction on tissue plasminogen activator (t-PA) antigen and PAI have been inconclusive (Palareti *et al.*, 1994; Hankey *et al.*, 1997).

Conclusion

For overweight subjects, reduction in body-weight leads to changes in most measures of haemostasis, rheology and fibrinolysis and improves CVD risk factors. Red cell aggregation decreases by about 2.5% and plasma viscosity by 2% per kilogram body-weight lost.

Weight loss and cardiovascular symptoms: angina

Angina is the most reliably diagnosed symptom of CVD, provided standard

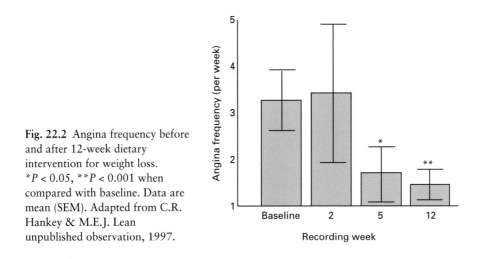

Fig. 22.2 Angina frequency before and after 12-week dietary intervention for weight loss. *P < 0.05, **P < 0.001 when compared with baseline. Data are mean (SEM). Adapted from C.R. Hankey & M.E.J. Lean unpublished observation, 1997.

criteria are used. In patients with known and stable angina, a drastic change in diet, together with a number of other interventions can reduce angina frequency after a 1-year period of dietary education (Ornish *et al.*, 1990). The intervention group lost weight from 91 to 81 kg over 12 months and had a 17% reduction in total serum cholesterol together with evidence of atheroma regression. Over this period of weight reduction other improvements were a reduction in both symptoms of angina (91%), and increase in exercise frequency (33%). Interpretation is complicated since the control group, who had no improvements in angina, were very much lighter than the intervention group. A single-stranded study of weight loss in overweight angina subjects found significant reductions in self-reported angina frequency after weight loss when compared with baseline (C.R. Hankey & M.E.J. Lean unpublished observation, 1997) (Fig. 22.2). It has recently been reported that close to 40% of obese angina patients do not have significant coronary artery disease, so benefit from weight loss might be expected without invoking atheroma regression (Bahadori *et al.*, 1996).

Conclusion

It seems likely that moderate intentional weight loss will improve the frequency of anginal pain, though further controlled studies are required.

Weight loss and atheroma regression

A number of studies in addition to that of Ornish *et al.* (1990) have investigated the possibility of reducing atheroma either by dietary intervention alone or together with medication. All published studies to date have reported reduction to varying degrees in the atheromatous plaques of those with established disease. The progression of coronary disease on the basis of serial angiograms was measured in 300 patients 21 months apart (Kramer *et al.*, 1983). They recognized that angiographic analyses were complicated by a number of biases which involved both under- and over-reporting.

The study of Ornish *et al.* (1990) showed important (8.8%) reductions in atheroma in a treatment regimen which included weight loss in subjects with coronary atherosclerosis while controls increased their atheroma by 8.0%. As part of the St Thomas's Atherosclerosis Regression Study (STARS) the effect of a 27% fat diet alone or diet plus cholestyramine on the coronary arteries of patients with coronary disease was investigated (Watts *et al.*, 1992). Those subjects whose BMI was > 25 kg/m^2 were advised on energy restriction to decrease body-weight. Computerized coronary angiograms were evaluated 3 years apart and the effect of different interventions compared. The proportions of patients who showed progression of coronary artery narrowing was 15% in the diet alone group, 12% in the diet and cholestyramine group, and 46% in the control group. The proportion of patients who showed an increase in luminal diameter were 38% in the diet group, 33% in the diet and cholestyramine group and 4% in the controls. Dietary change thus significantly retarded overall progression of disease, and diet and cholestyramine increased the luminal diameter.

Not all studies of atheroma regression documented weight loss (Brown *et al.*, 1990) but the treatments used—cholestyramine, colestipol, niacin and ileal bypass surgery—are all likely to have produced weight loss, and this could have played a part in the success for atheroma reduction. There is increasing speculation that the benefits of 'atheroma regression' actually reflect a change in plaque composition, or plaque stabilization. Weight loss may have a part in this.

Conclusion

There is sufficient evidence to make the suggestion that weight loss may offer benefits for atheroma regression or plaque stabilization. It is difficult to impart alterations solely to changes in body-weight when clearly many other complex interventions, which perhaps themselves were influencing body-weight, were being used. A specific intervention study on weight loss would be valuable.

Weight loss and effects on endocrine changes of obesity

A very wide range of endocrine changes are associated with overweight, and many benefit from weight loss. In particular the elevated sex hormone binding globulin (SHBG) in the polycystic ovary syndrome shows a tendency towards normalization, associated with improved insulin sensitivity (Friedman & Kim, 1985). Improvements have been demonstrated in endocrine and ovarian function in obese women with polycystic ovary disease after weight loss (Kiddy et al., 1992). Thirteen of the 24 women with mean weight 91.5 kg reduced their body-weight by 5% or more, and 11 of these achieved normal menstruation patterns. However, no improvements were seen in those who failed to reduce their body-weight by less than 5%. These findings confirm the earliest findings (Mitchell & Rogers, 1953) who showed dramatically the benefit of quite modest weight loss in obese amenorrhoeic women. After 7 kg loss from a baseline 98 kg menses returned to all women.

The impact of weight loss on a range of diseases was studied (Williamson et al., 1995). A striking reduction in incidence of the hormone-related cancers: prostrate in men, uterus and breast in women was shown. A weight loss of 0.5–8.6 kg decreased fully adjusted mortality by close to 55%, and a loss of greater than 9 kg reduced mortality by 40%. Reduced aromatase activity after weight loss, reducing androgen in women and oestrogen in men, is a possible mechanism.

Conclusion

Weight reduction can have marked influences on the endocrine system. Weight loss as a first measure to combat polycystic ovary syndrome is to be advocated before commencing other therapies.

Weight loss and psychiatric disorders

Many overweight patients exhibit features of depression, and clinical depression regularly occurs in the overweight, though research has reported that obese people are not psychiatrically different from non-obese people (Berman et al., 1993). In contrast, it has been proposed that the depression and poor self-esteem in some overweight subjects may be the result of living in a society who consider overweight and hold those who are overweight in poor regard (Stunkard & Wadden, 1992). Depression is often attributed to overweight and weight loss attempts using slimming regimens and physical activity are used to try to overcome it. On the other hand, starvation is known to cause apathy and depression and patients eat to overcome depression.

A wide range of theories have been discussed in relation to the psychological states and eating habits of the overweight. In practice these have been related to patterns of restrained eating also observed in those of healthy weight (Herman & Polivy, 1980), binge eating and bulimia (Pyle et al., 1981) and contempt of body image. It has been concluded (Stunkard & Wadden, 1992) that these effects are most likely to be consequences of the prejudice and discrimination that are suffered by the overweight in society. However, although no clear psychological characteristics have been observed in the overweight, particular characteristics have been associated with different behaviours. Binge eating has been associated with failure in weight management studies (Spitzer *et al.*, 1992).

The effects of personality disorder were investigated on the efficacy of weight loss in a study when either a behavioural programme or a liquid diet were offered to participants (Berman *et al.*, 1993). Those assessed and found to be free of personality disorder lost significantly more weight than those with a disorder on the liquid diet (5.3 vs 1.6 kg), though the opposite was the case in the behavioural programme (3.4 vs 4.5 kg).

Antidepressant drugs, particularly tricyclic antidepressants and phenothiazines often increase appetite and cause weight gain.

The use of behavioural therapy, which aims to challenge any of the psychological barriers to effective weight management, has been adopted by many therapists (Perri *et al.*, 1992). The use of behavioural therapy has been shown to be at least as effective as more conventional dietetic approaches, possibly as it offers practical strategies to overcome psychological barriers to weight loss (Perri *et al.*, 1992). The evaluation of mood and general psychiatric state during weight management and after weight loss have generated conflicting results (Wadden *et al.*, 1996). The earlier studies which have examined the effects of weight loss on mood before during and immediately after weight loss have tended to show falls in mood (Smoller *et al.*, 1987). This is probably partly due to the use of assessment methods which have rested on clinical opinion rather than the use of standardized assessment tools, and the numerous measures made, rather than one made before and after weight loss. The degree of improvement is also variable, as often those subjects involved in studies are themselves quite depressed and as such less likely to show radical improvements in mental state. Frequently, the desire to lose weight and apparent failure (or failure to recognize the value of relatively modest loss) of continual dieting has led many overweight people to even lower levels of self-esteem and self-worth (Wilson, 1993).

Conclusion

Overweight *per se* may be influential in developing some of the psychological characteristics that have been observed in overweight people. Although no clear pattern of psychological attributes have been identified in the overweight, weight loss and gain can be as a result of psychiatric disorders. Achieving intentional weight loss may facilitate improvements in some psychiatric disorders, possibly by improving the social pressures felt by overweight people. A review of this field has recently shown that weight loss in those 20% or greater overweight is usually associated with an improvement in mood when treated with diet and lifestyle information. It concluded that a 10% reduction in body-weight would be associated with improvements in both physical and psychological health.

Weight loss and other physical effects

Weight loss and gallstone development

An increased frequency of gallstones in the obese is well documented (Bray, 1985) and suggested to be secondary in importance as complications only to diabetes mellitus in their detrimental effects on health. In the Framingham Study, persons who were greater than 20% above their median weight for height had about twice the risk of developing gallstone disease when compared with those persons with less than 90% of their weight for height (Friedman *et al.*, 1966).

Weight loss appears not to help in gallbladder disease, although it made surgery easier (Everhart *et al.*, 1993). Gallbladder disease may indeed be exacerbated by weight loss (Sichieri *et al.*, 1991) and the main role of weight management remains primary prevention. The risk factors for gallstones were assessed in 457 subjects who entered a 520 kcal/day weight-control programme (Yang, 1992). During 16 weeks of rapid weight loss incidence of gallstones was 11%. There was no difference between males and females in prevalence of silent gallstones, but a higher actual incidence of gallstones in females (62%) and for males (33%).

Conclusion

Increased body-weight increases the risks of gallstones, and weight management is the only prevention. Subclinical disease may become apparent during weight loss.

Weight loss osteoarthritis and joint pain

It is widely accepted that weight reduction advice is appropriate to those overweight with arthritis as an increase in body-weight may be expected to add additional trauma to the weight-carrying joints. The effect of weight loss on the relief of joint pain in the morbidly obese was investigated (BMI $> 35 \, kg/m^2$) with encouraging results (McGoey *et al.*, 1990). Pain in the lower back, ankles and feet were all improved on moderate (6–10 kg) weight loss.

Conclusion

Moderate weight loss is likely to improve osteoarthritis and joint pain.

Hyperuricaemia and gout

Often intermingled with the incidence of joint and general structural pain is the development of gout. In the Framingham study, 33–45 years olds had increases in fasting uric acid levels with elevated body-weight (Kannel *et al.*, 1971). The relationship of gout with obesity is well known (Bray, 1985) but the effects of weight loss appear not to be documented. Uric acid may be acutely elevated during energy restriction, and acute gout occurs during weight loss with malignancies, so there may be mechanisms for increasing gout in predisposed individuals.

Conclusion

More evidence is required to illustrate whether the elevations in uric acid in the overweight are returned to normal after effective weight management, or whether there are clinical improvements in gout.

Weight loss and liver function

Changes in liver morphology, with fatty changes and portal infiltration related to abnormal liver function tests, have been documented in severely obese subjects, and are common in poorly controlled NIDDM. There are no conclusive data to relate this state to the overall health of the individual (Andersen *et al.*, 1984). Liver function usually returns to normal after weight loss which may be fairly minor. A study of liver biopsy in 41 subjects following a weight loss of 41 kg (BMI reduction by 27%) achieved by gastroplication and then VLCD was completed (Andersen *et al.*, 1991). Significant improvements were found in the fatty changes of the liver, but there were some signs of slight portal inflammation. Following ileal bypass surgery, liver disease and cirrhosis developed probably as a consequence of bacterial overgrowth in a blind loop.

Conclusion

The overall clinical implications of these obesity-related fatty changes in the liver remain open to speculation. It seems probable that minor weight loss is sufficient to correct them.

Weight loss and respiratory effects: sleep apnoea and pulmonary insufficiency

Shortness of breath is one of the commonest symptoms of the overweight, both

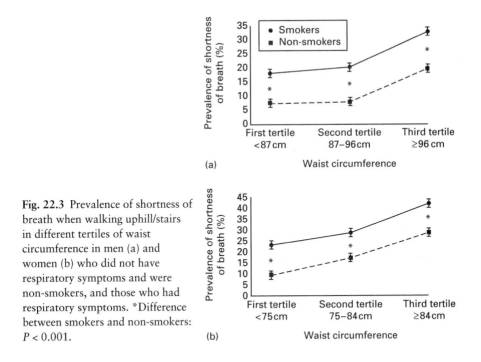

Fig. 22.3 Prevalence of shortness of breath when walking uphill/stairs in different tertiles of waist circumference in men (a) and women (b) who did not have respiratory symptoms and were non-smokers, and those who had respiratory symptoms. *Difference between smokers and non-smokers: $P < 0.001$.

through aggravation of underlying pulmonary disease and as a direct symptom. In those without pulmonary disease symptoms are worse with more marked obesity as shown by an increased waist circumference (T.S. Han, H.A. Smith, M.E.J. Lean & J.C. Seidell unpublished observation, 1997) (Fig. 22.3). Anecdotally, quite minor weight loss is sufficient to improve these symptoms but formal research trials are lacking.

Many abnormalities are seen in the measurements of pulmonary function in obese persons indicating an impairment in work capacity, and hypoventilation particularly during sleep. There are detrimental effects from overweight on chest expansion in partnership with an increase in the body's oxygen requirement at rest and the greater workload of physical activity (Bray *et al.*, 1985). The results of 22% weight loss following gastric banding in 34 otherwise healthy women were investigated with respect to pulmonary function. An improvement in pulmonary function was observed following weight reduction, with both a decrease in ventilatory demands and a moderate increase in ventilatory capacity (Sugermann *et al.*, 1986).

The extreme and potentially life-threatening condition of sleep apnoea in the obese incorporates physical effects from adipose accumulation, in neck and abdomen, and may also include a disorder of the respiratory control centre. A study of 12 morbidly obese men found that the loss of 42% body-weight offered significant reduction in the frequency of disordered breathing (Harman *et al.*,

1982). A weight loss of 9% overall was achieved, from 106.2 kg in a 15-subject study (Smith *et al.*, 1985). Important improvements were achieved in the apnoea frequency of these subjects, without any changes in the frequency of sleep apnoea in the control patients. Between the extremes of these two studies lie the results of Rubinstein *et al.* (1988). In overweight patients (eight men and four women) with BMI 41 kg/m^2, pulmonary function and other relevant sleep data were measured before and after the reduction of body-weight by 22%. An improvement in specific measurements in pharyngeal and glottic function (30–50%) were seen with weight loss. These results suggested improvement in sleep apnoea may have been achieved by an improvement in pharyngeal function. An editorial (Harman, 1986) summarized the benefits of weight loss on the respiratory insufficiency of obesity as being due to reductions in both increased chest pressure and upper airway restriction.

Conclusions

Weight loss in the obese can improve general measures of pulmonary function. Sleep apnoea can be improved by weight loss, and extreme weight loss is not always necessary.

Reflux oesophagitis and dyspepsia

Hiatus hernia, and consequent reflux oesophagitis are common in the overweight. The role of weight loss and/or cimetidine in the management of reflux oesophagitis, for a study period between 8 and 12 weeks was examined (Murray *et al.*, 1991). Similar weight loss of 7% (5.5 kg) was achieved for both groups. Both groups showed improvements, with no additional benefit attributable to the use of cimetidine. This study describes itself as the first to demonstrate that weight loss has a beneficial effect on the treatment of reflux oesophagitis. In contrast, obese patients with mean BMI was 31.4 kg/m^2 were examined. After a 6-month dietary intervention reducing weight by 10.8 kg no benefit in frequency of oesophageal reflux was observed (Kjellin *et al.*, 1995).

Conclusion

There is some evidence to support weight loss and improvements in reflux oesophagitis.

Obesity and urinary incontinence in women

Urinary incontinence is associated with obesity in many cases, and reduction in body-weight in the overweight with urinary incontinence has been recommended as beneficial. However, the prevalence of incontinence in the obese and overweight is poorly documented. A U.S. study examined the relationship between obesity and incontinence in 368 incontinent women who presented at urodynamic clinics over a 2-year period. They were compared with a non-obese urology clinic population (Dwyer *et al.*, 1988). Following full clinical and urodynamic assessment 63% were diagnosed as having genuine stress incontinence, and within this group, obesity >20% above IBW was significantly more common than in the general population. Other women (23%) were diagnosed as having an earlier form of urological weakness (detruser instability) and their BMI was seen to increase with age and the number of previous incontinence operations and parities. Another study found an increased BMI to be correlated with a positive clinical stress test, suggesting a direct relationship with urinary incontinence (Kolbl & Riss, 1988).

Role of overweight in the prognosis of incontinence was considered as part of a postal questionnaire examining the use of physiotherapy in the treatment of stress incontinence (Mantle *et al.*, 1991). Obesity was among a number of factors considered as bad prognostic features. The BMI was found to affect adversely the success of a range of surgical procedures used for the treatment of incontinence (Brieger & Korda, 1992).

The effect of surgically induced weight loss on lower urinary tract function in obese women was studied (Bump *et al.*, 1992). Thirteen subjects underwent comprehensive evaluation of urinary tract function before and 1 year after. After a 33% weight reduction (BMI was reduced from 49 SD 7.9 to 33.1 SD 6.7 kg/m²) a number of important improvements were seen in a range of bladder health measures and further incontinence therapy was unnecessary. In a similar study, amongst obese women who reduced body-weight by 33%, stress incontinence fell from 62 to 11% (Deitel *et al.*, 1988). It has been suggested that urinary incontinence is an important criterion to indicate obesity surgery, perhaps at a lower BMI than would normally be considered (Deitel & Shahi, 1992).

Conclusion

Urinary stress incontinence may be present in up to 60% of obese women. Weight loss is beneficial in achieving a major reduction in urinary incontinence in obese women.

Weight loss, mortality and weight cycling

Weight loss and regain is likely to be something to which humans are reasonably well adapted through evolution. 'Weight cycling' of this kind which occurs with fluctuations in food supply may, however, be different to the modern conditions of obesity and inactivity with episodic dietary restriction. Current statistics on the number of adults trying to follow a weight-reducing diet are alarming. The figures for the U.K. suggest up to 35% of adults are engaged in some form of slimming behaviour at any one time (Kent & Bowyer, 1992) and in the U.S.A. up to 40% of adult women and 20% of adult men (Williamson *et al.*, 1992). Given that the U.K. population is becoming more overweight, this evidence warns that large numbers of adults are, repeatedly in adult life, within cycles of slimming and weight regain.

The reductions in all the major risk factors for CVD would suggest that weight loss should ultimately lead to increased survival. Self-reported weight loss in a number of large observational studies appears to have adverse effects on survival, even amongst the overweight. There are also suggestions from retrospective studies that potential hazards exist from 'weight cycling', i.e., reported fluctuations in adult weight, with increases in heart disease risk and BMI, but the evidence supporting these claims remains weak and confounded. In the Western Electric study of self-reported weight change (Hamm *et al.*, 1989), 5% of the study group were considered as weight changers (a gain and a loss of 10% body-weight) within a 10-year period. The 98 men considered to be weight changers showed a significant 50% higher mortality from CVD and cancer than the remaining group. A number of other epidemiological and cohort studies with longitudinal survival data have been used to assess the disease associations of reported weight changes. The limitation of this approach is that weight loss may have been after intentional slimming, or it may have reflected the presence of a disease which would shorten survival.

The NHANES study identified obesity as a risk factor for mortality though found no benefit from reported weight loss for the whole population. The first NHANES study cohort (1971–1975) was followed and those subjects surviving to 5 years post-study for the cohort aged between 45 and 74 years at admission (Pamuk *et al.*, 1992). For those with a BMI between 26 and 29 kg/m^2, weight loss increased their risk of death even after adjustment for age, race, smoking habit, parity and pre-existing illness. Those subjects who lost 15% or more of their maximum weight had twice the mortality of those who only reduced their body-weight by 5%. At BMI > 29 kg/m^2 mortality was increased in proportion with weight lost for women. Other subjects may have lost weight intentionally precisely because of disease development, but remain at high risk from that disease even after weight loss.

The effect of body-weight change on longevity in the cohort of Harvard University alumni was investigated (Lee & Paffenbarger, 1992). Self-reported weights and health and activity questionnaires were completed at two weighed periods 11 years apart. The lowest mortality was found in those maintaining a stable weight. Both weight loss and gain were associated with significantly increased mortality from all causes. The effect of weight changes on mortality in the MRFIT cohort of over 10 000 men of mean BMI 27.7 kg/m² was examined over a 7-year period (Blair *et al.*, 1993). Mortality once more was found to be lowest in those whose weight remained stable, irrespective of smoking habit. The strongest associations were seen with 1 SD of weight change and death in the two lowest tertiles of BMI. There was no association with weight change in the heaviest tertile of the group. The results of the principal studies examining the issue of weight loss and mortality have recently been summarized, and concluded that the highest mortality rates do occur in the adult who has either gained or lost excessive amounts of body-weight (Andres *et al.*, 1993). The lowest mortality rates are usually associated with modest weight gains.

These data highlight interpretational difficulties with self-reported weight loss which may not have been intentional. Inadvertent weight loss usually indicates some subclinical disease process. The limited evidence on intentional weight loss is more reassuring but still incomplete. A study reported the intentional weight loss in 28 000 healthy non-smoking women showed a mean reduction of 9.1 kg was associated with a 25% reduction in all-cause, cardio-vascular and cancer mortalities (Williamson *et al.*, 1995). Similar benefits from weight loss of any amount in people who already had symptoms of obesity-related diseases were also shown. On the other hand, intentional weight loss under 9.1 kg appeared to increase mortality in uncomplicated individuals. Information on intentional weight loss in men is awaited.

Effects of weight cycling on body composition and energy expenditure

It has been proposed that 'weight cycling' may change body composition, and increases the percentage of body fat, and decreases the fat-free mass (FFM) (Prentice *et al.*, 1992). However, scant evidence to support this hypothesis has been found (National Task Force, 1994). Visceral fat deposition was not influenced by a history of weight cycling (Rebuffe-Scrive *et al.*, 1994). No effect of 'weight cycling' on total body fat, fat distribution or resting energy expenditure was found (Wing *et al.*, 1992b). This challenged the hypotheses that weight changes are related to metabolic changes or disease activity. To date no evidence exists to support that increased weight cycling leads to an elevation in percentage body fat.

Dieting, weight loss and subsequent weight regain, i.e., weight cycling, has been proposed to lead to a permanent decrease in basal metabolic rate. The theory is appealing as it supports the observation that the majority of successful slimmers fail to maintain their weight losses long term. However, the majority of studies (National Task Force, 1994) have been unable to establish a lower metabolic rate in those who had undergone weight cycling when the results were corrected for the differing body compositions. Further research on the other components of energy expenditure are required.

Psychological characteristics associated with weight cycling

Brownell and Rodin (1994) posed many as yet unanswered questions concerning weight cycling and suggested an equal prevalence of cycling in both males and females of both normal and increased body-weight. They also proposed that weight cycling may be associated with negative psychological and behavioural influences on lifestyle, the principal factors being binge eating, depression and life dissatisfaction. No consistent findings relating weight cycling behaviour and psychological characteristics have emerged, though very few completed studies exist. Individuals with a history of weight cycling have been shown to have greater number of psychopathologies in comparison with those who were weight stable, independent of BMI (Foreyt et al., 1995). Two recent reviews have supported these findings (National Task Force, 1994; Rebuffe-Scrive et al., 1994).

Conclusion

The health influences of reported fluctuations in body-weight in population studies are probably dominated by the presence of disease, either as a cause of weight fluctuations or as a reason for intentional weight loss (which did not completely reverse the associated risks). The evidence on intentional weight loss or slimming under advice supports advocating moderate weight loss in adults using conventional diets, with increased survival particularly in those with existing obesity-related disease such as NIDDM.

Potential health hazards of weight loss

Weight gain is the result of relative overeating in response to a highly complex system of psychological and social pressures, and reversing this process without resolving the psycho-social issues introduces stress. The sequence of adverse developments during starvation were described as depression, apathy, inactivity and cognitive impairment, infertility in women and impotence in men (Keys et al., 1950). A number of physical changes also occur during enforced weight reduction. Changes in the skin and hair loss are common, particularly with extreme dietary regimens such as VLCD. A comprehensive review of the evidence regarding the development of gallstones reported that after weight loss through dietary intervention the development of gallstones increased up to 22% (Everhart, 1993). Above 24% weight loss following diet there was a threefold increase in gallstone development. With weight loss greater than 45%, 60% patients developed either gallstones or gallbladder sludge (Shiffman *et al.*, 1991).

The area of weight reduction and seizure incidence, principally with respect to the use of VLCD regimens, was discussed by Kaufman *et al.* (1990). Their review was based on three clinical cases, each of whom were described as being at risk of seizure by electroencephalography. The weight loss preceding the incidence of seizure was 5%. These changes are recognized as cautions in the use of VLCD.

Bone mass is responsive to changes in body mass and is elevated in the overweight. Decreasing bone mass with weight loss has been demonstrated, but as overweight subjects returned to their prediet weight, the bone mass followed these patterns (Compston *et al.*, 1992). On the other hand, it has been found that weight regain was not accompanied by a complete restoration of bone mass (Avenell *et al.*, 1994). These findings are supported by the work of Fogelholm *et al.* (1997).

Starvation regimens have been largely dismissed as potentially dangerous, and have received little attention in the recent literature. Starvation entailing a daily energy deficit of 2500–2700 kcal will achieve a loss of about 3–4 kg per week. Tissue composition lost in starvation represents about 50% lean muscle and 50% adipose tissue, and thus presents difficulties from alteration in body composition (Garrow, 1988). Starvation runs increased risks of unexpected death even before body-weight reaches a minimal healthy weight (Garnett *et al.*, 1969). The profound psychological and physical effects of starvation were documented in detail in the classic work of Keys *et al.* (1950). The most likely causes of sudden death on use of starvation diets were either underlying heart disease exacerbated by the loss of heart muscle on starvation (Garnett *et al.*, 1969) or the development of ventricular arrhythmia secondary to the elevation of free fatty acids characteristic in starvation situations (Garrow *et al.*, 1989; Drott & Lundholm, 1992).

Conclusion

A number of potential hazards have been associated with weight loss, but they are relatively uncommon, and unlikely to out-weigh benefits, or frequently to account for a general impairment of quality of life.

Summary

Within the whole landscape of health consequences from overweight, weight loss as a result of intentional slimming results in predictable reduction in risk for vascular disease. Benefits and also health improvements are seen from a wide range of other specific weight-related conditions as well as more 'minor' symptoms including excess sweating and dyspepsia/indigestion.

A wide range of other physical disorders have been associated with overweight and obesity, although they have been less frequently studied than the cardiovascular-related effects. The relative scarcity of reports on these conditions in relation to body-weight change may reflect both the difficulty in measurements and possibly the considerable time period required to trace physical changes in these systems. Some common physical symptoms associated with obesity such as breathlessness, dyspepsia and profuse sweating are rarely described other than anecdotally. However, improvement in these symptoms are often the earliest and most predictable benefit to patients following weight loss. These improvements point to major reductions in health service demands.

The hazards of weight loss are principally related to underlying disease, or the result of inappropriate restrictions in energy intake. Intentional weight loss has been shown to offer considerable health benefits, which support population and other approaches to retard increases in the epidemic of obesity.

Overall good clinical evidence supports anecdotal evidence in justifying weight loss to improve health and reduce health costs.

References

Andersen, P., Nilsen, D.W.T., Bechkmann, S.L., Holme, I. & Hjermann, I. (1988) Increased fibrinolytic potential in healthy coronary high risk individuals. *Acta Medica Scandanavia* **22**, 499–506.

Andersen, T. & Gluud, C. (1984) Liver morphology in morbid obesity: a literature study. *International Journal of Obesity* **8**, 97–106.

Andersen, T., Glkuud, F., Franzmann, M.B. & Christofferson, P. (1991) Hepatic effects of dietary weight loss in morbidly obese patients. *Journal of Hepatology* **12**, 224–229.

Andres, R., Muller, D.C. & Sorkin, J.D. (1993) Long term effects of change in body weight on all-cause mortality: a review. *Annals of Internal Medicine* **119**, 737–743.

Avenell, A., Richmond, P.R., Lean, M.E.J. & Reid, D.M. (1994) Bone loss associated with a high fibre weight reduction diet in postmenopausal women. *European Journal of Clinical Nutrition* **48**, 561–566.

Bahadori, B., Neuer, E., Schumacher, M. *et al.* (1996) Prevalence of coronary-artery disease in obese versus lean men with angina-pectoris and positive exercise stress test. *American Journal of Cardiology* **77**, 1000–1001.

Barrett-Conner, E. (1985) Obesity, atherosclerosis and coronary artery disease. *Annals of Internal Medicine* **103**, 1010–1019.

Barrett-Connor, E., Suarez, L., Khan, K.T. & Criqui, M.D. (1984) Epidemiology of obesity and NIDDM. *Epidemiological Reviews* **11**, 172–181.

Baron, J.A., Schori, A., Crow, B., Carter, R. & Mann, J.I. (1989) A randomised controlled trial of low carbohydrate and low fat/high fibre diets for weight loss. *American Journal of Public Health* **76**, 1293–1296.

Bennett, N., Dodd, T., Flatley, J., Freeth, S. & Bolling, K. (1995) *Health Survey for England 1993*, Series H5 No. 3. London: HMSO.

Berman, W.H., Berman, E.R., Heymsfield, S., Fauci, M. & Ackerman, S. (1993) The effect of pscyhiatric disorders on weight loss in obesity clinic patients. *Behavioural Medicine* **18**, 167–172.

Bitzen, P.O., Melander, A., Schersten, B. & Svensson, M. (1988) Efficacy of dietary regulation in primary health care patients with hyperglycaemia detected by screening. *Diabetic Medicine* **5**, 634–639.

Björntorp, P. (1990) Obesity and adipose tissue distribution as risk factors for the development of disease—a review. *Infusiontherapie* **17**, 24–27.

Blair, S.N., Shaten, J., Brownell, K., Collins, G. & Lissner, L. (1993) Body weight change, all cause mortality in the multiple risk factor intervention trial. *Annals of Internal Medicine* **119**, 749–757.

Blonk, M.C., Jacobs, M.A.J.M., Biesheuvel, E.H.E., Weda-Manak, W.L. & Heine, R.J. (1994) Influences of weight loss in type 2 diabetic patients: little long term benefit from group behaviour therapy and exercise training. *Diabetic Medicine* **11**, 449–457.

Bottiger, L.E. & Carlson, L.A. (1982) Risk factors for death for males and females. *Acta Medica Scandinavia* **211**, 437–442.

Bray, G.A. (1985) Complications of obesity. *Annals of Internal Medicine* **103**, 1052–1062.

Brieger, G. & Korda, A. (1992) The effect of obesity on the outcome of successful surgery for genuine stress incontinence. *Australian and New Zealand Journal of Obstetrics and Gynaecology* **32**, 71–77.

Brown, G., Albers, J.J., Fisher, L.D.M. *et al.* (1990) Regression of coronary artery disease as a result of intensive lipid lowering therapy in men with high levels of apolipoproteinaemia. *New England Journal of Medicine* **323**, 1289–1298.

Brownell, K.D. & Rodin, J. (1994) Medical, metabolic and psychological effects of weight cycling. *Archives Internal Medicine* **154**, 1325–1330.

Bump, R.C., Sugerman, H.J., Fantl, J.A. & McClish, D.K. (1992) Obesity and lower urinary tract function in women: effect of surgically induced weight loss. *American Journal Obstetrics and Gynaecology* **167**, 392–399.

Chan, J.M., Rimm, E.B., Colditz, G.A., Stampfer, M.J. & Willett, W.C. (1994) Obesity, fat distribution, and weight gain as risk factors for clinical diabetes in men. *Diabetes Care* **17**, 961–969.

Colditz, G.A., Willett, W.C., Rotnitzky, A. & Manson, J.E. (1995) Weight gain as a risk factor for clinical diabetes in women. *Annals of Internal Medicine* **122**, 481–486.

Compston, J.E., Laskey, M.A., Croucher, P.I., Coxon, A. & Krietzman, S. (1992) Effect of diet induced weight loss on total body bone mass. *Clinical Science* **82**, 429–432.

Connacher, A.A., Jung, R.T., Mitchell, P.E.G., Ford, A.P., Leslie, P. & Illingworth, P. (1988) Heterogeneity of noradrenergic thermic responses in obese and lean humans. *International Journal of Obesity* **12**, 267–276.

Culter, J.A. (1991) Randomised clinical trials of weight reduction in non hypertensive persons. *Annals of Epidemiology* **1**, 363–370.

Davis, B.R., Blaufox, M.D., Oberman, A. *et al.* (1993) Effect of weight reduction by dietary intervention in overweight persons with mild hypertension. *Archives of Internal Medicine* **153**, 1773–1782.

Dattilo, A.M. & Kris-Etherton, P.M. (1992) Effects of weight reduction on blood lipids and lipoproteins: a meta analysis. *American Journal of Clinical Nutrition* **56**, 320–328.

Den Besten, C., Vansant, G., Weststraete, J.A. & Deurenberg, P. (1988) Resting metabolic rate and diet induced thermogenesis in abdominal and gluteal femoral obese women before and after weight reduction. *American Journal of Clinical Nutrition* **47**, 840–847.

Dennis, K. & Goldberg, A.P. (1993) Differential effects of body fatness and body fat distribution on risk factors for cardiovascular disease in women. *Arteriosclerosis and Thrombosis* **13**, 1487–1494.

Department of Health (1994) *Diet and Cardiovascular Disease*. London: HMSO.

Dietel, M. & Shahi, B. (1992) Morbid obesity: selection of patients for surgery. *Journal of the American College of Nutrition* **11**, 457–462.

Dietel, M., Stone, E., Kassam, H.A., Wilk, E.J. & Sutherland, D.J.A. (1988) Gynaecological-obstetric changes after loss of massive excess weight following bariatric surgery. *Journal of the American College of Nutrition* **7**, 147–153.

Drott, C. & Lundholm, K. (1992) Cardiac effects of calorie restriction-mechanisms and potential hazards. *International Journal of Obesity* **16**, 481–486.

Dwyer, P.L., Lee, E.T.C. & Hay, D.M. (1988) Obesity and urinary incontinence in women. *British Journal of Obstetrics and Gynaecology* **95**, 91–96.

Ernst, E. (1990) Plasma fibrinogen an independent cardiovascular risk factor. *Journal of Internal Medicine* **227**, 365–372.

Ernst, E. & Matrai, A. (1987) Normalisation of hemorheological abnormalities during weight reduction in obese patients. *Nutrition* **3**, 337–339.

Ernst, E., Weihmayr, T.H., Matrai, A. & Resch, K.L. (1989) Changes in blood rheology of grossly obese individuals during a very low calorie diet. *International Journal of Obesity* **13** (suppl. 2), 167–168.

Everhart, J.E. (1993) Contributions of obesity and weight loss to gallstone disease. *Annals of Internal Medicine* **119**, 1029–1035.

Finer, N., Finer, S. & Naoumova, R.T. (1992) Diet therapy after very low calorie diets. *American Journal of Clinical Nutrition* **1s**, 195s–198s.

Fogelholm, M., Sievanen, H., Heinonen, A. *et al.* (1997) Association between weight cycling history and bone mineral density in premenopausal women. *Osteoperosis International* **7**, 354–358.

Foreyt, J.B., Brunner, R.L., Goodrick, G.K., Cutter, G., Bronwell, K.D. St Jeor, S.T. *et al.* (1995) Psychological correlates of weight fluctuation. *International Journal of Eating Disorders* **17**, 263–275.

Friedman, C.I. & Kim, M.H. (1985) Obesity and it's effect on reproductive function. *Clinical Obstetrics and Gynaecology* **28**, 645–663.

Friedman, G.D., Kannel, W.B. & Dawber, J.R. (1966) The epidemiology of gallbladder disease: observations from the Framingham study. *Journal of Chronic Disease* **19**, 273–292.

Garrison, R.J. & Castelli, W.P. (1985) Weight and 30 year mortality of men in the Framingham study. *Annals of Internal Medicine* **103**, 1006–1009.

Garrow, J. (1988) *Obesity and Related Diseases*. London: Churchill Livingstone.

Garrow, J.S. & Summerbell, C. (1995) Meta-analysis: effect of exercise, with and without dieting on the body composition of overweight subjects. *European Journal of Clinical Nutrition* **49**, 1–10.

Garrow, J.S., Webster, J.D., Pearson, M., Pacy, P.J. & Harpin, G. (1989) Inpatient-outpatient randomised comparison of Cambridge diet versus milk diet in 17 obese women over 24 weeks. *International Journal of Obesity* **13**, 521–529.

Garnett, E.S., Barnard, D.L., Ford, J., Goodbody, R.A. & Woodhouse, M.A. (1969) Gross fragmentation of cardiac myofibrils after therapeutic starvation for obesity. *Lancet* **i**, 914–916.

Goldstein, D.J. (1992) Beneficial health effects of modest weight loss. *International Journal of Obesity* **16**, 397–415.

Gregory, J., Forster, K., Tyler, H. & Wiseman, M. (1990) *The dietary and nutritional survey of British adults: a survey of the dietary behaviour, nutritional status and blood pressure of adults aged 16–64 living Britain*. London: OPCS, HMSO.

Gris, J.C., Schved, J.F., Feugeas, O. *et al.* (1990) Impact of smoking, physical training and weight reduction on FVII, PAI-1 and haemostatic markers in sedentary men. *Thrombosis and Haemostasis* **64**, 516–520.

Hadden, D.R., Montgomery, D.A.D., Skelly, R.J. *et al.* (1975) Maturity onset diabetes mellitus: response to intensive dietary management. *British Medical Journal* **iii**, 276–278.

Hamm, P., Shekelle, R.B. & Stamler, J. (1989) Large fluctuations in body weight during young adulthood and the 25 year risk of coronary disease in men. *American Journal of Epidemiology* **129**, 312–318.

Hankey, C.R., Rumley, A., Lowe, G.D.O., Woodward, M. & Lean, M.E.J. (1997) Moderate weight reduction improves red cell aggregation and factor VII activity in overweight subjects. *International Journal of Obesity* **21**, 644–650.

Harman, E.M., Wynne, J.W., Block, A.J. & Malloy-Fischer, L. (1982) Sleep disordered breathing and oxygen desaturation in obese patients. *Chest* **79**, 256–260.

Harman, E.M. & Block, A.J. (1986) Why does weight loss improve the respiratory insufficiency of obesity. *Chest* **90**, 153–154.

Henry, R.R., Scheaffer, L. & Olefsky, J.M. (1985) Glycaemic effects of intensive care caloric restriction and isocaloric refeeding in noninsulin-dependent diabetes mellitus. *Journal of Clinical Endocrinology and Metabolism* **61**, 917–925.

Herman, C.P. & Polivy, J. (1980) Restrained eating. In: Stunkard, A.J. (ed.) *Obesity*. Philadelphia: W.B. Saunders.

Higgins, M., Kannel, W., Garrison, R., Pinsky, J. & Stokes, J. (1988) Hazards of obesity—the Framingham experience. *Acta Medica Scandinavia* **723**, 23–26.

Higgins, M., D'Agostino, R., Kannel, W. & Cobb, J. (1993) Benefits and adverse effects of weight loss: observations from the Framingham study. *Archives of International Medicine* **119**, 758–763.

Holbrook, T.L., Barrett-Connor, E. & Wingard, D.L. (1989) The association of lifetime weight and weight control patterns with diabetes among men and women in the adult community. *International Journal of Obesity* **13**, 723–729.

Houmard, J.A., McCulley, C., Roy, L.K., Bruner, K.R., McCammon, M.R. & Israel, R.G. (1994) Effects of exercise training on absolute and relative measurements of regional adiposity. *International Journal of Obesity* **18**, 243–248.

James, W.P.T., Mascie-Taylor, G.C.N., Norgan, N.G., Bistrain, B.R., Shetty, P.S. & Ferro-Luzzi, A. (1994) The value of arm circumference measurements in measuring chronic energy deficiency in third world adults. *European Journal of Clinical Nutrition* **48**, 883–894.

Kaufman, M.A. & Bhargava, A. (1990) Dietary weight reduction and seizures. *Neurology* **40**, 1905–1906.

Kanaley, J.A., Andersen-Reid, M.L., Oenning, L., Kottle, B.A. & Jensen, M.D. (1993) Differential health benefits of weight loss in upper body and lower body obese women. *American Journal of Clinical Nutrition* **57**, 20–26.

Kannel, W.B., Garcia, M.J., McNamara, P.M. & Pearson, G. (1971) Serum lipid precursers of coronary heart disease. *Human Pathology* **2**, 129–151.

Kent, A. & Bowyer, C. (1992) When weight gets out of control. *Doctor* May, 48–49.

Keys, A., Brozek, J., Henschel, A., Mickelson, O. & Taylor, H. (1950) *The Biology of Human Starvation*. Minneapolis: The University Minnesota Press.

Kiddy, D.S., Hamilton-Fairley, D., Bush, A. *et al.* (1992) Improvement in endocrine and ovarian function during dietary treatment of obese women with polycystic ovary syndrome. *Clinical Endocrinology* **36**, 105–111.

Kjellin, A., Ramel, S., Rossner, S. & Thor, S. (1995) Gastrophageal reflux in obese patients is not affected by weight reduction. *International Journal of Obesity* **19**, 305.

Koivisto, V.A. & Defronzo, R.A. (1984) Exercise in the treatment of type II diabetes. *Acta Endocrinologia* **262** (suppl.), 107–111.

Kolbl, H. & Riss, P. (1988) Obesity and stress urinary incontinence. Significance of indices of relative weight. *Urologia Internationalis* **43**, 7–10.

Kramer, J.R., Kitazume, H., Proudfit, W.L., Matsuda, Y., Williams, G.W. & Sones, F.M. (1983) Progression and regression of coronary atherosclerosis: relation to risk factors. *American Heart Journal* **105**, 134–139.

Law, M.R., Frost, C.D. & Wald, N.J., (1991a) By how much does dietary salt reduction lower blood pressure? I, II, III. *British Medical Journal* **302**, 811–824.

Law, M.R., Frost, C.D. & Wald, N.J. (1991b) Analysis of data from trials of salt restriction. *British Medical Journal* **302**, 819–824.

Lean, M.E.J., Powrie, J.K., Anderson, A.S. & Garthwaite, P.H. (1990) Obesity weight loss and prognosis in type 2 Diabetes. *Diabetic Medicine* **7**, 228–233.

Lean, M.E.J., Han, T.S. & Morrison, C.E. (1995) Waist circumference as a measure for indicating need for weight management. *British Medical Journal* 311, 158–161.

Lee, I.M. & Paffenbarger, R.S. (1992) Change in body weight and longevity. *Journal of the American Medical Association* 268, 2045–2049.

Marckmann, P., Sandstrom, B. & Jespersen, J. (1993) Favourable long-term effect of a low-fat/high-fiber diet in human coagulation and fibrinolysis. *Arteriosclerosis and Thrombosis* 13, 505–511.

Manning, R.M., Jung, R.T., Leese, G.P. & Newton, R.W. (1995) The comparison of four weight reducing strategies aimed at overweight diabetic patients. *Diabetic Medicine* 12, 409–415.

Manson, J.E., Colditz, G.A., Stampfer, M.J. *et al.* (1990) A prospective study of obesity and risk of CHD in women. *New England Journal Medicine* 322, 882–889.

Manson, J.E., Willett, W.C., Stampfer, M.J. *et al.* (1995) Body weight and mortality among women. *New England Journal Medicine* 333, 677–685.

Mantle, J. & Versi, E. (1991) Physiotherapy for stress incontinence: a national survey. *British Medical Journal* 302, 753–755.

McGoey, B.B., Deitel, M., Saplys, R.J.F. & Kliman, M.E. (1990) Effect of weight loss on musculoskeletal pain in the morbidly obese. *Journal of Bone and Joint Surgery* 72B, 322–323.

Meade, T.W., Imeson, J. & Stirling, Y. (1987) Effects of changes in smoking and other characteristics on clotting factors and the risk of ischaemic heart disease. *Lancet* 31, 986–988.

Meade, T.W., Ruddock, V., Stirling, Y., Chakrabarti, R. & Miller, G.J. (1993) Fibrinolytic activity, clotting factors, and long term incidence of ischaemic heart disease in the Northwick Park Heart Study. *Lancet* 11, 342–345.

Murray, F.E., Ennis, J., Lennon, J.R. & Crowe, J.P. (1991) Management of reflux oesophegitis: role of weight loss and cimetidine. *Irish Journal of Medical Science* 160, 2–4.

Must, A., Jacques, P.F., Dallal, G.E. Bajema, C.J. & Dietz, W.H. (1992) Long term morbidity and mortality of overweight adolescents. A follow-up of the Harvard Growth Study of 1922 to 1935. *New England Journal of Medicine* 327, 1350–1355.

National Task Force on the Prevention and Treatment of Obesity (1994) Weight cycling. *Journal of American Medical Association* 272, 1196–1202.

Oberman, A., Wassertheil-Smoller, S., Langford, H.G. *et al.* (1990) Pharmacologic and nutritional treatment of mild hypertension: changes in cardiovascular risk status. *Annals of Internal Medicine* 112, 879–883.

Ornish D., Brown, S.E., Scherwitz, B. *et al.* (1990) Can lifestyle changes reverse coronary heart disease. *Lancet* 336, 129–133.

Palareti, G., Legnani, C., Poggi, M. *et al.* (1994) Prolonged very low calorie diet in obese subjects reduces factor VII and PAI but not fibrinogen levels. *Fibrinolysis* 8, 16–21.

Pamuk, E.R., Williamson, D.F., Madans, J., Serdula, M.K., Kleinman, J.C. & Byers, T. (1992) Weight loss and mortality in a national cohort of adults, 1971–1987. *American Journal of Epidemiology* 136, 686–697.

Perri, M.G., Nezu, A.M. & Viegner, B.J. (1992) *Improving the Long Term Management of Obesity.* New York: Willey Bioscience.

Phinney, S.D., Tang, A.B., Waggoner, C.R., Tezanos, R.G. & Davis, P.A. (1991) The transient hypercholesterolaemia of major weight loss. *American Journal of Clinical Nutrition* 53, 1404–1410.

Pories, W.J., MacDonald, K.G., Flickinger, E.G. *et al.* (1992) Is type II diabetes mellitus (NIDDM) a surgical disease. *Annals of Surgery* 215, 633–643.

Prentice, A.M., Jebb, S.A., Goldberg, G. *et al.* (1992) Effects of weight cycling on body composition. *American Journal of Clinical Nutrition* 56, 209s–216s.

Poggi, M., Palareti, G., Biagi, R. *et al.* (1994) Prolonged very low calorie diet in highly obese subjects reduces plasma viscosity and red cell aggregation but not fibrinogen. *International Journal of Obesity* 18, 490–496.

Pyle, R.L., Mitchell, J.E. & Eckert, E.D. (1981) Bulimia: a report of 34 cases. *Journal of Clinical Psychiatry* 42, 60.

Rebuffe-Scrive, M., Hendleer, R., Bracero, N., Cummings, N., McCarthy, S. & Rodin, J. (1994)

Biobehavioural effects of weight cycling. *International Journal of Obesity* **18**, 651–658.

Reisin, E., Abel, R., Modan, M., Silverberg, D.S., Eliahou, H.E. & Modan, B. (1978) The effect of weight loss without salt restriction on the reduction in blood pressure in overweight hypertensive patients. *New England Journal of Medicine* **298**, 1–6.

Rissanen, A., Pietinen, P., Siljamaki-Ojansuu, U., Piirainen, H. & Reissel, P. (1985) Treatment of hypertension in obese patients: efficacy and feasibility of weight and salt reduction programs. *Acta Medica Scandinavia* **218**, 149–156.

Rogers, J. & Mitchell, G.W. (1952) The relation of obesity to menstrual disturbances. *New England Journal of Medicine* **247**, 53–56.

Rubinstein, I., Colapinto, N., Rotstein, L.E., Brown, I.G. & Hoffstein, V. (1988) Improvement in upper airway function after weight loss in patients with obstructive sleep apnea. *American Review of Respiratory Disease* **138**, 1192–1195.

Sattar, N. Tan, C.E., Han, T.S. *et al.* (1998) Association of indices of adiposity with atherogenic lipoprotein subfractions. *International Journal of Obesity* (in press).

Sichieri, R., Everhart, J.E. & Roth, H. (1991) A prospective study of hospitalisation with gallstone disease among women. Role of dietary factors, fasting period and dieting. *American Journal of Public Health* **81**, 880–884.

Shiffman, M.L., Sugerman, H.J., Kellum, J.M., Brewer, W.H. & Moore, E.W. (1991) Gallstone formation after rapid weight loss: a prospective study in patients undergoing gastric bypass surgery for treatment of morbid obesity. *American Journal of Gastroenterology* **86**, 1000–1005.

Skender, M.L., Goodrick, G.K., Del-Junco, D.J. *et al.* (1996) Comparison of 2 year weight loss trends in behavioural treatments for obesity, diet exercise and combination interventions. *Journal of the American Dietetic Association* **4**, 342–346.

Smith, P.L., Gold, A.R., Meyers, D.A., Haponik, E.F. & Bleecker, E.R. (1985) Weight loss in mild to moderately obese patients with obstructive sleep apnea. *Annals of Internal Medicine* **103**, 850–855.

Smoller, J.W., Wadden, T.A. & Stunkard, A.J. (1987) Dieting and depression: a critical review. *Journal of Psychosomatic Research* **31**, 429–440.

Sonne-holme, S., Sorensen, T.I.A., Jensen, G. & Schnohr, P. (1989) Independent effects of weight change and attained body weight on prevalence of arterial hypertension in obese and non-obese men. *British Medical Journal* **299**, 767–770.

Sönnichsen, A.C., Richter, W.O. & Schwandt, P. (1992) Benefit from hypocaloric diet in obese men depends on the extent of weight loss regarding cholesterol, and on a simultaneous change in body fat distribution regarding insulin sensitivity and glucose tolerance. *Metabolism* **41**, 1035–1039.

Spitzer, R.L., Devlin, M., Walsh, B.T. Hasin, D. *et al.* (1992) Binge eating disorders: a multi-site field trial of diagnostic criteria. *International Journal of Eating Disorders* **11**, 191–203.

Stunkard, A.J. & Wadden, T.A. (1992) Psychological aspects of severe obesity. *American Journal of Clinical Nutrition* **55** (suppl. 2), 524S–532S.

Sugerman, H.J., Fairman, R.P., Baron, P.L. & Kwentus, J.A. (1986) Gastric surgery for respiratory insufficiency of obesity. *Chest* **90**, 81–86.

Svedsen, O.L., Hassager, C. & Christiansen, C. (1994) Six months' follow up on exercise added to a short term diet in overweight postmenopausal women—effects on body composition, resting metabolic rate, cardiovascular risk factors and bone. *International Journal of Obesity* **18**, 692–698.

UKPDS (1995) Relative efficacy of randomly allocated diet, sulphonylurea insulin or metformin in patients with newly diagnosed non-insulin dependent diabetes. *British Medical Journal* **310**, 83–88.

UKPDS (1990) UK Prospective Diabetes Study 7. Response of fasting plasma glucose to diet therapy in newly presenting type II diabetic patients. *Metabolism* **39**, 909–912.

van Gaal, L., Wauters, M.A. & De Leeuw, I. (1997) The beneficial effects of modest weight loss on cardiovascular risk factors. *International Journal of Obesity* **21** (suppl. 1), s5–s9.

Vessby, B., Boberg, M., Karlstrom, B., Lithell, H. & Werner, I. (1984) Improved metabolic control in overweight diabetic patients. *Acta Medica Scandinavia* **216**, 67–74.

Wadden, T.A., Steen, S.N., Wingate, B.J. & Foster, G.D. (1996) Psychosocial consequences of weight reduction: how much weight loss is enough? *American Journal of Clinical Nutrition* **63** (suppl.), 461–465.

Wassertheil-Smoller, S., Blaufox, M.D., Oberman, A.S., Langford, H.G., Davis, B.R. & Wylie-Rosett, J. (1992) The trial of antihypertensive interventions and management TAIM study. Adequate weight loss, alone and combined with drug therapy in the treatment of mild hypertension. *Archives of Internal Medicine* **152**, 131–136.

Watts, N.B., Spanheimer, R.G., Digirolamo, M. *et al.* Prediction of glucose response to weight loss in patients with non-insulin-dependent diabetes mellitus. *Archives of Internal Medicine* **150**, 803–806.

Weinsier, R.L., James, R.D., Darnell, B.E. *et al.* (1992) Lipid and insulin concentration in obese postmenpausal women: separate effects of energy restriction and weight loss. *American Journal of Clinical Nutrition* **56**, 44–49.

Williamson, D.F., Serdula, M.K., Anda, R.F., Levy, A. & Byers, T. (1992) Weight loss attempts in adults, goals, duration, and rate of weight loss. *American Journal of Public Health* **82**, 1251–1257.

Williamson, D.F., Pamuk, E., Thun, M., Flanders, D., Byers, T. & Heath, C. (1995) Prospective study of intentional weight loss and mortality in never smoking US white women. *American Journal of Epidemiology* **141**, 1128–1141.

Wilson, G.T. (1993) Relation of dieting and voluntary weight loss to psychological functioning and binge eating. *Annals of Internal Medicine* **119**, 727–730.

Wing, RR. (1992a) Behavioural treatment of severe obesity. *American Journal of Clinical Nutrition* **55** (suppl. 2), 545s–551s.

Wing, R.R. (1992b) Weight cycling in humans: a review of the literature. *Annals of Behavioural Medicine* **14**, 113–119.

Wing, R.R., Shoemaker, M., Marcus, M.D.M., McDermott, M. & Gooding, W. (1990) Variables associated with weight loss and improvements in glycaemic control in type II diabetic patients. *Archives of Internal Medicine* **147**, 1749–1753.

Wing, R.R., Jefferey, R.W., Burton, L.R., Kuller, L.H. & Folsom, A.R. (1992) Change in waist-hip ratio with weight loss and its association with change in cardiovascular risk factors. *American Journal of Clinical Nutrition* **55**, 1086–1092.

Wing, R.R., Blair, E., Marcus, M., Epstein, L.H. & Harvey, J. (1994) Year-long weight loss treatment for obese patients with type II diabetes: does including an intermittent very-low-calorie diet improve outcome. *American Journal of Medicine* **97**, 354–359.

Wolf, R.N. & Grundy, S.M. (1983) Influence of weight reduction on plasma lipoproteins in obese patients. *Arteriosclerosis* **3**, 160–169.

Yang, H., Peterson, G.M., Roth, M.P., Schoenfield, L.J. & Marks, J.W. (1992) Risk factors for gallstones during rapid weight loss. *Digestive Disease Science* **37**, 912–918.

CHAPTER 23

Public Health Strategies and the Economic Costs of Obesity

AILA RISSANEN

Introduction

Obesity is a well-recognized health hazard, with up to one-half of the cases of chronic disabling conditions such as diabetes, hypertension and osteoarthritis being attributable to excess body-weight. For the obese person, overweight denotes an increased risk of chronic disabling conditions, lowered quality of life and loss of earnings. For the society, obesity is a major economic burden, accounting currently for about 4–8% of the total health care expenditure. The indirect costs arising from loss of productivity may be even higher. In view of the high and still increasing prevalence of obesity, the ageing populations of affluent countries are facing an increasing burden of chronic diseases with high social and economic cost.

The short-term benefits of reducing excess weight are well-documented for persons with chronic diseases. Improved health and quality of life and savings in medical expenditure could therefore be expected by weight loss. Lifestyles combining regular exercise with low-fat diet should be promoted to treat overweight as well as to prevent weight gain. Preventive measures should be supported by all levels of public policy. Special attention should be paid to high-risk groups of weight gain, including persons who plan to stop smoking and those with a family history of obesity and related metabolic disorders.

The prevalence and determinants of obesity

The prevalence of obesity is high and increasing steadily in Westernized countries. Approximately 20–50% of adults in these countries are overweight (body mass index (BMI) 25–30 kg/m²) and 5–20% are distinctly obese (BMI > 30 kg/m²). The prevalence of overweight and obesity has increased by 10–40% during the last decade (World Health Organization, 1997) (Table 23.1). Obesity and weight gain in adulthood are most common among people from the lowest social classes (Rissanen et al., 1991), and the gap between the classes may be widening (Pietinen et al., 1996).

Table 23.1 Prevalence and time trends of obesity (BMI > 30 kg/m^2) prevalence in some European countries.

Population	Year	Age group	Prevalence of obesity (%)	
			Men	Women
U.K.	1980	16–64	6	8
	1986–87		7	12
	1994		13	16
Finland	1978–89	20–75	10	10
	1985–87		12	10
	1991–93		14	11
Netherlands	1987–91	20–59	7	9
	1993		8	10
	1994		10	11
Sweden	1980–81	16–84	4.9	8.7
	1988–89		5.3	9.1

There is some uncertainty about the aetiology of this escalating trend. While the role of genetic susceptibility to weight gain is well documented, it is clear that the primary causes of the problem must lie in the exposure to environmental conditions that promote positive energy balance (James, 1995; Prentice & Jebb, 1995). A sedentary lifestyle and high-fat diet are likely to be the major determinants of weight gain in susceptible individuals.

The habitual diet in many Western countries has changed considerably in the last decades. The overall intake of energy has decreased, but the relative proportion of fat in the diet has increased (Prentice & Jebb, 1995). The obvious paradox of increasing obesity in the face of decreased energy intake suggests that energy expenditure has declined faster than energy intake, thus leading to an overconsumption of energy relative to a greatly reduced requirement.

A profound change has occurred in societal patterns of physical activity in the last few decades, as people have adopted increasingly sedentary lifestyles in which motorized transport, mechanized equipment and energy-saving appliances have reduced the need for even moderate activity at work and at home. The diminished demands of energy in the sedentary every-day life of most people are only partially compensated by an increase of active leisure pursuits, which has been documented in recent years (Fogelholm et al., 1996).

As judged from the steadily increasing average BMI of children and adults in most populations, there is a small energy surplus in the daily life of most people. In this kind of environment favouring weight gain, even small and temporary perturbations of energy balance such as pregnancy and smoking

Table 23.2 Relative risk of weight gain of 5 kg or more in 5 years according to selected demographic and behavioural factors in adult Finns. From Rissanen *et al.* (1991).

	Women	Men
Level of education		
Basic	1.0	1.0
Intermediate	0.9	0.8
High	0.5	0.8
Marital status		
In stable relationship	1.0	1.0
Married during the last 5 years	2.1	1.8
Widowed during the last 5 years	0.5	0.7
Divorced during the last 5 years	1.2	1.1
Smoking		
Non-smoker	1.0	1.0
Regular smoker	1.2	1.1
Started smoking in the last 5 years	0.5	0.7
Quitted smoking in the last 5 years	1.7	3.3
Alcohol		
None or moderate	1.0	1.0
> 300 g/month	1.3	1.4
Leisure time physical activity		
Frequent	1.0	1.0
Occasional	1.5	1.5
Rare	1.6	1.9
No. of childbirths in the last 5 years		
None	1.0	
One	1.2	
Two or more	1.7	

cessation (Rissanen *et al.*, 1991; Flegal *et al.*, 1995) may result in permanent increase in the prevalence of overweight of the population. Table 23.2 summarizes the main determinants of weight gain in 5 years in a large cohort of adult Finns (Rissanen *et al.*, 1991).

Health risks of obesity and consequences of weight loss

Risks of obesity

Overweight is a major health hazard, increasing morbidity, mortality and

Table 23.3 Relative risk and population attributable fractions of some diseases in overweight (BMI > 27 kg/m^2) French persons. From Levy *et al.* (1995). The prevalence of overweight (BMI > 27 kg/m^2) is assumed to be 16.7%. The attributable fraction relates to the relative risk of a person to contract the disease. The attributable fraction is calculated from the formula $AF = P \times (RR - 1)/1 + P \times (RR - 1)$, where P is the prevalence of obesity and RR is the relative risk of contracting the disease.

	Relative risk	Population attributable fraction (%)
NIDDM	16.7	66
Gallstones	10.0	52
Coronary heart disease	3.3	22
Hypertension	4.3	29
Breast cancer	1.3	6
Colon cancer	1.3	4

disability of obese persons. It favours the development of chronic conditions such as non-insulin-dependent diabetes mellitus (NIDDM), hypertension, coronary heart disease, stroke, gallbladder disease, osteoarthritis, certain types of cancer, disturbances in pulmonary and reproductive function and sleep. Considerable proportion of these common diseases could have been prevented if obesity did not exist. This is exemplified by the fractions of these diseases attributable to overweight in a French study (Levy *et al.*, 1995), shown in Table 23.3.

Modest overweight has little impact on mortality, but it strongly predicts severe functional impairment (Fig. 23.1). A quarter of all premature disability pensions from cardiovascular and musculoskeletal causes in Finnish women and half as many in men can be attributed to overweight alone (Rissanen *et al.*, 1990). In addition to the increased risks of morbidity and mortality, overweight persons are likely to have a compromised quality of life and face discrimination in most areas of social life (Sarlio-Lähteenkorva *et al.*, 1995).

Consequences of weight reduction in overweight persons

Weight loss improves many of the metabolic abnormalities associated with overweight as well as the obesity-related functional impairments. Most patients with NIDDM and about half of obese hypertensive patients can discontinue their medication after adequate weight loss. Even modest weight loss is beneficial (Goldstein, 1992). It can also prevent obesity-related functional impairments. For instance, weight loss of about 5 kg may be sufficient to reduce the risk of symptomatic osteoarthritis of the knee by over 50% (Felson *et al.*, 1992). Weight loss may also improve psychosocial functioning and mood of overweight persons

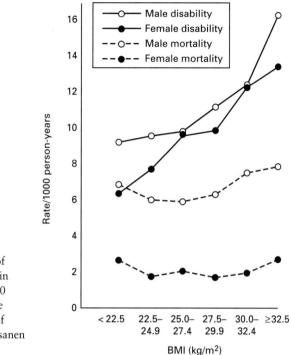

Fig. 23.1 Age-adjusted rates of work disability and mortality in 19 000 Finnish men and 12 000 women aged 25–64 at baseline during an average follow-up of more then 10 years. From Rissanen *et al.* (1990).

(Sarlio-Lähteenkorva *et al.*, 1995). It is likely that many of the well-documented beneficial effects of weight loss achieved by current treatments are not permanent, because weight loss is seldom maintained.

Data on long-term consequences of weight loss on health of obese persons are still scanty. The most compelling evidence of the benefits of sustained weight loss derive from the preliminary results from the ongoing Swedish Obese Subjects (SOS) Study. This study shows dramatic improvement of the health of severely obese persons after surgically induced weight loss (Sjöström *et al.*, 1995). For instance, the 2-year incidence of NIDDM in obese patients who had lost substantial amounts of weight after surgery was only 3/100 (incidence of 0.2%) of that of equally obese controls without weight loss. However, most epidemiological studies of weight and longevity, many of which are beset with methodological problems, have observed little overall survival advantage for obese persons who have lost weight, with the lowest mortality rates in persons maintaining stable weight (Williamson & Pamuk, 1993).

In view of the impressive gains from weight loss and the often disappointing long-term results of treatment of obesity, there is an urgent need for effective prevention and for improved management programmes for better weight control and maintenance of weight loss at the population level.

The economic costs of obesity

Overweight and obesity have sizeable economic consequences. The most commonly used approach to estimate the costs of obesity in society is to measure the value of resources used or lost because of this condition. Direct costs are the medical costs of diagnosis, treatment and management of diseases attributable to obesity. These costs could have been prevented if obesity did not exist. Indirect costs reflect the value of loss of productivity due to obesity. The limited data available at present suggest that about 4–8% of total health care expenditure in affluent countries can be attributable to obesity.

Direct costs

The excess use of medical care and associated costs due to overweight and obesity in the Netherlands were estimated using data on large population surveys from 1981 to 1989 (Seidell & Deerenberg, 1994). The health care costs included reported consultations of general practitioners and medical specialists, hospital admissions and use of prescribed drugs. The fraction of consultations of general practitioners attributable to obesity/overweight was about 3–4%. For hospitalizations, the respective attributable fractions were 3% for obesity and 2% for overweight. The excess use of medications by obese and overweight people was most conspicuous. It was estimated from these data that the direct costs of excess weight are about 4% of the total health care costs in the Netherlands. This is of the same order of magnitude as the health care costs attributable to cancers.

The direct costs of obesity in France in 1992 were estimated by the identification of the costs of personal health care, hospital care, physician services and drugs for diseases with well-established relationship with obesity, including NIDDM, hypertension, hyperlipidaemia, coronary heart disease, stroke, venous thrombo-embolism, osteoarthritis of the knee, gallbladder disease and certain cancers (Levy et al., 1995). The proportion of these diseases attributable to obesity (defined by the cut-off point of BMI = 27kg/m^2) ranged from about 25% for hypertension and stroke to about 3% for breast cancer (see Table 23.3). The direct costs of obesity were estimated to correspond to about 2% of the expenses of the French health care system. Costs of hypertension represented 33% of the total direct costs of obesity.

The Australian Institute of Health and Welfare estimated that in 1989 the health care costs resulting from obesity (BMI > 30kg/m^2) accounted for about 4% of pharmaceutical expenditure, 2% of the cost of medical consultations and 1.6% of the recurrent hospital expenditure (Segal et al., 1994). Overall, at least 2% of total recurrent health expenditure of some major obesity-related diseases (NIDDM, coronary artery disease, hypertension, gallstones and cancers of the breast and colon) could be attributed to obesity. This is equal to 86% of the health care costs used for the management of alcohol-related diseases and 71% of the costs for the management of tobacco-related disease in Australia.

The impact of obesity on several indicators of health care utilization was assessed among 10 000 adult Finns in the National Survey on Health and Social Security in 1987. The excess health care utilization was mainly due to an increased need for medication, the cost of which increased by about 120% when BMI increased from 25 to 40 kg/m². It was estimated that if all Finns were of normal weight, the annual savings would be of the same order of magnitude as if all smokers in Finland were to permanently stop smoking.

In the U.S.A., the total costs attributable for the major disease conditions due to obesity were calculated to represent 5.5% of the total cost of illness in 1986 (Colditz, 1992). About 57% of the costs of NIDDM, 19% of the costs of cardiovascular diseases, 26% of those for hypertension and about 2.5% of the costs of cancers were estimated to be attributable to obesity.

Perhaps the most compelling data regarding the costs of obesity come from preliminary observations from an ongoing nation-wide intervention study (the SOS Study), showing dramatic reductions in the incidence of obesity-related diseases in severely obese persons after surgical weight loss (Sjöström et al., 1995). There were three- to 23-fold decreases in the 2-year incidence of cardiovascular risk factors in obese subjects with weight loss as compared to subjects with stable weight. In particular, the reduction for the incidence of diabetes was reported to be about 17-fold. These findings suggest that impressive savings of the treatment costs of common diseases are achievable by effective treatment of severely obese persons.

Most of the available estimates of health care costs are based on cross-sectional data of selected obesity-related diseases. They do not include the costs of many of the diseases and conditions caused or worsened by obesity, such as the extra costs resulting from obesity-related complications of surgery and pregnancy. For instance, it was recently calculated that the hospitalization costs during pregnancy are more than twofold among overweight and obese French mothers, compared to the costs of pregnancies of normal-weight French women (Galtier-Dereure et al., 1995). The presented estimates on the direct costs of obesity are thus likely to under-estimate the magnitude of the true costs and of the savings achievable by the reduction of the prevalence of obesity in the society.

Indirect costs

Loss of productivity due to premature death and disability from illness associated with obesity are considerable. Only limited data on these indirect costs are available, but they are likely to be greater than the direct medical costs of excess weight.

In a recent study of Swedish women aged 30–59 years, approximately 10% of the total cost of loss of productivity due to sick-leave and disability pensions were estimated to be related to obesity and obesity-related diseases (Narbro *et al.*, 1996). The frequency of sick-leave was reported to be 1.5–1.9 times higher in obese women (mean BMI 39 kg/m²) compared with women in the general Swedish population. The rate of premature disability pensions was reported to be increased fourfold among the obese women.

In a large prospective Finnish study, obesity was associated with a twofold increased risk of premature work disability in men, and a 1.5-fold greater risk in women (Rissanen *et al.*, 1990). Most of the premature pensions attributable to obesity were due to cardiovascular and musculoskeletal diseases. A quarter of all disability pensions from these diseases in women and half as many in men were attributable to overweight and obesity alone.

The future of the societal costs of obesity

Any change in the prevalence of obesity will have a major impact on the consumption and cost of medical care in society, and even minor decline in the prevalence can be expected to result in substantial savings of the limited health care resources. Obesity represents a major avoidable contribution to the costs of illness in affluent countries. However, no such cost-containing prospects are evident. The prevalence of obesity is increasing. As advancing medical care reduces premature mortality of obese persons, the number of survivors with chronic diseases and premature disabilities will increase. The ageing populations of the Western world are thus facing a mounting burden of costs arising from the sequelae of excess weight.

To reverse the increasing trend, effective measures are needed to manage and prevent obesity.

Public health strategies to weight control

Despite the recognition of overweight and obesity as a major public health problem, few data exist about public health approaches to solving it. A systematic review of the public health dimensions of excess weight is under way by the International Task Force on Obesity (World Health Organization, 1997).

Public health approach to weight management

Given the large number of patients in need of medical care because of excess weight, the management of almost all overweight and obese patients should be centred in the primary health care, community or commercial sectors. The information about the management of obesity in these settings is scarce. There is an obvious need for well-planned strategies for obesity management in primary and community care. One of the first such approaches is the National Clinical Guidelines of Scotland (SIGN, 1996). A staged procedure for weight management in primary care proposed by this recommendation is presented in Chapter 15 (see Fig. 15.5).

The priority in obesity management in primary care should be in weight management with risk factor reduction, so that the focus shifts from short-term approaches to induce major weight loss into long-term weight management with an overall improvement of risk factors, functional capacity and well-being.

Weight management advice aiming at modest weight loss and its maintenance should therefore be an integral part of the treatment of all overweight and obese patients with obesity-associated conditions such as hypertension, dyslipidaemia, hyperglycaemia or osteoarthritis. The weight of these patients should be regularly monitored during clinic visits.

Professional awareness of the need to monitor weight of patients seeking medical care should be promoted in primary health setting. Weight or BMI and preferably also waist measurement should be routinely recorded as part of ordinary medical care. In particular, weight surveillance and preventive advice should be integrated routinely into clinical management of patients who have a history or a family history of overweight or related disorders.

Prevention of weight gain and overweight

The average BMI of most populations continues to rise despite the growing awareness of obesity as a health and social problem. The attempts to prevent overweight and obesity have thus far not proven to be successful, and this has been accompanied by a proliferation of seemingly ineffective commercial methods and business activities aiming at weight control (Levy & Heaton, 1993).

In public health terms, prevention encompasses two kinds of approaches: a general preventive approach to reduce the risk of weight gain in the population at large or the population strategy and targeted measures for those at greatest risk of becoming obese. These two strategies are not mutually exclusive but should complement each other.

The public health approach

It is most important that measures are taken to prevent the population in general becoming fatter. This is probably best achieved by promoting healthy eating and physical activity at all levels of public policies, including education, transportation, health, other public services, agriculture and food production.

Physical activity. In view of the central role played by the decline of daily physical activity in the observed weight gain of most Westernized populations, promoting opportunities for habitual physical activity is of prime importance. Examples of ways to promote access and affordability to exercise include city planning with provision of safe footpaths, cycle routes and cycle parking facilities, and improved public transport service with financial incentives for its use, possibly with disincentives for private car use, especially if supported by appropriate traffic regulations, speed limits, etc. The recommendations of James (1995) concerning daily physical activity in the prevention of obesity in the U.K. are summarized in Table 23.4.

There is also a need to increase the amount of leisure and sporting activity in many sectors of the population. The recommendations of James (1995) are listed in Table 23.5.

Diet. Public health strategies to promote healthy eating may also need to involve political issues at a variety of levels in the society, including food manufacturing, pricing and labelling, and agricultural policies. There could also be control of sales conditions and advertising practices of high-fat, nutritionally low-value foods. The recommendations of James (1995) concerning dietary issues in the prevention of obesity in the U.K. are presented in Table 23.6.

Public health education. Public health education is a necessary component in all preventive strategies. In particular, programmes targeting young people can

Table 23.4 Recommendations for active living in the prevention of obesity. From James (1995).

1   Long-term planning of town and city centres should encourage and sometimes require a progressive increase in walking and cycling
2   Measures are needed to encourage walking and cycling as means for travel for short journeys. These measures include:
    (a) Traffic speed limits
    (b) Traffic calming
    (c) Traffic banning in some areas
    (d) Provision of safe footpaths and cycle routes
    (e) Provision of safe cycle parking facilities
    (f) Special measures to improve access to low-cost reflective bands and cycle helmets
    (g) Financial incentives for walking, cycling, public transport
    (h) Disincentives for car use

Table 23.5 Recommendations for sport and leisure time activity in the prevention of obesity. From James (1995).

---

1   Targets for physical activity need to be defined for different groups of people which specify the time spent in different levels of activity
2   Pre-school facilities should encourage active play
3   Schools should emphasize the fun and health benefits of sport and active leisure for all, and allow experience of a wide range of sports
4   Schools should encourage activity outside school by
   (a) encouraging walking and cycling for transport and leisure
   (b) provide links to clubs and community activities
   (c) re-evaluating the payment and hours of work of teachers involved in extracurricular sport

5   Work places should encourage
   (a) awareness of health targets
   (b) sport/leisure participation by provision of facilities and opportunities
   (c) walking, cycling and public transport for work-related journeys

6   Local authorities should encourage access to leisure facilities, and make special provisions for:
   (a) mothers with babies and small children
   (b) children and adolescents
   (c) the elderly
   (d) the unemployed
   (e) GP prescription referrals
   (f) those who are unfit or overweight or unfamiliar with facilities; these groups need a sympathetic approach

---

Table 23.6 Recommendations concerning dietary issues in the prevention of obesity. From James (1995).

---

1   Concerted effort to reach the 35% fat target in the U.K.
2   The fat content of food to be displayed in government, local authorities and work canteens
3   Targets to be displayed in public eating facilities
4   Accentuate the drive to reduce the fat content of foods
5   Nutritional information for customers to be developed in a more easily understood form with simple visual cues
6   Standard set for nursery, school and hospital meals
7   Schools should teach:
   (a) skills to use a wide range of foods
   (b) healthy nutrition and active lifestyle across the curriculum and by example and practice
8   All primary care workers need to be taught the new concepts of energy balance and a healthy nutrition and active lifestyle. Their skills in using this knowledge need to be evaluated once a system for evaluating new procedures has been developed

---

be expected to be fruitful. However, few data are available on the benefits of such programmes. It seems likely that education on how to change behaviours have limited utility if not supported by public policies that make these changes easy in every-day life. In addition, education may help in changing the environment, if people develop greater awareness of the extent to which environmental factors and habits contribute to health.

Community campaigns and media. The effect of community-based programmes to prevent weight gain have been examined in several large-scale community programmes of health promotion. Although the prevention of obesity has not been the primary target of any of these programmes, they have contained multifaceted projects to control obesity. The Stanford Community projects relied on an intensive media campaign, community organizations, work-site treatments, face-to-face contact and a variety of community events (Farquhar *et al.*, 1990). The North-Karelia Study was a 5-year programme of an ambitious and largescale involvement of all communities in the county of North Karelia, Finland. The intervention including primary health care, work-sites, schools, a variety of community activities, the media and the chain of local food production and supply (Puska *et al.*, 1983). These programmes achieved a reduction of coronary risk factors other than obesity, suggesting that community campaigns alone may have little effect on obesity. However, it is possible that effectiveness of such programmes can be improved if modern technology and media are utilized to specifically address the needs of the various segments of the population such as those with little education.

High-risk-group approach

Certain groups of the population are known to be particularly vulnerable for weight gain and for the ill-effects of excess weight. Preventive programmes tailored to the specific needs may therefore be warranted to prevent the occurrence and sequelae of weight gain in these high-risk groups.

High-risk groups who might be targeted for special help are listed in Table 23.7. One of the most important groups for prevention are the offspring of parents who are obese. These persons have about twice the risk of obesity as compared to the offspring of lean parents. A second important target group for prevention are the members of families with a history of type 2 diabetes. This disease is highly heritable, but clinical disease emerges usually only when obesity or sedentary lifestyle is present. At least half of the cases of adult onset diabetes could be prevented if weight gain was prevented. Special attention should similarly be paid to the weight development of families with one or more members with hypertension or dyslipidaemia, as weight gain is likely to increase the

Table 23.7 High-risk groups for targeted preventive approach.

Children of families with members with distinct overweight
Persons with a family history of type 2 diabetes
Persons with a family history of hypertension or dyslipidaemia
Subjects planning to give up smoking
Women entering pregnancy with a BMI $> 25 \, \text{kg/m}^2$

chances of getting the disease for persons with a familial tendency for these disorders.

The risk of weight gain is known to be increased in physiological transition periods of life such as the menopause and pregnancy. As pregnancy is one of the established determinants of female obesity, a targeted approach to prevent excessive weight gain is recommended for women who enter pregnancy with a BMI over $25 \, \text{kg/m}^2$. Similarly, the risk of weight gain is increased with smoking cessation, which reduces energy expenditure by about 9% and often results in weight gain within 6 months. Therefore, targeted programmes should be implemented to prevent weight gain in adolescents and adults planning to give up smoking.

References

Colditz, G.A. (1992) The economic costs of obesity. *American Journal of Clinical Nutrition* 55, 503–507.

Farquhar, J.W., Fortmann, S., Flora, J.A. *et al.* (1990) Effect of community-wide education on cardiovascular risk factors; The Stanford Five-City Project. *Journal of the American Medical Association* 264, 359–365.

Felson, D.T., Zhang, Y., Anthony, J.M., Naimark, A. & Anderson, J.J. (1992) Weight loss reduces the risk for symptomatic knee osteoarthritis in women. *Annals of Internal Medicine* 116, 535–539.

Flegal, K.M. (1995) The influence of smoking on the prevalence of overweight in the United States. *New England Journal of Medicine* 333, 1165–1170.

Fogelholm, M., Männistö, S., Vartiainen, E. & Pietinen, P. (1996) Determinants of energy balance and overweight in Finland 1982 and 1992. *International Journal of Obesity* 20, 1097–1104.

Galtier-Dereure, F., Montpeyroux, F., Boulot, P., Bringer, J. & Jaffiol, C. (1995) Weight excess before pregnancy: complications and cost. *International Journal of Obesity* 19, 443–448.

Goldstein, D.J. (1992) Beneficial health effects of modest weight loss. *International Journal of Obesity* 16, 397–415.

James, W.P.T. (1995) A public health approach to the problem of obesity. *International Journal of Obesity* 19 (suppl. 3), S37–S45.

Levy, A.S. & Heaton, A.W. (1993) Weight control practises of U.S. adults trying to lose weight. *Annals of Internal Medicine* 119 (part 2), 661–666.

Levy, E., Levy, P., Le Pen, C. & Basdevant, A. (1995) The economic costs of obesity: the French situation. *International Journal of Obesity* 19, 790–792.

Narbro, K., Jonsson, E., Larsson, B., Waaler, H., Wedel, H. & Sjöström, L. (1996) Economic consequences of sick-leave and early retirement in obese Swedish women. *International Journal of Obesity* 20, 895–903.

Obesity. Reversing the Increasing Problem of Obesity in England. A report from the Nutrition and Physical Activity Task Forces, Department of Health 1995.

Pietinen, P., Vartiainen, E. & Männistö, S. (1996) Trends in body mass index and obesity among adults in Finland from 1972 to 1992. *International Journal of Obesity* 20, 114–120.

Prentice, A.M. & Jebb, S.A. (1995) Obesity in Britain: gluttony or sloth? *British Medical Journal* 311, 437–439.

Puska, P., Salonen, J. & Nissinen, A. (1983) Change in risk factors for coronary heart disease during 10 years of community intervention programme: North Karelia Project. *British Medical Journal* 287, 1840–1844.

Rissanen, A., Heliövaara, M., Knekt, P., Reunanen, A., Aromaa, A. & Maatela, J. (1990) Risk of disability and mortality due to overweight in a Finnish population. *British Medical Journal* 301, 835–837.

Rissanen, A., Heliövaara, M., Knekt, P., Reunanen, A. & Aromaa, A. (1991) Determinants of weight gain and overweight in adult Finns. *European Journal of Clinical Nutrition* 45, 419–430.

Sarlio-Lähteenkorva, S., Stunkard, A. & Rissanen, A. (1995) Psychosocial factors and quality of life in obesity. *International Journal of Obesity* 19 (suppl. 6), S1–S5.

Scottish Intercollegiate Guidelines Network. (1996) *Obesity in Scotland. A National Clinical Guideline*. Edinburgh: SIGN publication 8.

Segal, C.L., Cartre, R. & Zimmet, P. (1994) The cost of obesity. The Australian perspective. *PharmacoEconomics* 5 (suppl. 1), 45–52.

Seidell, J.C. & Deerenberg, I. (1994) Obesity in Europe. Prevalence and consequences for use of medical care. *PharmacoEconomics* 5 (suppl. 1), 38–44.

Sjöström, L., Narbro, K. & Sjöström, D. (1995) Costs and benefits when treating obesity. *International Journal of Obesity* 19 (suppl. 6), S9–S12.

Williamson, D.F. & Pamuk, E.R. (1993) The association between weight loss and increased longevity. A review of the evidence. *Annals of Internal Medicine* 119, 731–736.

World Health Organization (1997) Prevention and management of the global epidemic of obesity. Geneva: WHO. (In preparation.)

Index